# BIOARTIFICIAL ORGANS II

## TECHNOLOGY, MEDICINE, AND MATERIALS

ANNALS OF THE NEW YORK ACADEMY OF SCIENCES
*Volume 875*

# BIOARTIFICIAL ORGANS II
## TECHNOLOGY, MEDICINE, AND MATERIALS

*Edited by David Hunkeler, Aleš Prokop, Alan D. Cherrington, Ray V. Rajotte, and Michael Sefton*

*The New York Academy of Sciences*
*New York, New York*
*1999*

⊗*The paper used in this publication meets the minimum requirements of the American National Standard for Information Sciences—Permanence of Paper for Printed Library Materials, ANSI Z39.48-1984.*

**Cover:** The art on the softcover version of this volume highlights the work of Anthony Sun and Philippe Morel. Some of it appears in black and white in the paper by Zhou *et al.* (pp. 208–218).

**Library of Congress Cataloging-in-Publication Data**

Bioartificial organs II : technology, medicine, and materials / edited by David Hunkeler ... [et al.]
p. cm. — (Annals of the New York Academy of Sciences ; v. 875)
Includes bibliographical references and index.
ISBN 1-57331-194-4 (cloth : alk. paper). — ISBN 1-57331-195-2 (paper : alk. paper).
1. Artificial organs Congresses. 2. Biomedical materials Congresses. 3. Medical innovations Congresses. I. Title: Bioartificial organs 2. II. Title: Bioartificial organs two. III. Series.
[DNLM:1. Artificial Organs Congresses. 2. Biocompatible Materials Congresses. 3. Bone Substitutes Congresses. 4. Liver, Artificial Congresses. 5. Pancreas, Artificial Congresses. 6. Skin, Artificial Congresses. W1 AN626YL v.875 1999]
Q11.N5 vol. 875
[RD130]
500 s
[610'.28]—DC21
DNLM/DLC
for Library of Congress 99-26595
CIP

GYAT / PCP
*Printed in the United States of America*
**ISBN 1-57331-194-4** (cloth)
**ISBN 1-57331-195-2** (paper)
**ISSN 0077-8923**

ANNALS OF THE NEW YORK ACADEMY OF SCIENCES

*Volume 875*
*June 18, 1999*

# BIOARTIFICIAL ORGANS II[a]
## TECHNOLOGY, MEDICINE, AND MATERIALS

*Editors and Conference Organizers*
DAVID HUNKELER, ALEŠ PROKOP, ALAN D. CHERRINGTON,
RAY V. RAJOTTE, AND MICHAEL SEFTON

*Sponsor*
ENGINEERING FOUNDATION

CONTENTS



[a]This volume is the result of a conference entitled **Bioartificial Organs II: Technology, Medicine and Materials,** which was sponsored by the Engineering Foundation and held between July 18–22, 1998 in Canmore (Banff) Alberta, Canada.

**Part III. Encapsulation: Fundamentals and Applications**



**Part IV. Islet Isolation, Transplantation and the Bioartificial Pancreas**



**Part V. Biological Aspects**

## Part VI. Bioartificial Liver



## Part VII. Skin, Bone, Cartilage and Craniofacial Issues

**Financial assistance was received from:**

- BAXTER HEALTHCARE CORPORATION
- ENGINEERING FOUNDATION
- JUVENILE DIABETES FOUNDATION
- NATIONAL INSTITUTES OF HEALTH
- NATIONAL SCIENCE FOUNDATION
- NEW YORK ACADEMY OF SCIENCES
- ROCHE/BOEHRINGER MANNHEIM
- WHITAKER FOUNDATION

*This volume is dedicated to our friend and colleague Horst Dautzenberg, his wife Karin, brother Herbert, and the rest of his family. Horst, who participated actively in BIO+AO II, tragically passed away several days afterwards owing to complications arising from minor surgery.*

*We will miss you Horst.*

# Acknowledgments

This book would not have been possible without the meticulous and diligent efforts of Ingrid Margot, who edited each of the chapters, communicated with the authors and referees, and interfaced with the publisher. That she did all this ahead of schedule is a commentary of her excellence. We all know how frustrating this task can be, and Ingrid carried it out with the most pleasant demeanor one could imagine. Without her, the organizers would have been lost, and we are indebted to her dedication. Joyce Hitchcock and Bill Boland of the New York Academy of Sciences contributed extensively to the formulation, structure and publishing of the book. I would also like to thank José Maria Hernández Gil for his cover layouts along with Anthony Sun and Philippe Morel, whose work is highlighted on these photos. Those who participated in the chapter peer review process are thanked, anonymously. Your tireless and prompt work is much appreciated.

Barbara Hickernell, of the United Engineering Foundation, contributed so much to the conference organization, site selection and funding. We are deeply thankful of her efforts over the past five years with the Bioartificial Organs series, along with her associates Donna Romano and Rosa Landinez. Allen Laskin, the conference liaison, is also acknowledged for his program input. The conference site organization was expertly handled by Antionette Chartier.

The four co-chairs, Aleš Prokop, Allan Cherrington, Ray Rajotte and Michael Sefton, contributed endlessly over the two years this conference was being organized. I would also like to thank all the session chairs, speakers and chapter contributors who made, first the conference, and now the book, so successful. Allan Cherrington's tireless work on the awards committee is graciously acknowledged. Many of us would not have been in Banff were it not for the last minute flight organization of Rosa Landinez and Nancy Hunkeler. Artur Bartkowiak's coordination of the poster portion of the program was of invaluable assistance. Ray Rajotte, and his secretary Colleen Ruptash, are thanked for handling of all the local details.

Bioartificial Organs II was funded by generous donations from the United Engineering Foundation, New York Academy of Sciences, National Science Foundation, National Institutes of Health, Whitaker Foundation, Juvenile Diabetes Foundation International, Boehringer Manheim and Baxter Healthcare Corporation. A surplus from BIO+AO I, organized by Aleš Prokop, also contributed.

Bioartificial Organs III: Tissue Sourcing, Immunoisolation, and Clinical Trials, will be held in Davos, Switzerland October 7–11, 2000. Further information can be obtained from Ingrid Margot: +41-21-693-3692 (voice); +41-21-693-5690 (fax); ingrid.margot@epfl.ch (e-mail); or through the UEF web site: http://www.uefoundation.org.

DAVID HUNKELER
*16 January 1999*

# Introduction

*Bioartificial Organs II: Science, Medicine and Technology* attracted ninety-four participants, from fifteen countries and five continents, to Banff, Alberta, Canada. The five days of July 18–22, 1998, united forty-seven academics, twenty-nine industrialists, including eleven directors, CEOs and Vice-Presidents, as well as eighteen representatives from hospitals, national and international institutes, and funding agencies. The balance between medical professionals and biologists, material scientists, and engineers ensured a vigorous week of debates, which have already spawned some international initiatives and collaborations.

The conference began with an opening lecture by Joseph Kennedy on novel polymeric structures for immunoisolation based on carbocationic polymerizations. Fritz Bach of Harvard then gave the Plenary Dinner Talk, outlining his call for a moratorium on whole organ xenotransplantation. Between these excellent discussions, and the Closing Lecture by Gail Naughton, President of Advance Tissue Sciences, thirty- five oral presentations and twenty posters were presented. An afternoon panel discussion on Scale Up was also well attended. The eight sessions, which clustered founders and newcomers, researchers and inventors, clinicians and managers, included:

- Novel Materials and Clinical Applications
- Bioartificial Pancreas
- Tissue Sources: Xeno- versus Allografts
- Processing and Technology
- Oral and Craniofacial Issues
- Molecular Aspects in the Prevention and Recognition of New Materials
- Bioartificial Liver: Implants and Extracorpeal Cellular Devices
- Bioartificial Skin, Bone and Cartilage

The issues of appropriate tissue selection, including neonatal sources, was discussed in depth as were cell, in particular pancreatic islet, cryopreservation techniques. Phase II/III clinical trials of the bioartificial liver, injectable bioartificial cartilage, bioartificial skin, and modified hemoglobin blood substitutes were also outlined. In addition to the papers presented herein, BIO+AO II has been summarized in *Nature Biotechnology*[1] and has encouraged development of a unified platform on the safe and responsible development of immunoisolated xenografts.[2] The banquet was highlighted by Clark Colton's Lifetime Achievement Award for developments in the mechanistic understanding and mass transfer characteristics of bioartificial organs, the nutrient ingress and egress fluxes needed for cell viability, as well as the modeling and prediction of key device design parameters.

DAVID HUNKELER
*May 19, 1999*

[1] HUNKELER, D. 1999. Chameleons: bioartificial organs transplanted from research to reality. Nature Biotechnol. **17:** 335.

[2] HUNKELER, D., A. SUN, D. SCHARP, G. KORBUTT, R. RAJOTTE, R. GILL, R. CALAFIORE & PH. MOREL. Risks involved in the xenotransplantation of immunoisolated tissue. Nature Biotechnol. In press.

# Bioartificial Organs

## Risks and Requirements

DAVID HUNKELER

*Laboratory of Polymers and Biomaterials, Swiss Federal Institute of Technology, CH-1015, Lausanne, Switzerland*

### INTRODUCTION

The development of therapies based on bioartificial organs requires the appropriate tissue, material, and process selections. While the requirements for tissue engineered products, such as bioartificial skin and cartilage, differ from immunoisolation-based devices such as the bioartificial liver and pancreas, six key issues must be addressed, concomitantly, as one integrated clinical feedback with basic research and product development. These are summarized below.

#### *Appropriate Material Selection*

Sterilizability, residual endotoxin level and biocompatibility[1,a] are generally categorized as material preparation and purification operations. While their requirements are well documented[1] they are not usually coupled with questions related to quality control and raw material sourcing. Specifically, as bioartificial organs move into commerce[2] a consistent set of polymeric precursors will be required. Therefore, while tissue engineered products based on polylactic-co-glycolic acid can be regulated via the synthesis procedure, as can hollow fibers based on acrylics, diffusion chambers and microcapsules made of or filled with naturally occurring polysaccharides present challenges in terms of batch to batch repeatability. Recent innovations in controlled degradation of polyanions, such as alginate and carrageenans, as well as chitosan based polycations are discussed in the third chapter of Part II (Novel Materials) of this book. It is anticipated that only through the development of processes which regulate molecular parameters, principally the molar mass distribution and charge spacing, along with preparation protocols, which govern rheological and interfacial properties, and purification methods, can biomaterials be commercially applied as bioartificial organs. Material selection, therefore, relies on information related to the ability to purify polymer solutions via filtration, and centrifugation, the sterilizability of materials by irradiation and autoclaving, as well as endotoxin deactivation or removal. The use of blends or copolymers has also been shown to offer advantages in simultaneously controlling membrane properties such as permeability and mechanical strength.[3]

[a]Williams' Dictionary of Biomaterials, to be published in 1999 defines material biocompatibility as its ability to perform with an appropriate host response in a specific application.

### *Appropriate Tissue Sourcing and Harvesting*

The ethical issues related to tissue selection will be debated in the discussion section of this chapter. However, with the exception of autografts, which have a limited use in bioartificial organs (for example the re-transplantation of encapsulated islets from non-diabetic patients having full or partial pancreatotomies) tissue selection remains controversial. For several potential bioartificial organs the amount of allograft tissue available is significantly below demand and, as is the case for whole organ transplants, most national waiting lists are in the thousands for the kidney, liver, and pancreas. The ultimate substitution with xenografts or genetically modified cells is a topic of investigation and several sections of this monograph detail recent advances (Part IV: Islet Isolation, Transplantation and the Bioartificial Pancreas). To date xenograft-based bioartificial organs have had outstanding early successes[4] followed by two decades of minimal advancement. As a community, the physicians and biologists involved in tissue harvesting and selection need to assess contradictory data. For example, certain hormones secreted from discordant xenografts, such as porcine insulin, can be genetically quite similar to what is indigenously produced by the host (porcine insulin and human insulin differ by only one amino acid). However, in the case of porcine islets, tissue fragility is extreme and the xenotransplant cannot, despite the presence of a ingress- and egress-specific membranes, hide the graft from the host. Therefore, methods to improve graft survival, such as co-culture, and co-immobilization with various tissues, are viewed as possible means to induce a local immune protection (Part V: Biological Aspects). Clearly, this implicates transplant site selection as well as device recoverability. The latter presents a tradeoff between vascularization, to improve the supply oxygen and nutrients, and retrievability (Part III: Encapsulation).

### *Appropriate Process Selection*

The process of producing bioartificial organs is clearly a function of device geometry, with the appropriate material and method of preparation closely coupled.[5] Processes can vary from extrusion (liquid-liquid and liquid-air[6]) to spinning disks and mechanical cutting of fluid streams to generate discrete microcapsules. The tradeoffs associated with various immunoisolation technologies is treated in Part III (Encapsulation) with the aspects of the enzymatic process of cell harvesting, and tissue digestion, covered in Part IV. Clearly, the bioartificial organ, as a process, involves the synchronization of biological, technological and material quality control protocols. While this is not expected to be insurmountable, it has not been addressed to date.

### *Clinical Adaptability of the Device*

An aspect not normally addressed in bioartificial organ development is the ability to design materials which can cross platforms following clinical feedback. For example, most polysaccharides function only as components of microcapsular systems based on polyelectrolyte complexation, a reaction between oppositely charged molecules. The potential to use such systems in various transplantation sites is often limited by an inability to cast hollow fibers or structurally satisfactory flat membranes from the same material. This problem is exacerbated for typical phase inversion membranes which serve well in macro-sized bioartificial organs (e.g., Hybrid Bioartificial Pancreas) but cannot be formulated into microcapsules, and the acrylic hollow fibers which are easy to co-extrude, though only in a tubular configuration. Therefore, a hollow fiber based bioartificial pancreas, which may work intraperitoneally, would be impossible to inject intraportally in the liver. The development of novel materials which do not require device definition prior to clinical evaluation relieves several design constraints and, for the first time, provides surgeons with site-independent device alternatives (Part II).

### *Development of Science and Products*

Technology management requires the coordination of science, both existing and emerging, with product and process development, and marketing. For bioartificial organs this is complicated by the clinical trial sequence required to obtain regulatory approval. Although not specifically part of this compilation volume, BIO+AO II's Scale-Up panel discussion revealed that start-ups could technologically advance faster then the science justified and that this disequilibrium rippled through to the large corporate and venture capital supporters, often transiently destabilizing stock price. The predictability of marketing products, without regulatory approval, as well as the challenges in coordinating biological, material science and engineering activities, renders commercial biotechnology volatile at the best of times. Bioartificial organ development has not been an exception for the cartilage, skin and liver products (Parts VI and VII) in clinical trials, nor should one expect it to be for the next generation of devices treating other hormone deficient, or neurodegenerative, diseases.

### *Adequately Addressing Risks*

Bioartificial organs, as a therapy, present clinical risks. On a product level, technological development is coupled with financial and marketing uncertainties related to Phase I/II/III trials. Societal and ethical risks include those related to the use of xenografts. Recently Bach and Fineberg have called for a moratorium on xenotransplantation[7] which comprises four points:

- Public risk requires a public mechanism.
- Public risk requires an iterative legislation.
- Individual informed consent will have to be modified to include patients close relatives and sexual partners.
- Viruses can overcome the species barrier (e.g., return to pigs after infecting humans).

The discussion section of this chapter summarizes a response from eight participants at the BIO+AO II conference distinguishing the risks in whole-organ and immunoisolated xenotransplantation, as well as recommending a course of action.[8]

## DISCUSSION[b]

The authors of a recent paper[8] have noted the relevance of Bach and Fineberg's moratorium[7] to whole-organ transplantation and agreed, in general, with their first two statements, although the third point could be applied less strictly for immunoisolated xenografts for reasons that will be further elaborated herein. The following section is a verbatim copy of parts of the jointly issued response to the call for a moratorium.

*"Bach himself has noted that there has never been a reported case of a human infected with a porcine-derived pathogen due to porcine tissue exposure. Furthermore, as previously discussed, two recent studies clearly demonstrate no evidence of PERV infection following short[9] and long term[10] exposure to porcine tissues. As such, the risk is a potential risk and not a documented one. Therefore, society is put in the position to calculate an undefined risk. This is clearly distinct from defined infections transmitted by organ/tissue allografts. While this seems to reflect positively on cellular xenograft transplantation, we must remain concerned with our ability to limit exposure of the host to a potential porcine-derived pathogen. Since we do not know what the actual threat is, with some exceptions such as PERVs, it is difficult to quantify the risks, although one may speculate that an immune barrier will prevent egress of a pathogen to the recipient. In any case, the risks of whole-organ and cellular transplantation clearly differ, and the respective technologies should be examined and regulated (legislatively) separately. Bioartificial organs should follow a cautious path of implementation, as will be outlined in the recommendations section of this chapter.*

*A more general issue is that Bach and Fineberg's argument must also make the case that patient infection is due specifically to porcine xenografts. Since we raise, slaughter and eat pigs, our societal exposure to porcine tissues is considerable, including the aforementioned porcine tissue transplants. We have also implanted diabetics with porcine pancreatic extracts, prior to the development of genetically engineered human insulin, as well as porcine islets, and have no evidence of zoonoses contracted by this route. Thus, from a safety point of view (i.e., moratorium), one needs to argue that contracting a porcine-derived pathogen, if via a xenograft, could not also occur via another route (e.g., food supply).*

*Furthermore, the Karolinska Institute in Stockholm has grafted fetal pig islets into patients with insulin dependent diabetes mellitus while undertaking general immunosuppression.[11] Recently, the sera from these patients has been sent to the Center for Disease Control in Atlanta, GA. Although little, if any, function of the fetal tissue was detected, the naked islets caused no contamination, following intrahepatic implantation, in patients.*

*Cellular immunoisolated xenografts entail less risk than does whole-organ transplantation, since bioartificial organs are:*

- *Viral protective: membrane controls ingress/egress*
- *Antigen blocking: surface modifications change the host-contacting surface,*

[b]The text in the discussion is a highly condensed, verbatim, version of a paper, in press, used with permission of the publisher.[8] The DISCUSSION is not presented as the author of this chapter's sole work and full reference is given to all co-authors.

*blocking the antigen attachment-endothelial cell activation-hyperacute rejection cascade*

- *Retrievable: immunoisolation devices/bioartificial organs can be designed for retrievability*
- *Isolating: macro/micro device cascades can be constructed to provide cell isolation*
- *Controllable: cells can be genetically modified with suicide genes*
- *Robust: the transplantation site can be varied for bioartificial organs (e.g., use an immunoprivileged site)*

*Additionally, risk assessment can be performed prior to transplantation for cellular grafts such as islets. Indeed, preliminary evaluations have already been carried out, with extracorporeal xenograft-based bioartificial livers (BAL) in Phase III clinical trials (Part VI of this Book). Although the FDA has approved the use of the BAL as a bridge for comatose patients awaiting whole-organ transplantation, we believe that less threatening diseases require a cautious approach to implementation. Moreover, a clinical evaluation of cellular xenotransplantation should proceed only after it has been demonstrated that autografts and allografts of the bioartificial organ in question (e.g., pancreas, parathyroid) are safe and effective. Specifically, the authors of this paper advocate the systematic development of cellular xenotransplantation and application of bioartificial organs."*

## RECOMMENDATIONS

(1) *Research* on xenotransplantation in concordant and discordant animal models should proceed.
(2) Cellular xenograft transplantation should follow the *clinical* demonstration of concept and evaluation of bioartificial organ function in auto- and *allo*grafts.
(3) Cellular- and whole-organ xenotransplants involve unique recipient and societal risks and should, therefore, be regulated independently.
(4) The risks of cellular xenotransplantation can be assessed without threatening the public health. The proposed moratorium on whole-organ xenotransplantation should not be extended to xenograft-based bioartificial organs.[8]

## REFERENCES

1. Prokop, A. & T. Wang. 1997. Purification of polymers used for fabrication of an immunoisolation barrier. Ann. N.Y. Acad. Sci. **831:** 223–231.
2. Hunkeler, D. Chameleons: bioartificial organs move from the clinic to the market. Nature Biotechnol. In press.
3. Prokop, A., D. Hunkeler, M. Haralson, S. Dimari & T. Wang. 1998. Water soluble polymers for immunoisolation II: evaluation of multicomponent encapsulation systems. Adv. Polym. Sci. **136:** 55.
4. Lim, F. & A.M. Sun. 1980. Microencapsulated islets as bioartificial endocrine pancreas. Science **210:** 908.

5. RENKEN, A. & D. HUNKELER. 1998. Polimery **9:** 530.
6. HUNKELER, D. 1997. Polymers for bioartificial organs. Trends Polym. Sci. **5:** 286.
7. BACH, F. H. & H.V. FINEBERG. 1998. Call for moratorium on xenotransplants. Nature **391:** 326.
8. HUNKELER, D., A. SUN, D. SCHARP, G. KORBUTT, R. RAJOTTE, R. GILL, R. CALAFIORE & PH. MOREL. Risks Involved in the xenotransplantation of immunoisolated tissue. Nature In press.
9. PATIENCE, C., G.S. PATTON, Y. TAKEUCHI, R.A. WEISS, M.O. MCCLURE, L. RYDBER & M.E. BREIMER. 1998. Lancet **352:** 699.
10. HENEINE, W.H., A. TIBELL, M.W. SWITZER, P. SANDSTROM, G.V. ROSALES, A. MATHEWS, O. KORSGREN, L.E. CHAPMAN, T.M. FOLKS & C.G. GROTH. 1998. Lancet **352:** 695.
11. GROTH, C.G., O. KORSGREN, A. TIBELL, *et al.* 1994. Lancet **344:** 1402.

# Control of Complement Activities for Immunoisolation

HIROO IWATA,[a] YOSHINOBU MURAKAMI, AND YOSHITO IKADA

*Institute for Frontier Medical Sciences, Kyoto University, 53 Kawahara-cho, Shogoin, Sakyo-ku, Kyoto 606, Japan*

**ABSTRACT: Immunoisolation of cells by semipermeable membranes is a most promising approach to transplant xenogeneic cells. Although membranes which allow xenotranplantation have been reported, ambiguity remains as to their long term effectiveness. In this review, we would like to reconsider the immuno-isolative effectiveness of membranes reported from the standpoint of permeability and present our strategy to prepare membranes that can realize long-term functioning of xenograft. There are distinct different types of semipermeable membranes, hydrogel membranes and ultrafiltration membranes. Studies on their permeability indicated that neither of these membranes effectively fractionate solutes on the basis of molecular size under a diffusion-controlled process, nor thus can they immuno-isolate xenograft for a long time. Humoral immunity including antibodies and complement proteins is suspected of playing a major role in the rejection of xenografts. Control of complement cytolytic activities, not antibody permeation, may be a key factor determining the fate of the xenograft enclosed in membranes. We found that the microbead containing poly(styrene sulfonic acid) can consume complement cytolytic activities and thus can effectively protect xenogeneic islets of Langerhans in diabetic mice from the humoral immunity.**

## INTRODUCTION

Various endocrine diseases, such as insulin-dependent diabetes mellitus and parkinsonism, have had experimental and clinical recovery by transplantation of bioactive molecules releasing cells enclosed in a semipermeable membrane.[1,2] The principle of immunoisolation is shown in FIGURE 1. Oxygen and nutrients should be supplied at a sufficiently high rate through the membrane, though components of the host immune system should be prevented from ingress by semipermeability of the membrane. The properties required for the semipermeable membranes used in cell transplantation highly depend on the source of cells: allo- or xenogeneic.

An allograft is a graft between genetically different individuals within one species, while a xenograft is a graft between individuals from different species. It is believed that the predominant cause of allograft rejection is activation of cellular immunity by interactions of host T cells with a graft, while humoral immunity including antibodies and complement proteins is thought to play a major role in the rejection of xenografts.[3] For the allograft applied to a recipient without preformed antibodies, a membrane which can mechanically inhibit the contact of host immune

[a]To whom all correspondence should be addressed: +81-75-751-4119 (voice); +81-75-751-4144 (fax); iwata@frontier.kyoto-u.ac.jp (e-mail).

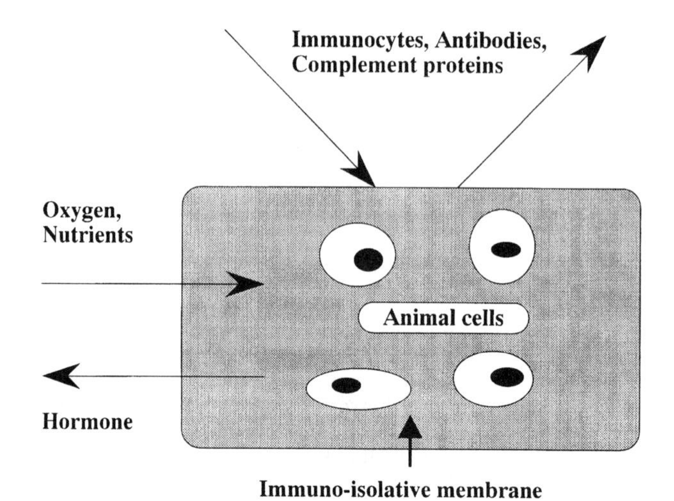


**FIGURE 1.** Schematic illustration of the immunoisolation principle.

cells with the graft is expected to effectively protect the graft from rejection. Such a membrane is not hard to be developed.[4–6] For xenografts, the semipermeable membrane must be designed to be highly permeable to low molecular weight molecules, but be able to prevent permeation of high molecular weight biomolecules, such as antibodies and complement proteins for a long time. The development of an immuno-isolative membrane that is applicable to xenografts is challenging, because of shortage of allogeneic donors. Although various membranes which allow xenotranplantation have been reported,[7–10] there is still ambiguity in their long-term effectiveness.

In this review, we will reconsider the immuno-isolative effectiveness of membranes reported from the standpoint of permeability, and present our strategy to develop the membrane applicable to xenograft.

## TRADITIONAL STRATEGY FOR IMMUNOISOLATION

There are distinct different types of semipermeable membranes, hydrogel membranes and ultrafiltration membranes, which have been employed (since the early 1970s) for immuno-isolation of xenografts. For both types of barriers, immuno-isolative efficacy has been believed to be attained by separating molecules according to their molecular size. In the hydrogel membrane, the increase in the solute molecular weight results in reduction in the diffusion coefficient due to interaction of the solute molecule with the hydrogel network. Ultrafiltration membranes are microporous in character and mechanically sieve molecules according to their molecular weight. In this part, the immuno-isolative efficacy of these two types of membranes is discussed from the stand point of permeability.

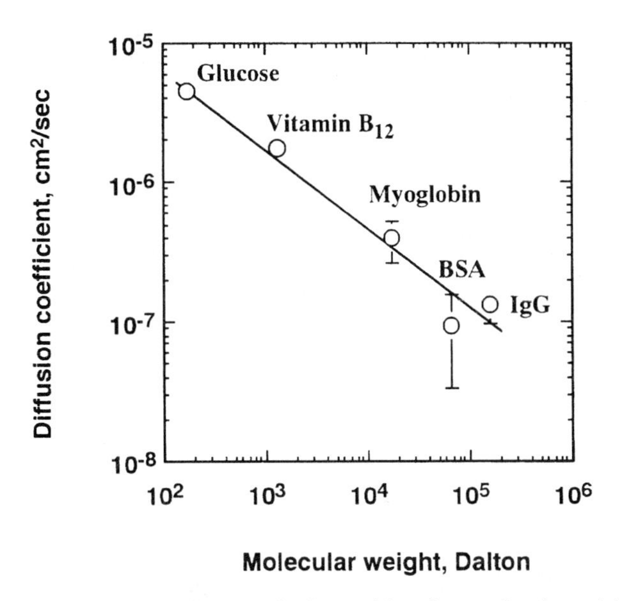


**FIGURE 2.** Diffusion coefficients of solutes with various molecular weights through a 5% agarose hydrogel.

### *Hydrogel Membrane*

A hydrogel membrane does not have distinct molecular weight cut-off and its selectivity is characterized by the diffusion coefficient of solutes. We have employed a 5% agarose hydrogel to immuno-isolate islets of Langerhans (islets).[11] The diffusion coefficients of solutes through the layer of 5% agarose hydrogel are shown in FIGURE 2.[12] Apparently, the increase in the molecular weight results in reduction in the diffusion coefficient. This is probably due to more prominent interaction of the solutes with the agarose network. However, most of xenogeneic recipients with microencapsulated hamster islets in 5% agarose hydrogel could not demonstrate normoglycemia for more than ten days.[11] The agarose gel can not effectively protect xenogeneic cells from the humoral immunity.

The time during which a solute diffuses through a microbead with thickness of L and then reaches to the cell surface is roughly expressed by:

$$t = \langle L^2 \rangle / 6D \qquad \textbf{(1)}$$

where $D$ is the diffusion coefficient of the solute through the hydrogel.[13] The diameter of the microbeads used in the islet transplantation is less than 1 mm. The diffusion coefficient of immunoglobulin G (IgG) through the 5% agarose hydrogel is an order of $10^{-7}$ cm$^2$/sec. Equation **(1)** predicts that it takes less than one day until IgG permeates through the microbead and reaches the surface of the islet. This calculation was confirmed using microencapsulated Protein A-Sepharose beads, which specifically bind IgG. When IgG diffuses into the agarose microbeads, the IgG attaches to and is immobilized onto the Protein A-Sepharose beads. The immobilized IgG

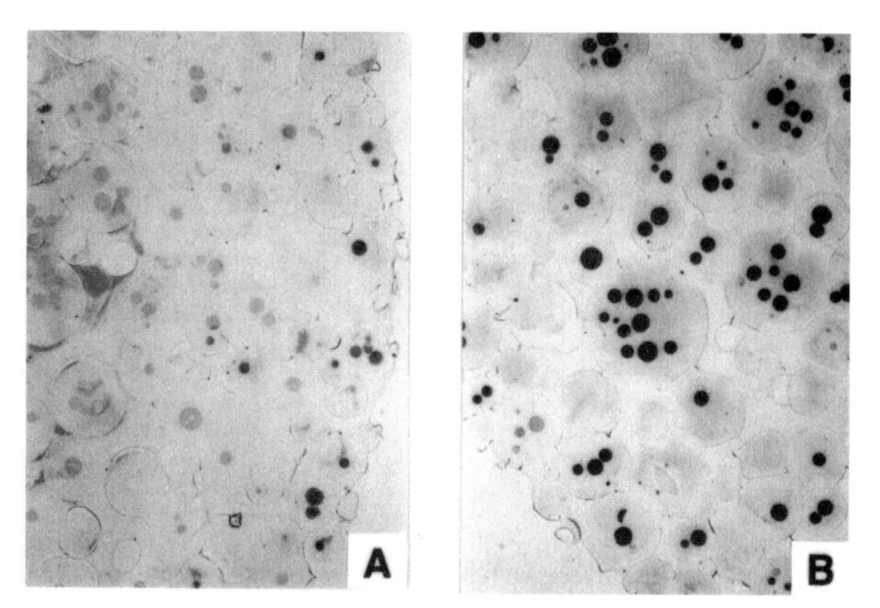


**FIGURE 3.** Permeation of immunoglobulins (IgG) through 5% agarose microbeads. When IgG diffuses into the agarose microbead, the IgG attaches to and is immobilized onto the Protein A-Sepharose beads. The immobilized IgG is visualized by immuno-staining. **(A)** one day incubation, **(B)** five days incubation.

was visualized by immuno-staining. The Protein A-Sepharose beads were stained lightly after 1 day and deeply after 5 days of incubation in rabbit serum, as is apparent from FIGURE 3.[14] This fact indicates that the agarose microbead retarded the permeation of IgG, but was unable to prevent the permeation of IgG for longer than several days.

The diffusion coefficient of IgG through the microbead should be less than 10–13 cm$^2$/sec to prolong the time more than 1 year during which IgG reaches the surface cells. However, it is extremely difficult to render the diffusion coefficient of IgG through the hydrogel membrane less than 10–13 cm$^2$/sec, simultaneously maintaining the rapid insulin release in response to high glucose stimulation.

### *Ultrafiltration Membranes*

The other type of membranes that has been used for immunoisolation is an ultrafiltration membrane. Ultrafiltration membranes with a nominal cut-off molecular weight of around 50 kD have been preferentially used to prepare devices for immunoisolation,[15] because it has been believed that the membrane allows passage of oxygen and nutrients, but restrict passage of antibodies of which molecular weights are higher than 150 kD. The representative membrane employed is Amicon's XM-50 membrane made of poly(acrylonitrile-co-vinyl chloride). Researchers working on bioartificial organs have believed that the solute permeability through a membrane determined by pressure-driven sieving experiments can predict its immuno-isolative

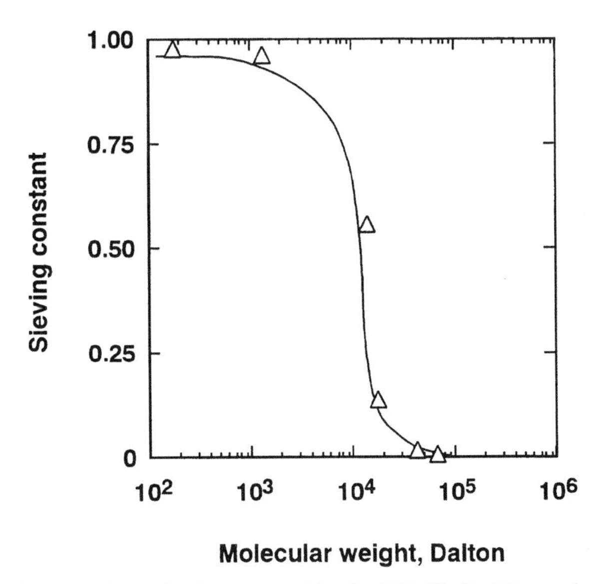


**FIGURE 4.** The solute rejection curve of the the XM-50 ultrafilter under the pressure-driven process.

efficacy.[10] However, it makes no sense because the fractionation efficiency of a membrane is known to highly depend on separation processes employed.[16]

*In vitro* permeation studies of solutes through the XM-50 membrane were performed under both pressure-driven filtration and concentration-driven permeation processes.[12] The solute selectivity under the pressure-driven filtration is given by sieving constant $\phi$ defined by

$$\phi = C_f / C_s \quad (2)$$

where $C_f$ is the concentration of a small volume of filtrate and $C_s$ is the simultaneous concentration of the filtering solution. The sieving constants of solutes with various molecular weights through the XM-50 membrane are plotted in FIGURE 4. The XM-50 membrane could reject 44.8% of lysozyme (MW = 14.3 kD) and 99.4% of bovine serum albumin (MW = 69 kD) in the filtration solutions, thereby effectively fractionating the solutes according to their molecular weights near 50 kD by ultrafiltration as claimed in the supplier's catalog.

When a device made of a XM-50 membranes is implanted, molecules permeate through the membrane driven by the concentration difference. In the *in vivo* situation, oxygen, nutrients, and immune competent proteins are afforded from the blood. They diffuse through several layers including the blood vessel wall, the host extra vascular space, the semipermeable membrane, and the hydrogel layer surrounding the cells as schematically shown in FIGURE 5(A). Thus, in *in vitro* permeation studies, the membrane was sandwiched with 5% agarose hydrogel layers, as illustrated in FIGURE 5(B), to mimic the *in vivo* diffusion process. The solute in the high concentration compartment was allowed to diffuse through the agarose hydrogel layer,

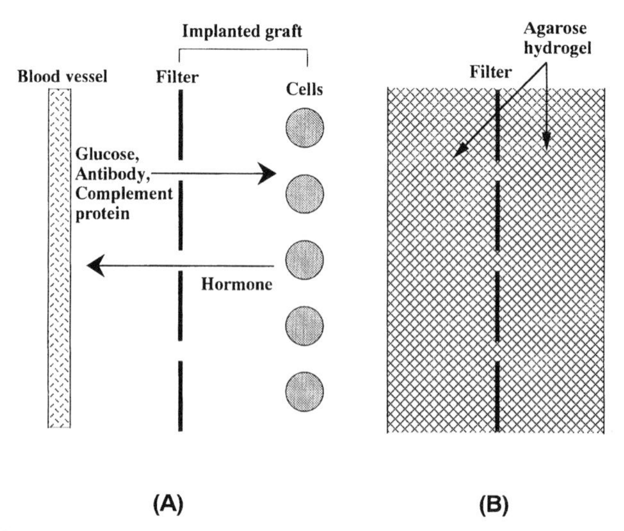


**FIGURE 5.** Model representation for diffusive permeation of solutes in the environment of an implanted graft **(A)** and a composite filter setup to simulate the *in vivo* diffusive permeation **(B)**.

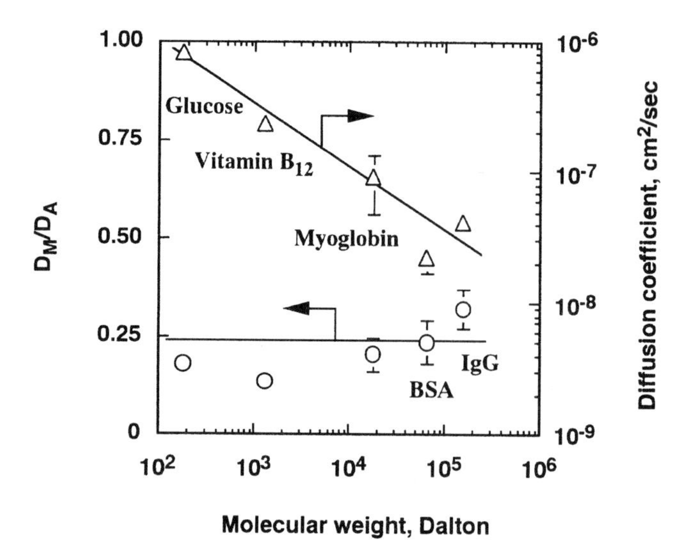


**FIGURE 6.** Diffusion coefficients of solutes with various molecular weights through the three-layered composite consisting of agarose hydrogel layers and the XM-50 filter. The ratios of the diffusion coefficient through the three-layered composite (DM) to that of the agarose hydrogel layer alone (DA), DM/DA, are also shown.

the XM-50 membrane, and then the other agarose hydrogel layer faced to the low concentration compartment. FIGURE 6 shows the diffusion coefficient of solutes through the three-layer composite membrane. Obviously, the diffusion coefficient decreases with the increase in the molecular weight of the solutes. FIGURE 6 also contains the ratio of the diffusion coefficient through the three-layered composite (DM) to that through the agarose hydrogel layer alone (DA) to extract the effect of the XM-50 membrane. The presence of the XM-50 membrane reduced the solute diffusion coefficients to approximately one fourth of those through the agarose hydrogel alone. However, appreciable dependence of the DM/DA ratio on the solute molecular weight was not observed. These findings indicate that the XM-50 membrane cannot fractionate the solutes on the basis of molecular size under the diffusion-controlled process.

These contradictory results shown in FIGURES 4 and 6 can be explained by accumulation of rejected proteins at the membrane surface under the pressure-driven process.[16] As Probstein *et al.*[17] proposed, a ultrafiltration membrane is actually a hybrid consisting of the original filter and the boundary layer in series, promoting rejection of a second partially rejected solute. However, such a hybrid layer might not be built up in the concentration-driven process because of low protein permeation rates, thereby limiting the fractionation efficiency of macrosolutes.

Dionne *et al.*[18] studied the transport characteristics of a membrane which is a hollow fiber made of poly(acrylonitrile-co-vinyl chloride) with the nominal molecular weight cut-off of 80 kD. Its chemical nature and membrane microstructure have resemblance to the XM-50 membrane. They also claimed that the standard pressure-driven measurements are inadequate to predict the rate or selectivity in diffusion-based devices and its diffusive transport properties must be determined for a membrane to be used for immunoisolation.

The ultrafiltration membrane, such as XM-50 membrane, loses the molecular size cut-off property in the diffusion-driven process. It can not protect xenografts by fractionating microsolutes and immune biomacromolecules according to their molecular weight. It seems to us that the immuno-isolative efficiency of the XM-50 membrane has been overemphasized by many researchers, because they have relied on data obtained from the pressure-driven ultrafiltration studies. It can be summarized that neither ultrafiltration membranes nor hydrogel membranes can immuno-isolate xenografts for periods which one would anticipate to require for a viable encapsulated cell therapy.

## COMPLEMENT FOR IMMUNOISOLATION

Various devices prepared using the XM-50 membrane and the agarose hydrogel have been employed for transplantation of xenogeneic islets into diabetic animals. The blood glucose level has been found to be normalized by the devices for periods of many months. One example is shown in FIGURE 7.[11] The network structure of an agarose hydrogel membrane was rendered dense by increasing the concentration of agarose. Although the diffusion coefficient of IgG in 7.5% agarose hydrogel is only one half of that in 5% agarose hydrogel, recipients that received 1500 of microencapsulated hamster islets in 7.5% agarose gel demonstrated 49, 63, and >100 (4 mice) days normoglycemic periods, respectively. Islet xenotransplantation in mice was possible using the microbead made of higher concentration agarose. This result

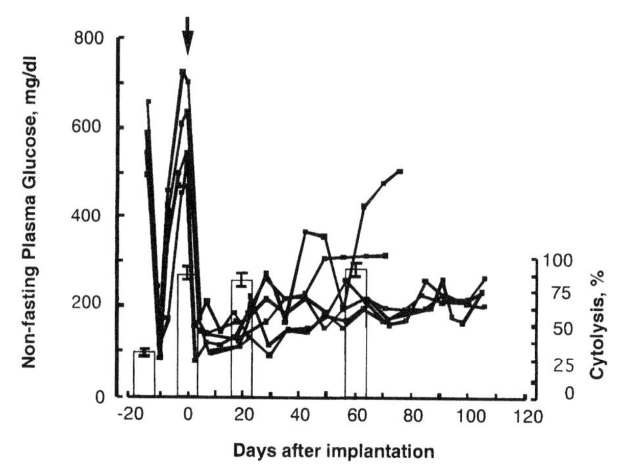


**FIGURE 7.** Changes in the nonfasting plasma glucose levels of diabetic BALB/c mice after intraperitoneal implantation of 1000 hamster islets enclosed in 7.5% agarose microbeads. Recipients were sensitized with implantation of native hamster islets at day −14. At day 0, microencapsulated islets were implanted. This figure also contains anti-hamster antibody levels.

conflicts with the prediction from the calculation using Equation **(1)** mentioned above.

### *Retardation of Permeation of Complement Proteins*

Antibody binding to the antigens on the xenogeneic cell surface alone cannot give lethal damage to the islet cells. For destruction of the xenogeneic cells, complement should be activated by antigen-antibody complexes on the cell surface. The contradictory results between the membrane permeability and its immuno-isolative effect on xenografts might be explained by the high instability of some complement proteins, such as C1, C2, and C5.[19] Complement proteins take certain time to permeate through the membrane and to reach the cell surface. It might be expected that some labile complement proteins are denatured and thus lose the cytolytic activity during permeation.

Stability of complement was simply studied by incubating serum from various animal species at 37°C for certain periods of time.[14] FIGURE 8 shows the plot of their hemolytic complement titers (CH50) as a function of the incubation time at 37°C. As can be seen, complement is rapidly inactivated following the pseudo first-order kinetics, irrespective of animal species. The inactivation kinetics is roughly expressed by:

$$\text{Inactivation rate} = -d(\text{CH50})/dt = k_1(C_0 - C_t) \qquad \textbf{(3)}$$

where $k_1$ is the rate constant of the pseudo first-order kinetics, $C_0$ is the initial CH50 value of individual serum or plasma, and $C_t$ is the CH50 value at time $t$. The $k_1$ values are tabulated in TABLE 1. It also represents the incubation periods during which the complement cytolytic activity decreased to one hundredth of the initial activity. All

**TABLE 1.** Rate constants of complement inactivation, $k_1$, and the incubation periods during which the complement activity decreased to one hundredth of the initial activity, $P_1/100$, for different sera and plasmas

| | $k_1$ day$^{-1}$ | $P_1/100$ days |
|---|---|---|
| Human plasma | 0.390 | 11.8 |
| Human serum | 0.507 | 9.1 |
| Dog serum | 0.369 | 12.5 |
| Guinea pig serum[a] | 4.76 | 1.0 |
| Rat plasma | 0.742 | 6.2 |
| Rat serum | 1.61 | 2.9 |

[a] Guinea pig serum was obtained from Organon Teknika Corp., PA.

of sera from various species lost the cytolytic complement activity during a few days incubations at 37°C.

These results suggest that the stability of complement proteins, not the antibody permeation, may be a key factor determining the fate of the xenogeneic cells in the agarose microbeads. Ideally, the complete exclusion of antibodies or complement proteins is required to realize the xenotransplantation. However, if the high instability of complements is considered, in practice, retardation of complement protein per-

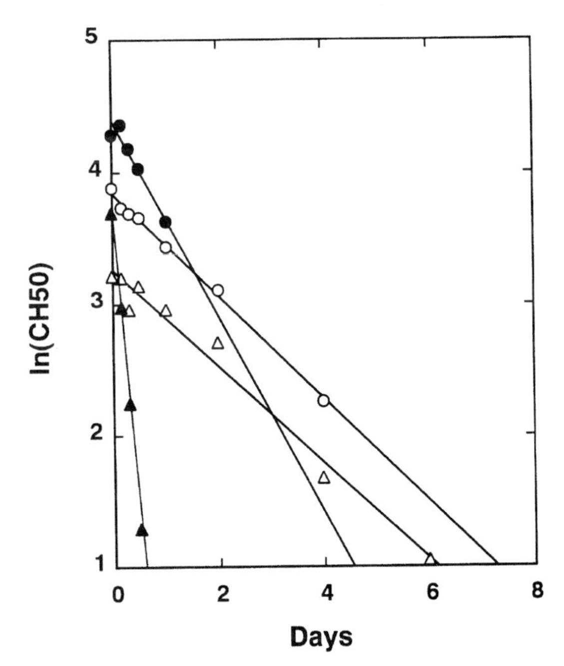


**FIGURE 8.** Time dependence of consumption of hemolytic complement activity (CH50) *in vitro* at 37°C. (O), Human plasma; (Δ), dog serum; (●), rat plasma; and (▲), guinea pig standard complement.

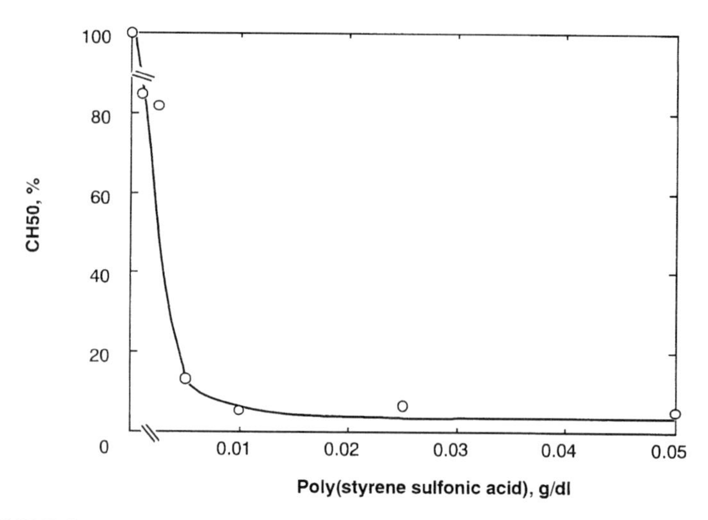


**FIGURE 9.** Effect of the addition of PSSa to serum on the hemolytic complement activity (CH50).

meation by the membrane for some periods during which the lytic activity of complements is destroyed is sufficient for immunoisolation.

### *Membrane Consuming Complement Cytolytic Activity*

The stability of complement proteins highly depends on species as shown in TABLE 1 and even on strains in the same species.[20] Since human and canine complements are more stable than those of rodents, membranes that can actively inhibit complement cytolytic capabilities are required to realize xenotransplantation in these recipients.

#### *Poly(styrene sulfonic acid) for Xenotransplantation*

Various polymers are known to interact with complement proteins. Hemodialysis membranes bearing hydroxyl groups, such as the regenerated cellulose, cellulose acetate, and poly(ethylene-co-vinyl alcohol) activate the complement system through the alternative pathway.[21] Other polymers carrying sulfonic acid or sulfate groups also strongly interact with complement proteins, resulting in a decrease of the cytolytic complement activity.[22] From these complement-interacting polymers, we selected poly(styrene sulfonic acid) (PSSa), since this is one of the most potent polymers that can consume cytolytic complement activities as will be discussed below and is miscible with agarose that we have employed for the preparation of the microbeads.[23,24]

The effect of PSSa on the complement cytolytic activity was examined by adding a certain amount of PSSa to human serum.[25] FIGURE 9 shows hemolytic complement titers (CH50) of the serum after incubation in the presence of PSSa at 37°C for 30 min. Apparently CH50 drastically decreased with the increasing PSSa concentra-

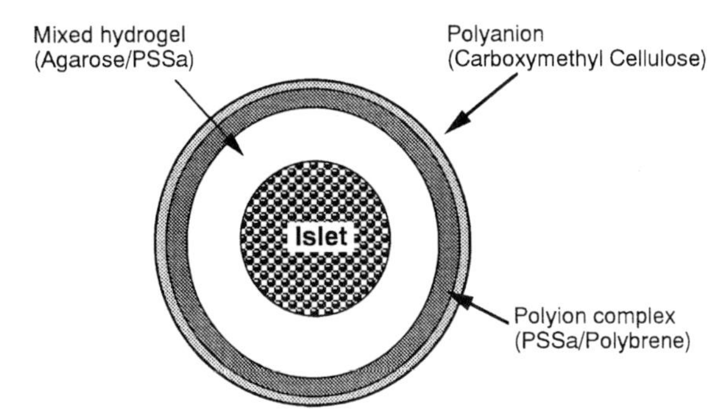


**FIGURE 10.** Schematic representation of the agarose/poly(styrene sufonic acid) (PSSa) microbead.

tion. An addition of $1 \times 10^{-2}$ g of PSSa to 100 ml of serum was enough to destroy the total hemolytic complement activity in the serum.

The structure of the agarose microbead containing PSSa and molecular structure of the polymers used are illustrated schematically in FIGURES 10 and 11, respectively. The microbead is composed of an agarose/PSSa mixed gel in which the PSSa is dissolved in the molecular network of the agarose hydrogel. A polyion complex layer is formed between the polyanionic PSSa and the polycationic polybrene at the periphery of the microbead to confine the PSSa molecules within the microbead. The

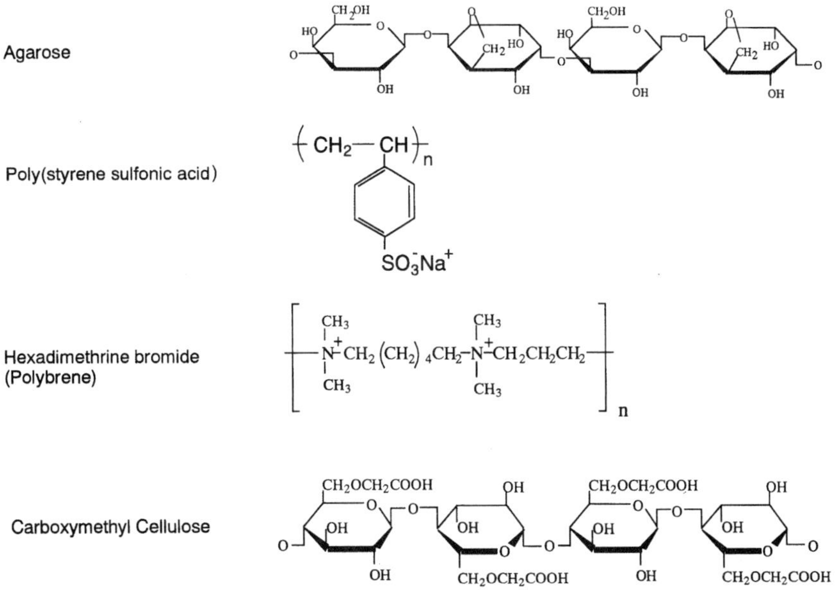

Agarose

Poly(styrene sulfonic acid)

Hexadimethrine bromide
(Polybrene)

Carboxymethyl Cellulose

**FIGURE 11.** Molecular structures of polymers used for preparing agarose/PSSa microbead.

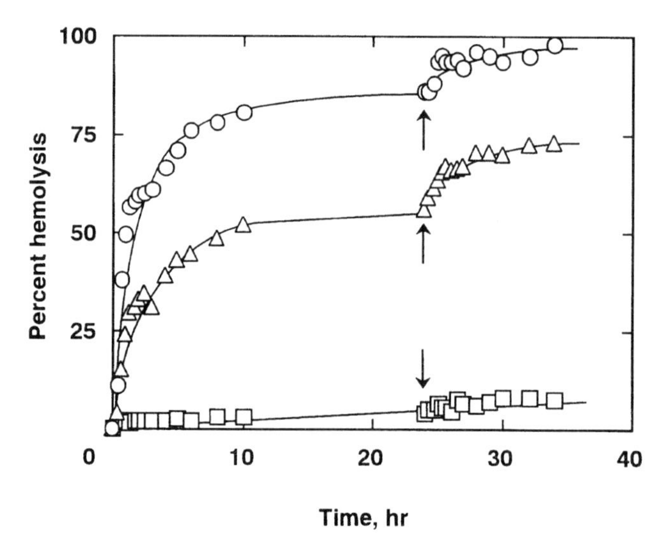


**FIGURE 12.** Time course of the percentage hemolysis of sensitized sheep erythrocytes (EA) encapsulated in various microbeads (incubation: in 10% human serum). (O), 2.5 wt% agarose microbead; (Δ), 5.0 wt% agarose microbead; and (□), 5.0 wt% agarose/5.0 wt% PSSa microbead. Arrows indicate the change of serum solution.

surface of the microbead is further coated with carboxymethyl cellulose to give tissue compatibility to the microbead.

The protective effect of the microbeads containing PSSa from the complement attack was assessed using sensitized sheep erythrocytes (EA) carrying antigen-antibody immune complexes on the cell surface.[25] Following microencapsulation, EA was incubated in the human serum. If active complement proteins permeate through the microbead, EA cells are lysed and release hemoglobin into the serum. The percentage hemolysis calculated from the released hemoglobin is plotted against the incubation period in FIGURE 12. As can be seen, the EA in the agarose microbeads without PSSa were lysed and released hemoglobin into serum. This means that the permeation of active complement proteins could not be prevented by the agarose hydrogel. On the other hand, quite low hemoglobin release was observed from EA when the agarose microbeads contained PSSa. It seems probable that during permeation of complement proteins through the agarose/PSSa microbeads, some of them were consumed or deactivated as a result of the interaction with PSSa. Therefore, complement proteins no longer destroyed the cell membrane, even when they reached the surface of EA.

The immuno-isolative effectiveness of the agarose/PSSa microbead was also examined by xenotransplantation of hamster islets to streptozotocin-induced diabetic BALB/c mice.[23] One thousand of hamster islets that were enclosed in 5% agarose/10% PSSa microbeads were implanted into the peritoneal cavity. Nonfasting plasma glucose changes are shown in FIGURE 13. The plasma glucose levels of the all recipients remained normal for more than 50 days after implantation. The microbead containing PSSa can effectively protect xenogeneic islets from the humoral immunity.

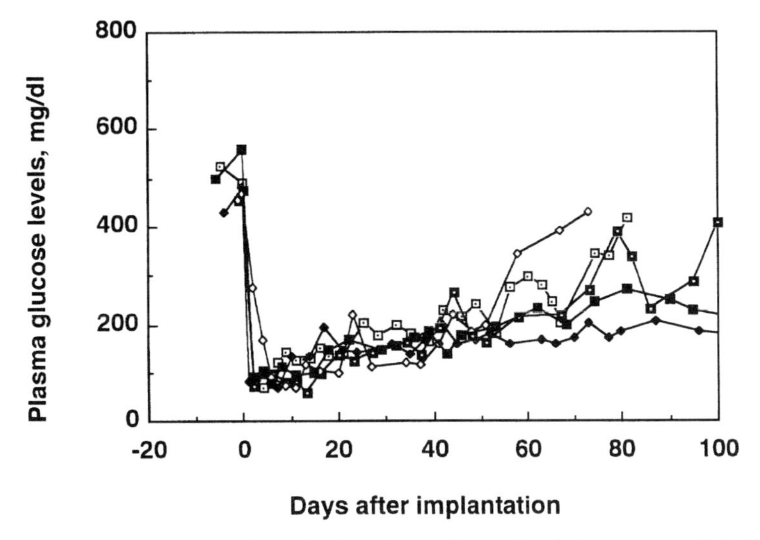


**FIGURE 13.** Changes in the nonfasting plasma glucose level of streptozotocin-induced diabetic BALB/c mice after intraperitoneal implantation of 1000 hamster islets enclosed in 5% agarose/10% PSSa microbeads.

*Interaction Mechanism of PSSa with the Complement System*

We were studying in some detail the interaction of PSSa with the complement system to make clear the mechanism of the immuno-isolative function of the agarose/PSSa microbead.[26]

Activation pathways of the complement system are shown in FIGURE 14. The hemolytic complement titer (CH50) of serum drastically decreased after incubation in the presence of PSSa at 37°C for 30 min as shown in FIGURE 9. The amounts of C3a and Bb generated in it is plotted against the PSSa concentration in FIGURE 15. As the PSSa concentration in serum increased, the amounts drastically increased. The fact indicates that activation of the alternative pathway was accelerated by addition of PSSa. The alternative pathway of the complement system is primarily down-regulated by accelerating the dissociation of C3 convertase, C3bBb, by factors *H* and *I*. Isoelectric focusing electrophoresis of the PSSa added serum demonstrated that the factor *H* band shifted to the cathode side compared with that in normal serum without PSSa. Factor *H* has more negative charges in the PSSa added serum than that in the native serum by forming a complex with PSSa. This fixation must lead to blockage of the regulatory function of factor *H*, resulting in escape of C3 convertase, C3bBb, from the inactivation action of regulatory factors *H* and *I*. Thus, component C3 and factor B are extensively activated in the fluid-phase C3b-dependent amplification system of the alternative pathway. The key component, C3, for complement cytolytic activities is consumed and lost during the activation. That resulted in no activation of the cytolytic phase even through the classical pathway, since the activation pathways of complement are a sequentially acting, multistep cascade and C3 locates at the confluence of the alternative and classical pathways.

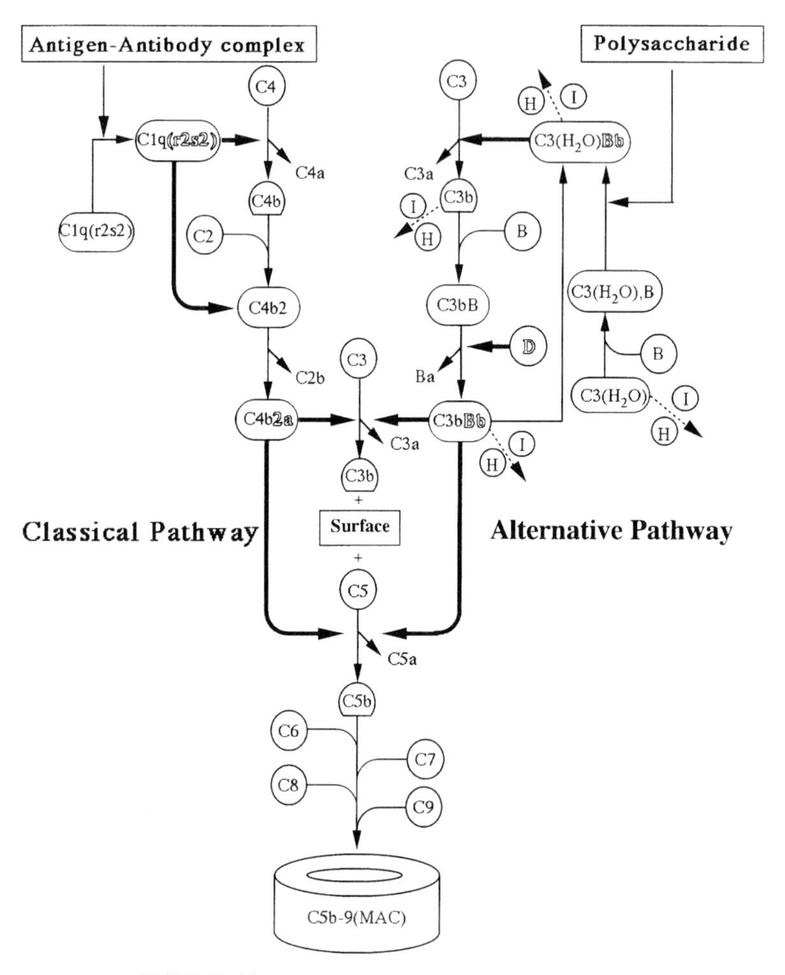


**FIGURE 14.** The activation pathways of complement.

The activation process of the classical pathway is initiated by binding of C1q to the Fc portion of IgM and IgG integrated within immune complex. The inhibitory effect of PSSa on C1 was studied using intermediate erythrocytes, EAC1, that is, sensitized erythrocytes (EA) carrying the complement component C1 on the surface. The EAC1 cells were incubated in PSSa solutions at 30°C for 15 min and PSSa removed by washing with Veronal buffer saline. The EAC1 cells treated with PSSa were exposed to the C1 deficient human serum or normal human serum. The hemolysis percentage sharply decreased in the PSSa density range from 0.01 to 0.1 g/1.5 $\times 10^9$ cells in the C1 deficient serum as shown in FIGURE 16. The EAC1 cells treated with PSSa could not be lysed when exposed to serum without C1. On the other hand, they were effectively hemolysed in the normal serum. These facts suggest that the C1 interacting with the immune complex on the erythrocytes was removed by exposure of the EAC1 to the PSSa solution. On the other hand, the denuded immune com-

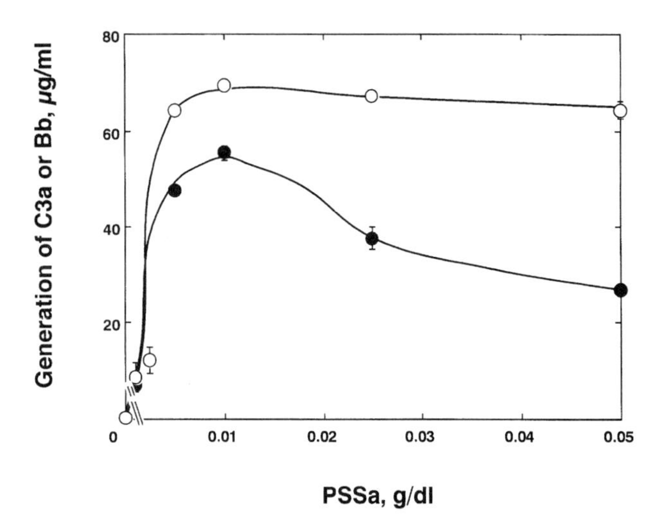


**FIGURE 15.** Generation of C3a and Bb fragments upon addition of PSSa into normal human serum. After 30 min of incubation of serum at 37°C in the presence of different amounts of PSSa, the amount of C3a and Bb generated was determined by ELISA. (O), C3a; (●), Bb.

plex could immobilize C1 again and initiated the complement cascade resulting in hemolysis in the normal human serum.

There is uncertainty in the long-term immuno-isolative effectiveness of the microbead containing PSSa through inhibition of C1 and factor H activities. When PSSa solution is added to serum, PSSa will interact with cationic components of the complement system, such as C1q and factor H, probably through polyion complex formation. If this is only one way for PSSa to interact with complement components, the microbead containing PSSa will lose potential to inhibit complement cytolytic activity after a certain time, since PSSa will be saturated with C1q and H and other cationic proteins that are continuously supplied by the recipient. Although there are a number of studies on the interaction between sulfonated or sulfated polyanions and the complement system, there are still ambiguities in mechanism. For example, some studies demonstrated the inhibition of complement activation by dextran sulfate,[27] while others showed the activation of complement by this polymer.[28] More detailed and well-organized studies are needed to make clear the mechanism of PSSa effects on the complement functions. There is another possibility for a long-term functioning of xenogeneic grafts enclosed in the agarose/PSSa microbeads. Graft accommodation, which is defined as the survival of a graft in the face of normal complements and antibodies, might occur after hyperacute graft rejection is shirked by the PSSa action.

A number of studies have demonstrated the inhibition of complement activation by polyanions. Neither an ultrafiltration membrane nor a hydrogel membrane can immuno-isolate xenografts for a long time, as mentioned above. We believe that the microbeads containing polyanion which can effectively regulate the complement function is the most promising approach to realize clinical xeno-islet transplantation.

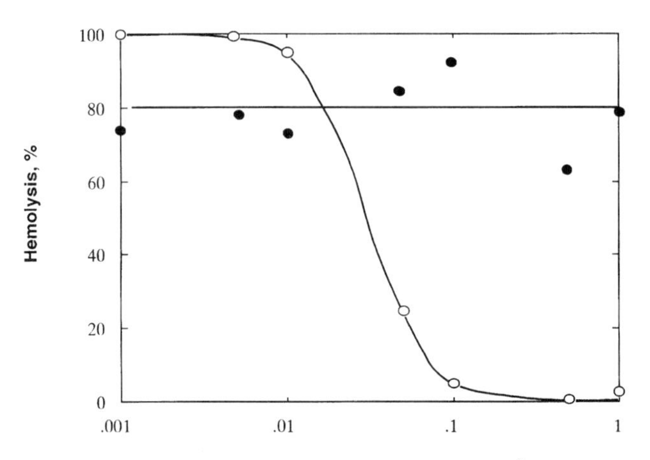


**FIGURE 16.** Effect of PSSa on the activation of the classical passway. Sensitized erythrocytes (EA) carrying complement component C1, EAC1, were incubated in the presence of PSSa at 30°C for 15 min. After thoroughly washing, the EAC1 cells were exposed to C1 deficient human serum or normal human serum. (O), in C1 deficient human serum; (●), normal human serum.

## REFERENCES

1. Soon-Shiong, P., R.E. Heintz, N. Merideth, Q.X. Yao, Z. Yao, T. Zheng, M. Murphy, M.K. Moloney, M. Schmehl, M. Harris, *et al.* 1994. Insulin independence in a type 1 diabetic patient after encapsulated islet transplantation. Lancet **343:** 950–951.
2. Aebischer, P., M. Goddard, A.P. Signore & R.L. Timpson. 1994. Functional recovery in hemiparkinsonian primates transplanted with polymer-encapsulated PC12 cells. Exp. Neurol. **126:** 151–158.
3. Paul, L.C. 1991. Mechanism of humoral xenograft rejection. *In* Xenotransplantation. D.K.C Cooper, E. Kemp, K. Reemtsma & D.J.G. White, Eds. : 47-67. Springer-Verlag. Berlin, Heidelberg.
4. O'Shea, G.M, M.F. Goosen & A.M. Sun. 1984. Prolonged survival of transplanted islets of Langerhans encapsulated in a biocompatible membrane. Biochim. Biophys. Acta **804:** 133–136.
5. Sullivan, S.J, T. Maki, K.M. Borland, M.D. Mahoney, B.A. Solomon, T.E. Muller, A.P. Monaco & W.L. Chick. 1991. Biohybrid artificial pancreas: long-term implantation studies in diabetic, pancreatectomized dogs. Science **252:** 718–721.
6. Iwata, H., T. Takagi, H. Amemiya, H. Shimizu, K. Ymashita, K. Kobayashi & T. Akutsu. 1992. Agarose for a bioartificial pancreas. J Biomed. Mater. Res. **26:** 967–977.
7. Maki, T., I. Otsu, J.J. O'Neil, K. Dunleavy, C.J. Mullon, B.A. Solomon & A.P. Monaco. 1996. Treatment of diabetes by xenogeneic islets without immunosuppression. Use of a vascularized bioartificial pancreas. Diabetes **45**(3)**:** 342–347.
8. Sun,Y., X. Ma, D. Zhou, I. Vacek & A.M. Sun. 1996. Normalization of diabetes in spontaneously diabetic cynomologus monkeys by xenografts of microencapsulated porcine islets without immunosuppression. J. Clin. Invest. **98**(6)**:** 1417–1422.

9. LANZA, R.P., D.ECKER, W.M. KUHTREIBER, J.E. STARUK, J. MARSH & W.L.CHICK.1995. A simple method for transplanting discordant islets into rats using alginate gel spheres. Transplantation **59:** 1485–1487.
10. COLTON, C.K. & E.S. AVGOUSTINIATOS. 1991. Bioengineering in development of the hybrid artificial pancreas. J. Biomech. Eng. (Trans. ASME) **113:**152–170.
11. IWATA, H., K. KOBAYASHI, T. TAKAGi, T. OKa, H. YANG, H. AMEMIYA, T. TSUJI & F. ITO. 1994. Feasibility of agarose microbeads with xenogeneic islets as a bioartificial pancreas. J. Biomed. Mater. Res. **28:** 1003–1011.
12. IWATA, H., N. MORIKAWA & Y. IKADA. 1996. Permeability of filters used for immunoisolation. Tissue Eng. **2:** 289–298.
13. ATKINS, P.W. 1994. 24.12 Diffusion probabilities. *In* Physical Chemistry, 5th Ed. : 854-855. Oxford University Press. Oxford.
14. IWATA, H., N. MORIKAWA, T. FUJII, T. TAKAGI, T. SAMEJIMA & Y. IKADA. 1995. Does immunoisolation need to prevent the passage of antibodies and complements?. Transplant Proc. **27:** 3224–3226.
15. ARCHER, J., R. KAYE & G. MUTTER. 1980. Control of streptozotocin diabetes in Chinese hamsters by cultured mouse islet cells without immunosuppression: a preliminary report. J. Surg. Res. **28:** 77–85.
16. INGHAM, K.C., T.F. BUSBY, Y. SAHLESTROM & F. CASTINO. 1980. Separation of macromolecules by ultrafiltration: Influence of protein adsorption, protein-protein interactions, and concentration polarization. *In* Ultrafiltration Membranes and Applications. Polymer science and technology, Eds. A.R. Cooper, Ed.: 141–158. Plenum Press. New York.
17. PROBSTEIN, R.F., W.F. LEUNG & Y. ALLIANCE. 1979. Determination of diffusivity and gel concentration in macromolecular solutions by ultrafiltration. J. Phys. Chem. **83:** 1228–1232.
18. DIONNE, K.E, B.M. CAIN, R.H. LI, W.J. BELL, E.J. DOHERTY, D.H. REIN, M.J. LYSAGHT & F.T. GENTILE. 1996. Transport characterization of membranes for immunoisolation. Biomaterials **17:** 257–266.
19. KITAMURA, H. Personal communication.
20. HITSUMOTO, Y. Personal communication.
21. DEPPISCH, R., H. GOEHL, E. RITZ & G.M. HAENSCH. 1998. Complement activation on artificial surfaces in biomedical therapies. *In* The Complement System, 2nd rev. ed. K. Rother, G.O. Till, G.M. Haensch, Eds : 487–504. Springer-Verlag. Berlin Heidelberg.
22. PANGBURN, M.K. 1998. Alternative pathway: activation and regulation. *In* The Complement System, 2nd rev. edit. K. Rother, G.O. Till, G.M. Haensch, Eds.: 93–115. Springer-Verlag. Berlin Heidelberg.
23. TAKAGI, T., H. IWATA, H. TASHIRO, T. TSUJI & F. ITO. 1994. Development of a novel microbead applicable to xenogeneic islet transplantation. J. Controlled Release **31:** 283–291.
24. IWATA, H., T. TAKAGi, K. KOBAYASHI, T. OKA, T. TSUJI & F. ITO. 1994. Strategy for developing microbeads applicable to islet xenotransplantation into a spontaneous diabetic NOD mouse. J. Biomed. Mater. Res. **28:** 1201–1207.
25. MORIKAWA, N., H. IWATA, T. FUJII & Y. IKADA. 1996. An immuno-isolative membrane capable of consuming cytolytic complement proteins. J. Biomater. Sci-Polym. Ed. **8:** 225–236.
26. MURAKAMI, M., E. KITANO, H. IWATA, H. KITAMURA & Y. IKADA. In press.
27. WUILLEMIN, W.A., H. TE-VELTHUIS, Y.T. LUBBERS, C.P. DE-RUIG, E. ELDERING & C.E. HACK. 1997. Potentiation of C1 inhibitor by glycosaminoglycans: dextran sulfate species are effective inhibitors of in vitro complement activation in plasma. J-Immunol. **159:** 1953–1960.
28. BURGER, R., U. HADDING, H.U. SCHORLEMMER, V. BRADE & D. BITTER-SUERMANN. 1975. Dextran sulphate: a synthetic activator of C3 via the alternative pathway. I. Influence of molecular size and degree of sulphation on the activation potency. Immunology **29:** 549–554.

# Designing Biomaterials to Direct Biological Responses

KEVIN E. HEALY,[a] ALIREZA REZANIA, AND RANEE A. STILE

*Division of Biological Materials, Northwestern University Medical School, 311 East Chicago Avenue, Chicago, Illinois 60611-3008, USA*

*Department of Biomedical Engineering, McCormick School of Engineering and Applied Science, Technological Institute, Evanston, Ilinois 60201, USA*

**ABSTRACT: We have set forth a design strategy for creating biomimetic materials that direct the formation of tissue surrounding implants or regeneration within porous scaffolds. Our studies have established that heterogeneous mimetic peptide surfaces (MPS) containing both the -RGD- (cell-binding) and -FHRRIKA- (putative heparin-binding) peptides, unique to BSP, in the ratio of 75:25 (MPS II) or 50:50 (MPS III) proved to be more biologically relevant and specific for RCO cell function. The initial response of human osteoblast-like cells to these surfaces was mediated by the collagen ($\alpha_2\beta_1$) and vitronectin receptors ($\alpha_v\beta_3$), whereas the vitronectin receptor alone dominated longer-term events (> 30 min). MPS II and III surfaces enhanced cell spreading and long-term events such as mineralization of the extracellular matrix compared to homogenous peptide surfaces and controls. Furthermore, extensive mineralization of the ECM deposited by RCOs occurred when the peptide was coupled to an interfacial interpenetrating polymer network (IPN) that resisted protein deposition (i.e., non-specific adsorption) and fouling. Work on thermo-reversible P(NIPAAm-*co*-AAc) hydrogels demonstrated the ability to create materials that can be delivered to the body in a minimally invasive manner and support tissue regeneration. These hydrogels can be modified to incorporate biofunctional components such as the biomimetic peptides, theoretically enhancing their ability to foster tissue regeneration. These results suggest that biomaterials can be engineered to mimic ECM components of bone (e.g., various organs) by grafting peptides in the appropriate ratios of the cell and heparin-binding domains, and ultimately modulate the expression of the osteoblast cell phenotype. Approaches similar to the one presented in this work can be used to design materials for hybrid artificial organs and other tissues.**

## INTRODUCTION

New classes of materials are being designed to control cell behavior and subsequently direct the formation of organ specific tissue. As early as the late first century AD synthetic materials have been used as functional dental implants with surprisingly simple techniques (e.g., wrought iron).[1] Although this false tooth is a remarkable example of an ancient functional implant in direct apposition with the tissue of the surrounding organ (i.e., osseointegration with bone), the biological interface be-

[a]Author for correspondence: Division of Biological Materials, Northwestern University, 311 East Chicago Avenue, Ward Bldg. 10-116, Chicago, IL 60611-3008; 312-503-4735 (voice); 312-503-2440 (fax); kehealy@nwu.edu (e-mail).

tween an implant and the host tissue is still considered as a major source of failure for most hybrid artificial organs and medical devices. When a material comes in contact with biological systems, initial events are dominated by protein adsorption, and platelet, blood and inflammatory cell adhesion. These events constitute what is regarded as the native response to the material and do not represent the optimal behavior between a material and host tissue. In the case of dental, craniofacial, and orthopedic implants, a major drawback to implant operations is the recuperation period needed before the patient is able to load the implant. A significant reduction in the time needed for adequate interfacial bonding between the implant and the surrounding tissue could reduce prolonged hospitalization associated with the procedure, decrease disability before function is restored, decrease morbidity, increase function, and ultimately lead to making therapies more widely available.

A design strategy for creating biomimetic materials that direct tissue regeneration either on solid implant surfaces or within porous bodies is delineated in FIGURE 1. The approach depicted is general for materials capable of regeneration of various tissues; however, specific reference is made to regeneration of bone and cartilage. A common theme in engineering cell and tissue behavior at device surfaces is to modify the material to selectively interact with a specific cell type through biomolecular recognition events. Thus, the first step in the process is the rational design of a biomolecular component of the material. A large variety of biological functions can be built into hybrid materials including: ligands for engagement with cell-surface receptors; enzymes to catalyze reactions; drugs for site-specific delivery; plasmid vectors for cell transfection; and, antibodies for analyte detection or chelation.[2] Materials modified in this manner can be used in sensors, diagnostic assays, drug delivery devices, separation and purification systems, hybrid artificial organs and devices, and medical and dental implants. Regarding materials for hybrid artificial organs, implants, and tissue engineering, covalent immobilization of peptides containing the adhesion domains of extracellular matrix (ECM) proteins to the base material is a promising approach.[3–7] These interactions are mediated by cell surface receptors, such as integrins and transmembrane proteoglycans, which bind to the peptide presenting the specific domain of the ECM protein. We refer to this approach as *biomimetic modification* or *engineering* of the material.

The central hypotheses of biomimetic surface engineering are that monolayer (i.e., one molecular layer) coatings of biologically active peptides affect cell attachment to the materials, and that surfaces or three-dimensional structures modified with these peptides preferentially induce tissue formation consistent with the cell type seeded on the device. To test these hypotheses one can employ computer-aided chemistry to optimize the structure-activity relationships between the peptides and a specific type of cell (e.g., osteoblasts, chondrocytes), and subsequently synthesize surfaces containing covalently immobilized peptides amenable for testing cell behavior (e.g., adhesion, proliferation, and phenotypic expression). Knowledge gained from these two dimensional experiments can be utilized to synthesize new materials that exploit these signals in three dimensions on either implants or within porous scaffolds. Ideally, tissue either formed surrounding the implant or within the porous scaffold would be directed by the biological signal present.

In this manuscript we address components of the strategy portrayed in FIGURE 1 to synthesize biomimetic materials. Although this design cycle has not been com-

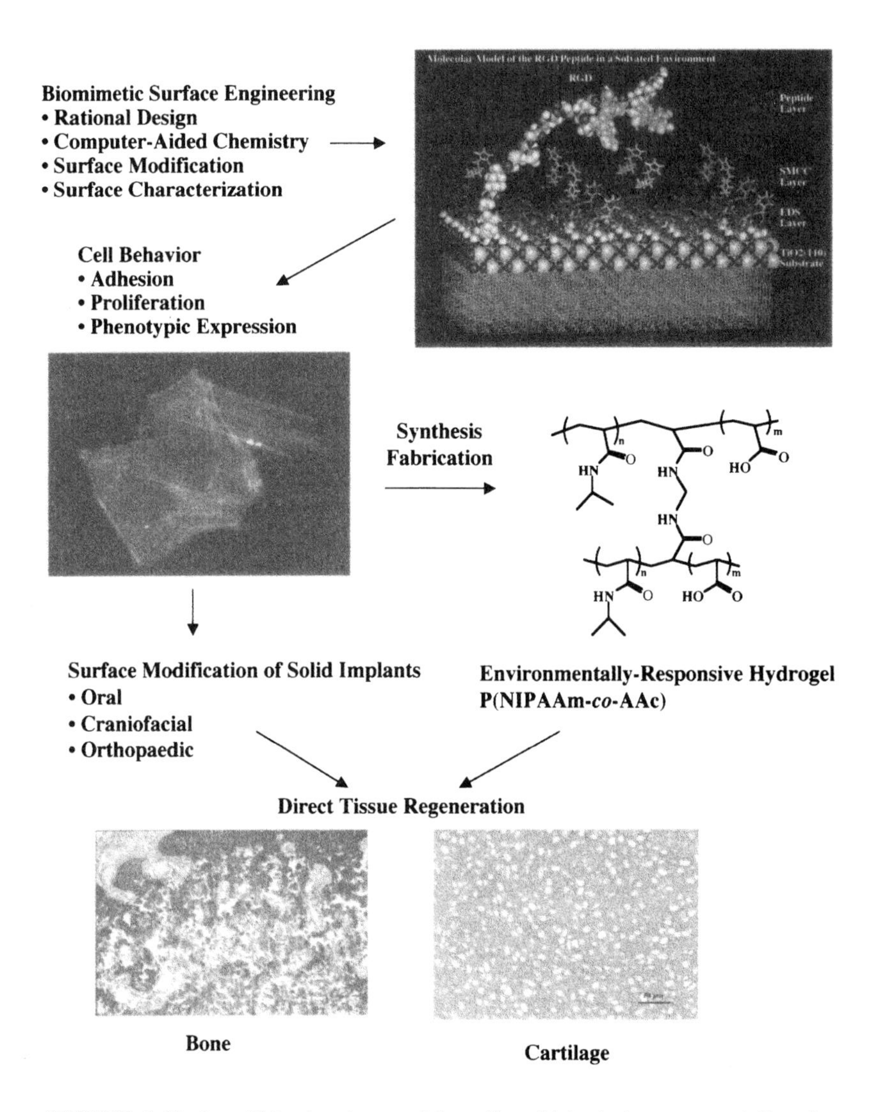


**FIGURE 1.** Design of biomimetic materials to direct biological responses. A flowchart of a design strategy for creating biomimetic materials that direct tissue regeneration either on solid implant surfaces or within porous bodies. The strategy is depicted for materials that foster bone and cartilage regeneration, but is sufficiently general as an outline for creating similar materials for the regeneration of other tissues. The figure points out a common theme in design and synthesis of bioactive materials: that a biomolecular signal can be incorporated directly into the material. Materials modified in this manner can be used in various devices including sensors, artificial organs, and medical and dental implants. The histological sections shown in this figure were obtained from either experiments addressing *in vivo* bone regeneration using porous bioabsorbable poly(D,L-lactide-co-glycolide)[31] or cartilage growth *in vitro* empolying P(NIPAAm) hydrogels.[25]

pleted to date, it represents a clear path for the creation of a generation of materials that can regulate tissue formation. In this report we: summarize our data testing the aforementioned hypotheses of biomimetic surface engineering; discuss preliminary data on injectable thermo-reversible hydrogels amenable to biomimetic modification; and, discuss future directions regarding the synthesis of bio- and environmentally responsive polymers useful for bone and cartilage regeneration.

## BIOMIMETIC SURFACE ENGINEERING

### *Design and Synthesis of Mixed Peptide Surfaces*

The central objective of biomimetic surface engineering for bone regeneration is to examine whether monolayer coatings of bioactive peptides affect bone cell adhesion and preferentially induce mineralization of the synthesized ECM on the modified materials. This objective was tested by designing model biomimetic surfaces containing different ratios of both the Arg-Gly-Asp (-RGD-) and heparin-binding domains of bone sialoprotein (BSP) capable of controlling mammalian cell behavior. We chose BSP since it is the major noncollagenous protein in bone and it has been shown to have a degree of specificity in human and rat osteoblast attachment.[8–10] Recently, BSP has been shown to have potential osteoinductive properties.[11]

The choice of making biomimetic surfaces containing two distinct binding domains of an ECM protein was based on our assessment of the literature. The most extensively used cell-binding domain to enhance cell adhesion onto biomaterial surfaces is the -RGD- sequence. However, other non-RGD containing cell-binding domains exist, such as Tyr-Ile-Gly-Ser-Arg (-YIGSR-) and Ile-Lys-Val-Ala-Val-(IKVAV) in laminin, Arg-Glu-Asp-Arg-Val (-REDRV-) and Leu-Asp-Val (LDV) in fibronectin, Asp-Gly-Glu-Ala- (DGEA) in collagen I, and various heparin-binding domains. However, previous data implicate the heparin-binding domain of adhesive ECM proteins, such as fibronectin, as a cofactor in promoting cell adhesion and spreading.[12–15] Studies by Dalton *et al.*[12] and Woods *et al.*[13] demonstrated that a more "complete" cell response (e.g., cell attachment, spreading, formation of discrete focal contacts, and organized cytoskeletal assembly) was obtained by providing the cell with both the cell binding (-RGD- containing) and heparin-binding domains of fibronectin. Thus, peptide sequences from both the cell binding and heparin binding domains of BSP were employed in our work.

Initial experiments analyzing cell behavior on biomimetic surfaces were performed with surfaces modified with peptides using organosilane chemistry. Based on our assumption that monolayer coatings dominate cell behavior, biological modifications were performed on quartz and $SiO_2$ substrates; however, the coupling methodology was easily transferable to implant materials (e.g., titanium). The immobilization strategy involved coupling of an aminofunctional organosilane (*N*-(2-aminoethyl)-3-aminopropyl-trimethoxysilane) to the metal oxide surface (i.e., $SiO_2$/Si and $TiO_2$/Ti) and derivitizing the terminal amine to a maleimide functional surface by coupling a heterobifunctional crosslinker (4-(*N*-maleimidomethyl) cyclohexane-1-carboxylate). The maleimide terminated surfaces were then used to couple a peptide from the cell-binding domain of bone sialoprotein CGGNGEP**RGD**-TYRAY via the thiol group on the terminal cysteinyl residue in the peptide.[6,16,17]

This methodology ensures that the molecule can freely interact with the cell-surface receptors and that the orientation of the coupled peptide is known in reference to the substrate. In addition to the RGD-containing peptide, a consensus peptide sequence of the heparin-binding domain, -Phe-His-Arg-Arg-Ile-Lys-Ala- (-FHRRIKA-), found within BSP was coupled to the surface. The CGGFH**RRIK**A peptide consists of a segment that includes clusters of basic and hydrophobic amino acids to form the consensus sequence, X**BB**X**B**X [where X = hydrophobic and B = basic]. Mimetic peptide surfaces (MPS) were made as homogenous layers and in mixed layers with the RGD: FHRRIKA peptides in ratios of 25:75 (MPS I), 75:25 (MPS II), and 50:50 (MPS III).

In addition, we have designed and synthesized interfacial interpenetrating polymer networks (IPNs) that resist protein deposition (i.e., non-specific adsorption) and fouling, and can be modified to tether bioactive groups such as the aforementioned peptides that mimic cell binding domains found in BSP. Coupling the peptide to a material that resists non-specific protein adsorption (e.g., the native response) maintains the activity of the molecule even in complex protein-containing biological environments.[3,7] The IPN was created by sequential photoinitiated synthesis of a thin layer of poly(acrylamide) [P(AAm)] followed by a secondary photoinitiation step using poly(ethylene glycol) [PEG] based monomers to create the network. Tethering of the peptide from BSP, CGGNGEP**RGD**TYRAY, was accomplished as described elsewhere.[7] All surfaces were characterized by contact angle measurements, spectroscopic ellipsometry, and X-ray photoelectron spectroscopy to confirm the presence of the peptides and their surface density, ~ 4–6 pmol/cm$^2$.[16–18]

## OSTEOGENIC CELL BEHAVIOR ON BIOMIMETIC SURFACES

### *Cell Adhesion and Morphology on Mixed Peptide Surfaces*

The morphology, extent of spreading, number, and strength of adhesion of primary rat calvaria osteoblast-like cells (RCOs) were examined on mimetic peptide and clean surfaces. Isolation of RCOs was modeled after methods described by Whitson *et al.*[19–21] The morphology and measured area of RCOs on the -RGD-, mixed RGD:FHRRIKA monolayers, FHRRIKA, -RGE- control surfaces (non-active peptide), and clean substrates after 4 h to 4 d were significantly different (Kruskal-Wallis analysis of variance by ranks). For example, after 2 h of incubation, the mean area of examined cells was significantly higher on the -RGD- compared to the -RGE- ($p < 0.00005$) and clean ($p < 0.00005$) surfaces. RCOs proliferated and reached confluence by 4 d for RGD, MPS II and MPS III surfaces. The rate to confluence was slower on the other surfaces: FHRRIKA, MPS I, and clean substrates. Inhibition assays, exposing cells to peptides prior to plating, confirmed the mechanism of attachment was due to the peptide immobilized on the surface. GAG lyases (heparinase I and chondroitinase ABC) were included in the cell medium to test the inhibition power of such enzymes on RCO attachment and spreading to -FHRRIKA- immobilized surfaces. Exposing cells to either heparinase, chondroitinase ABC, or both, to degrade cell surface proteoglycans, showed markedly decreased cell attachment and spreading. The inhibition assays confirmed the cell behavior was in direct response to the biomimetic modification of the surface.

### *Focal Contact Formation and Cytoskeletal Organization*

The degree of focal contact formation following 4 h of incubation on the peptide-grafted surfaces was examined by visualizing fluorescent staining of vinculin. The -RGD-, MPS I, II, and III surfaces all exhibited a significant number of discrete focal contact sites on the periphery of the fixed cells. Furthermore, there was no observable difference between the extent and location of vinculin staining on the -RGD-containing surfaces. Discrete vinculin staining was also observed on fixed cells attached to clean surfaces in the presence of 15% fetal bovine serum (FBS). However, there was no focal contact formation observed on -FHRRIKA-, -RFHARIK-, and -RGE- grafted surfaces. The extent of cytoskeletal organization was examined by staining for F-actin using rhodamine-phalloidin. There was extensive formation of thick microfilament bundles, extending across the length of spread cells, by cells on -RGD-, MPS II, and MPS III surfaces. Spread cells on MPS I surfaces exhibited fewer thick microfilament bundles compared to -RGD-, MPS II, and MPS III surfaces. Also, very few actin filaments were observed on -FHRRIKA- grafted surfaces. The attached cells on negative controls, -RGE- and -RFHARIK-, surfaces showed no cytoskeletal organization. Cells attached to clean surfaces in the presence of 15% (FBS) also exhibited extensive formation of thick microfilament bundles throughout the cell area. These results demonstrate that the -RGD- signal was required for prominent formation of focal contacts and cytoskeletal organization, and that the -FHRRIKA- peptide by itself promoted cell spreading, but was insufficient for focal contact formation and cytoskeletal organization.

### *Degree of Mineralization*

The extent of mineralized ECM formed on peptide-grafted surfaces was examined by Von Kossa staining of surfaces following 24 d of incubation in mineraliza-

**TABLE 1.** The fraction (%) of the surface covered by a mineralized matrix after 24d incubation *in vitro*[a]

| Surface | %Mineralized area |
|---|---|
| Clean | 0.2 ± 0.1 |
| Clean+FBS | 13.3 ± 0.6 |
| RGE | 4.1 ± 0.3 |
| FHRRIKA | 8.2 ± 0.5 |
| RGD | 24.0 ± 2.2 |
| MPS I | 24.8 ± 1.4 |
| MPS II | 31.0 ± 1.4 |
| MPS III | 29.9 ± 2.5 |

[a]The extent of mineralization was determined using the standard von Kossa stain and digital image acquisition and analysis. All surfaces were exposed to identical culture conditions.[17]

tion media.[20] After 24 d in culture the surface area covered by mineralized tissue was significantly different on the various surfaces. MPS II and MPS III surfaces promoted significantly ($p < 0.05$) larger areas of mineral deposits followed by MPS I > -RGD- > clean with FBS in media > -FHRRIKA- ≫ -RGE- ≫ clean. These findings indicated that the surfaces containing the proper ratio of -RGD-:-FHRRIKA- provided the osteoblast-like cells with signals that allowed both integrin and proteoglycan mediated adhesion, which resulted in significant and rapid expression of a mineralized ECM on the surface.

A non-adhesive IPN copolymer of acrylamide, ethylene glycol, and acrylic acid P(AAm-*co*-EG/AAc) was successfully functionalized with the biomimetic RGD peptide to test the efficacy of the peptide in the presence of serum proteins.[7,22] Biomolecular recognition processes were established with the RGD-IPN, while the system retained the ability to minimize non-specific protein binding interactions. Cells attached to RGD-IPN substrates at levels significantly greater than on RGE modified control, clean quartz, or unmodified IPN surfaces both in the presence and absence of FBS in the media (MANOVA, $p < 0.0002$, Post-hoc Newmann-Keuls). Cells maintained in media containing 15% FBS proliferated, exhibited nodule formation, and formed a mineralized ECM with the addition of β-glycerolphosphate to the media. Cell cultures tested positive for both membrane bound alkaline phosphatase, and mineralized tissue formation occurred over the entire RGD modified surfaces (Von Kossa). These combined staining results convey that the peptide modified coating was able to sustain viable cells, promote growth, and phenotypic expression.

### *Integrin Subunits Responsible for Adhesion of Human Derived Osteoblasts*

We have identified the integrin subunits responsible for initial adhesion and spreading of human osteoblast-like cells (HTOs) on peptide-modified surfaces (RGD, FHRRIKA, and MPS II). A panel of monoclonal antibodies against human $\alpha_1$, $\alpha_2$, $\alpha_3$, $\alpha_4$, $\alpha_5$, $\beta_1$, $\alpha_v$, and $\alpha_v\beta_3$ were used to identify the subunit(s) most dominant in mediating short term cell adhesion to the peptide surfaces. Anti-$\alpha_2$, anti-$\beta_1$, and anti-$\alpha_v$ significantly ($p < 0.05$) diminished cell attachment to RGD containing surfaces following 30 min of incubation. Following 4 h of incubation on RGD-grafted surfaces, immunostaining of these integrin subunits revealed discrete localization of the $\alpha_v$ subunit to the cell periphery similar to focal contact points, whereas the $\alpha_2$ and $\beta_1$ subunits showed very diffuse staining throughout the cell. A radial flow apparatus[23] was used to determine the effect of anti-integrin antibodies on the strength of cell detachment following 10 min of incubation on peptide grafted surfaces. The strength of detachment from RGD containing surfaces was significantly reduced ($p < 0.05$) in the presence of anti-$\alpha_2$, anti-$\alpha_v$, or anti-$\beta_1$ compared to control (preimmune mouse IgG). Furthermore, none of the antibodies used had any significant influence in mediating cell attachment to homogenous FHRRIKA-grafted surfaces. These results demonstrate that initially (> 30 min) HTO attachment to RGD containing surfaces was mediated by both the collagen receptor, $\alpha_2\beta_1$, and vitronectin receptor, $\alpha_v\beta_3$, whereas the vitronectin receptor governed longer term events (> 30 min). The importance of temporal differential usage of integrins in mediating bone cell attachment to RGD immobilized surfaces represents a potential strategy for engineering materials with built in surface specificity to cell adhesion.

## ENVIRONMENTALLY RESPONSIVE HYDROGELS AS SCAFFOLDS FOR TISSUE ENGINEERING

### *Synthesis of Injectable Poly(N-isopropylacrylamide)-based Thermo-reversible Hydrogels*

Having identified both the activity and mechanisms of interaction between the biomimetic surfaces and osteogenic cells, the next step in the outlined design strategy was to either create peptide-modified implant surfaces or materials for graft replacement. This section discusses the component of our work that addresses the need for materials that promote the regeneration of either bone or cartilage using the principles of tissue engineering.[24] We are trying to design and synthesize materials that contain biomimetic features and can be seeded with the patient's cells for implantation to replace missing or damaged bone or cartilage. Materials designed using this approach should also be minimally invasive and amenable to existing arthroscopic procedures.

Model injectable hydrogels that support cell growth and tissue formation *in vitro* were synthesized using the thermo-responsive polymer, poly(*N*-isopropylacrylamide) [P(NIPAAm)]. P(NIPAAm) is water-soluble at room temperature (RT) and phase-separates from water at a lower critical solution temperature (LCST) of approximately 32°C.[26] Aqueous P(NIPAAm) solutions turn cloudy above the LCST because the hydrophobic groups in the polymer chain form insoluble aggregates.[27] A schematic representation of the phase behavior of P(NIPAAm) chains and hydrogels is shown in FIGURE 2. The phase separation is reversible, and P(NIPAAm)

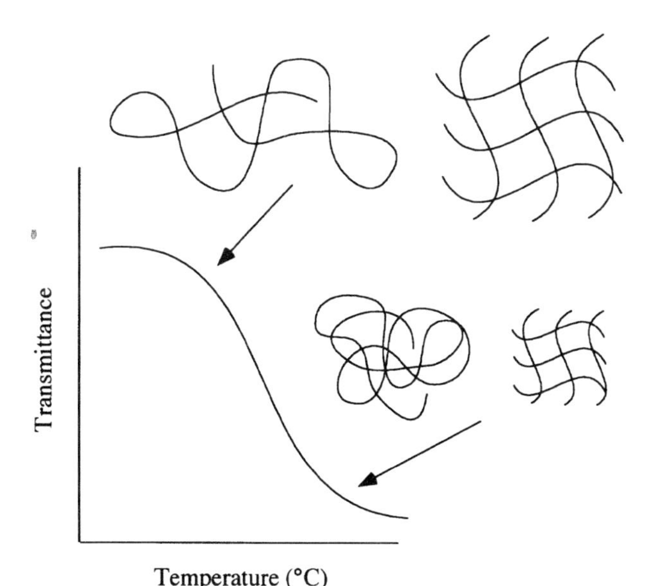


**FIGURE 2.** A schematic representation of a typical transmittance versus temperature curve for P(NIPAAm) chains and hydrogels, and a depiction of the phase change behavior of P(NIPAAm) chains and hydrogels at specific points in the transition (adapted from Hoffman[28]).

chains will redissolve in water as the temperature is lowered below the LCST.[28] P(NIPAAm) hydrogels demonstrate a reversible volume phase transition at the LCST and collapse as the temperature is increased above the LCST.[29,30] This unique phase behavior in water imparted both injectability and *in situ* stabilization to P(NIPAAm)-based matrices. As the highly hydrated three-dimensional (3D) network of the P(NIPAAm) hydrogel resembles the structure of the extracellular matrix (ECM) of tissues such as bone and articular cartilage, bovine articular chondrocytes were seeded into the injectable hydrogels and their response was studied *in vitro*.

In one injectable system, NIPAAm monomer and *N,N′*-methylenebisacrylamide (BIS) crosslinker (0.11–0.16% w/w NIPAAm) were polymerized in ultrapure (UP) water. A second injectable scaffold was synthesized with the addition of a comonomer, acrylic acid (AAc) [P(NIPAAm-*co*-AAc)]. Hydrogels containing NIPAAm, AAc (2.6% w/w total monomer), and BIS (0.16–0.20% w/w total monomer) were polymerized in phosphate-buffered saline (PBS). Following polymerization, both the P(NIPAAm) and P(NIPAAm-*co*-AAc) hydrogels were washed thoroughly in UP water to extract unreacted compounds.

### *Characterization of the P(NIPAAm)-based Hydrogels*

Qualitatively, the loosely crosslinked P(NIPAAm) and P(NIPAAm-*co*-AAc) hydrogels were readily injectable through a small diameter aperture (2 mm) and did not exhibit appreciable macroscopic fracture during injection. At RT, the hydrogels were colorless, transparent, and extremely pliable. When heated to 37°C, the P(NIPAAm) hydrogel collapsed extensively, released a large fraction of pore water, and turned opaque. The P(NIPAAm-*co*-AAc) hydrogels also experienced a phase transition when heated to 37°C, but were much less pliable than at RT. These hydrogels demonstrated a minimal volume change and maintained their shape well.

The polymer chemistry of the hydrogels was verified with solid-state $^1$H-magic angle spinning (MAS)-nuclear magnetic resonance (NMR) spectroscopy. The hydrogels were further characterized by determining the LCST with a UV-Vis spectrophotometer, calculating the water content (porosity) at RT (≈22°C) and 37°C via a freeze-drying technique, estimating the change in volume between RT and 37°C with a water displacement method, and studying the rheology with an oscillating rheometer.

The chemical structures of the P(NIPAAm) and P(NIPAAm-*co*-AAc) hydrogels were verified with the $^1$H-NMR spectroscopic analyses. Although a very small amount of residual NIPAAm monomer appeared to be present in the P(NIPAAm) hydrogel, no residual reaction components (e.g., NIPAAm or AAc) were present in the P(NIPAAm-*co*-AAc) hydrogel. The LCST of the P(NIPAAm) hydrogel was determined to be 31.2 ± 0.8°C, while the LCST of the P(NIPAAm-*co*-AAc) hydrogel was found to be 34.4 ± 0.5°C ($p < 0.01$). The water content of the P(NIPAAm) hydrogel at RT was initially 91.5 ± 0.8% and increased to 95.3 ± 0.8% after 6 days of swelling in PBS ($p < 0.01$). When the P(NIPAAm) hydrogel was heated to 37°C, the water content was initially 43.7 ± 7.7% and increased to 67.8 ± 11.9% after 6 days of swelling in PBS ($p < 0.01$). At RT, the water content of the P(NIPAAm-*co*-AAc) hydrogel was 92.6 ± 0.7% and was not affected significantly by swelling in PBS. When the P(NIPAAm-*co*-AAc) hydrogel was heated to 37°C, the water content was initially 93.3 ± 5.4% but decreased to 74.0 ± 8.4% when the hydrogel was swollen in PBS for

6 days prior to heating ($p < 0.01$). The change in volume exhibited by the P(NIPAAm) hydrogel decreased from 92% to 96% after 6 days of swelling ($p < 0.01$). The P(NIPAAm-*co*-AAc) hydrogel demonstrated an initial change in volume of $+5.3 \pm 6.1\%$, but collapsed $17.3 \pm 6.1\%$ and $41.3 \pm 4.6\%$ after 3 and 6 days of swelling, respectively ($p < 0.01$). It is important to note that the water content of the P(NIPAAm-*co*-AAc) hydrogel at 37°C was significantly higher than the water content of the P(NIPAAm) hydrogel at 37°C ($p < 0.01$). In addition, the P(NIPAAm-*co*-AAc) hydrogel demonstrated significantly less volume change than the P(NIPAAm) hydrogel when heated from RT to 37°C ($p < 0.01$). Finally, the P(NIPAAm-*co*-AAc) hydrogel became significantly more rigid when heated from RT to 37°C, as indicated by a significant increase in complex modulus determined from oscillatory rheometry studies.

### *Chondrocyte Growth and Viability* in Vitro *and* in Vivo

As a first step in evaluating these hydrogels for use in dental, craniofacial, and orthopedic applications, bovine articular chondrocytes were seeded into the hydrogels and cultured *in vitro*. We chose to use chondrocytes in our initial experiments, since the cell's phenotype is maintained by allowing the cell to attain a round morphology within a three-dimensional substrate. Since the P(NIPAAm-*co*-AAc) hydrogel was not yet functionalized with a biomimetic signal, it was capable of promoting the round morphology of the chondrocytes. *In situ* fluorescent viability studies and histological analyses were performed on the cell-loaded constructs. Bovine articular chondrocytes seeded into the hydrogels were viable for at least 28 days of *in vitro* culture, based on the *in situ* fluorescent studies. In addition, the cells maintained a round morphology throughout the course of the study, a typical indication of the differentiated chondrocyte phenotype. Histologically, the tissue formed in the hydrogels resembled native articular cartilage and was composed of individual cells surrounded by an ECM containing sulfated polysaccharides (i.e., sulfated glycosaminoglycans). The presence of sulfated glycosaminoglycans is another marker of the differentiated chondrocyte phenotype. Based on these observations, the hydrogel characterization data, and the fact that the carboxylic acid group in AAc can be easily funtionalized for targeting more cell-specific applications, P(NIPAAm-*co*-AAc) hydrogels have the potential to be used as synthetic scaffolds for articular cartilage and bone regeneration.

## FUTURE DIRECTIONS

### *Synthesis of Bio- and Environmentally Active Polymers*

The current state of our research program put us into position to complete the design cycle for creating materials that begin to direct tissue formation. We will test the ability of our current peptide modifications to promote bone regeneration. We are currently conducting studies comparing the effectiveness of the mimetic peptide surfaces (MPS II or III) on materials (e.g., titanium) that model craniofacial and orthopedic implants, and within the P(NIPAAm-*co*-AAc) hydrogels. Using similar chemistry, coatings of the P(AAm-*co*-EG/AAc) IPN grafted to metallic implants, and the P(NIPAAm-*co*-AAc) hydrogel can be modified with the heterogeneous mimetic peptide combination containing -RGD- (cell-binding) and -FHRRIKA- (putative heparin-binding). Positive results from these studies should set the stage for new classes of biomimetic materials useful for other applications in tissue engineering and the design of artificial organs.

## ACKNOWLEDGMENTS

This research was supported in part by NIH R01 AR43187, NIH T32 DE07042, and The Whitaker Foundation.

## REFERENCES

1. Crubezy, E., P. Murail, L. Girard & J.-P. Bernadou. 1998. False teeth of the Roman world. Nature **391:** 29.
2. Hoffman, A. S. 1992. Molecular bioengineering of biomaterials in the 1990s and beyond: a growing liaison of polymers with molecular biology. Artificial Organs **16:** 43–49.
3. Drumheller, P.D., D.L. Elbert & J.A. Hubbell. 1994. Multifunctional poly(ethylene glycol) semi-interpenetrating networks as highly selective adhesive substrates for bioadhesive peptide grafting. Biotechnol. Bioeng. **43:** 772–780.
4. Massia, S.P. & J.A. Hubbell. 1991. An RGD spacing of 440 nm is sufficient for integrin ($\alpha5\beta3$-mediated fibroblast spreading and 140 nm for focal contact and stress fiber formation. J. Cell. Biol. **114:** 1089–1100.
5. Massia, S..P. & J.A. Hubbell. 1992. Vascular endothelial cell adhesion and spreading promoted by the peptide REDV of the IICS region of plasma fibronectin is mediated by intgerin $\alpha_4\beta_1$. J. Biol. Chem. **267:** 14019–14026.
6. Rezania, A., C.H. Thomas, A.B. Branger, C.M. Waters & K.E. Healy. 1997. The detachment strength and morphology of bone cells contacting materials modified with a peptide sequence found within bone sialoprotein. J. Biomed. Mater. Res. **37:** 9–19.
7. Bearinger, J.P., D.G. Castner & K.E. Healy. 1998. Biomolecular modification of p(AAm-co- EG/AA) IPNs supports osteoblast adhesion and phenotypic expression. J. Biomater. Sci. Polymer Edn. **9:** 629–652.
8. Bianco, P., L.W. Fisher, M.F. Young, J.D. Termine & P.G. Robey. 1991. Expression of bone sialoprotein (BSP) in developing human tissue. Calcif. Tissue. Int. **49:** 421–426.
9. Mintz, K.P., W.J. Grzesik, R.J. Midura, P.G. Robey, J.D. Termine & L.W. Fisher. 1993. Purification and fragmentation of nondenatured bone sialoprotein: evidence for a cryptic, RGD-resistant cell attachment domain. J. Bone. Min. Res. **8:** 985–995.
10. Somerman, M.J., L.W. Fisher, R.A. Foster, J.J. Sauk. 1988. Human bone sialoprotein I and II enhance fibroblast attachment in vitro. Calcif. Tissue. Int. **43:** 50–53.
11. Wang, J., J.G. Kennedy, J.R. Kasser, M.J. Glimcher & E. Salih. 1998. Novel bioactive property of purified native bone sialoprotein in bone repair of a calvarial defect. Transactions of the 44th annual Orthopaedic Research Society Meeting **23-2:** 1007.
12. Dalton, B.A., C.D. McFarland, P.A. Underwood & J.G. Steele. 1995. Role of the heparin binding domain of fibronectin in attachment and spreading of human bone-derived cells. J.Cell. Sci. **108:** 2083–2092.
13. Woods, A., J.R. Couchman, S. Johansson & M. Hook. 1986. Adhesion and cytoskeletal Organisation of fibroblasts in response to fibronectin fragments. EMBO. J. **5:** 665–670.

14. PULEO, D.A. & R. BIZIOS. 1991. RGDS tetrapeptide binds to osteoblasts and inhibits fibronectin-mediated adhesion. Bone **12:** 271–276.
15. LATERRA, J., J.E. SILBERT & L.A. CULP. 1983. Cell surface heparan sulfate mediates some adhesive responses to glycosaminoglycan-binding matrices, including fibronectin. J. Cell. Biol **96:** 112–123.
16. REZANIA, A., R. JOHNSON, A.R. LEFKOW & K.E. HEALY. 1999. Bioactivation of metal oxide surfaces: I. Surface characterization and cell response. Langmuir. Submitted.
17. REZANIA, A. & K.E. HEALY. 1999. Biomimetic peptide surfaces that regulate adhesion, spreading, cytoskeletal organization, and mineralization of matrix deposited by osteoblast-like cells. Biotech. Progress. **15:** 19–32.
18. REZANIA, A. & K.E. HEALY. 1999. Integrin subunits responsible for adhesion of human osteoblast-like cells to RGD containing surfaces. J. Orthop. Res. In press.
19. WHITSON, S.W., M.A. EHITSON, D.E. BOWERS & M.C. FALK. 1992. Factors influencing synthesis and mineralization of bone matrix from fetal bovine cells grown in vitro. J. Bone. Min. Res. **7:** 727–741.
20. HEALY, K.E., C.H. THOMAS, A. REZANIA, J.E. KIM, P.J. MCKEOWN, B. LOM & P.E. HOCKBERGER. 1996. Kinetics of bone cell organization and mineralization on materials with patterned surface chemistry. Biomaterials **16:** 195–208.
21. THOMAS, C.H., C.D. MCFARLAND, M.L. JENKINS, A. REZANIA, J.G. STEELE & K.E. HEALY. 1997. The role of vitronectin in the attachment and spatial distribution of bone-derived cells on materials with patterned surface chemistry. J. Biomed. Mater. Res. **37:** 81–90.
22. BEARINGER, J.P., D.G. CASTNER, S.L. GOLLEDGE, A. REZANIA, S. HUBCHAK & K.E. HEALY. 1997. P(AAm-*co*-EG) interpenetrating polymer networks grafted to oxide surfaces: Surface characetrization, protein adsorption, and cell detachment studies. Langmuir **13:** 5175–5183.
23. REZANIA, A., C. H. THOMAS & K. E. HEALY. 1997. A probabilistic approach to measure the strength of bone cell adhesion to chemically modified surfaces. Ann. Biomed. Eng. **25:** 190–203.
24. Langer, R., J.P. Vacanti. 1993. Tissue engineering. Science **260:** 920–926.
25. STILE, R.A., W.R. BURGHARDT & K.E. HEALY. 1999. Synthesis and characterization of injectable Poly(*N*-isopropylacrylamide)-based hydrogels that support tissue formation in vitro. Macromolecules. In press.
26. HESKINS, M. & J.E. GUILLET. 1968. Solution properties of poly(*N*-isopropylacrylamide). J. Macromol. Sci. Chem. Edition **A2:** 1441–1455.
27. CHEN, G. & A.S. HOFFMAN. 1995. Graft copolymers that exhibit temperature-induced phase transitions over a wide range of pH. Nature **373:** 49–52.
28. HOFFMAN, A.S. 1991. Environmentally sensitive polymers and hydrogels: "Smart" biomaterials. MRS Bulletin **16:** 42–46.
29. HIROKAWA, Y. & T. TANAKA. 1984. Volume phase transition in a nonionic gel. J. Chem. Phys. **81:** 6379–6380.
30. HOFFMAN, A.S., A. AFRASSIABI & L.C. DONG. 1986. Thermally reversible hydrogels: II. Delivery and selective removal of substances from aqueous solutions. J. Controlled Release **4:** 213–222.
31. WHANG, K., K.E. HEALY, D.R. ELENZ, *et al.* 1999. Engineering bone regeneration with bioabsorbable scaffolds with novel microarchitecture. Tissue Eng. **5:** 35–51.

# New Microcapsules Based on Oligoelectrolyte Complexation

ARTUR BARTKOWIAK[a] AND DAVID HUNKELER

*Laboratory of Polymers and Biomaterials, Department of Chemistry, Swiss Federal Institute of Technology, CH-1015 Lausanne, Switzerland*

**ABSTRACT: A new one-step microencapsulation procedure has been developed. For the alginate/oligochitosan system the molar mass of the chitosan is a key parameter in the formation of stable, elastic capsules with high modulus. Furthermore, the selection of an optimum molar mass provides an additional degree of freedom, permitting the simultaneous regulation of mechanical properties and permeability without the need for multicomponent organic-inorganic chemistries as have been previously employed. The effects of molar mass of chitosan, its concentration, the alginate molar mass and its metal salt on the preparation, physical properties, and release characteristics of the capsules have been studied.**

## INTRODUCTION

Over the past two decades a variety biologically active species have been immobilized or encapsulated, ranging from enzymes for bioreactors and biosensors[1] to hepatocytes for the treatment of liver failure.[2] Microencapsulated cells, in general, have potential for the treatment of diseases requiring enzyme or endocrine replacement as well as in nutrient delivery of enzymes and bacteria. Encapsulation is, furthermore, employed in various industries including food,[3] agriculture,[4] and biotechnology,[5] the latter of which is clearly a high value-added application. A particular case of encapsulation involves immunoisolation of mammalian cells for the generation of bioartificial organs.

A wide variety of approaches, based on various polymer chemistries, processes for membrane formation and encapsulation technologies have been evaluated. These have been summarized in a recent review.[6] Other than some innovative chemistries introduced by Sefton[7] and Dautzenberg,[8] who employed, respectively, phase inversion and complex coacervation to form the capsular membranes, the overwhelming majority of the literature over the past two decades has utilized the alginate/poly-L-lysine polyelectrolyte symplex system.[9] Generally, multivalent ions such a calcium or barium are used to gel the alginate. These solid beads are then coated with a solution of an oppositely charged polyelectrolyte (poly-L-lysine). The beads are converted into a permeable capsule by liquefying the gel, usually via the addition of the chelating agent such as ethyleneditetracetic acid or sodium citrate.

While Sun, who pioneered the alginate/poly-L-lysine chemistry,[10] was successful, originally in rodents and more recently in larger animal discordant xenografts,

[a]e-mail: Artur.Bartkowiak@epfl.ch

many authors have failed to repeat his results. Further disadvantages of the alginate/poly-L-lysine system include the present cost of the polycation and the limited mechanical properties and biocompatibility reported by some groups.[11] Moreover, the reproducibility of the capsule properties of both polymers is still questionable, owing to the batch to batch changes in properties. Therefore, modification of this chemistry has been extensively investigated, where metal cations other than $Ca^{2+}$ [12] and poly(amino acids) other than poly-L-lysine[13] have been employed. Poly-L-lysine can be also replaced by other polycations, with the chitosan found to be a good substitute. This natural occurring polysaccharide exhibits various biological activities and many attempts have been made to apply it as a biomaterial.[14]

They are many "so-called" chitosan/alginate capsules described in the academic literature,[15] with the first attempt to replace poly-L-lysine with chitosan having been reported by Rha *et al.* in 1984.[16] Such capsules can be produced by a one-step procedure, where alginate is dropped into the calcium/chitosan solution, or in two steps where alginate/calcium preformed beads are subsequently coated with chitosan.[15]

Several of the preparation methods for preparing alginate/$Ca^{2+}$/chitosan capsules have been patented.[17–19] However, all techniques employ high molar mass polymers (greater than 10 kD) with reactions carried out below a pH of 6.6 to ensure chitosan solubility. Furthermore, the replacement of PLL by chitosan does not significantly improve capsule mechanical properties nor does it permit the control of membrane molar mass cut-off.

The capsule membrane formation involves a salt bond formation between two oppositely charged polymers during the diffusion of chitosan macromolecules into the wide pore alginate/$Ca^{2+}$ gel bead matrix. However, in the absence of the addition of calcium cations, very thin and fragile membranes are formed owing to the slow diffusion of polycation. The authors believe that this limitation can be overcome by employing a lower molar mass chitosan, in analogy to the cellulose sulfate/pDADAMC system introduced by Dautzenberg.[8]

The objective of our investigation has been the evaluation of the effect of chitosan molar mass (<100 kD) on mechanical properties and permeability of binary alginate/chitosan microcapsules.

It will be shown in this paper that the control of the molar mass (MM) of the polyelectrolytes is a key parameter in the formation of stable capsules.[20] Furthermore, the selection of an optimum MM provides an additional degree of freedom to the binary polyelectrolyte complexation, permitting the simultaneous regulation of mechanical properties and permeability without the need for multicomponent organic–inorganic chemistries as have been previously employed.

## EXPERIMENTAL

### *Materials*

#### *Alginate*

Alginate Keltone HV (lot. 46592A: $M_n$ = 300 kD and polydispersity of 2.3) was obtained from Kelco/NutraSweet (San Diego, CA, USA). Molar masses were inferred from (gel permeation chromatography) measurements on a Shodex OHpak

SB-804 HQ stationary phase using 0.1 M aq. $Na_2SO_4$ as a mobile phase. A relative calibration curve based on pullulan standards (PSS, Mainz, Germany) was employed.

*Chitosan*

Chitosan samples with different molar masses (1–100 kD) were obtained in controlled radical degradation by hydrogen peroxide (0.8–6.4 mMol/g of polysaccharide) at 80°C[21,22] of chitosan HMW (Aldrich, Buchs, Switzerland, Lot. 06026MN with degree of deacetylation 86.2%). Molar masses of chitosan samples were estimated by GPC measurements using the Shodex OHpak SB-804 HQ and 0.5 M acetic acid/0.5 M sodium acetate buffer system, which is recommended by Showa-Denko Company (Tokyo, Japan).[23] Pullulan and polyethylene glycol standards (PSS, Mainz, Germany) were used for column calibration and as relative references for MM calculation. All other reagents were of analytical grade.

### *Microcapsule Preparation*

Capsules were formed from a pair of oppositely charged polysaccharides, where a 0.75–1.5% aqueous sodium alginate was prepared in deionized water, 0.9% NaCl, or a 1% aq. mannitol solution. Approximately 2 mL of this solution was introduced into a 5 mL disposable syringe with a 0.4 mm flat-cut needle (Becton Dickinson AG, Basel, Switzerland). The droplets were sheared off for 30 sec (kdScientific syringe pump, Bioblock Scientific, Frenkendorf, Switzerland: flow rate 1 mL/min) into 20 mL of 1% chitosan (molar mass varied between 1–100 kD) solution when the pH was adjusted to 6.5 with 1 M NaOH. The microcapsules produced (1–3 mm in diameter) were allowed to harden for 30 minutes, filtered and rinsed with solvent used for preparation of polysaccharide solutions. Each process was repeated 3–4 times with collected microcapsules (more than 2 mL in volume) stored at 4°C. The entire capsule formation procedure described herein has been performed at ambient temperature.

### *Permeability Measurements*

Two mL of microcapsules were placed in a 10 mL recipient bath. Two mL of a 0.1% polymer standard solution (glucose plus four dextrans 4–110 kD), in 0.9% NaCl, was added under agitation. Aliquots were withdrawn at various times and injected into a liquid chromatograph equipped with a Shodex SG-G and SB-803 HQ columns. The eluent was 0.9% NaCl applied at a flow rate of 0.5 mL/min. The polymer concentration was proportional to the height of the detected chromatographic peak and solute diffusion was calculated with respect to the initial standard concentration. In this study the cut-off of microcapsules was defined as the lowest molar mass of dextran for which solute diffusion was smaller than 2% after a contact time of 32 minutes.

### *Mechanical Characterization*

Microcapsules were tested on a Texture Analyzer (TA-2xi, Stable Micro Systems, Godalming, UK). The apparatus consists of a mobile probe moving vertically at a constant velocity. The capsules were compressed at 0.1 mm/sec speed until bursting

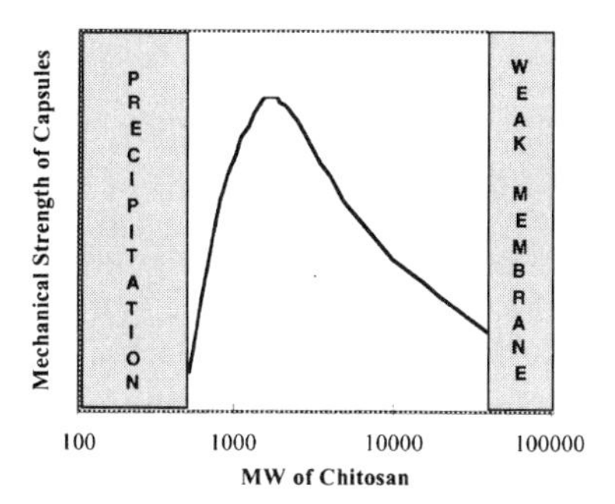


**FIGURE 1.** Mechanical properties of alginate/chitosan capsules as a function of the chitosan molar mass.

occurred. The force exerted by the probe on the capsule was recorded as a function of the displacement (compression distance), therefore leading to a force vs. strain curve. Twenty capsules per batch were analyzed in order to obtain statistically relevant data.

## RESULTS

Chitosans of various molar masses were prepared by controlled radical degradation method using continuous addition of hydrogen peroxide at 80°C from 0.5 to 4 hours. All samples have similar polydispersity of MM (1.5–1.6) and degrees of deacetylation (80–84%).

The effect of chitosan molar mass on the relative mechanical strength of the prepared chitosan-alginate capsules, measured by their bursting force, is illustrated in FIGURE 1. Mechanical properties of capsules are strong function of the chitosan molar mass. Below approximately 600–1000 daltons, precipitates are formed (no microcapsules). In the few seconds after the reaction the alginate drop surface is covered with a milky, non-transparent, unstable membrane, which during the reaction transforms into the white precipitate. Apparently, the oligochains (2–6 monomeric units) are to short to react with more than one alginate chain and, therefore, do not function as crosslinkers and consequently do not create stable membranes.

Above a molar mass of 30 kD the membranes are quite thin and have weak mechanical properties. Generally capsules are so fragile that after removing the surrounding solution they rupture under their own weight.

Dautzenberg *et al.* described membrane formation of two oppositely charged polyelectrolytes as a two-step process.[24] This begins with the spontaneous creation of a solid-like precipitate at the droplet surface as the result of the phase separation process. After this initial step the inner-direction build-up of membrane is observed. This process is diffusion-controlled, where the polycation penetrates through the membrane formed in the first step. When the cut-off of the primary membrane is too low the polycation molecules are not able to diffuse through. This is the case when chitosan of molar mass higher than 30 kD was used.

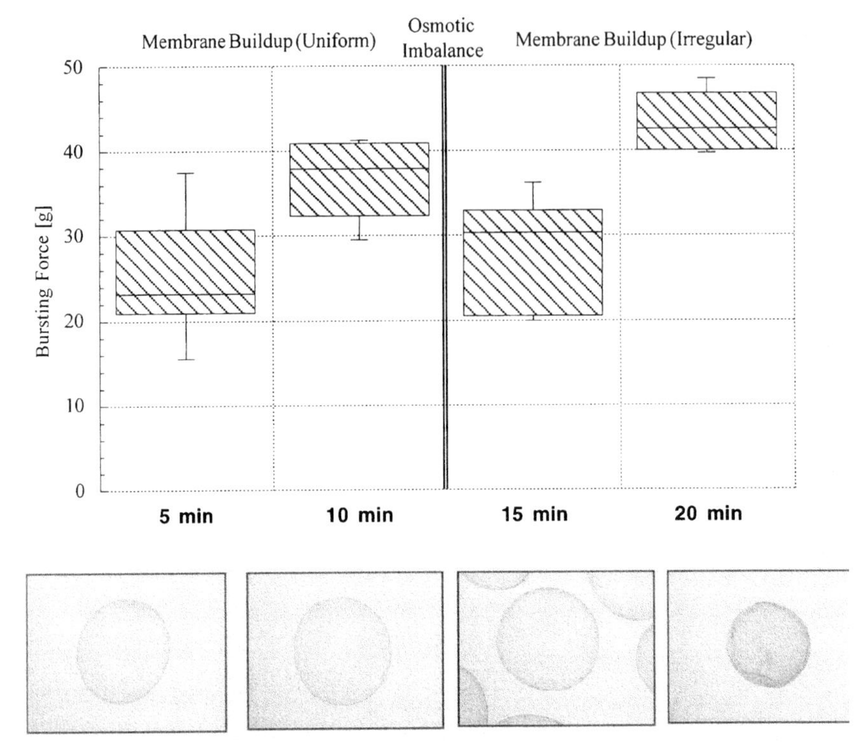


**FIGURE 2.** Influence of reaction time on alginate/chitosan capsule mechanical resistance (chitosan 2.5 kD, reaction time 5–20 min, 1.25–1.75 mm in diameter). The vertical line refers to the "osmotic imbalance" between solution interior and exterior to the capsules. The horizontal lines in the "box" represent the average values of the bursting forces.

Between the molar mass extremes mentioned above, stable capsules are generated with a maximum strength at a chitosan molar mass of 2000–3000 daltons. The capsule mechanical strength is one of the most important features for practical purposes. With reduction of the chitosan molar mass below 30 kD, the formation of capsules with increasing membrane thickness and mechanical properties is observed. Similarly the molar mass of chitosan employed in the encapsulation procedure was determined to by a key factor in the alginate/$Ca^{2+}$/chitosan capsule formation.[25] However, in that case the optimum molar mass for stable capsules formation was in the range of 160–330 kD. This difference is caused by immobilization of alginate by calcium cations in the form of porous gel matrix. The decrease of membrane stability observed for molar mass below 2000 is a consequence of the participation of precipitation process in alginate/chitosan membrane formation.

All reactions described in this paper were carried out at pH 6.5, which is a limit of chitosan solubility. However, oligochitosans below 8–10 kD are soluble above pHs of 7.0. The new binary capsules with good mechanical properties can be formed up to a pH of 7.4, which will be detailed elsewhere.[26] The ability to produce capsules under neutral and slightly basic conditions is a strong advantage of the newly devel-

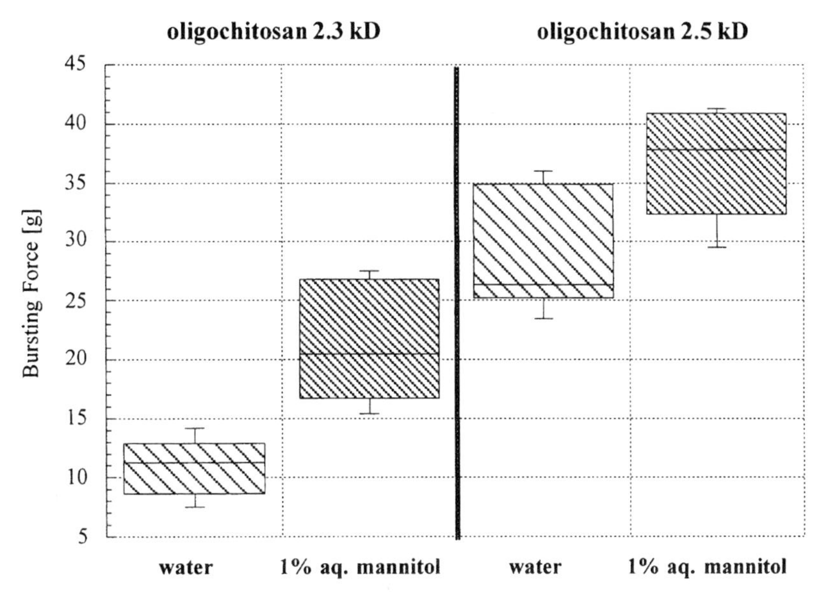


**FIGURE 3.** Mechanical resistance of capsules prepared in pure water and 1% mannitol solution (chitosan 2.3 and 2.5 kD, reaction time 10 min, 1.25–1.75 mm in diameter).

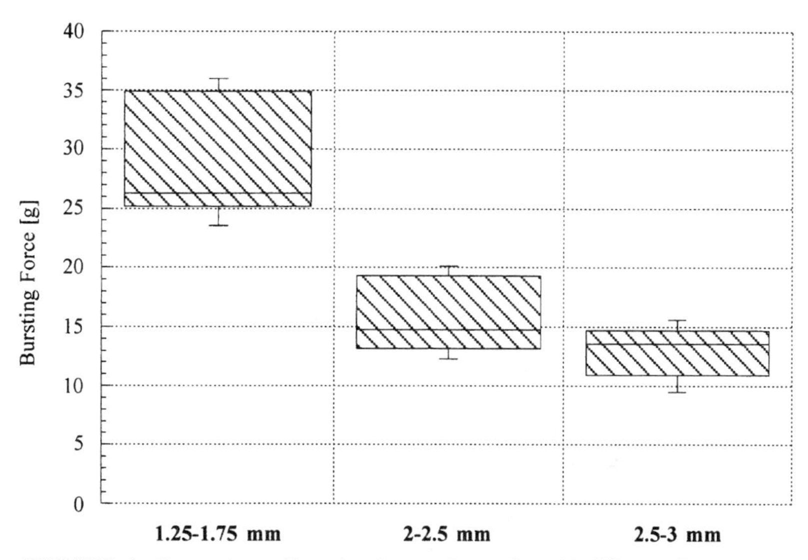


**FIGURE 4.** Comparison of bursting forces of capsules with different diameters (chitosan 2.5 kD, reaction time 10 min).

oped method, since the alginate/$Ca^{2+}$/chitosan-based capsules can only be produced up to a pH of 6.6. Since several types of biologically active species, including mam-

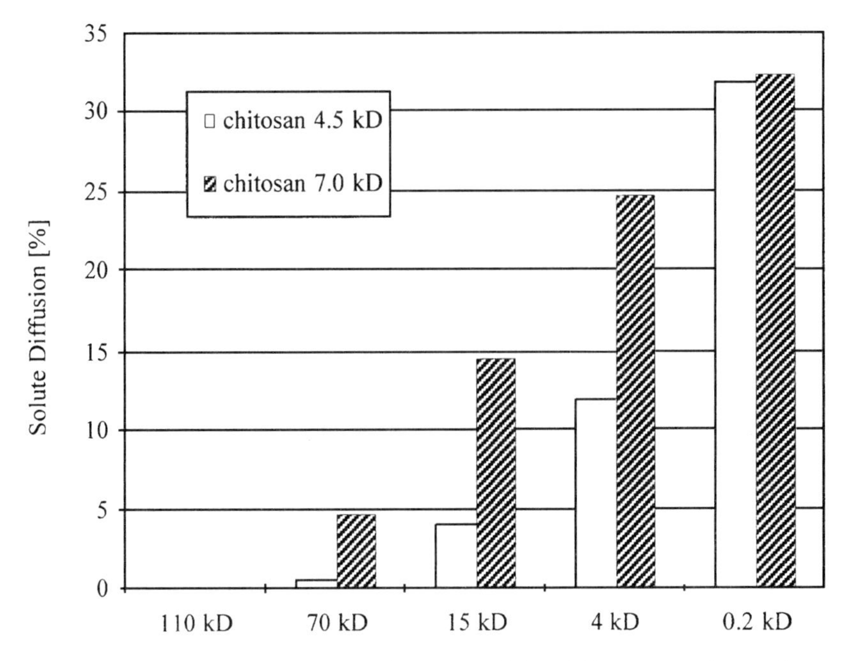


**FIGURE 5.** Diffusion of dextrans through an alginate/chitosan capsule membrane. Comparison of capsules obtained with chitosan of different molar masses (reaction time 30 min). The ingress was measured after a contact time of 32 min.

malian cells, require a pH range between 7 and 7.4 for culture, the new encapsulation procedure described herein is evidently much more robust over a practical range.

The mechanical properties of the capsules vary remarkably as a function of the reaction conditions. The molar mass of chitosan, and the reaction time, have been found to be of the greatest importance for the process of capsule formation. Generally, the mechanical strength of the capsules increases with progressing reaction time owing to the growth of the capsule wall thickness (FIG. 2). The significant drop in mechanical stability and surface deformation after ten minutes of reaction are the result of differences in osmotic pressure between solution interior and exterior to the capsules (osmotic imbalance). The wall morphology not only changes according to the progressing conversion of the polyelectrolytes, but also because of the osmotic effects caused by the counterions of the separated polyelectrolytes. A reduction of the capsule volume due to the osmotic draining of water plays an important part in capsule stability and porosity. This negative effect can be reduced by introduction non-reactive low molar mass osmotic pressure modifiers such as mannitol. The capsules synthesized in the presence of 1% mannitol solution have improved mechanical properties (FIG. 3) with the mechanical strength depending strongly on the size of the capsules (FIG. 4). Larger capsules with higher volume/surface ratios are less resistant than the smaller capsules.

Porosity, like mechanical resistance, depends on the thickness and morphology of the capsule wall. Lower cut-offs are obtained after longer reaction times and using

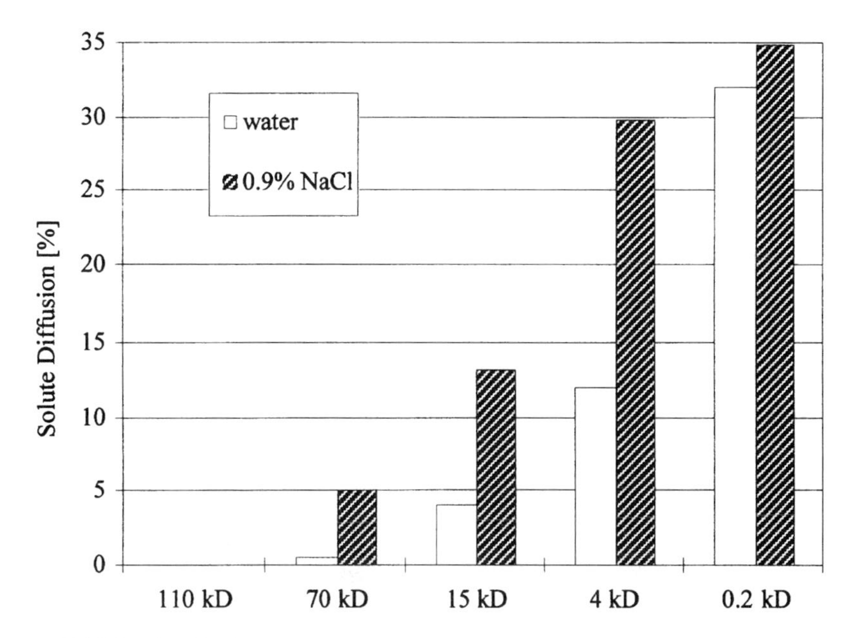


**FIGURE 6.** Diffusion of dextrans through an alginate/chitosan capsule membrane. Comparison of capsules prepared in water and in salt solution (chitosan 4.5 kD, reaction time 30 min). The ingress was measured after a contact time of 32 min.

chitosan of higher molar masses (FIG. 5). For the chitosan of 4.5 kD the membrane molar mass cut-off is approximately 70 kD while for a chitosan of 7 kD it is 110 kD. Surprisingly, no significant difference in the permeability of alginate/$Ca^{2+}$/chitosan capsules, prepared with chitosan of the $M_v$ = 160–310 kD, was observed.[25]

The presence of the low molar mass salt (0.9% NaCl) during the binary capsule formation accelerates the diffusion of the oligocations and leads to thicker capsule walls. Therefore, the capsule has less stability and a more porous membrane (FIG. 6). This difference can be explained by shielding effect of the sodium cations during the polyelectrolytes complex formation. At low alginate concentration the membrane growth occurs more rapidly than at higher concentrations. The oligocations can penetrate more easily through less concentrated polyanion solutions and create thicker and less dense membranes. Consequently, the final capsules are more porous and have higher cut-offs (FIG. 7).

## CONCLUSIONS

A new generation of microcapsules can be prepared by utilizing a polyelectrolyte complexation reaction between two oppositely charged polysaccharides, one of which is oligomeric.[20] The resulting microcapsules have good mechanical properties and, more significantly in relation to the existing literature, can be applied up to a pH of 7.5. The latter is a necessity of other competing technologies, with bead formation accomplished with the addition of simple electrolyte, normally a divalent

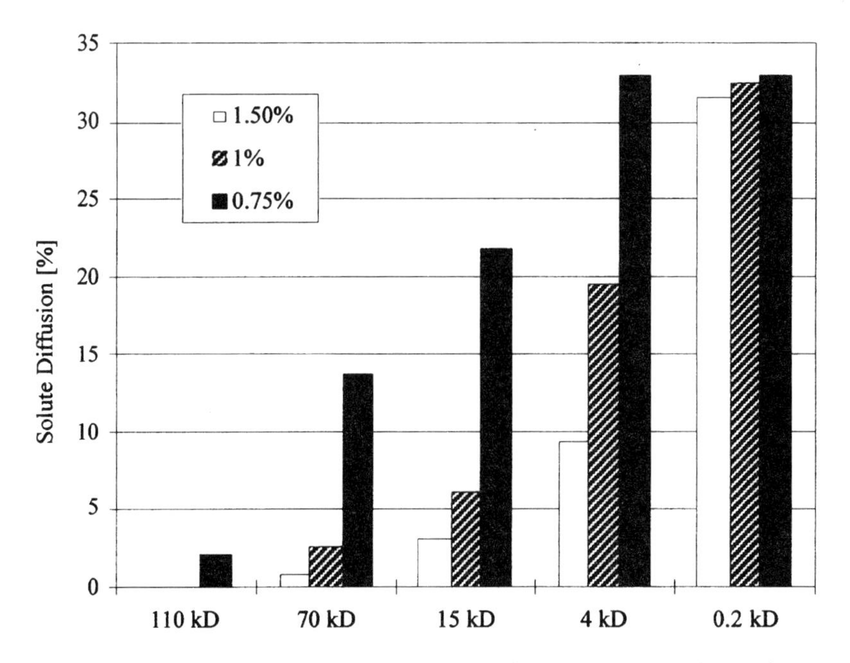


**FIGURE 7.** Diffusion of dextrans through an alginate/chitosan capsule membrane—different alginate concentrations (chitosan 2.7 kD, reaction time 30 min). The ingress was measured after a contact time of 32 min.

salt. The novel technology forms a membrane directly between two oppositely charged polyelectrolytes in solution in the absence of simple electrolyte. The new capsule is unique relative to most polyelectrolyte complex systems in that it involves a single step process to generate the membrane and microcapsule, avoiding the formation of a bead as a precursor. The molar mass of the "outer" polymer has been optimized so as to permit the formation of mechanically stable capsules. Specifically, chitosan oligomers with molar masses between 2 and 20 kD are favored. These are envisioned to have applications in the bioencapsulation field in general, pertaining specifically to the pharmaceutical, food and cosmetic industries, as well as in biomedical transplants.

## REFERENCES


1. Parthasarathy, R.V. & C.R. Martin. 1994. Synthesis of polymeric microcapsule arrays and their use for enzyme immobilization. Nature **369:** 298–301.
2. Sun, A.M., Z. Cai, Z. Shi, F. Ma & G.M. O'Shea. 1987. Microencapsulated hepatocytes: an in vitro and in vivo study. Biomater. Artif. Cells Art. Org. **15:** 1483–1496.
3. Perols, C., B. Piffaut, J. Scher, J.P. Ramet & D. Poncelet. 1997. The potential of enzyme entrapment in konjac cold-melting gel beads. Enzyme Microbial Technol. **20(1):** 57–60.
4. Chung, Y.C., C.P. Huang & C.P. Tseng. 1997. Biotreatment of ammonia from air by an immobilized *Arthobacter oxydans* CH8 biofilter. Biotechnol. Prog. **13(6):** 794–798.

5. CHANG, T.M.S. 1995. Artificial cells with emphasis on bioencapsulation in biotechnology. Biotechnol. Annu. Rev. **1:** 267–295.
6. HUNKELER, D. 1997. Polymers for bioartificial organs. Trends Polym. Sci. **5:** 286–293.
7. SEFTON, M.V. 1989. Blood, guts and chemical engineering. Can. J. Chem. Eng. **67:** 705–712.
8. DAUTZENBERG, H., F. LOTH, J. POMMERENING, K.-J. LINOW & D. BARTSCH. 1984. Microcapsules and process for the production therefore, UK Patent Application no. 135 954 A.
9. SUN, A. M. 1997. Microencapsulation of cells, medical applications. Ann. N.Y. Acad. Sci. **831:** 271–279.
10. LIM, F. & A.M. SUN. 1980. Microencapsulated islets as bioartificial endocrine pancreas. Science **210:** 908–910.
11. DE VOS, P. *et al.* 1997. Effect of alginate composition on the biocompatibility of alginate-polylisine microcapsules. Biomaterials **18:** 273–278.
12. ZEKORN, T. *et al.* 1992. Barium-alginate beads for immunoisolated transplantation of islets of Langerhans. Transplant. Proc. **24:** 937–939.
13. BASTA, G. *et al.* 1996. J. Ultrastructural examination of pancreatic islet containing alginate/polyaminoacidic coherent microcapsules. Submicrosc. Cytol. Pathol. **28:** 209–213.
14. SHIGEMASA, Y. & S. MINAMI. 1995. Biotech. Genetic Rev. **13:** 383.
15. YAO, K. *et al.* 1995. Microcapsules and microspheres related to chitosan. J.M.S.-Rev. Macromol. Chem. Phys. **C35(1):** 155–180.
16. RHA, C. *et al.* 1984. Biotechnology of Marine Polysaccharides, R.R. Colwell, E.R. Pariser & A.J. Sinskey, eds. Washington: Hempshire Publishing Corp. 283.
17. RHA, C. 1985. Process for encapsulation and encapsulated active material system. European Patent Application no.0 152 898.
18. RHA, C. 1988. Encapsulated active material system. US Patent 4,749,620.
19. DALY, M.M., R. KEOWN & D.W. KNORR. 1989. Chitosan alginate capsules. US Patent no. 4,808,707.
20. BARTKOWIAK, A. & D. HUNKELER. 1998. UK Patent Application no. GB-A-9814619.4.
21. MULLAGALIEV, I.R. *et al.* 1995. Degradation of chitosan in the presence of hydrogen peroxide. Poklady Akademii Nauk. **345(2):** 199–204.
22. BARTKOWIAK, A., *et al.* 1998. Abstract Book of Second International Symposium on Polyelectrolytes, 14. Inuyama, Japan. 31 May–3 June.
23. http://www.sdk.co.jp/shodex/english/dc030605.htm.
24. DAUTZENBERG, H. *et al.* 1996. Immobilisation of biological matter by polyelectrolyte complex formation. Ber. Bunsenges. Phys. Chem. **100:** 1045–1053.
25. MCKNIGHT, C.A. *et al.* 1988. Synthesis of chitosan-alginate microcaapsule membrane. J. Bioact. Comp. Polym. **3:** 334–354.
26. BARTKOWIAK, A. & D. HUNKELER. Alginate-ologoohitoson microcapsules: a mechanistic study relating membrane and capsule properties to reaction conditions. In preparation.

# Development of Cellulose Sulfate-based Polyelectrolyte Complex Microcapsules for Medical Applications

HORST DAUTZENBERG,[a,g] UTE SCHULDT,[a] GERD GRASNICK,[a] PETER KARLE,[b] PETRA MÜLLER,[e] MATTHIAS LÖHR,[c] MIREIA PELEGRIN,[d] MARC PIECHACZYK,[d] KERSTIN V. ROMBS,[e] WALTER H. GÜNZBURG,[b] BRIAN SALMONS,[e] AND ROBERT M. SALLER[e,f]

[a] *University of Potsdam, Germany*

[b] *Institute of Virology, University of Veterinary Sciences, Vienna, Austria*

[c] *Universitätsklinik Rostock, Germany*

[d] *Institut de Génétique Moleculaire de Montpellier, France*

[e] *Bavarian Nordic Research Institute, Germany*

**ABSTRACT: Microencapsulation, as a tool for immunoisolation for allogenic or xenogenic implants, is a rapidly growing field. However most of the approaches are based on alginate/polylysine capsules, despite this system's obvious disadvantages such as its pyrogenicity. Here we report a different encapsulation system based on sodium cellulose sulfate and polydiallyldimethyl ammonium chloride for the encapsulation of mammalian cells. We have characterized this system regarding capsule formation, strength and size of the capsules as well as viability of the cells after encapsulation. In addition, we demonstrate the efficacy of these capsules as a "microfactory" *in vitro* and *in vivo*. Using encapsulated hybridoma cells we were able to demonstrate long-term release of antibodies up to four months *in vivo*. In another application we could show the therapeutic relevance of encapsulated genetically modified cells as an *in vivo* activation center for cytostatic drugs during tumor therapy.**

## INTRODUCTION

As long as forty years ago Chang proposed microencapsulation as a possible tool to create artificial organs.[1] Owing to the lack of mild procedures for preparing microcapsules, all attempts to encapsulate viable cells or sensitive biological material without serious damage failed in the beginning. It took almost 30 more years until a breakthrough was achieved by Lim and Sun,[2] who invented the now well-known Alginate/L-Polylysine (ALG/PLL) procedure and described the first successful immobilization of islets of Langerhans. Since then, numerous groups all over the world have been dealing with cell encapsulation in either its biotechnological or medical aspects. In the meantime, the ALG/PLL procedure has been continuously improved and other gentle encapsulation procedures based on different polymers were estab-

[f]Corresponding author: Bavarian Nordic Research Institute, Fraunhofer Str.18b,D-82152 Martinsried Germany; +49-89-85651351 (voice); +49-89-85651333 (fax); saller@bavarian-nordic.de (e-mail).

[g]Deceased.

lished. For example Sefton[3] suggested microencapsulation in polyacrylates, Zekorn[4] recommended the entrapment into beads of Barium-alginate without subsequent membrane formation by additional treatment, and Hunkeler *et al.* proposed a modified ALG procedure.[5] However, almost all research activities focused on the optimization of ALG/PLL system using islets of Langerhans as the main subject of investigation. In the meantime first successful results from clinical trials using ALG/PLL encapsulated Langerhans Islets were reported by American[6] and Italian[7] research teams. Although the published data provide strong evidence for a successful clinical application in the future, there are many problems which need to be overcome before this system can be considered as a therapy for diabetes. These problems are due to islet cells being very sensitive to any kind of stress as well as to the capsules themselves.

One of the most serious problems in the development of a reproducibly sterile microcapsule is the quality of the raw material. Since alginate is a natural product recovered from seaweed, significant batch to batch differences exist. Furthermore, alginate is often contaminated with pyrogenic or even toxic side products at ppm levels which are very difficult to remove or to deactivate. In addition the preparation of these ALP/PLL capsules is fairly complex, requiring a multistep procedure, comprising an ionotropic gelation of pre-shaped droplets of raw alginate solution by $Ca^{2+}$-ions, the formation of a polyelectrolyte complex (PEC) layer at the surface by treatment of the gel beads with PLL (or other suitable polycation solutions), and finally the reliquification of the capsule core by an ion exchange substituting $Ca^{2+}$ ions with $Na^{+}$. The latter can be accomplished by treating the beads with sodium citrate solution. The properties of the final resulting polyelectrolyte complex microcapsules (PECMC) depend on several process variables, which are difficult to control individually. Prokop *et al.*[8] recently compared the most relevant encapsulation procedures regarding their performance and their suitability for the encapsulation of islets. They were able to overcome some restrictions limiting the original ALG/PLL procedure by adding a second polyanion like NaCS to the alginate solution and using polycations of lower molecular weight, e.g., polymethylene-co-guanidine hydrochloride. This resulted in the production of gel beads with a defined membrane thickness.

In the early 1980s the authors of this chapter developed a procedure for the preparation of PECMC[9,10] that we believe to be advantageous relative to the ALG/PLL method. As we observed, PECMC can be prepared directly in a one step-procedure from suitable oppositely charged polyelectrolytes by introducing droplets of a solution containing one of the reaction components into a solution of the other reaction component, preferably by using the polyanion as core material. In collaboration with several other institutions we studied the applicability of this encapsulation method to different types of sensitive biological matter, such as proteins, enzymes, cell fragments micro-organisms, mammalian cells or tissue.[11–15] Sodium cellulose sulfate (NaCS) and Poly (diallyldimethylammonium chloride) (PDADMAC) proved to be the best polymer combination and allowed, after streamlining of their molecular parameters, the preparation of microcapsules with outstanding mechanical properties under physiological reaction conditions. Initially all experiments were performed with NaCS samples prepared homogeneously according to a method described by Wagenknecht *et al.*[16] with linters as cellulose starting material and a mixture of $SO_2$/

$N_2O_4$/DMF (dimethylformamide) as a sulfating medium. After realizing that this kind of synthesis is not very practical, we looked for other NaCS sources and possibilities to prepare NaCS of the required quality. However all commercially available products did not meet the requirements for using them as reaction components in microencapsulation. Finally we succeeded in creating a heterogeneous sulfating process[17] that led to cellulose sulfate samples of sufficient quality. In this process a reaction mixture of *n*-propanol and sulfuric acid served as sulfating medium and agent. Our initial efforts were mainly centered on biotechnological usage of this encapsulation process, although encouraging results were obtained in encapsulation of islets, thyroid tissue, hepatocytes, embryos and other sensitive biological material relevant for medical application. Recently, very promising results have been achieved regarding the encapsulation of various genetically modified cells of different origin. During the last years all methods necessary for a sufficiently comprehensive characterization of the polyionic reaction components as well as for the determination of relevant capsule properties (capsule size, mechanical strength, residual polymer inside the capsule, membrane properties, such as morphological structure, permeability, or cut-off) have been elaborated. The process of capsule formation has been studied in detail. Relationships between the course of capsule formation and capsule properties on one hand and the polymer chemical features of the starting polyelectrolytes as well as the process variables, like reaction time, temperature, polymer and salt concentrations, influence of components derived from culture media on the other hand have been elucidated. This information provided a useful basis for the establishment and optimization of the process of capsule formation under different conditions and for adapting capsule properties to various fields of application.[18–21] The capacity of PEC formation for encapsulation has been confirmed by independent investigations of other research groups.[22,23]

This optimized system now has a variety of different applications. One of our main focuses is applications in the biomedical field, since in principle, the system can be applied for extracorporal usage or *in vivo* as implants for short- as well as long-term purposes. In this chapter we report the characterization and optimization of the NaCS/PDADMAC encapsulation system for biomedical purposes and two potential clinical applications.

## MATERIALS AND METHODS

### *General*

Sodium cellulose sulfate (FIG. 1a) served as polyanion and poly(diallyldimethylammonium chloride) (FIG. 1b) as polycation. The NaCS solution was used to build the capsule core and the PDADMAC solution as a precipitation bath delivering the second reaction component for PEC formation at the surface of the droplets, thus forming the capsules by covering the droplets with a solid membrane. The PDAMAC used was selected from a series of technical batches from Katpol/Wolfen tested in model experiments. In order to assure a supply of NaCS of reproducible quality and with good capsule forming properties, the heterogeneous laboratory synthesis was standardized and transferred to a semi-technical scale in a small enterprise. A special type of standard linters from Hercules was used as initial cellulose

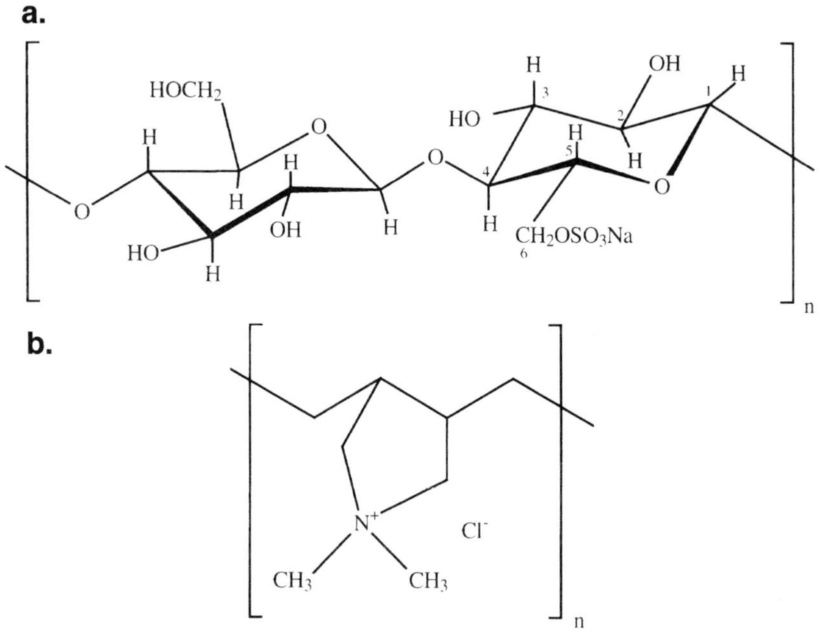

**FIGURE 1.** Chemical structure of the poly electrolytes used for encapsulation. **a:** Sodium cellulose sulfate (NaCS); **b:** Poly(diallyldimethylammonium chloride) (PDADMAC).

material. Later on NaCS was obtained from Bavarian Nordic. The polyelectrolytes were characterized by common analytical methods as well as by gel permeation chromatography (GPC), NaCS additionally by polarography and by Fourier transformation infrared spectroscopy (FTIR) analysis.

### *Capsule Formation, and Encapsulation*

Droplet generation was performed by a newly developed device from Inotech.[24]

### *Characterization of Capsules*

Size and shape of capsules were checked under a light microscope. Viability of encapsulated cells was evaluated using the Live/Dead Viability/Cytotoxicity kit according to the manufacturers instructions (Molecular probes, L-3224).

### *Tissue Culture and Culturing of Capsules* in Vitro

Cell lines and capsules were cultured under standard tissue culture conditions. Adherent cells were incubated in Dulbecco's modified eagle medium (DMEM) in the presence of 10% FCS. Encapsulated hybridoma cells were incubated in RPMI medium in the presence of 10% FCS.

### *Toxicity Studies*

A group of 5 male and 5 female animals were injected intraperitoneally with a nominal level of 2000 mg/kg body weight of ground capsule material and observed for a period of 14 days. Animals were killed at the end of the observation period and subjected to necroscopic examination.

### *Animals*

Nude mice (CD-1 nu/nu) were obtained from Charles River, Germany. C3H mice were obtained from Harlan Nassan s.r.l. Corezzana (Mi), Italy (IFFA-CREDO).

### In Vivo *Experiments*

*Pancreas*

$1 \times 10^6$ cells of the human pancreatic adenocarcinoma derived cell line PaCa-44 (ATCC) were injected subcutaneously into the flanks of nude mice in order to establish tumors. 20-40 capsules were applied through a 21G needle in the tumor. Animals were treated with 100 mg/kg body weight ifosfamide every third day for 2 weeks. To prevent urotoxicity, the same dosage of sodium 2-mercaptoethansulfonate (MESNA; Asta Medica) was administered at the same time with the same dosage i.v. into the tail vein.

*Antibody Release*

Six to 20 capsules were implanted into anesthesized 6-week-old C3H mice either intraperitoneally or subcutaneously. For detection of the monoclonal antibody (Mab) Tg 10, mice were bled, clotted blood samples were centrifuged and serum was tested for the presence of Tg 10 in an ELISA.[25]

## RESULTS

The aim of this work was to establish an encapsulation system based on NaCS/ PDADMAC as reaction components of PECMC formation, which is efficient, reproducible, and optimized for a biomedical application. This demanded the establishment of a reliable basis for delivering the raw materials in sufficient amounts and reproducible standard quality. A combination of compatible polyelectrolytes has been identified which gave rise to capsules of sufficient quality regarding size, mechanical stability and viability of encapsulated cells.

### *Optimization of the Encapsulation Procedure*

The selection of materials and the optimization of the reaction conditions were based on results obtained with model capsules of about 3 mm in diameter. The present development aimed at capsules of about 600 μm in diameter (d). A reduction of the capsule diameter by a factor of 5 means that the capsule volume is lowered by a factor of 125 from about 15 μl to about 0.1 μl. Furthermore it implies that the amount of NaCS available per surface area for membrane formation is decreased by a factor of 5 (proportional to d) and consequently also limits the maximum mem-

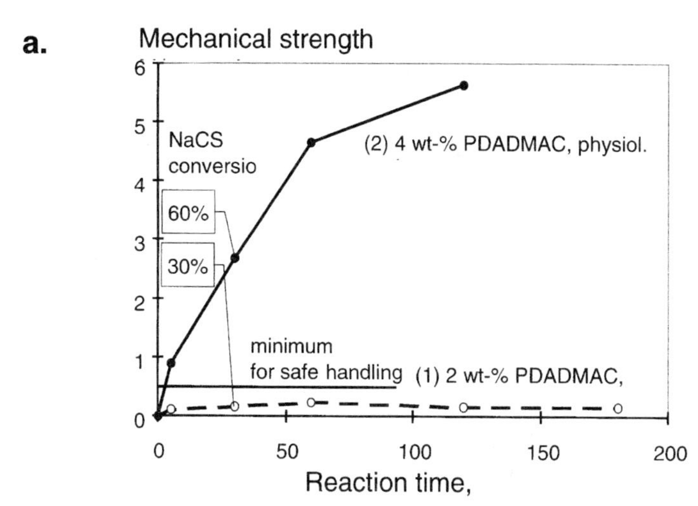


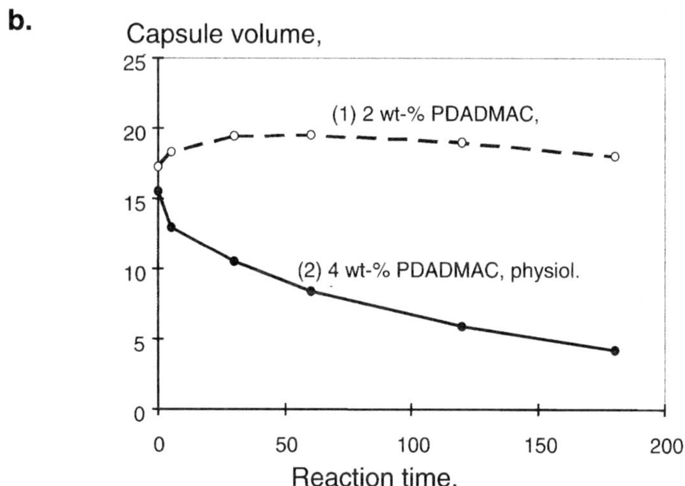


**FIGURE 2.** Capsule properties versus reaction time (4 wt-% NaCS, standard quality, technical PDADMAC sample, M = 8000 Dalton, room temperature). **a:** Mechanical strength; **b:** Capsule volume.

brane thickness to a fifth in terms of that of the larger capsules. According to the mechanism of capsule formation described earlier[20, 21] mass transport processes play an important part in the capsule wall building and control. Osmotic conditions or in the presence of additional low molecular mass ions of the DONNAN equilibrium, established after the formation of a primary membrane at the droplet surface, also affect the course of the PEC formation at the reaction zone near to the interface and thus the capsule's properties. For evaluating a series of technical PDADMAC samples regarding their suitability for capsule preparation, the process of capsule formation was monitored for model capsules under different reaction conditions over reaction times up to 3 hours by following capsule size and strength. In addition, the rate of NaCS conversion has been measured in some of the capsules. A representative example of these experiments is depicted in FIGURE 2. These results clearly demonstrate that the process of capsule formation can proceed very differently even with the same polymers. Besides the polymer, chemical features of the polyelectrolytes the reaction conditions play a decisive part. As found earlier[20,21] outstandingly high mechanical strength can be achieved in presence of salt and at sufficiently high PDADMAC concentrations (FIG. 2, *upper curve*). As can be concluded from the figures, the effect is partly caused by an accelerated NaCS conversion. Under nonoptimized reaction conditions the membrane growth can even come to a total standstill thus leaving the capsules fragile with mechanical strengths below the level defined for safe handling. Nearly every kind of intermediate can occur between these two extremes. As FIGURE 2b shows, the capsule volume can drop from the beginning on or pass through a maximum with progressing reaction time. The capsules interact osmotically with their surrounding because of the semipermeability of the capsule wall. According to the osmotic pressure difference, mainly caused by the counterions of the non permeating polyions, between the interior and the exterior of the capsules in the beginning and its shift due to consumption of NaCS during the reaction, water either streams into or out of the capsules. The DONNAN equilibrium establishing in the presence of salt reduces the pressure differences and thereby affects the process of membrane formation.

The effect of salt on the capsule strength achieved after a certain reaction time depends on the PDADMAC concentration chosen in the experiment (FIG. 3). The mechanical strength increases with increasing PDADMAC concentration. The curve shows an S like shape especially in the absence of salt and less pronounced in presence of salt. This is probably caused by the DONNAN effect reducing osmotic pressure differences. As a result curves cross each other at a certain PDADMAC concentration, demonstrating that the presence of salt can have a major impact on the process of capsule formation.

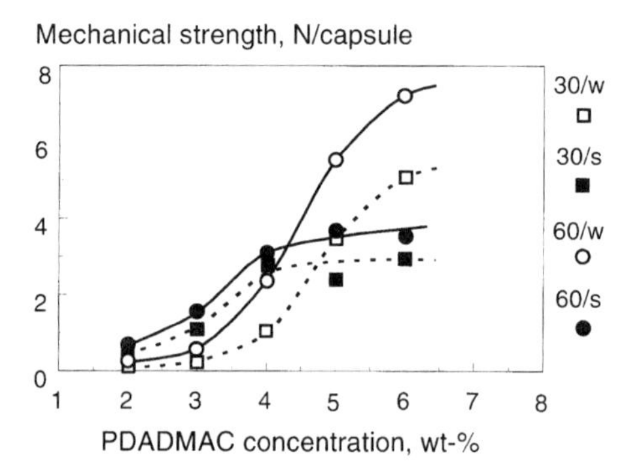


**FIGURE 3.** Mechanical strength of capsules versus PDADMAC concentration for different conditions of preparation (4 wt-% NaCS, standard quality PDADMAC sample, M = 32,000 Dalton, room temperature. Reaction conditions: reaction time/reaction medium. 30/w–30 min/water; 30/s–30 min/physiological NaCl; 60/w–60 min/water; 60/s–60 min/physiological NaCl).

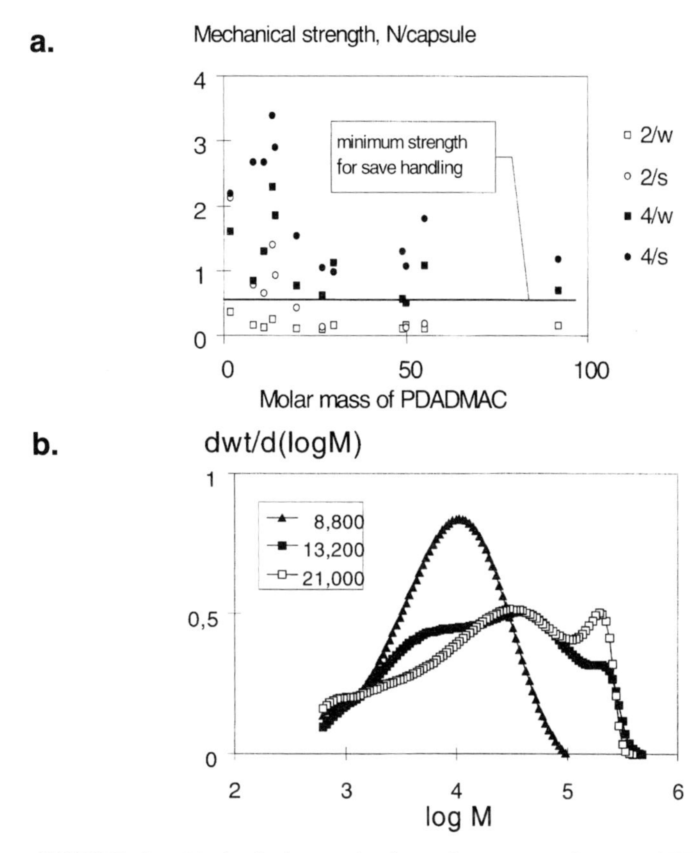


**FIGURE 4. a:** Mechanical strength of capsules versus molar mas of PDADMAC (4 wt-% NaCS, standard quality, techincal PDADMAC samples. Reaction conditions: PDADMACconcentration/reaction medium. 2/w–2 wt-% water; 2/s–2 wt-%/physiological NaCl; 4/w–4 wt-% water; 4/s–4 wt-%/physiological NaCl). **b:** Molecular weight distribution of selected technical PDADMAC samples measured by size exclusion chromatography. (Remark: the second maximum in MWD is probably caused by insufficient separation power in the region above 200kD of the column used; measurements with other columns are under way.)

FIGURE 4 shows the influence of PDADMAC samples varying in molar mass between approximately 2 and 100 kD on the mechanical strength of capsules (FIG. 4a). Although most capsules show a minimal strength required for safe handling above a critical concentration of PDADMAC, an optimum exists with samples of molar masses between 10 and 20 kD. One reason for this is the molecular weight distribution (MWD) of the PDADMAC. As depicted in FIGURE 4b the sample with M = 13 kD leads to best capsule properties because of the broadest MWD. This knowledge served as a basis for the appropriate combination of polymers and reaction conditions, leading to capsules adapted to biological requirements. It was found that in principle the qualitative correlations could be applied also to the production of

**TABLE 1.** Characteristics of NaCS based capsules

| Size | 0.7 mm +/– 0.1 |
|---|---|
| N° of cells/capsule | $1–2 \times 10^4$ |
| Viability | > 95% |

smaller capsules with two predicted exceptions: i) the reaction time was shorter (a few minutes instead of 30 to 60 minutes) and ii) while leaving the mechanical properties of the capsules generally unchanged the load-bearing capacity of the capsules falls to about a tenth due to the smaller capsule surface and the thinner capsule wall (data not shown).

### *Toxicology*

One of the major drawbacks of the NaCS-based encapsulation system was the lack of toxicological data. We evaluated our capsule material for the potential of causing acute toxicity to the recipient organism upon injection. The experimental set up was carried out in full compliance with the OECD guideline number 401. 2000 mg/kg body weight of ground capsule material, which is the maximum dosage for completely new test substances, has been injected into 10 immunocompetent mice. The animals were checked for weight loss, fever or any abnormal behavior, parameters that are accepted indicators for a reaction against the injected test substance. No acute toxicity of the material was detected in any of the animals.

### *Characterization of Optimized NaCS Capsules*

Capsules were produced using an semi-automatic encapsulation device based on the principle of a vibrating nozzle. It allows the production of mostly uniform beads of a defined size. It also allows the production of up to 2000 capsules per minute. The capsules are round (FIG. 5) and densely packed with cells (TABLE 1). The viability remains high for about 4 weeks and slowly decreases over time (FIG. 6). After 13 weeks about 5% of the encapsulated cells that were viable immediately after encapsulation were still alive. Surprisingly we did not observe a significant difference in viability after incubation at 37°C or 4°C. Interestingly we observed a migration of cells inside the capsule over time dependent on the cell type. Cells were equally distributed immediately after encapsulation but they migrate out of the center towards the membrane probably owing to a better nutrition situation close to the membrane (data not shown).

#### *Applications*

Microcapsules based on NaCS offer a variety of potential applications although the biomedical field can be considered as being of particular interest. So far the limited life span of encapsulated cells restricts the application to disease models not requiring an unlimited supply of the therapeutic agent. Two different models were chosen as target diseases and discussed in the following sections.

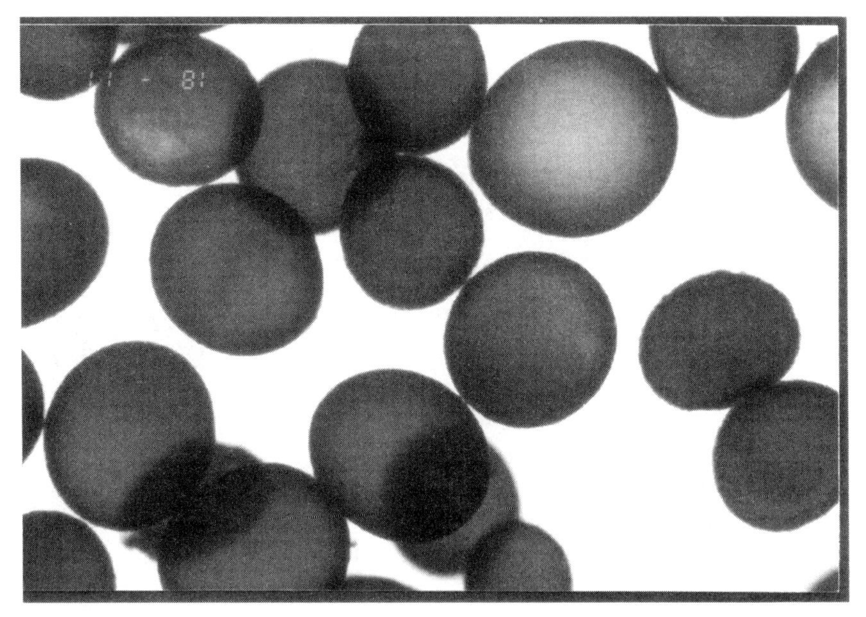

**FIGURE 5.** Empty capsules with an average diameter of 0.6 mm, produced as described in MATERIALS AND METHODS.

*Pancreatic Cancer*

Pancreatic cancer is responsible for every fourth cancer death in Germany. The incidence of this type of tumor is 0.01%[26] with an increasing rate. Tumors of the pancreas have a particular poor prognosis with an average survival rate of less than 2.5%, five years after diagnosis.[27] At the time of diagnosis the tumor very often has entered a stage which makes it inoperable. Unfortunately also the few cases allowing a surgical removal very often show a relapse. The current treatment is high dose chemotherapy the efficacy of which is limited by a number of factors, for example, the degree of sensitivity of the tumor and systemic toxicity of the cytostatic agent. One of the therapeutic agents which has been used for treatment of pancreatic cancer is ifosfamide (IFO). It is a prodrug, which is metabolized in the liver by cytochrome P450 converting the prodrug into phosphoramide mustard and acrolein that alkylate DNA and protein, respectively. As this alkylation is not specific to the tumor it causes considerable side effects in other cell types and organs such as the hematopoetic system as well as the brain[28] and therefore limits the dosage of the prodrug. The establishment of a second prodrug activation center in the vicinity of the tumor should improve the efficacy in targeting relatively high concentrations of the metabolites to the tumor. Simultaneously this approach should allow a reduction of the total body dose and therefore reducing the side effects to nontarget tissue.

A cell clone has been established, showing a high level of expression of the transfected cytochrome P450 gene (CYP450) determined in an indirect reporter assay.[24,29] This cell clone has been encapsulated and the production of CYP450 was

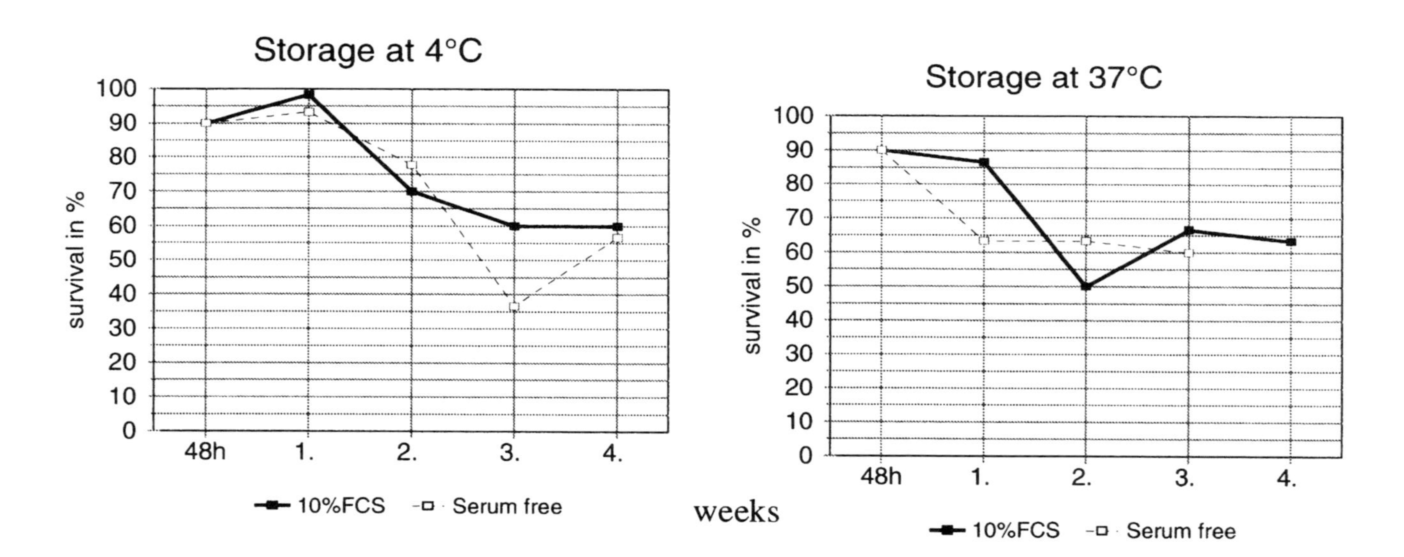


**FIGURE 6.** The viability of capsules harboring a 293 derivative cell line was studied over 4 weeks under normal tissue culture conditions (37°C and ±10% FCS) and at 4°C ±10% FCS. A slow but constant decrease in cell viability has been observed, but no significant difference was detectable between the different culture conditions.

**TABLE 2.** Enzyme activity test (pmol)

| Enzyme Activity Test | |
|---|---|
| $10^5$ cells (not encapsulated) | 0.17 |
| $10^5$ cells (encapsulated) | 0.16–0.23 |

analyzed as compared to non encapsulated cells in order to determine a potential effect of the capsule membrane on the rate of release of the activated metabolites. These experiments revealed no significant difference in activity between encapsulated and nonencapsulated cells (TABLE 2). In order to evaluate the therapeutic potential of this approach an *in vivo* nude mouse model has been established.[30] $1 \times 10^6$ cells of the human pancreatic cancer derived cell line PaCa-44 were injected subcutaneously into the animal in order to create a pancreatic tumor as a target for the capsules. At the time that the tumor had reached a volume of ~1 $cm^3$, 20–40 capsules were injected through a 21G needle directly into the tumor or in a distance of 1 cm from the tumor. The animals received IFO and MESNA to prevent urotoxicity. After two weeks of treatment a significant response could be detected in comparison to the various control groups which also showed a partial response upon IFO application (FIG. 7). This was expected since IFO, as such, causes a reduction of tumor burden due to the liver-mediated conversion.

### *Antibody Release*

Another potential application is the release of monoclonal antibodies from encapsulated hybridoma cells. This could be used not only as a delivery system for neutralizing antibodies for treatment of viral diseases but also as an adjuvant anti-cancer therapy after surgical removal of the primary tumor in order to eliminate residual tumor cells which often cause a relapse. Such a system also could be of interest to remove factors from the blood stream. The aim of this project was to demonstrate that

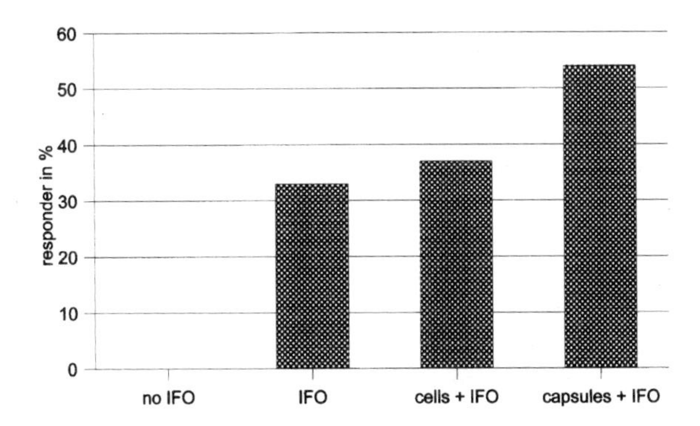


**FIGURE 7.** Twenty to 40 capsules were injected directly into a pre-inoculated human pancreatic tumor. IFO was administered i.p. every third day for two weeks. None of the animals receiving no treatment survived, whereas a 33% response has been observed after administration of IFO alone (conventional therapy).The highest response was shown in the group receiving capsules and IFO. Response was defined as reduction of tumor mass of >50%.

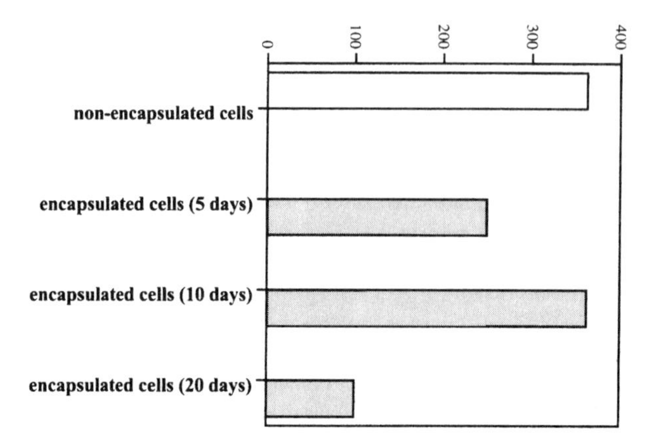


**FIGURE 8.** Twenty-five capsules containing Tg 10 hybridoma cells (mean of $2 \times 10^4$ cells per capsule) were cultured as described in MATERIAL AND METHODS. The culture medium was replaced every 24 hours and Tg 10 Mab concentration was assayed by ELISA. The production of Tg 10 Mab by nonencapsulated cells was compared to the Tg 10 Mab produced by encapsulated cells at several times after cell encapsulation.

long-term systemic delivery of monoclonal antibodies *in vitro* as well as *in vivo* from encapsulated cells is feasible.

Cells of a hybridoma cell line secreting a mouse monoclonal antibody (Mab) directed against the human thyroglobulin (Tg 10) were encapsulated and analyzed for antibody production after encapsulation.[31] Production and release of Tg10 from the capsules was detected by ELISA. Antibody could be detected in the medium over a period of 50 days *in vitro* with a peak after 10–12 days (FIG. 8). The drop in secretion correlated with the onset of cell death inside the capsule. However this does not imply a toxic effect of the capsule material on the encapsulated cells, as we found that non encapsulated Tg 10 cells also died under standard culture conditions without passaging.

In order to achieve a systemic delivery of Tg 10 for a maximum length of time we needed to determine whether the site of implantation has an impact on antibody release. Six to 20 capsules were implanted either in the peritoneal cavity or subcutaneously. Animals receiving capsules subcutaneously not only gave higher levels of Tg10 detected in the blood but also showed release of Tg 10 into the bloodstream for an elongated period of time (FIG. 9). Again, the highest values, 12.5 µg/ml, after subcutaneous implantation and 2.5 µg/ml after intraperitoneal implantation, respectively, were detected after 10 days followed by a steady decline probably correlating with cell death. Interestingly, Tg 10 could be detected up to 4 months (1 animal) after subcutaneous implantation, whereas no Tg 10 production was detectable after 50 days in animals having received capsules intraperitoneally.

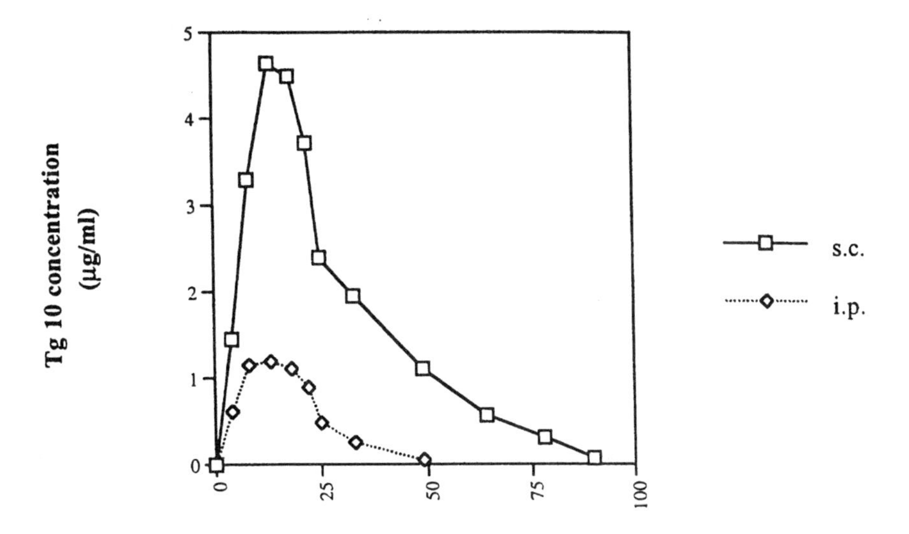


**FIGURE 9.** C3H mice were implanted with capsules containing Tg 10 hybridoma cells either subcutneously or intraperitoneally. Blood samples were retrieved at the indicated times and Tg 10 Mab concentration was assayed by ELISA. s.c. is the mean value of Tg 10 Mab concentration in the bloodstream of 6 mice implanted with capsules subcutaneously (3 mice implanted with 6 capsules and 3 mice implanted with 20 capsules). The highest Mab concentration detected was 12.5 μg/ml, obtained from a mouse with 20 capsules. i.p. is the mean value of Tg 10 Mab concentration in the bloodstream of mice implanted with capsules intraperitoneally (3 mice implanted with 6 capsules and 1 mouse implanted with 20 capsules). The highest Mab concentration detected was 2.5 μg/ml, obtained from the mouse implanted with 20 capsules.

## DISCUSSION

The project aimed at establishing a reproducible encapsulation system that could be used for the encapsulation of eucaryotic cells. Given the variability of the natural product a number of difficulties had to be overcome. The initial analysis of capsules were carried out on microcapsules having a diameter of about 3 mm. At that time it was very difficult to efficiently produce capsules with a diameter smaller than 1 mm. This limitation in size was due to the encapsulation system based on a laminar air jet flow. Furthermore NaCS based capsules produced with this technique also showed a variation in size which is not acceptable for many applications. Using the principle of a vibrating nozzle for the formation of droplets and undertaking fundamental changes in the encapsulation protocol, we were able to make capsules as small as 0.6 mm with little variation. Detailed polymer chemical analysis as well as investigation of the mechanical properties and the behavior of the encapsulated cells allowed us to set up a technology for the production of NaCS-based capsules which is fully controlled and can be manipulated for different purposes. It became obvious that there were clear criteria, especially for PDADMAC, that determine the size and strength of the microcapsules. Interestingly these parameters held true also after a fivefold reduction in size—only the reaction time of the two compounds could be dramatically reduced from more than one hour to a range of a few minutes. This again improves the viability of the encapsulated cells. Toxicological evaluation of ground empty capsules revealed no acute toxicity in mice even after high dose injection of the test substance.

Analysis of encapsulated cells demonstrated a viability of greater than 95% determined 48 hours after encapsulation *in vitro*. In fact we observed only a very moderate death rate resulting in about 5% viable cells after 13 weeks. Interestingly there appears to be a migration of cells inside the capsule into areas with the most favorable environment, i.e., under the capsule membrane. In the case of adherent growing cells we also observed a migration towards each other resulting in multiple cell aggregates. The data obtained in these studies created a promising basis for *in vivo* studies.

With the prolonged but still not unlimited viability of the encapsulated cells, short-term and middle-term applications were considered as being suitable to demonstrate their efficacy. Pancreatic cancer has been chosen as a model system. The standard chemotherapy using IFO so far suffers the problems of a limited dosage of the cytostatic drug due to side effects, the liver being the major site of activation of the prodrug, and a short half life of the active metabolites. Here we report the establishment of microfactories consisting of genetically engineered cell lines stably expressing CYP450.[24,32] We could show that there is virtually no difference in prodrug activation between nonencapsulated cells and the encapsulated homologue (TABLE 2). These microfactories were injected into pre-inoculated human pancreatic tumors in a nude mouse model in order to create a second center of activation at the site of the tumor. A significant improvement in killing of tumors could be demonstrated in the group of animals receiving encapsulated cells and IFO. However in a real clinical situation the capsules need to be placed in the pancreas, which is one of the most sensitive organs regarding physical stress or damage. Any kind of stress of the pancreas very often results in development of a pancreatitis which can be even life threatening. We, therefore, tested the effect of direct injection of capsules into the pancreas of immunocompetent animals. None of the animals developed a pancreatitis, the only effect being observed was a minor infiltration of granulocytes and lymphocytes in the vicinity of the capsules (data not shown). Based on these data, a clinical trial was initiated at the end of July 1998. In principle, this short-term application can be used for other tumors the therapy of which foresees the application of cytostatic prodrugs. At the moment our model may have an endpoint determined by the lifespan of the encapsulated cells, though it should allow several cycles of chemotherapy. This is particularly important in case of a relapse caused by residual cells not killed during the initial therapy.

In our second model we were able to demonstrate the release of a monoclonal antibody from encapsulated hybridoma cells that had been implanted in immunocompetent mice. A peak of antibody release was observed after about 2 weeks followed by a steady decrease. However Tg 10 could be detected up to 4 months after subcutaneous implantation. It turned out that the site of implantation had a major impact on the length of time in which release of antibody could be demonstrated. Implantation of capsules into the peritoneal cavity shortened the release of antibodies to a period of 55 days. The reason for this probably lies in the different rate of vascularization. No vascularization has been observed upon intraperitoneal implantation, whereas vascularization took place quickly after subcutaneous implantation. This situation did not change even after a 10-month follow up.[31]

In conclusion, our NaCS-based capsule technology probably is a relevant alternative to the already well-characterized ALG/PLL system. In particular the high mechanical stability and the quick production procedure show improvements to the ALG/PLL system. Interestingly the most limiting factor for a long-term application seems to be located on the cellular rather than on the polymer side. A big step progress towards an "*in vivo* microfactory" would be achieved if cell types with a long lifespan (e.g., primary fibroblasts or muscle cells) could be genetically engineered and encapsulated or cells inside the capsule could be prevented from proliferation without causing a shortening of lifespan, simultaneously.

## ACKNOWLEDGMENTS

A part of this work was supported by grants from the Bundesministerium für Bildung und Forschung, BOE 21-03113673.

## REFERENCES

1. Chang, T.M.S. 1997. Artificial cells and bioencapsulation in bioartificial organs. *In* Bioartificial Organs, Science: Medicine and Technology. A. Prokop, D. Hunkeler & A.D. Cherrington, Eds. Ann. N.Y. Acad. Sci. **831:** 249-259.
2. Lim, F. & A.M. Sun. 1980. Microencapsulated islets as bioartificial endocrine pancreas. Science **210:** 908-909.
3. Sefton, M.V. & W.T.K. Stevenson. 1993. Microencapsulation of live animal cells using polyacrylates. Adv. Polym. Sci. **107:** 145-198
4. Zekorn, T., A. Horcher, U. Siebers, G. Klöck, U. Zimmermann, K. Federlin & R.G. Bretzel. 1992. Barium-cross-linked alginate beads: a simple one-step-method for successful immuno isolated transplantation of islets of Langerhans. Acta Diabetologica **29:** 99-106.
5. Prokop, A., D. Hunkeler, A.C. Powers, R.R. Whitsell & T.G. Wang. 1998. Water soluble polymers for immunoisolation II: Evaluation of multicomponent microencapsulation systems. Adv. Polym. Sci. **136:** 53–73
6. Soon-Shiong, P., R. Heintz, N. Merideth, Q.X. Yao, Z. Yao, T. Zheng, M. Murphy, M.K. Molony, M. Schmehl, M. Harris, R. Mendez, R. Mendez & P.A. Sandford. 1994. Insulin-independence in a type I diabetic patient after encapsulated islet transplantation. Lancet **343:** 950–951.
7. Calafiore, R., G. Basta, G. Luca, C. Boselli, A. Bufalari, G.M. Giustozzi, L. Moggi & P. Brunetti. 1997. Alginate/polyaminoacidic coherent microcapsules for pancreatic islet graft immunoisolation in diabetic recipients. Ann. N.Y. Acad Sci. **831:** 313–322.
8. Prokop, A., D. Hunkeler, R.R. Whitesell & T.G. Wang. 1998. Adv. Polym. Sci. **136:** 53–73.
9. Dautzenberg, H., F. Loth, K. Pommerening, K.-J. Linow & D. Bartsch. 1984. Microcapsules and process for the production thereof. UK Patent Application, GB 2 135 954 A.

10. DAUTZENBERG, H., F. LOTH, K. FECHNER, B. MEHLIS & K. POMMERENING. 1985. Preparation and performance of symplex capsules. Makromol. Chem. Suppl. **9:** 211–217.
11. TORNER, H., P.M. KAUFFOLD, H. GÖTZE, H. KÖNIG, H. DAUTZENBERG & F. LOTH. 1986. Immobilisierung präimplantiver Säugetierembryonen durch Mikrokapsulierung. Arch. exper. Vet. med. Leipzig **40:** 541–547.
12. GEMEINER, P., V. STEFUCA, L. KURILLOVA, H. DAUTZENBERG, M. POLAKOVIC & V. BALES. 1991. Polyelcctrolyte complex capsules as a material for enzyme immobilization. Catalytic properties of lactate dehydrogenase. Appl. Biochem. Biotech. **30:** 313–324.
13. MERTEN, O.-W., H. DAUTZENBERG & G.E. PALFI. 1991. A new method for the Encapsulation of mammalian cells. Cytotechnology **7:** 121–130.
14. MANSFELD, J., M. FÖRSTER, T. HOFFMANN, A. SCHELLENBERGER & H. DAUTZENBERG. 1995. Coimmobilisation of Yarrowia lipolytica and invertase in polyelectrolyte complex capsules. Enzyme Microb. Technol. **17:** 11–17.
15. DAUTZENBERG, H., J. STANGE, S. MITZNER & B. LUKANOFF. 1996. Encapsulation by polyelectrolyte complex formation—a way to make hepatocyte cultures safe, efficient and on-line available. *In* Immobilised Cells, Basics and Applications. Progress in Biotechnology. Elsevier. Amsterdam, Lausanne, New York, Oxford, Shannon, Tokyo **11:** 181–.
16. WAGENKNECHT, W., B. PHILIPP & D. PLASCHNIK. 1981. Verfahren zur Herstellung von Polyhydroxypolymersulfatestern, insbesondere von Cellulosesulfat. DD-PS 152565.
17. LUKANOFF, B. & H. DAUTZENBERG. 1994. Natriumcellulosesulfat als Komponente für die Erzeugung von Mikrokapseln durch Polyelektrolytkomplexbildung. 1. Mitt. Heterogene Sulfatierung von Cellulose unter Verwendung von Schwefelsäure/Propanol als Reaktions medium und Sulfatiermittel. Das Papier **48:** 287–296.
18. DAUTZENBERG, H., G. HOLZAPFEL & B. LUKANOFF. 1993. Methods for a comprehensive characterisation of microcapsules based on polyelectrolyte complex formation. Biomater. Artif. Cells, Artif. Cells & Immob. Biotechnol. **21:** 399-405.
19. DAUTZENBERG, H., B. LUKANOFF, B. & K. NEUBAUER. 1995. Sodium cellulose sulfate as component for polyelectrolyte complex formation—preparation, characterisation, testing. *In* Cellulose and Cellulose Derivatives: Physico-chemical Aspects and Industrial Applications. J.F. Kennedy, G.O. Phillips, P.O. Williams, L. Piculell, Eds.: 435–444. Woodhead Publishing Ltd. Abington Hall, Abington, Cambridge CB1 6 AH, UK.
20. DAUTZENBERG, H., B. LUKANOFF, U. ECKERT, B. TIERSCH & U. SCHULDT. 1996. Immobilisation of biological matter by polyelectrolyte complex formation. Polyelectrolytes, Potsdam 1995, Ber. Bunsen Ges. Proc. **100** (6): 1045–1053.
21. DAUTZENBERG, H., G. ARNOLD, B. TIERSCH, B. LUKANOFF & U. ECKERT. 1996. Polyelectrolyte complex formation at the interface of solutions. Prog. Colloid & Polym. Sci. **101:** 149–156.
22. BADER, H., D. RÜPPELT, M. MAGERSTÄDT & A. WALSCH. 1987. Intelligente Mikrokapseln. Chem. Ind.
23. DYAKONOV, T.A., L. ZHOU, Z. WAN, B. HUANG, Z. MENG, X. GUO, H. ALEXANDER, W.V. MOORE & W.T.K. STEVENSON. 1997. Synthetic strategies for the preparation of precursor polymers and of microcapsules suitable for cellular entrapment by polyelectrolyte complexation of those polymers. Ann. N.Y. Acad. Sci. **831:** 72–85.
24. KARLE, P., P. MÜLLER, R. RENZ, R. JESNOWSKI, R.M. SALLER, K. VON ROMBS, H. NIZZE, S. LIEBE, W.H. GÜNZBURG, B. SALMONS & M. LÖHR, 1998. Intratumoral injection of encapsulated cells producing an oxazaphosphorine activating cytochrome P450 for targeted chemotherapy. Cancer Gene Therapy. In press.
25. DEL RIO, M., *et al.*, 1995. Idiotypic restriction of murine monoclonal antibodies to a defined antigenic region of human thyroglobulin. Immunol. Invest. **24:** 655–667.
26. HOWARD, T.J. 1996. Pancreatic adenocarcinoma. Curr. Probl. Cancer. **20:** 281–328.
27. ROSEWICZ , S. & B. WIEDEMANN. 1997. Pancreatic carcinoma. Lancet **349:** 485–489.
28. KUROWSKI, V. & W. WAGNER. 1993. Comparative pharmacokinetics of ifosfamide, 4-hydroxyifosfamide, chloroacetaldehyde, and 2- and 3-dechloroethylifosfamide

in patients on fractionated intravenous ifosfamide therapy. Cancer Chemother. Pharmacol. **33:** 36–42.

29. DONATO, M.T., M.J. GOMEZ-LECHON & J.V. CASTELL, 1993. A microassay for measuring cytochrome P450IA1 and P450IIB1 activities in intact human and rat hepatocytes cultured on 96-well plates. Anal Biochem. **213:** 29–33.
30. LÖHR, M., B. TRAUTMANN, S. PETERS, I. ZAUNER, S. LIEBE, G. KLÖPPEL & E.D. KREUSER. 1995. Expression and function of integrins in human pancreatic adenocarcinoma. Pancreas **12:** 248–259.
31. PELEGRIN, M., M. MARIN, D. NOEL, M. DEL RIO, R.M. SALLER, J. STANGE, S. MITZNER, W.H. GÜNZBURG & M. PIECHACZYK. 1998. Systemic long-term delivery of antibodies in immunocompetent animals using cellulose sulfate capsules containing antibody-producing cells. Gene Therapy **5:** 828–834
32. LÖHR, M., P. MÜLLER, P. KARLE, J. STANGE, S. MITZNER, R. JESNOWSKI, H. NIZZE, B. NEBE, S. LIEBE, B. SALMONS & W.H. GÜNZBURG. 1998. Targeted chemotherapy by intratumour injection of encapsulated cells engineered to produce CYP2B1, an ifosfamide activating cytochrome P450. Gene Therapy **5:** 1070–1078.
33. LÖHR, M., Z.T. BAGO, H. BERGMEISTER, M. CEIJNA, M. FREUND *et al.* 1999. Cell therapy using microencapsulated 293 cells transfected with a gene construct expressing CYP2B1, an ifosfamide converting enzyme, instilled intraarterially in patients with advanced-stage pancreatic carcinoma: a phase I/II study. J. Mol. Med. **77:** In press.

# Radiation Sterilization of a Bifunctional Cement Formulation of Hydroxilapatite-Plaster-Polymers

DIANELYS SAINZ VIDAL,[a,d] DANIA RODRIGUEZ NAPOLES,[a] GASTON FUENTES ESTEVEZ,[b] MERCEDES GUERRA,[a] WILLIAMS ARCIS SORIANO,[b] EDUARDO PEON AVES,[b] JOSE M. DIAZ ARGOTA,[b] AND DIONISIO ZALDIVAR SILVA[c]

[a]*Department of Radiobiology and Irradiation Techniques, CEADEN, Miramar, C. Habana, Cuba*

[b]*Department of Ceramics and Composites, BIOMAT, University of Havana, Cuba*

[c]*Department of Macromolecular Chemistry, BIOMAT, University of Havana, Cuba*

**ABSTRACT: A sterilization method based on the use of gamma ionizing radiation was applied to a cement formulation of hydroxilapatite, plaster and polymers to be used in bone restorations in dental, aesthetic, and neurological surgery. After the cement was exposed to a dose of 21.5 kGy it reached the sterility assurance level which was necessary for its employment in surgical applications as specified by International Standard ISO ordinate 11137: Radiation Sterilization of Health Care Products. No variation in the initial cement composition or processing parameters, such as working or setting time and molding quality was observed due to sterilization. Its characteristics as a drug delivery system were also not affected. Therefore, radiation sterilization provides a feasible alternative to conventional sterilization methods such as dry/wet heat and ethylene oxide.**

## INTRODUCTION

Ionizing radiation processing is an efficient technology for the sterilization of certain products which can not be treated by other methods since it offers advantages such as the possibility to sterilize at low temperatures as well as after packaging.[1] At present, radiation sterilization plants for medical equipment are operating successfully worldwide.[1] The cement of hydroxilapatite (HAP), plaster and polymers is a bifunctional formulation designed for filling bone defects and cystic cavities of various geometries, by the efficient use of the mass of bone growing inductor (HAP) contained in the mix. The material can also include an antibiotic that will be delivered into the organism at a controlled rate. This novel product will allow improved mechanical properties for traditional ceramics (powdered), an extension of the use of HAP to zones with high physical loads, and better manipulation and molding during surgery. Since the formulation contains sodium alginate, an organic compound, it is sensitive to contamination. In addition, it is not possible to sterilize it by heat,

[d]Corresponding author. Present address: Laboratory of Polymers and Biomaterials, Swiss Federal Institute of Technology, CH-1015, Lausaune, Switzerland.

which is usually employed for the sterilization of surgical material. Similarly, high temperatures have an adverse effect on several drugs. Given these constraints the aim of this work is to establish a required sterilization dose for this product as well as the verification that sterilization does not alter material properties.

## MATERIALS AND METHODS

### *Sterilization Dose Assessment*

In order to determine the sterilization dose, Method 1, described in ISO 11137 for the sterilization of health care products,[2] was followed. In accordance with the product characteristics, the Sterility Assurance Level (SAL) selected was $10^{-6}$ and the unit was taken as a Simple Item Portion (SIP).

#### *Bioburden Assessment*

For product bioburden determination 10 random samples (product units) of 1g from three different production batches were taken. Each sample was diluted in 99 ml of Soybean Casein Digest Broth (from Oxoid). Following this, three decimal dilutions in saline solution were made with 0.1 ml of each spread in Petri plates and incubated at 30°C for 5 days. Five replicates were performed. Finally, the colony counting was carried out in order to obtain the average bioburden per product unit. Microbial recovery was performed in several culture media and solutions such as plate count agar, nutrient agar, tryptone soy agar, tryptone soy broth, nutrient broth, buffer solution and saline solution (all the reagents were purchased from Oxoid).

#### *Verification Dose Experiment*

One hundred samples from the same production batch were selected and irradiated at the obtained verification dose (8.2 kGy). For the sterility assay, the irradiated samples were added to 10 ml of Soybean Casein Digest Broth and incubated at 30°C for 14 days in order to determine the number of samples with surviving microorganisms. As Method 1 indicates, if no more than two positive assays occur in 100 tested samples, the verification is acceptable. In our study no positives occurred.

### *Irradiation*

All the material used in the study was irradiated in a PX-gamma-30 facility, a laboratory irradiator with $^{60}Co$ sources, at the Center of Applied Studies to Nuclear Development (CEADEN), Havana, Cuba. The dose rate in the selected facility chamber point for each exposition was determined according to Prieto *et al.*[3] All the irradiations were made at 25 ± 1°C.

### *Analysis of Product Behavior Following Irradiation*

Samples of 2 g of bone cement (HAP, plaster, PVP, sodium alginate and gentamicin) were irradiated at six different doses (1, 5, 10, 15, 20, and 25 kGy). Following irradiation the following series of tests were performed.

*Handling*

The solid part of the material (HAP, plaster, PVP, sodium alginate and gentamicin) was mixed with the liquid part ($K_3PO_4$, 4%, sterile) in a rubber dentistry tray, by using a spatula. The material was molded to match a possible bone defect.

*Working and Setting Time*

The partial and total material setting times were assessed manually.

*Infrared Spectrometry*

Infrared spectra for the product samples not irradiated, and irradiated at 10 kGy and 25 kGy, before and after setting, were obtained. The spectra were registered using a Philips FTIR PU-9800 with a spectral range of 400–4000 $cm^{-1}$, employing KBr pellets.

## RESULTS

### *Sterilization Dose Assessment*

The main parameters employed in sterilization dose determination are shown in TABLE 1. The initial contamination of samples was found to amount to 120 cfu/g. The verification dose was found to be 8.2 kGy. The result of the sterility test was acceptable since none of the 100 samples showed positive growth of microorganisms. Regarding the required SAL ($10^{-6}$), the sterilizing dose was found to be 21.5 kGy.

**TABLE 1.** Principal parameters employed in the sterilization dose determination

| Parameter | Value |
|---|---|
| SAL | $10^{-6}$ |
| SIP | 1 |
| Average bioburden before irradiation | 120 cfu/g |
| Verification dose | 8.2 kGy |
| Sterility test result | Non Positive |
| Sterilization dose | 21.5 kGy |

### *Analysis of Product Behavior Following Irradiation*

The original properties of the cements, good handling and partial and total setting times, were maintained after irradiation. TABLE 2 shows the results of the previously

**TABLE 2.** Comparison of the results for handling and setting tests obtained before and after irradiation

| Stage | Molding (first 4 hours) | Medium Hardness (hours) | Total Hardness (hours) |
|---|---|---|---|
| Before irradiation | Good plasticity; no sticking or moisturizing; good shape preservation | >4 | ≃24 |
| After irradiation | Good plasticity; no sticking or moisturizing; good shape preservation | >4 | ≃24 |

mentioned study (in MATERIALS AND METHODS), which are important for good material aesthetics and for selection of the proper formulation for the type of bone lesion to be repaired.

### *Infrared Spectrometry*

Infrared spectra for the product samples not irradiated, and irradiated at 10 kGy and 25 kGy, before and after setting, are shown in FIGURES 1–6. Notice that, although in some cases certain functional groups peaks have changed slightly, there

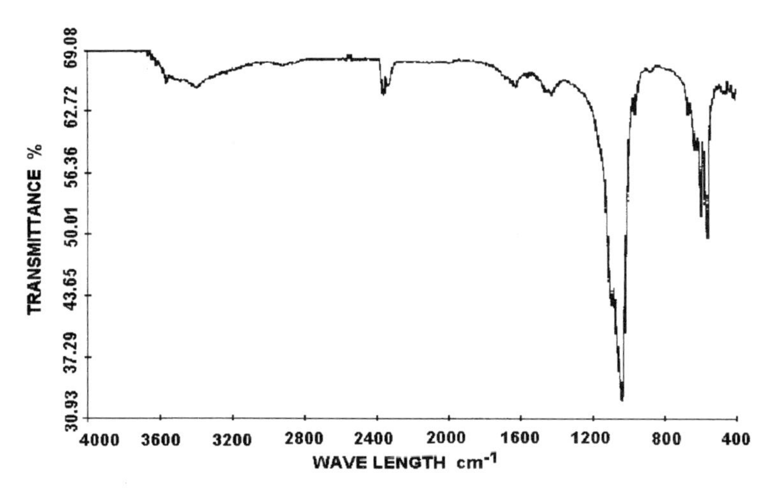


**FIGURE 1.** FTIR Spectra of irradiated cement prior to setting.

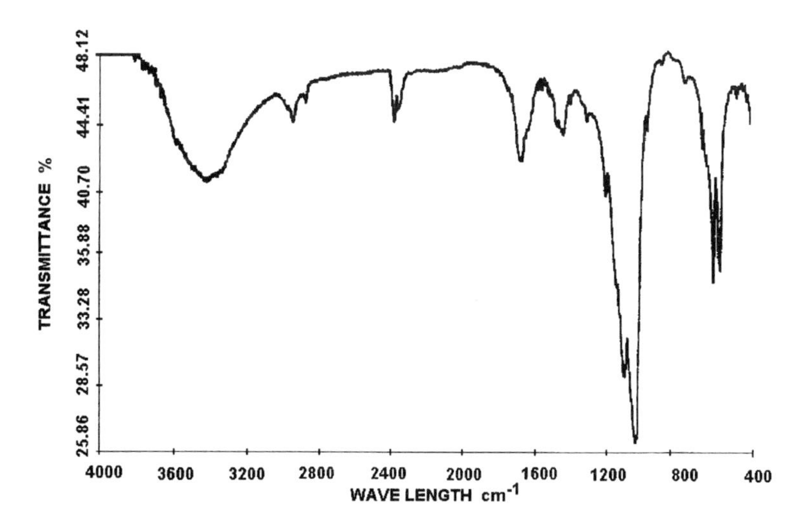


**FIGURE 2.** FTIR Spectra of non-irradiated cement after setting.

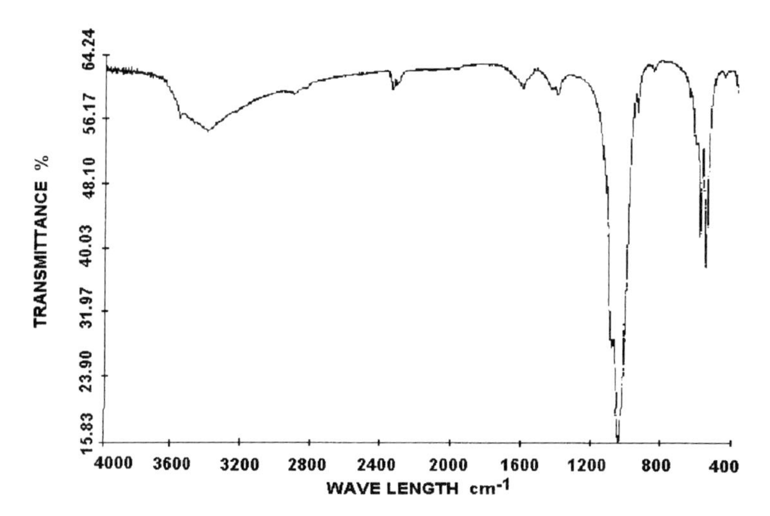


**FIGURE 3.** FTIR Spectra of cement irradiated to 10 kGy prior to setting.

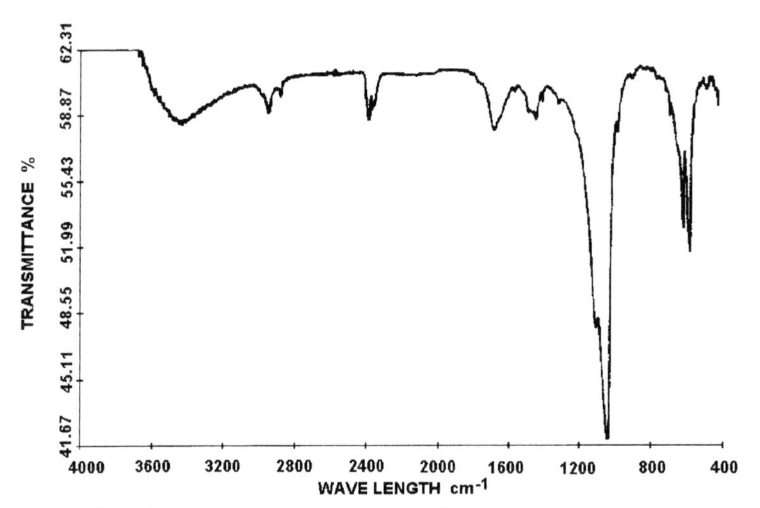


**FIGURE 4.** FTIR Spectra of cement irradiated to 10 kGy after setting.

are no major differences in the spectra, which supports the idea that no remarkable changes in cement composition due to irradiation have occurred.

## CONCLUSIONS

The value of the minimal absorbed dose required for achieving the sterility of a cement contaminated with the estimated bioburden was assessed to be 21.5 kGy. It was demonstrated that no variations in cement properties such as working time, set-

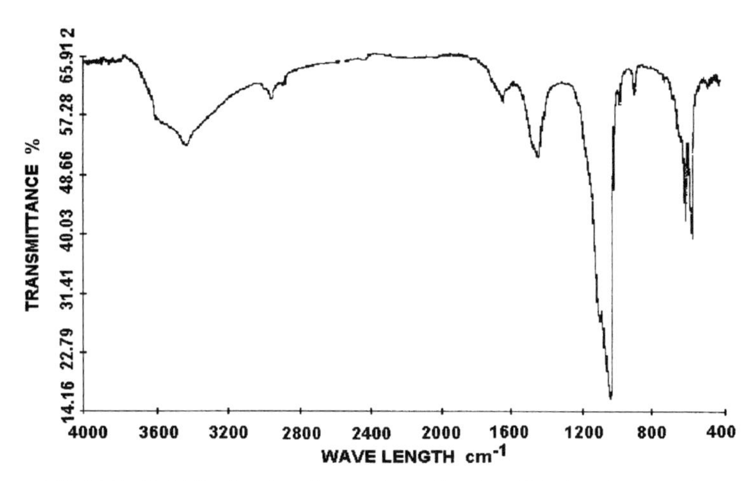


**FIGURE 5.** FTIR Spectra of cement irradiated to 25 kGy prior to setting.

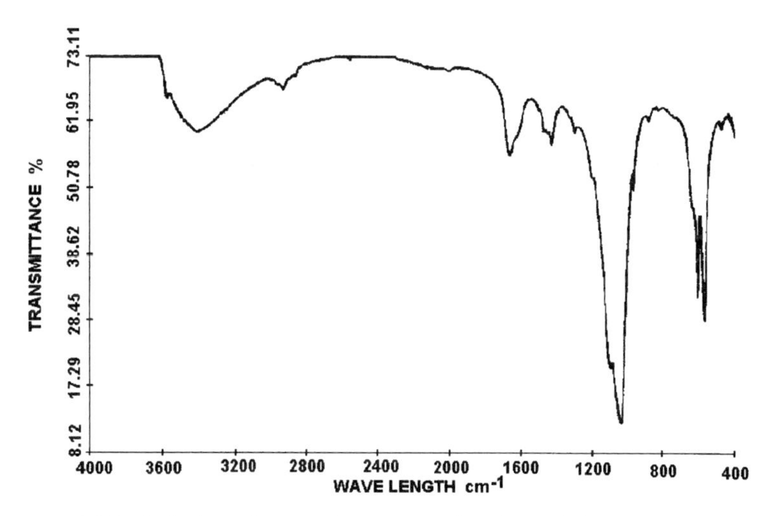


**FIGURE 6.** FTIR Spectra of cement irradiated to 25 kGy after setting.

ting time, and molding qualities occur and that there were no major changes from initial cement composition. The feasibility of the use of gamma radiation for bifunctional cement sterilization was, therefore, proven.

## REFERENCES

1. Advanced Radiation Chemistry Research: Current Status, IAEA/TECDOC/834, October 1995.
2. International Standards Organization. 1995. Sterilization of Health Care Products: Requirements for Validation and Routine Control/Radiation Sterilization. ISO/ 11137, Geneva, Switzerland.

3. Prieto Miranda, E.F., A. Chavez Ardanza, D. Sainz Vidal & G.I. Cuesta Fuente. Dosimetry for the Commissioning of the PX-Gamma-30 Irradiation Facility. In press.
4. Prieto, E.F., Norma Ramal NRIAL. 1991. Absorbed Dose Assessment using Fricke Dosimeter IIIA.
5. Ng, Q., L. Hien, X. Tham, N. Nagasawa, F. Yoshii *et al.* Effect of radiation depolymerized alginate on growth-promotion of plants. Submitted to J. Agric. Food Chem. Am. Chem. Soc., 1997.
6. Humphreys, G.R. & G.R. Howells. 1971. Carbohydrates Res. **16:** 63.
7. Dam, A.M., L.G. Gazso, S. Kaewpila & I. Mashek. 1995. Radiation sterilization dose calculation for heparin and aprotinin based on ISO Method 1. Int. J. Pharmaceutics **121**.

# Artificial Cells, Encapsulation, and Immobilization

THOMAS MING SWI CHANG [a]

*Artificial Cells and Organs Research Centre, Departments of Physiology, Medicine and Biomedical Engineering, Faculty of Medicine, McGill University, Montreal, Q.C., Canada H3G 1Y6*

**ABSTRACT: The basic principles of artificial cells, encapsulation and immobilization form the basis for a number of bioartificial organs. Hemoperfusion based on encapsulated adsorbent has been in routine clinical uses for many years to remove toxins or drugs from the circulating blood. Blood substitutes based on crosslinked hemoglobin or encapsulated hemoglobin are being developed and tested in phase II and Phase III clinical trials. Enzyme therapy using microencapsulated enzymes have been studied in animal studies and in a preliminary human study. Encapsulation or other ways of immobilization of cells are being developed extensively by many groups. This includes the encapsulation or immobilization of islets, hepatocytes and genetically engineered cells.**

## INTRODUCTION

The biological cell is an example of a naturally occurring system where enzymes and intracellular organelles are microencapsulated within the cell membrane. Semipermeable microcapsules have been prepared to retain biologically active materials while allowing some permeant molecules to cross the membrane.[1–3] These semipermeable microcapsules containing biologically active materials are sometime referred to as artificial cells.[3–5] Many types of biologically active materials can be microencapsulated individually or in combination ( FIG. 1). The permeability, composition and configuration of the membrane can be varied using different types of synthetic or biological materials. These possible variations in contents and membranes allow for variations in the properties and functions of these "artificial cells."

The membrane separates the encapsulated materials from the external system (FIG. 1). While retained inside the microcapsules, biologically active materials can act on smaller external molecules that can cross the membranes. Smaller molecules produced inside the microcapsules can also cross the membrane to enter the "extracellular environment". In this way, the enclosed material can be retained and separated from undesirable external materials like antibodies, tryptic enzymes and leukocytes (FIG. 1). At the same time, the large surface area and the ultrathin membrane allow permeant substrates and products to diffuse rapidly (FIG. 1). Ten ml of 20-micron diameter artificial cells have a total surface area of about 20,000 $cm^2$ which, therefore allows a rapid movement of permeant molecules across the membrane of the semipermeable microcapsules.

[a]Address for correspondence: 3655Drummond Street Montreal, Q.C., Canada H3G 1Y6; 1-514-398-4983(fax); artcell@physio.mcgill.ca (e-mail); http://www.physio.mcgill/artcell (web).

## MEDICAL AND BIOTECHNOLOGICAL APPLICATIONS

Encapsulation and immobilization have been used in a number of medical and biotechnological applications[3–5] as shown below.

- Artificial cells containing adsorbents are routinely used in hemoperfusion for the treatment of acute poisoning in children and adults.
- Artificial cells containing adsorbents are employed clinically in hemoperfusion to remove toxins and waste in liver failure patients as a partial artificial liver support. They are presently applied together with immobilized hepatocytes, as a bioartificial liver in clinical trial.
- Artificial cells containing enzymes delivered orally are being used for the removal of unwanted metabolites in inborn errors of metabolism. For example, the removal of phenylalanine in phenylketonuria based on the new finding of enterorecirculation of amino acids (being developed for clinical trial) and removal of hypoxanthine in hypxanthinemia (clinical trial).
- First generation blood substitutes in the form of cross-linked ultrapure hemoglobin has been developed. Ongoing Phase II to Phase III clinical trials infusing up to 5000ml in the case of polyhemoglobin are under assay.
- Second generation blood substitutes in the form of cross-linking hemoglobin (Hb), superoxide dismutase (SOD) and catalase (CAT) to form polyHb-SOD-CAT.
- Third generation blood substitutes in the form of liposome encapsulated hemoglobin or, more recently, biodegradable nanocapsules containing hemoglobin and enzymes to form a more complete artificial red blood cell.
- Encapsulated islets and other endocrine tissues: for diabetes and other endocrine diseases (in development for clinical trial).
- Encapsulated hepatocytes as bioartificial liver for implantation (experimental) and in hemoperfusion (clinical trial).
- Drug delivery systems are used for routine applications and in experimental protocols.
- Encapsulation of genetically engineered cells involves implantation (experimental), implantation with retrieval (clinical trial) and oral administration (being developed for clinical trial).
- Production of fine chemicals and biotechnological materials.
- Food and aquatic culture.
- Other biotechnological and medical applications in progress.

## HEMOPERFUSION

Microcapsules containing adsorbents[3] (FIG. 1) are now being used routinely in hemoperfusion for patients, especially for treating drug poisoning.[5,6] Hemoperfu-

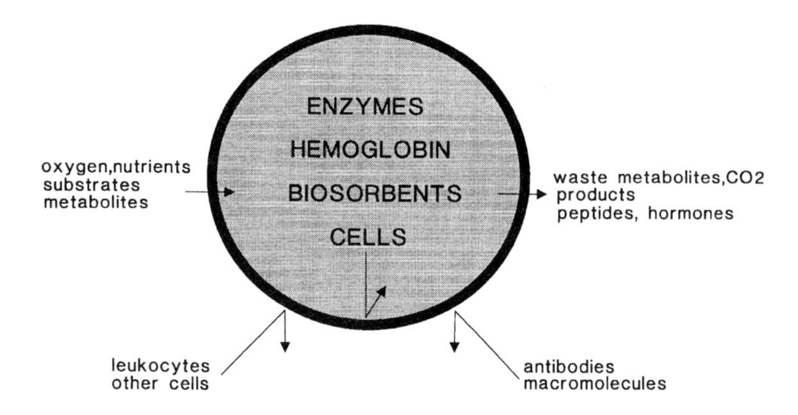


**FIGURE 1.** The principal functioning of encapsulated biologically active materials. The microcapsule membrane excludes external cells such as leukocytes and external macromolecules like antibodies and tryptic enzymes. At the same time it permits smaller molecules such as oxygen, nutrients, substrates to enter and be acted on by the enclosed materials. The egress of smaller molecules (e.g., peptides secreted by cells) produced by the enclosed material is also permitted. This results in immunoisolation of the encapsulated materials that can still continue to carry out their functions.

sion is a process in which blood perfuse through a column of biologically active particles. It has also been used as a partial artificial liver support system for the removal of toxic and unwanted metabolites in liver failure patients.[6] It is now being applied in combination with immobilized hepatocytes to form a more complete bioartificial liver.

## BLOOD SUBSTITUTES

Concern in regard to HIV in donor blood has stimulated the development of blood substitutes in the recent years.[7,8] When other approaches failed, investigators started to re-develop our earlier ideas.[1,3] The first approach at preparing modified hemoglobin blood substitutes was in the form of microencapsulated hemoglobin.[1] This has also been simplified into cross-linking hemoglobin together into polyhemoglobin[1,3] to form first generation blood substitute. These modifications prevent the hemoglobin, a tetramer, from breaking down into dimers in the circulation. There is no blood group antigens and crossmatching is not needed, thus allowing for ease of use in some surgery, emergencies, major disasters or wars. Blood substitutes can be stored for a long time in the lyophilized formed. What is very important is that they can be sterilized to remove infective microorganisms like HIV and hepatitits viruses.

The use of glutaraldehyde as a cross-linking agent to form polyhemoglobin[10] has been extensively developed.[7,8] Up to 5000 ml of glutaraldehyde cross-linked human polyhemoglobin has been infused safely into surgical patients in F.D.A. approved Phase III clinical trials by Gould's group.[11] Polyhemoglobin can circulate for about 24 hours after infusion and is therefore suitable only for short-term uses. This has been extended into other first-generation blood substitutes, for example, other cross-linked hemoglobin (intramolecular and conjugated) and also recombinant hemoglobin (internal fusing of 2 subunits).[7,8] These first generation blood substitutes contain only hemoglobin. Red blood cells contain important enzymes such as superoxide dismutase and catalase that are important in removing oxidants like superoxide and other free radicals that can cause tissue damage. In ischemic conditions encountered in hemorrhagic shock, stroke, mycardial infarction, infusion of the first-generation blood substitutes containing no enzymes can there result in reperfusion injury.[7,8] A second-generation blood substitute formed by cross-linking hemoglobin (Hb), superoxide dismutase (SOD) and catalase (CAT) into polyHb-SOD-CAT is being successfully developed to prevent these problems.[12] The first-generation and second-generation blood substitutes circulate for approximately 24 hours after infusion in the case of PolyHb, conjugated Hb and PolyHb-SOD-CAT and 10–12 hours for the others. As a result, they can only function for 24 hours as compared to about 30 days for donor blood. They are therefore more suitable for certain elective surgeries and also for emergencies. Microencapsulated hemoglobin is being developed as a third-generation blood substitute with a longer circulation time. The original idea of microencapsulated Hb[1,3] has been developed first into liposome-encapsulated hemoglobin.[13,14] A more recent development is the use of biodegradable polymeric nanocapsules to encapsulate hemoglobin and enzymes to form a more complete blood substitute.[15]

## ENZYME THERAPY

Artificial cells containing catalase (FIG. 1) have been implanted into acatalesemic mice, i.e., animals with a congenitical deficiency in catalase.[16] This replaces the deficient enzymes and prevents the animals from the damaging effects of peroxides. Artificial cells containing asparaginase implanted into mice with lymphosarcoma delayed the onset and growth of lymphosarcoma.[17] The single problem preventing the clinical application of enzyme artificial cells was the need to implant these artificial enzyme cells. An exciting solution to this problem is our recently finding that orally administered artificial cells containing xanthine oxidase can lower the high systemic levels of hypoxanthine in hypoxanthiuria in patients.[4] We also found that microencapsulated phenylalanine ammonia lyase given orally can lower the elevated phenylalanine levels in phenylketonuria rats.[4] Our recent finding shows that this is because of an extensive recycling of amino acids between the body and the intestine.[4] This procedure is now being developed for clinical trials.

## CELL ENCAPSULATION

We have microencapsulated cells and suggested that this approach can be used for immunoisolation of implants[2,3] via the exclusion of leukocytes and antibodies (FIG. 1). While inside the microcapsules, the cells continue to be supported by external oxygen and nutrients. Their secretions of lower molecular weights can diffuse out of the microcapsules to carry out their functions.[2–5] Microencapsulated cells are now being studied by many groups for the treatment of diabetes, liver failure and other conditions.[4,5,18–38] The ideal approach would be to encapsulate cells and implant these into the body for long-term functions. For example, a number of groups have implantation microencapsulated islets to maintain normal glucose levels in diabetic animals and also in diabetic patients in Phase I clinical trials.[18–21] Microencapsulated hepatocytes—when implanted—can lower the elevated bilirubin level in Gunn rats with an inborn error of bilirubin metabolism.[4] The transplanted, microencapsulated xenogenic cells are protected from immunorejection[4,18–21] owing to their separation from external leukocytes and antibodies.

These promising results described in the preceeding paragraphs have stimulated further research into the safety and long-term feasibility of microencapsulation with a view to clinical applications.[4,5,18–23] However, material biocompatibility and mass transfer are two of the important factors which have not received sufficient attention. For example, foreign body reaction with resulting fibrous reaction will decrease mass transfer of oxygen, nutrients, and metabolites and cause death of the encapsulated cells. Therefore, there is much research on improving the biocompatibility of microcapsules. Microcapsules can exclude leukocytes and antibodies, resulting in immune protection. This has already been demonstrated by several groups.[4,5,18–23] Some researchers are now looking into the more detailed aspects of immunoprotection. For instance, several researchers suggest that it is not sufficient just to exclude leukocytes and antibodies. They feel that if the implanted encapsulated cells are not "biocompatible" they can activate complements resulting in smaller complement components (e.g., C5a, C3a) that can enter the microcapsules to damage the enclosed cells.. For example, Hagihara *et al.*[24] studied the implantation of encapsulated β-endorphin secreting xenogeneic cells. They analyzed the ability of components of complement to penetrate the capsule membrane. In addition, activation of leukocytes may result in the secretion of cytokines that can also enter the implanted microcapsules to cause damage to the enclosed cells. These biocompatibility problems would require very delicate adjustment of membrane permeability to restrict complement components and cytokines and at the same time to allow the free diffusion of the factors secreted by the encapsulated cells. This may then limit the use of microencapsulated xenogeneic cells that secrete factors of larger molecular weights. The development of "biocompatible" materials is an extensive topic of investigation.[18–23] The elimination of foreign body reactions presents another challenge. This can result in fibrous and cell coating of the microcapsules resulting in marked decrease to mass transfer—initially for the larger molecules, and then later for oxygen, nutrients and other molecules. In preparing different types of microcapsules, it may be useful to have a screening method for analyzing the permeability of the microcapsule membrane to macromolecules with a wide range of molecular weight. The authors employ liquid chromatography to study variations in microcapsule membrane composition on the diffusion of larger molecules.[25] We have started with the use of dextran with a wide range of molecular weights to analyze the kinetics of mass transfer of large molecules. Since the mass transfer characteristics of dextran molecules may be different from biomolecules, we are now using biological proteins of different molecular weights to standardize this approach.

Several researchers look into other configurations for more immediately clinical applications. For example, Aebischer's ingenious use of capillary fibers to encapsulate cells has allowed his group to insert these subcutaneously into the cerebral spinal fluid on a short-term basis thus allowing them to remove and renew the fibers.[26] This would prevent the problem related to permanent retention of genetically engineered cells and other effects of long-term implantation. However, the fiber encapsulation and insertion approach is applicable to situations not requiring large amounts of encapsulated cells. Other groups use encapsulated cells in extracorporeal systems. A recent promising approach, for use under certain conditions, that does not require implantation or insertion is the oral administration of microencapsulated genetically engineered cells.

## ENCAPSULATION OF GENETICALLY ENGINEERED CELLS

### *Molecular Biology and Gene Therapy*

Advances in molecular biology have resulted in exciting possibilities for medical applications. One important area is gene therapy.[27,28] There are two main approaches in gene therapy, with the first very promising approach based on direct *in vivo* gene transfer to the host cells.[27,28] Another method involves the introduction of genetic materials *ex vivo* into cell cultures outside the body. The genetically engineered cells are subsequently transplanted.[28] This requires the use of autologous cells, i.e., cells obtained from the same patient. Clearly, it would be more convenient and enabling from a therapeutic viewpoint if other sources of cells could be employed. This need has stimulated the application of encapsulation of genetically engineered cells to protect cells from immune rejection after implantation.

There are two methods employed for the encapsulation of cells. The first involves the direct implantion of the microencapsulated, genetically engineered cells.[29–36] The results in animal studies have been promising with researchers continuing to study 1) the safety of injecting genetic engineered cells into the body and 2) the retention and biocompatibility of the injected microcapsules. A more recent finding has shown that microencapsulated genetically engineered cells, given orally, can function during their passage through the intestine prior to excretion in the stool.[37–38] Oral use would avoid the need to transplant the microencapsulated genetically engineered cells and solve the problems related to retention and biocompatibility. On the other hand, the oral approach is only suitable for those conditions where the substrates to be removed can equilibrate at a sufficient rate between the body compartment and the intestinal lumen. These include small molecules like urea and lipid- soluble molecules like hypoxanthine which can equilibrate rapidly between the circulating blood and the intestinal lumen. Also in this group are amino acids because they can equilibrate rapidly between the body and the intestinal lumen by the newly shown enterorecirculation route.[4,5]

### *Transplantation of Microencapsulated Genetically Engineered Cells*

As discussed in the preceeding section, the encapsulation of genetically engineered cells has been an active area of research for several bioartificial organs. For example, Sun's group[29] reported their study of microencapsulating mouse fibroblasts with a human growth hormone (hGH) fusion gene. They showed that after transplantation, the encapsulated genetically engineered cells remained viable. Human growth hormone (hGH) from these cells were secreted and delivered *in vivo*. When the encapsulated cells were recovered from implanted recipients, the cells continued to secrete hGH *in vitro*. Aebischer's group[30,31] encapsulated baby hamster kidney (BHK) cells inside hollow fibers for use in amyotrophic lateral sclerosis (ALS). ALS is a neurodegenerative disease where there is progressive loss of motoneurons leading to death in a few years. Ciliary neurotrophic factor (CNTF) has been investigated for potential use in ALS. However, it has a very short half-life and it is also difficult to administer to the central nervous system. They microencapsulated genetically engineered BHK cells containing the gene for human or mouse CNTF. These encapsulated cells released bioactive CNTF *in vitro*. When transplanted, they continued to release human or mouse CNTF. Implantation resulted in the rescue of 26–27% more motoneurons from axotomy-induced cell death when compared to those microcapsules containing parent BHK cells.

Saitoh *et al.*[32] encapsulated Neuro2A cells containing propiomelanocortin gene that released β-endorphin. These were encapsulated inside silicone microcapsules at a density of $5 \times 10^6$ gene/ml. They injected these into the cerebral spinal fluid of male Sprague-Dawley rats and used three tests for pain: the tail pinch test, the hot plate test, and electrical stimulation test. The results showed that rats implanted with encapsulated Neuro2A cells ($n = 6$) were significantly less sensitive to pain than control animals ($n = 8$). The analgesia induced by the encapsulated cells secreting β-endorphin could be attenuated by the opiate antagonist naloxone. Histology showed that the encapsulated cells survived for 1 month after implantation.

Okada *et al.*[33] microencapsulated SK2 hybridoma cells that secreted anti-hIL-6 monoclonal antibodies (SK2 mAb). They implanted these alginate-poly(L)lysine-alginate microcapsules intraperitoneally into human interleukin-6 transgenic mice (hIL-6 Tgm). They showed that implantation suppressed IgG1 plasmacytosis in the hIL-6 Tgm mice and the survival time of these mice increased significantly. Microencapsulated cells remained viable and continued to secrete SK2 mAb *in vivo* for at least 1 month after implantation. SK2 mAb was detected in the serum at concentrations of 3–5 mg/ml day 14 to day 50 after implantation. Implantation of free SK2 cells had no therapeutic effect on hIL-6 Tgm mice. P.L. Chang's group[34] encapsulated genetically engineered human factor XI–secreting mouse myoblasts for use in hemophilia B. They implanted these into allogeneic mice and showed the presence of human factor IX in the mouse plasma (4 ng/ml) for up to 14 days. However, after 3 weeks, antibodies to human factor IX increased and cleared human factor IX from the circulation of the implanted mice. Despite the fact that the encapsulated myoblasts retrieved up to 213 days after implantation were still viable and continued to secrete human factor IX *ex vivo*.

Date *et al.*[35] microencapsulated human baby hamster kidney fibroblasts that secrete nerve growth factor (BHK-hNGF). They co-implanted these with free rat adrenal medullary chromaffin cells into the striatum of hemi-parkinsonian rats. Those rats that received both encapsulated BHK-hNGF cells and free chromaffin cells showed decreases (39–56%) in apomorphine-induced rotational behavior. Histology showed that co-grafting with microencapsulated BHK/hNGF cells increased chromaffin cell survival by 20 times. On the other hand, survival was poor when free adrenal medullary chromaffin cells were implanted alone. After implantation, the retrieved microcapsules contained viable encapsulated BHK-hNGF cells that continued to release hNGF. They suggested the potential of using intrastriatal implantation of encapsulated hNGF-secreting cells to augment the survival of co-grafted chromaffin cells for hemi-parkinsonian rats.

Winn *et al.*[36] encapsulated xenogeneic cells genetically modified to secrete human nerve growth factor. They used this to promote the survival of axotomized septal cholinergic neurons. They implanted these encapsulated BHK cells into fimbria-fornix-lesioned rat brains. Studies showed that the encapsulated BHK cells continued to release human nerve growth factors 3 weeks after transplantation. There was significant protection of axotomized medial septal cholinergic neurons. Encapsulated cell survival was also confirmed by histology. The authors suggested the potential use of this to deliver other neurotrophic factors for different sites in the body.

### *Oral Administration of Microencapsulated Genetically Engineered Cells*

A number of problems still need to be resolved before transplantation of microencapsulated genetically engineering cells can be used clinically. These include the need to inject genetically engineered cells and the retention and biocompatibility of implanted microcapsules. The author's group have recently studied an oral approach to avoid the need for surgical interventions or transplantation.[37–38] Orally administered microcapsules containing genetically engineered cells pass through the intestine and are excreted in the stool (FIG. 2). Therefore, there is no retention in the body. On their passage through the intestinal tract, urea enters the microcapsules and is used in cell synthesis (FIG. 2).

The author's group initiated a feasibility study on the application of microcapsules on urea removal since only 15% of the world's uremic patients can afford dialysis therapy, an otherwise effective treatment.[39] Oral therapy consisting of a combination of adsorbents, osmotic agents and other oral agents.[39] The single major remaining obstacle was the lack of an effective oral method for urea removal. Advances in molecular biology have resulted in the availability of nonpathogenic genetically engineered microorganisms that can effectively convert urea into ammonia and then use the ammonia for cell synthesis.[40] Therefore, we have carried out research on microencapsulated genetically engineered nonpathogenic *E. coli* DH5 cells containing *K. aegrogens* urease gene for oral removal of urea in renal failure

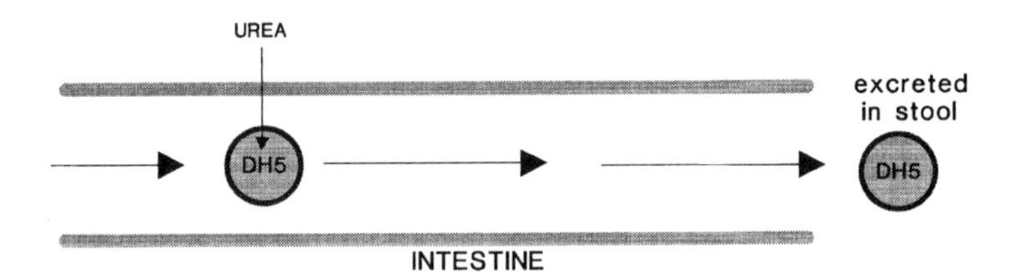


**FIGURE 2.** Oral administration of artificial cell microencapsulated *E. coli* DH5 cells. On their passage through the intestine they take up urea and use the urea-nitrogen for their cellular synthesis. The microcapsules are subsequently excreted in the stool together with the urea-nitrogen thus removing urea from the body.

rats. An optimized method to prepare alginate-polylysine-alginate microcapsules containing nonpathogenic *E. coli* DH5 cells with an average diameter of 500 ± 45 μm[41] was employed. There was considerable cell growth when incubated in plasma with high urea level as the cells used the urea-nitrogen as their nitrogen source for growth. Our single pool model shows that 8.60 grams of *E. coli* DH5 cells in the microcapsules can remove 99.99 % of the urea in a 40 liter pool with 100 mg/dl of urea ( equivalent to the removal of 40 g).[41] This is very striking when compared to other available urea removal systems. For instance, to remove the same amount of 40 grams of urea, 388 g of oxystarch or 1212 g of microcapsules containing urease-zirconium-phosphate[41] are required. Experimental renal failure rats were prepared by the surgical removal of one kidney and partial ligation of the other kidney.[37] Rats were partially nephrectomized so that they still had adequate control of water and electrolytes. The major changes in these renal failure rats were an elevation of urea and other waste metabolites. All the rats were placed on standard rat diet containing 22.5% of protein. We gave orally 11.15 ± 2.25 mg/kg body weight of log phase microencapsulated genetically engineered *E. coli* DH5 cells daily for 21 days to a group of renal failure rats. Their original plasma urea level of 52.08 ± 2.06 % mg was lowered and maintained at the normal range of 9.10 ± 0.71 % mg during the treatment period (FIG. 3).[37] A return to high urea level was observed when the treatment was stopped, showing that there was no significant retention of *E. coli* DH5 cells in the intestine. The microcapsules containing the *E. coli* DH5 cells and the urea-nitrogen were excreted in the stool. Calculations based on the result of this study showed that in a 70 kg patient we would only need to give 4 grams of *E. coli* DH5 cells each day. This therefore has the potential to help solve the single major obstacle of urea removal that has prevented the investigation of oral therapy for terminal renal failure in human. An evaluation of the safety of this therapy was carried out.

The body weight growth profile of different group of rats[42] was followed. The rat groups were designed with a degree of renal failure where the animals could still maintain control of water and electrolytes. Therefore, there was no body weight gain due to fluid accumulation. Thus, in the control renal failure rats receiving control microcapsules with no *E. coli* DH5 cells, the body weight decreased with time as the animals became sicker. On the other hand, the renal failure rats that received microencapsulated *E. coli* DH5 cells have the same weight gain profile as normal rats. This shows that microencapsulated nonpathogenic *E. coli* DH5 cells did not adversely disturb the growth of the renal failure rats. Instead, the growth of these renal failure rats paralleled the normal control animal. The survival results also showed that microencapsulated *E. coli* DH5 cells given orally increased the survival of renal failure rats when compared to the control renal failure rats.[42]

The effects of the escape or liberation of some of the encapsulated nonpathogenic *E. coli* DH5 cells on their passage through the intestine before being excreted in the stool was evaluated. To carry out the most severe test, we gave a second group of renal failure rats the same daily oral doses of *E. coli* DH5 cells, though all in all the free form for the same 21-day period. This provides a model to evaluate the complete liberation of the *E. coli* DH5 cells were to leak out during their passage through the intestine. The results obtained showed that even if all the *E. coli* DH5 cells were to have leaked out there was no adverse effect on the growth of the renal failure rats.[42]

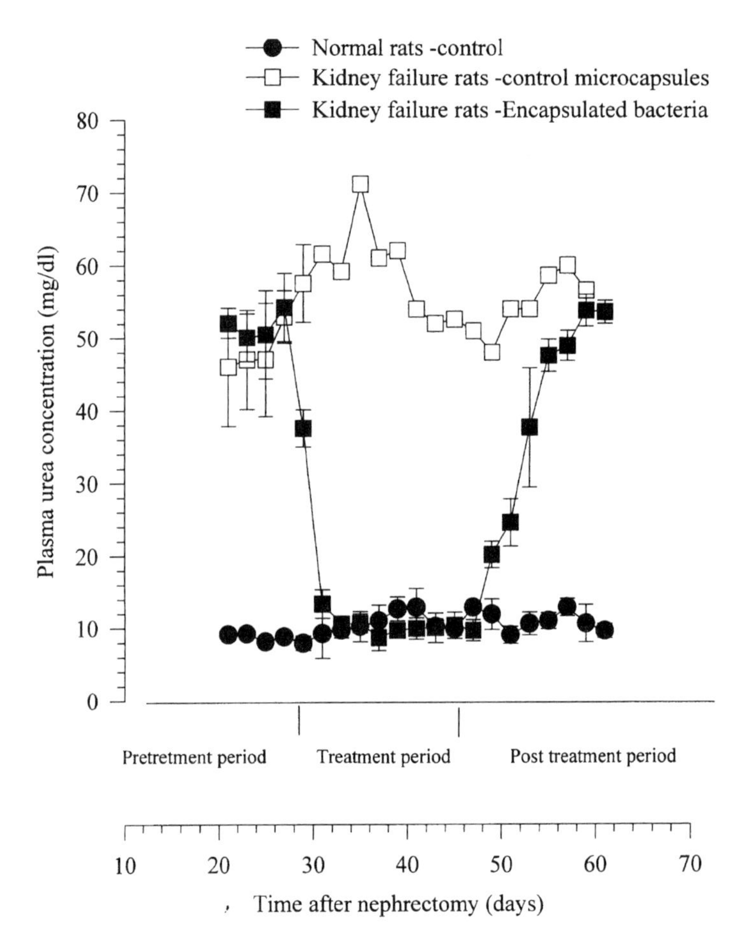


**FIGURE 3.** Results of oral administration of artificial cells microencapsulated *E. coli* DH5 in rats with kidney failure. In the rats with renal failure fed daily control microcapsules, the blood urea remained elevated. In the renal failure rats fed daily microencapsulated *E. coli* DH5 cells, the blood urea was lowered during the treatment period. The level is comparable to the normal level of the control normal group of rats. Once treatment is discontinued, the blood urea levels return to high uremic levels.

On the contrary, those receiving free *E. coli* DH5 cells gained weight at the same rate as normal animals and renal failure rats treated with oral microencapsulated *E. coli* DH5 cells. This does not mean that *E. coli* DH5 cells should be given orally in the free form. When free *E. coli* DH5 cells were used, some of them were retained in the intestine as shown our research.[37] Repeated large doses of the nonpathogenic free *E. coli* DH5 cells may change the normal intestinal flora. Furthermore, urea removal is based on the use of urea as nitrogen source by the encapsulated *E. coli* DH5 cells that are then excreted in the stool with its nitrogen content. If the *E. coli* DH5 cells stay in the intestine, we are not removing the urea-nitrogen. Failure to lower systemic urea levels by manipulations of intestinal microorganisms[43] may be related to the retention of the free microorganisms in the intestine so that the nitrogen source is retained in the body to be recycled. This approach has great potential for the removal of urea in chronic renal failure and could then complete the presently available oral therapy for uremia using adsorbents, ion-exchange resins, and osmotic agents. Their ability to remove ammonia[37] may also permit the application of microcapsules in chronic liver failure. This study also provides the potential basis for the use of oral microcapsules containing other types of nonpathogenic genetically engineered cells for other conditions. For instance, our research showed that the enterorecirculation of amino acids between the body amino acid pool and the intestinal content is very extensive.[4] This has already allowed the use of microcapsules containing enzymes to deplete specific elevated amino acids. One example is the use of microencapsulated phenylalanine ammonia lyase to lower the high systemic phenylalanine level in experimental phenylketonuria rats.[4] There are other medical conditions requiring the depletion of other specific amino acids. Enzymes are not stable and they are also expensive to extract and purified. The use of the presently available, or subsequently developed, genetically engineered cells to remove specific amino acids would be more practical.

## PRESENT STATUS AND FUTURE PERSPECTIVES IN CELL ENCAPSULATION

Long-term transplantation using microencapsulated cells could be an ideal situation, though material biocompatiability must improve before this can be realized. Meanwhile, several groups are looking into other configurations for more immediately clinical applications. For example, capillary fibers encapsulated cells can be inserted subcutaneously into the cerebral spinal fluid on a short-term basis and allowing them to remove and renew the fibers.[26] This would prevent the problem related to permanent retention of genetically engineered cells and other effects of long term implantation. However, the fiber encapsulation and insertion approach is applicable to situations not requiring large amounts of encapsulated cells. Another example is the seeding of hollow fibers with hepatocytes for extracorporeal use as bioartificial liver.[18] A more recent approach that does not required implantation or insertion is the oral administration of microencapsulated genetically engineered cells. However, this is only for use in certain conditions only. As in all medical therapies, the various problems will require divers solutions. The application of microencapsulated cells may be a flexible therapy for transplantation, subcutaneous insertion, extracorporeal perfusion, and oral administration.

## ACKNOWLEDGMENTS

The operating grants and career investigator award from the Medical Research Council of Canada and the Virage Centre of Excellence in Biotechnology award from the Quebec Minister of Education, Science and Technology are gratefully acknowledged.

## REFERENCES

1. CHANG, T.M.S. 1964. Semipermeable microcapsules. Science **146:** 524–525.
2. CHANG, T.M.S., F.C. MACINTOSH & S.G. MASON. 1966. Semipermeable aqueous microcapsules: I. Preparation and properties. Can. J. Physiol. Pharmacol. **44:** 115–128.
3. CHANG, T.M.S. 1972. Artificial Cells. Charles C Thomas, Publisher. Springfield, IL.
4. CHANG, T.M.S. 1995. Artificial cells with emphasis on bioencapsulation in biotechnology. Biotechnol. Annu. Rev. **1:** 267–295.
5. CHANG, T.M.S. 1997. Artificial Cells. *In* Encyclopedia of Human Biology. R. Dulbecco, Editor-in-Chief.**1:** 457–463. Academic Press. San Diego, CA.
6. CHANG, T.M.S. 1975. Microencapsulated adsorbent hemoperfusion for uremia, intoxication and hepatic failure. Kidney Int. **7:** S387–S392.
7. CHANG, T.M.S. 1997. Blood Substitutes: Principle, Methods, Products and Clinical Trials, Vol I. Karger. Basel.
8. CHANG, T.M.S., Ed. 1998. Blood Substitutes: Principles, Methods, Products and Clinical Trials, Vol. 2. Karger. Basel.
9. CHANG, T.M.S. 1998. Modified hemoglobin-based blood substitutes: crosslinked, recombinant and encapsulated hemoglobin. Vox Sanguinis **74**(Suppl. 2)**:** 233–241.
10. CHANG, T.M.S. 1971. Stabilisation of enzymes by microencapsulation with a concentrated protein solution or by microencapsulation followed by cross-linking with glutaraldehyde. Biochem. Biophys. Res. Commun. **44**(6)**:** 1531–1536.
11. GOULD, S.A., L.R. SEHGAL, H.L. SEHGAL, R. DEWOSKIN & G.S. MOSS. 1998. *In* Blood Substitutes: Principles, Methods, Products and Clinical Trials. T.M.S. Chang, Ed. **2:** 12–28. Karger. Basel.
12. D'AGNILLO, F. & T.M.S. CHANG. 1998. Polyhemoglobin-superoxide dismutase-catalase as a blood substitute with antioxidant properties. Nature Biotechnol. **16:** 667–671.
13. RUDOLPH, A.S., R. RABINOVICI & G.Z. FEUERSTEIN, Eds. 1997. Red Blood Cell Substitutes. Marcel Dekker, Inc. New York.
14. TSUCHIDA, E., Ed. 1995. Artificial Red Cells. John Wiley & Sons. New York.
15. CHANG, T.M.S. & W.P. YU. 1996. Biodegradable polymer membrane containing hemoglobin for blood substitutes. US Patent 5670173, September 23, 1997.
16. CHANG, T.M.S. & M.J. POZNANSKY. 1968. Semipermeable microcapsules containing catalase for enzyme replacement in acatalsaemic mice. Nature **218**(5138)**:** 242–245.
17. CHANG, T.M.S. 1971. The in vivo effects of semipermeable microcapsules containing L- asparaginase on 6C3HED lymphosarcoma. Nature **229**(528)**:** 117–118.
18. LANZA, R.P. & D.K.C. COOPER. 1998. Xenotransplantation of cells and tissues: application to a range of diseases, from diabetes to Alzheimer's. Mol. Med. Today **4:** 39–45.
19. PROKOP, A., D. HUNKELER & A.D. CHERRINGTON, Eds. 1997. Bioartificial Organs: Science, Medicine and Technology. Ann. N.Y. Acad. Sci. **831**.
20. SUN, A.M. 1997. Microencapsulation of Cells: medical applications. Ann. N.Y. Acad. Sci. **831:** 271–279.
21. COLTON, C.K. 1996. Implantable biohybrid artificial organs. Cell Transplant. **4:** 415–436.
22. DIONNE K.E., B.M. CAIN, R.H. LI, W.J. BELL, E.J. DOHERTY, D.H. REIN, M.J. LYSAGHT & F.T. GENTILE. 1996. Transport characterization of membranes for immunoisolation. Biomaterials **17:** 257–266.
23. PROKOP, A., D. HUNKELER, S. DIMARI, M.A. HARALSON & T.C. WANG. 1998. Water soluble polymers for immunoisolation I: complex coacervation and cytotoxicity. Adv. Polym. Sci. **136:** 2–51.
24. HAGIHARA, Y., Y. SAITOH, H. IWATA, T. TAKI, S. HIRANO, N. ARITA & T. HAYAKAWA. 1997. Transplantation of xenogeneic cells secreting beta-endorphin for pain treatment: analysis of the ability of components of complement to penetrate through polymer capsules. Cell Transplant. **6:** 527–530.

25. COROMILI, V. & T.M.S. CHANG. 1993. Polydisperse dextran as a diffusing test solute to study the membrane permeability of alginate polylysine microcapsules. Biomater. Artif. Cells Immun. Biotechnol. **21:** 427–444.
26. AEBISCHER, P., M. SCHLUEP, N. DEGLON, J.M. JOSEPH, L. HIRT, B. HEYD, M. GODDARD, J.P. HAMMANG, A.D. ZURN, A.C. KATO, F. REGLI & E.E. BAETGE. 1996. Intrathecal delivery of CNTF using encapsulated genetically modified xenogeneic cells in amyotrophic lateral sclerosis patients. Nat. Med. **2:** 696–699.
27. VERMA, I.M & N. SOMIA. 1997. Gene therapy—promises, problems and prospects. Nature **389:** 239–242.
28. REIMER, D.L., M.B. BALLY & S.M. SINGH. 1997. Human gene therapy: principles and modern advances. Biotechnol. Annu. Rev. **3:** 59–110.
29. BASIC, D., I. VACEK & A.M. SUN. 1996. Microencapsulation and transplantation of genetically engineered cells: a new approach to somatic gene therapy. Artif. Cells Blood Substit. Immobil. Biotechnol. **24:** 219–255.
30. TAN, S.A., N. DEGLON, A.D. ZURN, E.E. BAETGE, B. BAMBER, A.C. KATO & P. AEBIscher. 1996. Rescue of motoneurons from axotomy-induced cell death by polymer encapsulated cells genetically engineered to release CNTF, Cell Transplant. **5:** 577–587
31. ABISCHER, P., N.A. POCHON, B. HEYD, N. DEGLON, J.M. JOSEPH, A.D. ZURN, E.E. BAETGE, J.P. HAMMANG, M. GODDARD, M. LYSAGHT, F. KAPLAN, A.C. KATO, M. SCHLUEP, L. HIRT, F. REGLI, F. PORCHET & N. DE TRIBOLET. 1996. Gene therapy for amyotrophic lateral sclerosis (ALS) using a polymer encapsulated xenogenic cell line engineered to secrete hCNTF. Hum. Gene Ther. **1:** 851–860.
32. SAITOH, Y., T. TAKI, N. ARITA, T. OHNISHI & T. HAYAKAWA. 1995. Cell therapy with encapsulated xenogeneic tumor cells secreting beta-endorphin for treatment of peripheral pain. Cell Transplant. **Suppl. 1:** S13–S17.
33. OKADA, N., H. MIYAMOTO, T. YOSHIOKA, A. KATSUME, H. SAITO, K. YOROZU, O. UEDA, N. ITOH, H. MIZUGUCHI, S. NAKAGAWA, Y. OHSUGI & T. MAYUMI. 1997. Cytomedical therapy for IgG1 plasmacytosis in human interleukin-6 transgenic mice using hybridoma cells microencapsulated in alginate-poly(L)lysine-alginate membrane. Biochim. Biophys. Acta **1360** (1)**:** 53–63.
34. AL-HENDY, A., G. HORTELANO, G.S. TANNENBAUM & P.L. CHANG.. 1966. Growth retardation—an unexpected outcome from growth hormone gene therapy in normal mice with microencapsulated myoblasts. Hum. Gene Therap. Jan. **7**(1)**:** 61–70.
35. DATE, I., T. OHMOTO, T. IMAOKA, T. SHINGO & D.F. EMERICH. 1996. Chromaffin cell survival from both young and old donors is enhanced by co-grafts of polymer-encapsulated human NGF-secreting cells. Neuroreport **7**(11)**:** 813–818.
36. WINN, S.R., J.P. HAMMANG, D.F. EMERICH, A. LEE, R.D. PALMITER & E.E. BAETGE. 1994. Polymer-encapsulated cells genetically modified to secrete human nerve growth factor promote the survival of axotomized septal cholinergic neurons. Proc. Natl. Acad. Sci. USA **91**(6)**:** 2324–2328.
37. PRAKASH, S. & T.M.S. CHANG. 1996. Microencapsulated genetically engineered live *E. coli* DH5 cells administered orally to maintain normal plasma urea level in uremic rats. Nature Med. **2** (8)**:** 883–887.
38. CHANG, T.M.S. & S. PRAKASH. 1998. Therapeutic uses of microencapsulated genetically engineered cells. Mol. Med. Today. **4:** 221–227.
39. FRIEDMAN, E. A. 1996. Bowl as an artificial kidney. Am. J. Kidney Dis. **Dec.:** 521–528.
40. SCOOT, B., H. MULROONEY, P. STUART & R.P. HAUSSINGER'S. 1989. Regulation of gene expression and cellular localization of cloned *K. aerogens* urease. J. Gen. Microbiol. **135:** 1769–1776.
41. PRAKASH, S. & T.M.S. CHANG. 1995. Preparation and in-vitro analysis of engineered *E. coli* DH5 cells, microencapsulated in artificial cells for urea and ammonia removal. Biotechnol. Bioeng. **46:** 621–626.
42. PRAKASH, S. & T.M.S. CHANG. 1998. Growth and survival of renal failure rats that received oral microencapsulated genetically engineered *E. coli* DH5 cells for urea removal. Biomater. Artif. Cells Immobil. Biotechnol. **26:** 35–52.
43. WRONG, O.M., C.J. EDMONDS & V.S. CHADWICK, Eds. 1981. The Large Intestine. MTP Press. Lancaster.

# Physico-chemical and Mass Transfer Considerations in Microencapsulation

MATTHEUS F. A. GOOSEN[a]

*College of Engineering, Sultan Qaboos University P.O. Box 33, Muscat 123, Sultanate of Oman*

**ABSTRACT: To gain better insight into mass transfer problems in encapsulated cell systems requires a combination of experimental investigations and mathematical modeling. Specific mass transfer studies are reviewed including oxygen transfer in immobilized animal cell culture bioreactors, modeling of polymer droplet formation and encapsulated animal cell growth, and growth of somatic tissue encapsulated in alginate using electrostatics. Special emphasis is given to electrostatic droplet generation for cell immobilization.**

## INTRODUCTION

To be able to scale-up an encapsulated cell system, it is essential to have a good understanding of the oxygen/nutrient/cell product mass transfer process. Applied scientists and engineers are ideally suited for this task since they can combine experimental and theoretical/mathematical modelling studies to give a clearer insight into potential mass transfer bottlenecks.

Microencapsulation systems have found applications in a variety of areas, including encapsulated cell therapy,[1–4] immobilized biocatalysts,[5,6] and polymeric drug-delivery systems.[7,8] All areas, however, suffer from specific mass transfer problems. With drug-delivery systems, the release of the bioactive agent from the polymer matrix or capsule must be controlled so as to provide a constant steady release rate. In the case of immobilized cells, oxygen must be able to reach the viable cells at a sufficient rate to keep the cells alive, while the desired product, such as insulin in the case of diabetes treatment, must diffuse out of the capsule, along with low molecular weight waste products. With biocatalysts, whether they be enzymes or cells, the substrate must be able to reach the bead/capsule interior to allow the biochemical reaction to occur and the desired products must be able to diffuse out of the bead.

This paper will review specific mass transfer studies performed in our laboratory including oxygen transfer in immobilized animal cell culture bioreactors, modeling of polymer droplet formation and encapsulated animal cell growth, and growth of somatic tissue encapsulated in alginate using electrostatics. Experimental and theoretical/modelling studies will be combined in an attempt to give the reader a better insight into common mass transfer problems.

[a]Fax: (968)513-416; e-mail: theog@squ.edu.om (office); mattheus@gto.net.om (home).

## SCALE-UP OF IMMOBILIZED ANIMAL CELL CULTURE BIOREACTORS AND OXYGEN TRANSFER

Providing adequate oxygen to the cells without damaging them is perhaps the most important function of an animal cell bioreactor. In the operation of a bioreactor the gas to bulk liquid oxygen transfer is the only resistance which can be controlled. Varying the aeration rate will affect the gas to liquid oxygen transfer which in turn will affect the transfer of oxygen from the bulk liquid to the cell. Researchers have, therefore, focused on measuring the mass transfer coefficient $k_l a$, under various operating conditions, for the purpose of developing useful correlations that may be employed as scale-up criteria for animal cell bioreactors. A common technique used in dynamic $k_l a$ measurements involves deoxygenating the reactor contents.[9] Subsequently, gas of a different oxygen concentration is admitted and the oxygen profile is monitored.

### *Modeling the Oxygen Transfer Process*

It is not adequate simply to transfer sufficient oxygen to the bulk liquid culture medium in immobilized cell systems. Oxygen must also be transferred from the liquid to the cells. Consider for instance the transfer of oxygen from a gas bubble, through the culture medium to a microcapsule containing animal cells. The resistances to oxygen transfer from the gas phase to the inside edge of the microcapsule (i.e. gas to liquid, liquid to microcapsule, and trans-membrane resistance) (FIG. 1) can be added together resulting in the following expression for the resistance to oxygen transfer, R:[10,11]

$$R = \frac{1}{V_L k_l a} + \frac{1}{V_L k_s a} + \left( \frac{\frac{1}{r_o} - \frac{1}{r_i}}{4\pi n D_{o_2,m}} \right) \tag{1}$$

where $V_L$ is the volume of the liquid phase, $n$ is the number of microcapsules, $r_o$ and $r_i$ are the outside and inside radius of the microcapsule, respectively, $k_s a$ is the volumetric mass transfer coefficient from a liquid to a solid, and $D_{o_2,m}$ is the diffusivity of oxygen in the membrane.

Employing Fick's Law of Diffusion[12] it can be shown that the oxygen transfer rate from the gas phase to the inside edge of a microcapsule, $OTR_G$, is given by:

$$OTR_G = \left( \frac{1}{V_L k_l a} + \frac{1}{V_L k_s a} + \frac{\frac{1}{r_o} - \frac{1}{r_i}}{4\pi n D_{o_2,m}} \right)^{-1} (C^* - C_{i,m,i}) \geq Q = Q_{o_2} x \tag{2}$$

where $C^*$ is the oxygen concentration in equilibrium with the oxygen partial pressure in the gas phase, $C_{i,m,i}$, is the oxygen concentration on the inside of the membrane, $Q$ is the oxygen consumption rate of cells inside a microcapsule ($mgO_2$/Lhr), $Q_{o_2}$ is the oxygen consumption rate per cell, and $x$ is the cell density. To enable the cells in the microcapsule to survive, the oxygen transfer rate, $OTR_G$, must be greater

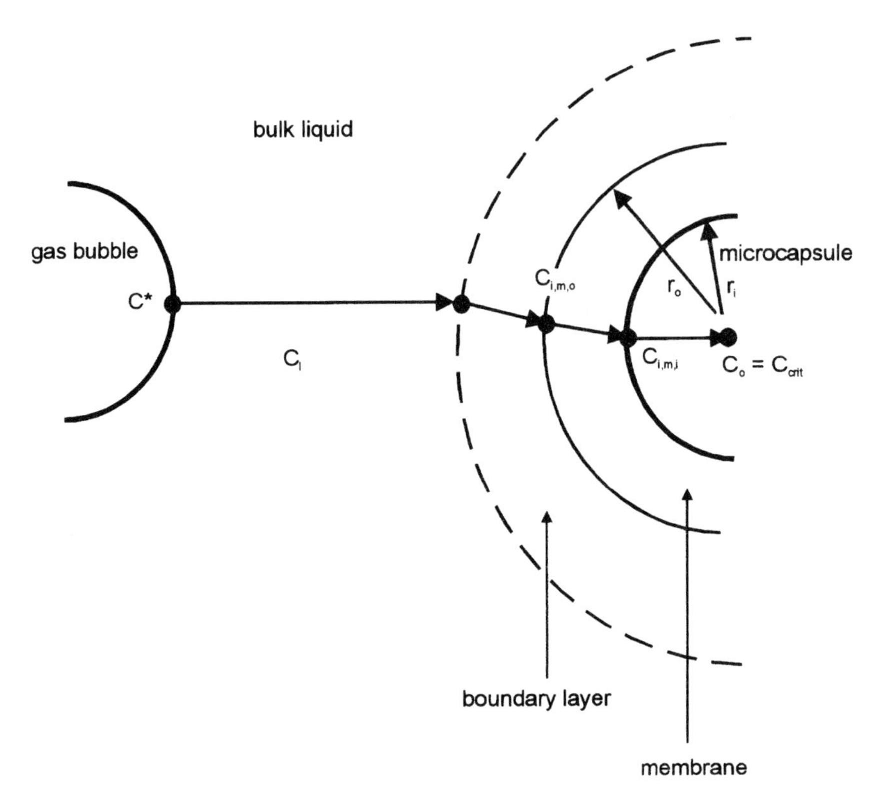


**FIGURE 1.** Schematic diagram of oxygen profile from gas bubble to center of microcapsule.[10]

than (or at least equal to) the oxygen consumption rate of cells inside the capsules, $Q$. Based on the work of Heath and Belfort[13] the oxygen concentration profile within a microcapsule can be represented by:

$$C_{i,\,m,\,i} - C_o = \frac{Q}{D_{O_2,\,a}}\frac{1}{6}r^2 \tag{3}$$

where $r$ is the radius of the alginate core. If the concentration of oxygen in the center of the microcapsules, $C_o$, is equal to a critical oxygen concentration, $C_{crit}$, the concentration of oxygen at the inner surface of the membrane, $C_{i,m,i}$, can be determined from Equation 3.

The performance of a one liter external-loop air-lift bioreactor was investigated by studying the gas-liquid oxygen transfer at various aeration rates (0.1 vvm to 1.06 vvm). The influence of suspended alginate beads on the hydrodynamics and mass transfer of the system was examined over a range of microbead loadings (0 to 25% by volume). The intent was to investigate the effect of using various concentrations of cell immobilization matrices on the physical properties of the system. A mathematical correlation was developed for expressing the dependence of $k_l a$ on aeration rate and microbead loading. A mathematical study of the mass transfer resistances from the gas phase to the interior of a microcapsule was also performed, using experimentally determined $k_l a$ values, to enable the determination of the maximum bioreactor microcapsule loading.

The oxygen probe time constant for our studies was $27 \pm 7$ sec and the maximum $k_l a$ value found was 0.00861 $sec^{-1}$. Since this is approximately equal to 1/5 $k_l a$, the oxygen probe response time was therefore not accounted for in the determination of the $k_l a$ values in our investigation. According to Van't Riet,[14] the response lag of an oxygen probe can be neglected if the oxygen probe time constant, $\tau_p$, is less than 1/5 $k_l a$.

To ensure that the $k_l a$ studies would be measuring the gas-to-liquid mass transfer coefficient and not the mass transfer from the gas to the interior of the bead, the $k_l a$ in the presence of alginate beads was compared to that in the presence of ion-exchange resin beads. The $k_l a$ for a 10% loading of alginate beads it was determined to be $31.7 \pm 0.7$ $h^{-1}$ and for a 10% loading of ion-exchange resin beads it was 31.4 $\pm$ 1.5 $h^{-1}$, at an aeration rate of 0.67 vvm. The $k_l a$ values are essentially equal. This suggested that the alginate beads were not acting as a "sink" for oxygen and that the desired quantity, gas-to-liquid mass transfer coefficient, was being measured.

### *Estimating the $k_l a$ Value in the Presence of Alginate Beads*

In two-phase (gas/liquid) systems such as bubble columns and airlift bioreactors, the $k_l a$ is usually found to be an exponential function of the superficial gas velocity as follows:[15]

$$k_l a = \alpha v_s^{\beta} \tag{4}$$

As a first approach to correlate the $k_l a$ values with an aeration term, the $k_l a$ values were plotted versus the normalized aeration rate, vvm (FIG. 2). In the presence of alginate beads, this resulted in a monotonic relationship, whereby increasing the percentage of beads in the reactor decreased the $k_l a$. It is important to note, however, that this was not valid in the absence of beads (i.e. 0% loading). For the range of aeration rates studied, at 0% bead loading, the bioreactor was predominantly operated under turbulent conditions (i.e., Re $\geq$ 4000). On the other hand, in the presence of beads, 10% to 25%, the bioreactor was mostly being operated in the transition zone. We can speculate that this could affect the $k_l a$ values. Using vvm instead of the superficial gas velocity accounted for the presence of "internals" (i.e., alginate beads) since vvm normalizes the gas flow rate with respect to the liquid volume. Correlating the $k_l a$ with vvm by performing a linear regression on the data and setting the constant equal to zero using the statistical package Minitab (Version 5.1.3, Copyright - Minitab, Inc., 1985) gave correlation coefficients ($R^2$ values) ranging from 64.6% for 0% bead loading to 84% for 15% bead loading. This was not considered to be a very good fit of the data because of the low $R^2$ values. Also, this did not give a single correlation that would account for the presence of the beads but rather a correlation for each bead loading was required.

To account for the presence of alginate beads, it was then proposed to add a term in the correlation. Thus, a concentration effect term, $C_E$, was introduced. To define

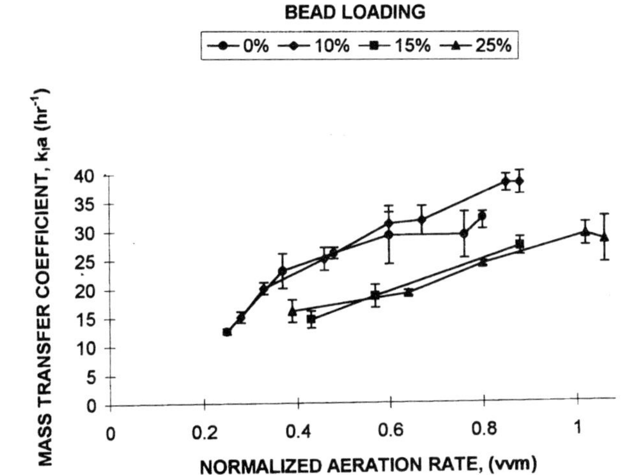


**FIGURE 2.** Mass Transfer Coefficient, $k_la$, versus Normalized Aeration Rate (adapted from refs. 10 and 11).

the concentration effect, Einstein's equation for the suspension of rigid spheres was used:

$$C_E = 1 + 2.5\varphi \tag{5}$$

where $\varphi$ is the volume fraction occupied by the spheres (i.e., alginate beads). A multiple linear regression using Minitab was used to correlate $k_la$ with vvm and $C_E$. This multiple linear regression resulted in the following expression:

$$\ln k_la = 4.10 + 0.803 \ln \text{vvm} - 1.67 \ln C_E \tag{6}$$

where $k_la$ has units of $h^{-1}$.

Rearranging Equation 6 into a more convenient form gave:

$$k_la = 60.34 \text{ vvm}^{0.803} C_E^{-1.67} \tag{7}$$

This correlation had a coefficient of 0.815 which was indicative of a good fit. There were no trends in the residual plots. Also, the T-ratios for the constant and coefficients in the correlation were very large which indicated that these parameters were significant to the model. It was, therefore, concluded that this regression line was adequate to explain the data. Equation 7, which was used to predict the $k_la$ value for a given aeration rate (vvm) and alginate bead loading, gave a good fit (FIG. 3).

When attempting to develop a correlation that can be used as a design parameter for bioreactor scale-up, a single correlation that can be applied to all systems is desirable. Correlations involving liquid velocity were not considered to be appropriate due to the dependence of the liquid velocity on the aeration rate. Although used successfully for describing two-phase systems,[16,17] correlations involving the gassed power per unit liquid or reactor volume ($P_g/VL$ and $P_g/V$, respectively) did not ac-

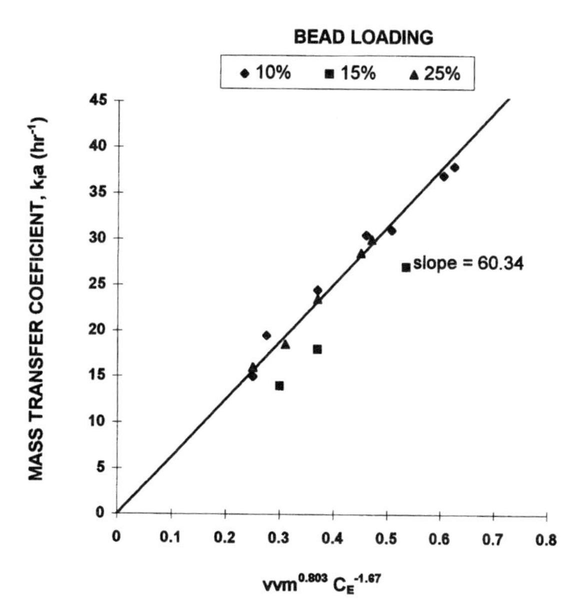


**FIGURE 3.** Correlation between Mass Transfer Coefficient, Normalized Aeration Rate and Bead Loading.[10]

count for the change in bulk fluid properties due to the presence of alginate beads. It is important to note that the correlation proposed (Equation 7) does not fit the $k_l a$ data when there are no beads present due to the turbulent flow regime at 0% bead loading.

### *Sensitivity of $k_l a$ to Microcapsule Loading*

For immobilized cell systems, such as microcapsules, ensuring adequate oxygen transfer from the gas phase to the liquid medium does not necessarily ensure that adequate oxygen will reach the immobilized cells. It is possible that the $k_l a$ may not be adequate for a certain microcapsule loading. A theoretical study was performed in our laboratory of oxygen transfer to cells immobilized in microcapsules in a bioreactor for various microcapsule loadings using Equations 2 and 3.[10] A schematic diagram of the oxygen concentration profile from a gas bubble to the center of a microencapsule is shown in FIGURE 1. Upon arbitrarily specifying the critical oxygen concentration in the center of the microcapsule, the rate of oxygen transfer from the gas phase to the inner surface of the microencapsule membrane ($OTR_G$, mg/h) for a certain microcapsule loading was compared to the oxygen demand of the cells ($Q_{O_2}x$) for the same microcapsule loading. The study was made for *Spodoptera frugiperda* (i.e., insect) cells cultivated in poly-1-lysine/alginate microcapsules at a maximum cell density of $8 \times 10^7$ *cells/mL capsules*.[18] An oxygen demand of $1.4 \times 10^{-10}$ *mmole $O_2$/cell hour* was assumed. These insect cells are usually cultivated at 27°C and 33°C. Therefore our study was performed at both temperatures.

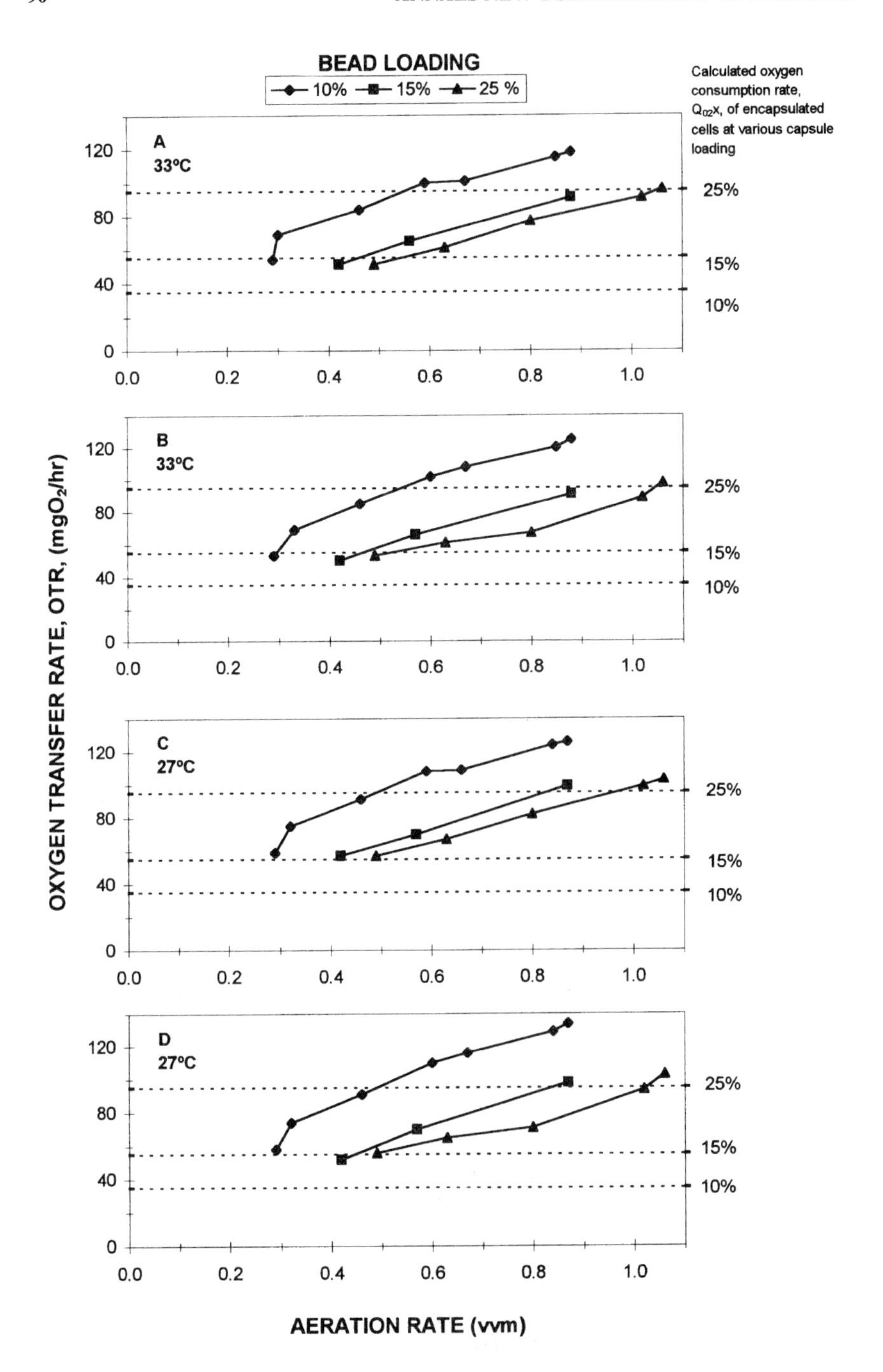
BEAD LOADING
10%
15%
25 %
Calculated oxygen consumption rate, $Q_{O2}X$, of encapsulated cells at various capsule loading
A
33°C
B
33°C
C
27°C
D
27°C
25%
15%
10%
OXYGEN TRANSFER RATE, OTR, (mgO$_2$/hr)
AERATION RATE (vvm)
0
40
80
120
0.0
0.2
0.4
0.6
0.8
1.0

It was necessary to estimate several of the parameters used to evaluate the oxygen transfer rate. The diffusivity of oxygen in sodium alginate (the immobilization agent inside the microcapsule) was estimated to be 86% of the diffusivity of oxygen in water (i.e., approximately the same as the diffusivity of oxygen in calcium alginate). According to King *et al.*,[18] the membrane is 5 μm thick and is composed of approximately 90% water. The diffusivity of oxygen through the membrane was therefore assumed to be equal to that of oxygen in water. A critical oxygen concentration in the center of the microcapsule was assumed to be 40% of air saturation.

FIGURE 4 shows the results for the oxygen transfer rate, *OTR* attainable for microcapsule loadings of 10, 15, and 25% at 33°C and 27°C as a function of the aeration rate. The terminal settling velocity was used to calculate the Reynold's number. Comparing FIGURES 4A and 4B, the latter uses the difference between the bead and liquid velocities (determined experimentally) to calculate the Reynold's number, and indicates that there is not much difference (at most 8%) between the two methods. This suggests that the terminal velocity may be used as a good approximation of the relative velocity between the bead and the liquid if it is not feasible to determine the liquid and bead velocities experimentally.

At 33°C, for 10% bead loading, the oxygen demand of the cells was achieved at 0.29 vvm, which is the minimum vvm for suspension of the beads (FIG. 4A). On the other hand, for 25% bead loadings a vvm of 1.06 is required to meet the oxygen demand of the cells. This is quite a high aeration rate thus it may not be feasible to operate at 25% bead loading. Decreasing the temperature to 27°C (FIGS. 4C and 4D) increased the oxygen transfer rate but only slightly (by approximately 8%). This was expected since a decrease in temperature increases the solubility of oxygen in the bulk liquid which increases the driving force for oxygen transfer. This, in turn, increases the oxygen transfer rate to the cells. The temperature did not, however, have a very significant effect on the oxygen transfer rate. These results suggest that for this bioreactor the cells will not be oxygen limited at microcapsule loadings of 10% and 15% (by volume). However, there is the potential for oxygen limitation at 25% microcapsule loadings if the reactor is not operated at a minimum aeration rate of 1.06 vvm.

## MATHEMATICAL MODELING OF POLYMER DROPLET FORMATION AND ENCAPSULATED ANIMAL CELL GROWTH

### *Modeling of Electrostatic Droplet Formation*

Droplet formation in the presence of an electric field has been analyzed previously.[19] If gravity were the only force acting on the meniscus of a droplet attached to the

---

**FIGURE 4.** Theoretical Oxygen Transfer Rate, *OTR*, as a function of Aeration Rate for encapsulated insect cells in bioreactor at 33°C using the Terminal Settling Velocity to calculate the Reynold's Number **(A)**; *OTR* at 33°C using the difference between the Bead Velocity and the Liquid Velocity to calculate the Reynold's Number **(B)**; *OTR* at 27°C using the Terminal Settling Velocity to calculate the Reynold's Number **(C)**; *OTR* at 27°C using the difference between the Bead Velocity and the Liquid Velocity to calculate the Reynold's Number **(D)**.[10]

end of a tube, large uniformly sized droplets would be produced. The gravitational force, $F_g$, pulling the droplet from the end of the tube is given by:

$$F_g = \frac{4}{3}\pi r^3 \rho g \tag{8}$$

where $\rho$ is the density of the polymer solution, $r$ is the droplet radius, and $g$ is the acceleration due to gravity. The capillary surface force, $F_\gamma$, holding the droplet to the end of the tube is given by:

$$F_\gamma = 2\pi r_o \gamma \tag{9}$$

where $r_o$ is the internal radius of the tube and $\gamma$ is the surface tension.

Equating the gravitational force on the droplet to the capillary surface tension force holding the droplet to the tube (i.e., extrusion orifice) gives:

$$r = \left(\frac{3r_o\gamma\rho g}{2}\right)^{1/3} \tag{10}$$

In the presence of an applied voltage, the electric force, $F_e$, acting along with the gravitational force, $F_g$, would reduce the critical volume for drop detachment resulting in a smaller droplet diameter. Equating the gravitational and electrical forces on the droplet to the capillary surface force, $F_\gamma$, yields:

$$F_\gamma = F_g + F_e \tag{11}$$

In the case of a charged needle, the stress produced by the external electric field at the needle tip is obtained by using a modified expression developed by De Shon and Carlson:[20]

$$F_e = 4\pi\varepsilon_o\left(\frac{V}{\mathrm{Ln}\left(\frac{4H}{r_o}\right)}\right)^2 \tag{12}$$

where $H$ is the distance between the needle tip and collecting solution, $V$ is the applied voltage, and $\varepsilon_o$ is the permittivity of the air.

The effect of applied potential on the droplet radius for a charged needle arrangement can be derived by substituting Equations 8, 9, and 12 into Equation 11:

$$r = \left(\left[\frac{3}{2\rho g}\right]\left[r_o\gamma - 2\varepsilon_o\left(\frac{V}{\mathrm{Ln}\left(\frac{4H}{r_o}\right)}\right)^2\right]\right)^{1/3} \tag{13}$$

Equation 10 was employed to calculate the microbead diameter in the absence of an applied voltage (i.e., 0 kV). The surface tension, $\gamma$, of the alginate solution was as-

**TABLE 1.** Comparison of experimental and calculated microbead diameter as a function of extrusion orifice size and applied potential

| Extrusion orifice diameter (microns) | Applied potential, $V$ (kV) | Microbead diameter (microns) | |
|---|---|---|---|
| | | Calculated[a] | Experimental[b] |
| 400 | 0 | 2600 | 2000 |
| 1000 | 0 | 3500 | 2800 |
| 1900 | 0 | 4400 | 3700 |
| 1900 | 5 | 4018 | 3500 |
| 1900 | 10 | 1680 | 1700 |

[a]Bead size at 0 kV was determined using Equation 3 and 5 and 10 kV using Equation 6.
[b]Bead size using 4% w/v non-autoclaved sodium alginate in water with an electrode distance of 6 cm and a 22 gage needle ($r_o = 500$ microns).

sumed to be 73 g/s$^2$ which is the value for water against air.[21] The density of the polymer solution was taken as 1 g/cm$^3$. In the presence of an applied voltage, Equation 13 was used to determine microbead size. The permittivity of air, $\varepsilon_o$, used in calculations was 1.0 g cm/s$^2$ kV$^2$. This value was estimated based on previous studies.[19]

Reasonably good agreement was obtained between calculated and experimental values of microbead diameter (TABLE 1).[22] For example, when the extrusion orifice diameter decreased from 1900 to 400 microns, the calculated bead diameters decreased from 4400 to 2600 microns, and the experimental values decreased from 3700 to 2000 microns. When the extrusion orifice diameter (i.e., syringe) was kept constant at 1900 microns and the applied voltage was increased from 0 to 10 kV, there was also a similar decrease in bead size from 4400 to 1690 microns for the calculated values and from 3700 to 1700 microns for the experimental values.

### *Development of a Mathematical Model for Animal Cell Growth in Microcapsules*

A mathematical model for animal cell growth in microcapsules was also developed and compared to experimental data.[23,24] There have been several attempts to address mathematical modeling of microcapsules. Mogensen and Vieth[25] studied the mass transfer properties of semi-permeable microcapsules. Their model did not account for any cell growth since they were dealing with enzymes. Heath and Belfort[13] also provided a mathematical treatment on microcapsules, entrapping biocatalysts, but again no cell growth was taken into account.

The derivation of our model was based on the case in which microcapsules with fluid intracapsular liquid were used in stationary culture. The characteristics of this scenario of cell growth in microcapsules is that the cells initially settle to the bottom of the capsules, and the cell population expands from the bottom up during the culture period. This cell population expansion in the capsules is accounted for in the model by a computation mechanism, which initializes the neighboring control volumes with cells when a control volume becomes overcrowded.

The model is made up of a set of differential balance equations of the following form:

$$\frac{\partial}{\partial t}(C_i \varepsilon) + \mathrm{div}(J_i) = S_i \quad \textbf{(14)}$$

where $C_i$ is the concentration of a nutrient such as glucose and glutamine in a microcapsule, $J_i$ is the diffusive flux of the nutrient, $S_i$ is the rate of consumption of the nutrient and $\varepsilon$ is the void fraction inside a microcapsule. Similar balance equations are written for the capsule membrane and the culture medium. The rate of cell growth is expressed as:

$$\frac{dX}{dt} = u(t - t_{\mathrm{lag}})\left[\mu X + \lambda \int_o^t X(\eta) d\eta\right] \quad \textbf{(15)}$$

where

$$u(t - t_{\mathrm{lag}}) = \begin{cases} 1 \text{ if } t > t_{\mathrm{lag}} \\ 0 \text{ if } t < t_{\mathrm{lag}} \end{cases} \quad \textbf{(16)}$$

$X$ is the cell density, $\mu$ is the specific growth rate, $t_{\mathrm{lag}}$ is the lag time and $\lambda$ is the cell death constant. Equation 15 describes the change in cell density from the beginning of the exponential growth phase to the end of the culture.[26] The lag phase can be included mathematically by introducing a step function. The lag time will have to be determined experimentally. Since in an unstructured model a cell is treated as a single-component body, Equation 15 is sufficient to characterize the growth of a cell population. The dependence of the specific growth rate ($\mu$) on nutrient concentration is expressed as:

$$\mu = \mu_{\mathrm{max}} \prod_{i=1}^{n} \left(\frac{C_i}{K_{C_i} + C_i}\right) \quad \textbf{(17)}$$

where $C_i$ is the concentration of rate limiting nutrient $i$; $K_{C_i}$ is the saturation constant for nutrient $i$; $n$ is the total number of rate limiting nutrients; $\mu_{\mathrm{max}}$ is the maximum specific growth rate. Frame and Hu[27] developed a contact-inhibition model to describe the dependence of specific growth rate on cell density:

$$\mu = \mu_{\mathrm{max}}\left[1 - \exp\left(-B\frac{X_{\mathrm{max}} - X}{X}\right)\right] \quad \textbf{(18)}$$

where $X_{max}$ is the maximum cell density and $B$ is an adjustable parameter. The degree of influence of cell density on $\mu$ depends on the value of $B$; if a relatively large value of $B$ is used, then the specific growth rate will remain more or less unaffected by the cell density until it is very close to $X_{max}$. Thus, the incorporation of Equation 17 into the kinetic expression with a large value of $B$ should allow us to control the cell density as it approaches the maximum cell density while leaving the specific growth rate unaffected during most of the culture. A complete expression for $\mu$ is therefore proposed as follows:

$$\mu = \mu_{max} \prod_{i=1}^{n} \left( \frac{C_i}{K_{C_i} + C_i} \right) \left[ 1 - \exp\left( -B \frac{X_{max} - X}{X} \right) \right] \quad \textbf{(19)}$$

The mechanism of cell population expansion may be treated in several ways. The mechanism that was adopted here conforms to the control-volume (CV) formulation. Cell growth in a neighboring CV may begin before the maximum cell density is reached. Equations 15 and 18 constitute the basic model equations for cell growth in this study. The rate of consumption of nutrient *i* by the cells (i.e., $S_i$) can be related to the rate of cell growth by the following equation:

$$S_i = \frac{1}{Y_{X/C_i}} \mu X u(t - t_{lag}) \quad \textbf{(20)}$$

where $Y_{X/C_i}$ is the yield factor for nutrient *i* to cells. Note that the term $S_i$ as expressed in Equation 19 is the rate of consumption of nutrient *i* based on a unit volume in the interior phase. Equation 19 also assumes a constant yield factor. For details on estimation of model parameters, solution of model equations, derivation of discretization equations, cell population expansion and the numerical solution algorithm see the paper by Yuet *et al.*[24]

Using this model the highest rate of growth ($\mu \leq 0.026\ h^{-1}$) was found in the boundary region at the top of the cell mass. This is the region which receives the most abundant supply of nutrients and oxygen, both from across the membrane and from the upper half of the capsule. The cells at the bottom of the capsule close to the membrane have virtually stopped growing since they have reached the maximum cell density and there is no more space available for further cell division. The cells at the central region of the population are probably suffering from the lack of nutrients and oxygen and therefore have only a very low specific growth rate ($0.0104 < \mu \leq 0.0156\ h^{-1}$).

The maximum oxygen concentration, which is found in the upper half of the capsule where no cells are present, is only about 0.066 mM, or 26% of the saturation value (0.25 mM). This value is very close to that in the external culture medium (0.068 mM). The low oxygen concentration should not be too surprising considering the low value of $k_l a$. The oxygen concentration within the cell mass itself is even lower, decreasing towards the centre of the cell mass. The distribution of oxygen within the cell population is mainly a result of the consumption of oxygen by the cells located in the outer layer of the capsule, as well as the reduced effective diffusivity through the cell matrix. The transport of oxygen into the microcapsules, however, does not seem to be limited as the concentration of oxygen in the upper half of the capsule is almost the same as that in the external medium. The lack of oxygen within the cell mass is therefore more likely caused by the high oxygen demand, which is in turn caused by the extraordinarily high intracapsular cell density particularly in the outer layer of the cell mass. Oxygen deficiency caused by high oxygen demand but not the diffusion limitation was also noted by other investigators.[28,29]

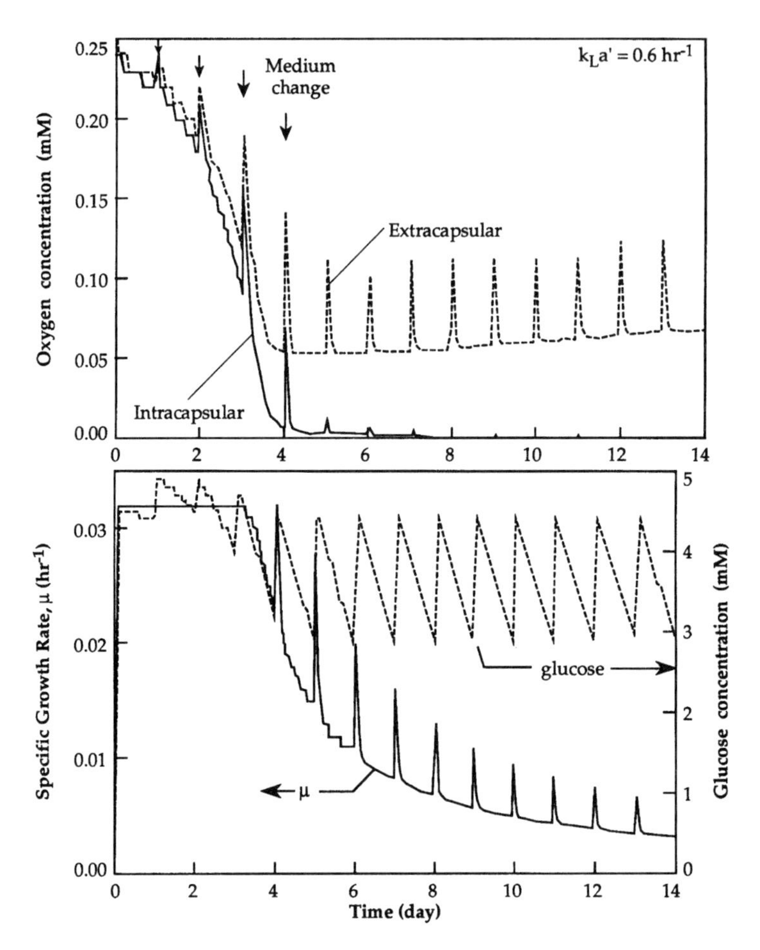


**FIGURE 5.** Simulated time-variation of oxygen concentration in the medium and the interior phase and the specific growth rate and intracapsular glucose concentration for $k_l a = 0.6\ h^{-1}$. Microcapsules with fluid intracapsular liquid in suspension. The medium is changed every 24 h.[24]

The distribution of cell density in the microcapsule at the end of the culture period shows that the highest density occurs close to the inner surface of the capsule membrane which confirms earlier experimental work.[18]

The scenarios of calcium alginate gel beds and microcapsules with fluid intracapsular liquid in suspension culture were simulated using the same model. In the case of calcium alginate gel beads, the diffusivities of nutrients in calcium alginate were taken as 75% of those in water; while in the two cases of fluid intracapsular liquid microcapsules suspension, $k_l a$ was taken as $0.6\ h^{-1}$ and $4.0\ h^{-1}$ separately. A $k_l a$ value of $4.0\ h^{-1}$ is more realistic since the culture medium has to be agitated (in a shake flask, for example) in order to keep the microcapsules in suspension; the value of 0.6 $h^{-1}$ was included for comparison. With $k_l a$ equal to $4.0^{-1}$, the cell density, after 14 days of culture, is approximately $1.4 \times 10^{i}$ cells $ml^{-1}$ while with $k_l a$ equal to 0.6 $h^{-1}$, the cell density reaches $7.1 \times 10^7$ cells $ml^{-1}$. The intracapsular cell density alone, however, does not provide a complete picture of what is actually happening in the microcapsule or the culture medium. A further examination of the oxygen and nutrient concentration in the system reveals a rather interesting situation regarding the effect of nutrients on the specific growth rate.

Let us take a brief look at the case where $k_l a$ is $0.6^{-1}$ (FIG. 5), keeping in mind that the medium is changed every 24 hours. During the first three days of culture, μ stays at about 0.032 $h^{-1}$ because of the abundant supply of oxygen and nutrients. In the meantime, however, the oxygen concentrations in the intracapsular region as well as in the medium are decreasing rapidly. At the beginning of day 4, there is a boost of oxygen concentration by the fresh supply of medium, which is saturated with oxygen. The oxygen concentration drops sharply during day 4, and by the end of the day, the intracapsular oxygen is reduced to 0.005 mM, while μ drops to about 0.023 $h^{-1}$. Beginning from day 5, the specific growth rate is boosted at the beginning of each day because of the addition of fresh medium. However, the growth rate drops abruptly during the first 4 or 5 hours owing to the rapid depletion of intracapsular oxygen. Neglecting the pulses, the specific growth rate decreases slowly from about 0.025 $h^{-1}$to about 0.004 $h^{-1}$ at the end of the culture. Note that the intracapsular glucose concentration never drops below 2.8 mM. This result suggests that from the second half of day 4 to the end of the culture, the cell growth in the microcapsule is limited by the lack of oxygen. We now conclude this chapter by looking at the encapsulation of plant cells using electrostatics.

## GROWTH OF SOMATIC TISSUE ENCAPSULATED IN ALGINATE USING ELECTROSTATICS

In recent articles,[30–33] the mechanism of alginate droplet information using an electrostatic droplet generator was investigated with a variable-voltage power supply. Animal cell suspensions were successfully extruded using the electrostatic droplet generator. The application of this technology to plant cell immobilization has only recently been reported.[11, 22, 33] A major concern in cell and bioactive agent immobilization has been the production of very small microbeads so as to minimize the mass-transfer resistance problem associated with large-diameter beads (>1000 μm). Klein *et al.*[34] reported production of alginate beads with diameters from 100 to 400 μm using compressed air to quickly pass the cell/gel solution through a nozzle. Few attempts have been made in the application of electric fields to the production of micron size polymer beads for cell immobilization.[35]

Somatic embryogenesis is a new plant tissue culture technology in which somatic cells (i.e., any cell except a germ or seed cell) are used to produce an embryo (i.e., plant in early state of development).[36] The technique of somatic embryogenesis in liquid culture, which is believed to be an economical way for future production of artificial seeds, may benefit from cell immobilization technology. Encapsulation may aid in the germination of somatic embryos by allowing for higher cell densities, protecting cells from shear damage in suspension culture, allowing for surface at-

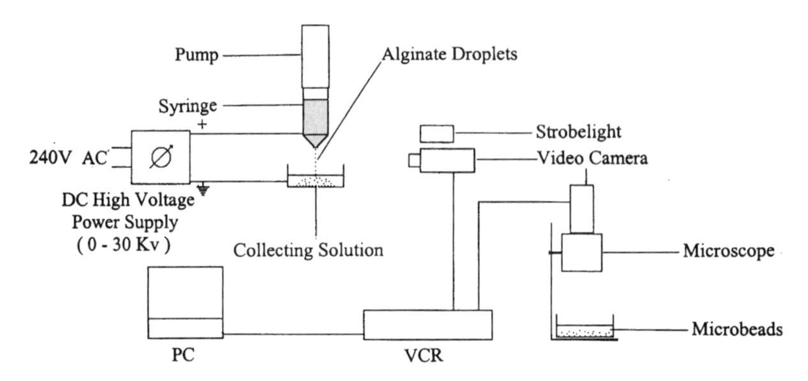


**FIGURE 6.** Effect of needle size on microbead diameter using variable high-voltage power supply (± SD).[33]

tachment in the case of anchorage dependent cells, and being very suitable for scale-up in bioreactors.

The long-term objective of the project reported in this section is the development of an economical method for the mass production of artificial seeds using somatic embryogenesis and cell immobilization technology. The short-term aim was to investigate the production of small alginate microbeads using an electrostatic droplet generator. Callus tissue from carnation leaves was also immobilized and cultured. The section starts with a detailed experimental description of electrostatic droplet generation for those not familiar with the technique[32] (FIG. 6).

### *Production of Alginate Beads Using Electrostatics*

Attach a syringe pump to a vertical stand. Use a 10 mL plastic syringe and 22- or 26-gage stainless steel needles. A variable high voltage (0–30 kV) power supply with low current (<0.4 mA) is required. We have used a commercial power supply model 230–30R from Bertan (Hicksville, NY). Prepare 1.5% (w/v) $CaCl_2$ in saline (0.85 g NaCl in 100 mL distilled water). Saline can be replaced with distilled water if an alginate solution without cells is being extruded. Place the $CaCl_2$ solution in a petri dish on top of an adjustable stand. The stand allows for fine- tuning of the distance between the needle tip and collecting solution. Prepare 1 to 4% (W/V) low viscosity sodium alginate by dissolving alginate powder with stirring in a warm water bath. Slowly add the 1 to 4 g sodium alginate to 100 mL warm saline solution (or distilled $H_2O$), stirring continuously. It may take several hours to dissolve all of the alginate. Add about 8 mL of the alginate solution to a 10-mL plastic syringe, put back the plunger, and attach the syringe to the upright syringe pump. Make sure that the stainless steel needle, 22 gage, is firmly attached and the syringe plunger is in firm contact with the movable bar on the pump. Position the petri dish (or beaker) containing $CaCl_2$ solution so that the needle tip is about 3 cm from the top of the $CaCl_2$ hardening solution. This is the primary reason for using an adjustable stand. Attach the positive electrode wire to the stainless steel needle and the ground wire to the collecting solution. The wires may need some additional support to prevent them from bending the needle. Switch on the syringe pump and wait for the first few drops to come out of the end of the needle. This could take a minute or two. Doing it this way also ensures that the needle is not plugged. After the first drop or two has been produced, switch on the voltage power supply. Make sure that the voltage is set low, <5 kV. If this is the first time that you have tried electrostatic droplet generation, raise the voltage slowly and observe what happens to the droplets. The rate at which they are removed from the needle tip increases until only a fine stream of droplets can be seen. The changeover from individual droplets to a fine stream can be quite dramatic. The most effective electrode and charge arrangement for producing small droplets is a positively charged needle and a grounded plate. Two other arrangements are also possible; positively charged plate attached to needle and positively charged collecting solution. Make sure that the positive charge is always on the needle. This ensures that the smallest microbead size is produced at the lowest applied potential. With a 22-gage needle and an electrode spacing of 2.5–4.8 cm there will be a sharp drop in microbead size at about 6 kV. This can be noticed visually by observing the droplets coming from the needle tip. Standard commercially available stainless steel needles can be employed. However, when going from a 22- to 26-gage (or higher) needle, needle oscillation may be observed. This needle vibration will produce a bimodal bead size distribution with one peak around 50 μm diameter beads and another around 200 μm.

If a syringe pump is not available, remove the syringe plunger and attach an air line with a regulator to the end of the syringe. The alginate extrusion rate can be controlled by varying the air pressure on the regulator.

Lumps of sodium alginate often form if the powder is added all at once to the warm saline. Sprinkle the alginate powder into the saline a small amount at a time with gentle mixing. Once it has dissolved (up to 1–2 h), allow the viscous solution to cool and then transfer it to several plastic test tubes, cap and store in the refrigerator until required. This prevents bacterial growth. If the alginate solution is very viscous, air bubbles will be trapped during stirring. These bubbles will disappear if the viscous solution is left to stand overnight.

If the needle is plugged, place it in dilute citrate solution for a few minutes. Passing a fine wire through the needle also helps. Resuspending cells in 1% (w/v) sodium alginate solution will dilute the alginate solution and could give tear-drop shaped capsules when the solution is extruded. To solve this problem, increase the concentration of sodium alginate solution to 3 or 4%.

Extrusion of alginate droplets using a 5.7 kV fixed-voltage power supply showed that there is a direct relationship between the electrode distance and the bead diameter. For example, at 10-cm electrode distance, the bead diameter was 1500 μm while at 2 cm it decreased to 800 μm. The greatest effect on bead diameter was observed between 2 and 6 cm electrode distance. While there was overlap in bead sizes between 6, 8, and 10 cm electrode distance, there was a significant difference (i.e., no overlap in SD) between bead sizes at 2 and 6-cm electrode distance. An inverse relationship between needle size and microbead diameter was observed. Aside from the 23-gage needle there was a significant difference between bead sizes produced by all needles (i.e., no SD overlap). As the needle size decreased from 19- to 26-gage, the bead size decreased from 1400 to 400 μm, respectively. These results support previous work reported by Bugarski *et al.*[31] The present investigation showed that the alginate concentration does not appear to be important due to overlapping

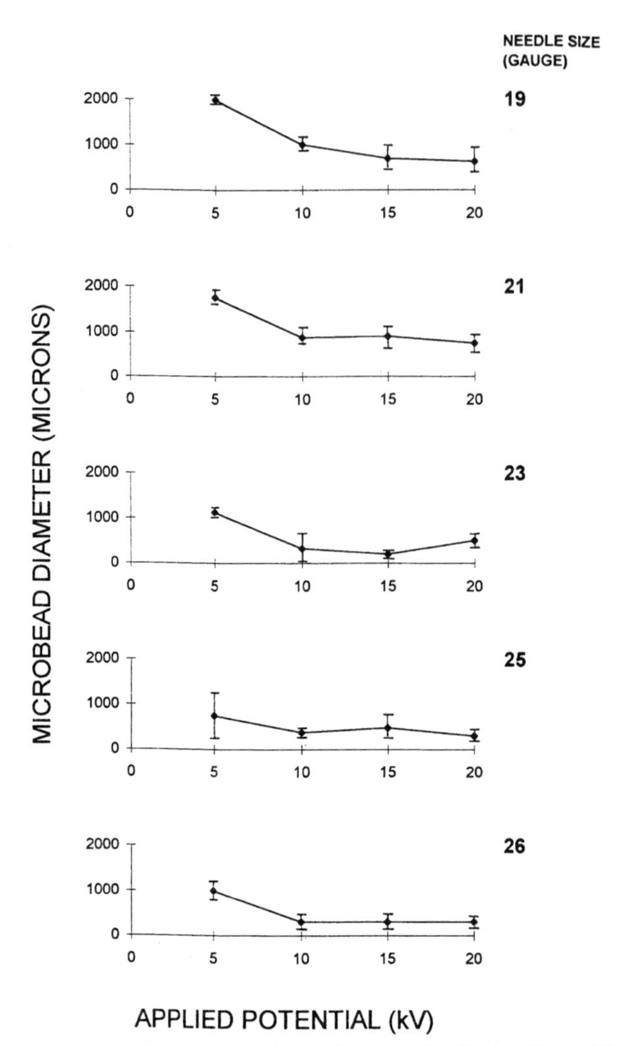


**FIGURE 7.** Callus cells from carnation leaf encapsulated using 4% (w/v) sodium alginate over a one month culture period on agar gel. *Top*: time zero; *middle*: two weeks; *bottom*: one month.

SD intervals for all data points. The bead diameter was found to be 800 μm at both 1% and 3% alginate concentration.

Looking more closely at the effect of needle size on bead diameter, as a function of applied potential (FIG. 7) we see that the decrease in microbead size was greatest between 5 and 10 kV for all needle gages tested. For example, when the applied potential was increased from 5 to 10 kV, the microbead diameter decreased from 2000 (±100) to 1000 (±150) μm and from 1000 (±150) to 250 (±125) μm for the 19-and 26-gage needles, respectively. The smallest bead, 200 (±80) μm, was produced with a 26-gage needle at 20 kV.

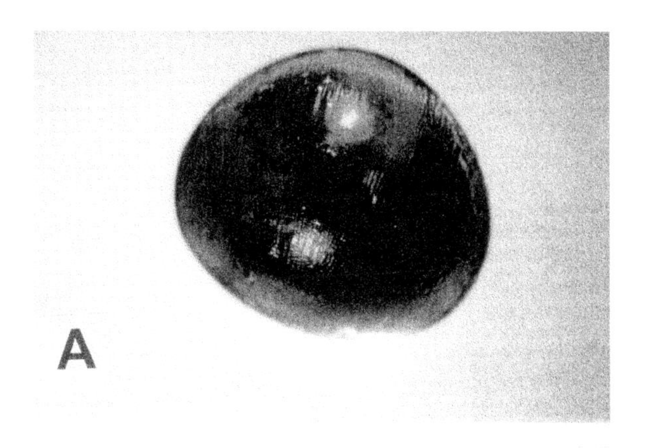


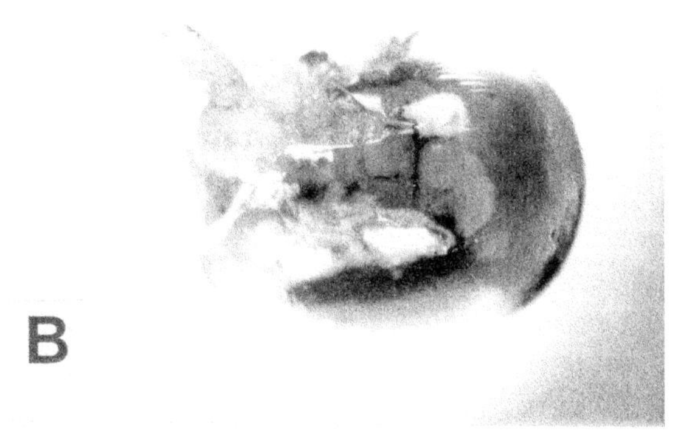


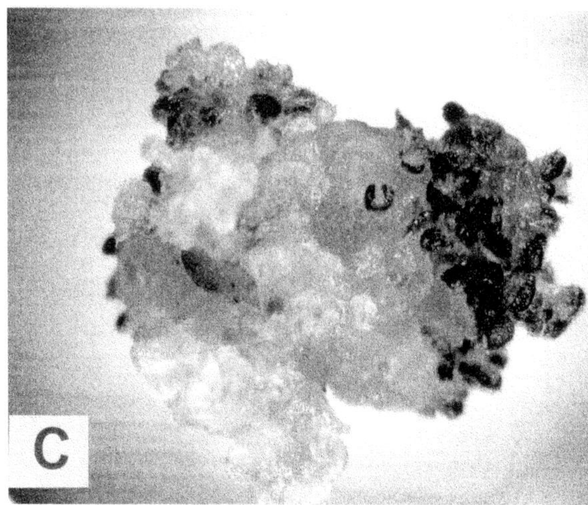


**FIGURE 8.** Callus cells from carnation leaf encapsulated using 4% (w/v) sodium alginate over a one month culture period on agar gel: *top*, time zero; *middle*, two weeks; *bottom*, one month.

### *Growth of Immobilized Callus Tissue*

Immobilized callus cells from carnation leaves retained viability as observed by cell growth and plantelet formation (FIG. 8). In a related study, Shigeta[37] was able to germinate and grow encapsulated somatic embryos of carrot using a 1% sodium alginate solution, as compared to a 2% alginate solution used in the present investigation. The main findings of the present experiment, though, indicate that somatic tissue can be electrostatically extruded and aseptically cultured while retaining viability.

Plantlets obtained from 4% alginate beads on agar, originally immobilized at 10 kV, 6 cm distance, were transferred to sterilized potting mixture at two months culture. The plantlets grew well and showed complete leaf and root development by four months.[22] Suspension culture of encapsulated somatic tissue was less successful. Piccioni[38] in a recent study investigated the growth of plantlets from alginate encapsulated micropropagated buds of M.26 apple rootstocks. He showed that the addition of growth regulators (e.g., indolebutyric acid) to the somatic tissue culture several days prior to the encapsulated, as well as the addition of the same regulators to the encapsulation matrix, improved the production of plantlets in suspension culture from 10% to more than 60%. We can speculate that culturing carnation leaf somatic tissue in the presence of growth regulators prior and during encapsulation may enhance the production of plantlets from suspension culture. Tissue from various types of plants, though, behave quite differently. For example, mulberry and banana plantlets were attained from alginate-encapsulated tissue without any specific root induction treatment[39,40] while Piccioni's apple rootstock buds required growth regulators.

Electrostatic droplet generation does not appear to have a negative impact on somatic tissue viability since cell growth and plantlet formation were observed. This is in agreement with similar studies reported for insect cells[41] and mammalian cells,[35] where it was shown that high electrostatic potentials did not affect cell viability. Finally, the technique has great potential in medicine for encapsulating genetically engineered cells[42] and in environmental engineering for removal of heavy metals from water using gel beads.[43]

## CONCLUDING REMARKS

The development of successful and well understood microencapsulated cell systems will necessitate close collaboration between scientists with different areas of expertise such as engineering, microbiology, biochemistry and medicine. Furthermore, to gain better insight into mass transfer problems in encapsulated cell systems requires not only experimental investigations but also mathematical modeling studies. As our knowledge of the physico-chemical characteristics of such systems increases, we can expect to see many new areas of application over the next decade.

## ACKNOWLEDGMENTS

The financial support of the Natural Science and Engineering Research Council of Canada, and Sultan Qaboos University, College of Agriculture (Grant AGBIOR

9505 to Mattheus Goosen) is gratefully acknowledged. The plant cell immobilization study was performed by H. Al-Hajry, S. Al-Maskari and L. Al-Kharousi (SQU). The assistance of Dr. O. El-Mardi in the plant tissue culture is also acknowledged.

## REFERENCES

1. COLTON. C.K. 1996. Engineering challenges in cell encapsulation technology. TIBTECH **14:** 158–162.
2. LANZA, R.P., J.L. HAYES & W.L. CHICK. 1996. Encapsulated cell technology. Nature Biotechnol. **14:** 1107–1111.
3. DE VOS, P. 1996. Association between capsule diameter, adequacy of encapsulation, and survival of microencapsulated rat islet allografts. Transplantation **62:** 893–899.
4. STEGEMANN, J.P. & M.V. SEFTON. 1996. Video analysis of submerged jet microencapsulation using HEMA-MMA. C. J. Chem. Eng. **74:** 518–525.
5. SVEC, F. & P. GEMEINER. 1995. Engineering aspects of carriers for immobilized biocatalysts. Biotechol. Gen. Eng. Rev. **13:** 217–235.
6. TAKIZAWA, S., V. ARAVINTHAN & K. FUJITA, 1996. Nitrogen removal from domestic wastewater using immobilized bacteria. Wat. Sci. Tech. **34** (1-2)**:** 431–440.
7. YAO, K., T. PENG, M. XU & C.YUAN. 1994. pH-Dependent hydrolysis and drug release of chitosan/polyether interpenetrating polymer network hydrogel Polymer Int. **34:** 213–219.
8. YAN, K.-H, W.P. GEUS, W. BAKKER, C.B.H.W. LAMER & H.G.M. HEIJERMAN. 1996. In vitro dissolution profiles of enteric-coated microsphere/microtablet pancreatin preparations at different pH values. Aliment Pharmacol Ther. **10:** 771–775.
9. LINEK, V., V. VACEK & P. BENES. 1987. A critical review and experimental verification of the correct use of the dynamic method for the determination of oxygen transfer in aerated agitated vessels to water, electrolyte solutions and viscous liquids. Chem. Eng. J. **34:** 11–34.
10. SHARP, N.A., A.J. DAUGULIS & M.F.A. GOOSEN. 1998. Hydrodynamic and mass transfer studies in an external-loop air-lift bioreactor for immobilized animal cell culture. Appl. Biochem. Biotechnol. **73** (1)**:** 57–77.
11. GOOSEN, M. F. A. 1999. Mass transfer in immobilized cell systems. *In* Handbook of Cell Encapsulation Technology and Therapeutics. W. M. Kuhtreiber, R. P. Lanza & W. L. Chick, Eds.: 18–28. Chap. 2. Birhäuser and Springer-Verlag.
12. MCCABE, W.L. & J.C. SMITH. 1985. Units of Chemical Engineering. McGraw-Hill. New York. p. 602.
13. HEATH, C. & G. BELFORT. 1987. Immobilization of suspended mammalian cells: analysis of hollow fiber and microcapsule bioreactors. Advances Biochem. Eng/ Biotechnol. **34:** 1–31.
14. VAN'T RIET, K. 1979. Review of measuring methods and results in nonviscous gas-liquid mass transfer in stirred vessels. Ind. Eng. Chem. Process Des. Dev. **18:** 357–364.
15. DECKWER, W.D., R. BURCKHART & R. ZOLL. 1974. Mixing and mass transfer in tall bubble columns. Chem. Eng. Sci. **29:** 2177–2188.
16. MOO-YOUNG, M. & J.W. BLANCH. 1983. Kinetics and transport phenomena in biological reactor design. Biochem. Eng.
17. SIEGEL, M.H. & J.C. MERCHUK. 1988. Mass transfer in a rectangular air-lift reactor: effects of geometry and gas circulation. Biotechnol. Bioeng. **32:** 1128–1137.
18. KING, G.A., A.J. DAUGULIS, P. FAULKNER & M.F.A. GOOSEN. 1987. Alginate-polylysine microcapsules of controlled membrane molecular weight cut-off for mammalian cell culture engineering. Biotechnol. Prog. **3:** 231–240.
19. BUGARSKI, B., B. AMSDEN, R.J. NEUFELD, D. PONCELET & M.F.A. GOOSEN. 1994. Effect of electrode geometry and charge on the production of polymer microbeads by electrostatics. C. J. Chem. Eng. **72:** 517–521.
20. DE SHON, E.W. & R. CARLSON. 1968. Electric field and model for electrical liquid spraying. J. Colloid Sci. **28:** 161–166.

21. WEAST, R.C. 1979. Handbook of Chemistry and Physics, 59th Ed. CRC Press Inc. Boca Raton, FL. p. F45.
22. AL-HAJRY, H.A., S.A. AL-MASKARY, L.M. AL-KHAROUSI, O. EL-MARDI, W.H. SHAYYA & M.F.A. GOOSEN. 1999. Growth of somatic tissue encapsulated in alginate using electrostatics. Biotechnol. Progress. Submitted for publication.
23. YUET, P.K., W. KWOK, T.J. HARRIS & M.F.A. GOOSEN. 1993. Mathematical modelling of immobilized animal cell growth: a comparison with experimental results. *In* Fundamentals of Animal Cell Encapsulation and Immobilization. M.F.A. Goosen, Ed. CRC Press. Boca Raton, FL. p. 79.
24. YUET, P.K., T. . HARRIS & M.F.A. GOOSEN. 1995. J. Artif. Cells, Blood Substitutes and Immobilization Biotechnol. **23:** 1.
25. MOGENSEN, A.O. & W.R. Vieth. 1973. Biotechnol. Bioeng. **15:** 467.
26. BAILEY, J.E. & D.F. OLLIS. 1986. *In* Biochemical Engineering Fundamentals, 2nd ed. J.E.B & D.F. Ollis, Eds., Chap. 7. McGraw-Hill Book Co. New York.
27. FRAME, K.K. & W.S. HU. 1988. Biotechnol. Bioeng. **32:** 1061.
28. CHANG, H.N. & M. MOO-YOUNG. 1988. Appl. Microbiol. Biotechnol. **29:** 107.
29. GOSMANN, B. & H. J. REHN. 1988. Appl. Microbiol. Biotechnol. **29:** 554.
30. BUGARSKI, B., J. Smith, J. Wu & M.F.A. GOOSEN. 1993. Methods of animal cell immobilization using electrostatic droplet generation. Biotechnol. Tech. **6** (9)**:** 677–682.
31. BUGARSKI, B., Q. LI, M.F.A. GOOSEN, D. PONCELET, R. NEUFELD & G. VUNJAK. 1994. Electrostatic droplet generation: mechanism of polymer droplet formation. Am. Inst. Chem. Eng. J. **40** (6)**:** 1026–1031.
32. GOOSEN, M.F.A., E.S.E. MAHMOUD, A.S. Al-GHAFRI, H.A. AL-HAJRI, Y.S. AL-SINANI & B. BUGARSKI 1996. Immobilization of cells using electrostatic droplet generation. *In* Methods in Molecular Biology: Immobilization Enzymes and Cells. G. Bickerstaff, Ed., Chap. 20: 167–174. Humana Press. Totowa, NJ.
33. GOOSEN, M.F.A., A.S. AL-GHAFRI, O. EL-MARDI, M.I.J. AL-BELUSHI, H.A. AL-HAJRI, E.S.E. MAHMOUD & E.C. CONSOLACION. 1997. Electrostatic droplet generation for encapsulation of somatic tissue: assessment of high voltage power supply. Biotechnol. Prog. **13** (4)**:** 497–502.
34. KLEIN, J., J. Stock & D.K. VORLOP 1993. Pore size and properties of spherical calcium alginate biocatalysts. Eur. J. Appl. Microb. Biotechnol. **18:** 86.
35. GOOSEN, M.F.A., G.M. O'SHEA, M.M. GHARAPETIAN & A.M. SUN. 1986. Immobilization of living cells in biocompatible semipermeable microcapsules: biomedical and potential biochemical engineering applications. *In* Polymers in Medicine. E. Chiellini, Ed.: 235. Plenum Publishing. New York.
36. TENG, W.-L., Y.-J. LIU, V.-C., TSAI & T.-S. SOONG 1994. Somatic embryogenesis of carrot in bioreactor culture systems. Hort. Sci. **29** (11)**:** 1349–1352.
37. SHIGETA, J. 1995. Germination and growth of encapsulated somatic embryos of carrot for mass propagation. Biotechnol. Tech. **10** (9)**:** 771–776.
38. PICCIONI, E. 1997. Plantlets from encapsulated micropropagated buds of M.26 apple rootstock. Plant Cell, Tissue and Organ Culture. **47:** 255–260.
39. BAPAT, V.A. & P.S. RAO. 1990. In vivo growth of encapsulated auxiliary buds of mulberry (*Morus indica*, L). Plant Cell Tissue Organ Cult. **20:** 60–70.
40. GANAPATHI, T.R., P. SUPRASANNA, V.A. BAPAT & P.S. RAO. 1992. Propagation of banana through encapsulated shoot tips. Plant Cell. Rep. **11:** 571–575.
41. KING, G.A., A.J. DAUGULIS, P. FAULKNER, D. BAYLY & M.F.A. GOOSEN. 1989. Alginate concentration a key factor in growth of temperature-sensitive insect cells in microcapsules. Biotechnol. Bioeng. **34:** 1085–1091.
42. CHANG, T.M.S. & S. PRAKASH. 1998. Therapeutic uses of microencapsulated genetically engineered cells. Mol. Med. Today **4** (5)**:** 221–227.
43. HAREL, P., L. MIGNOT, J.P. SAUVAGE & G.A. JUNTER. 1998. Cadmium removal from dilute aqueous solution by gel beads of sugar beet pectin. Industrial Crops and Products **7:** 239–247.

# *In Situ* Electrochemical Oxygen Generation with an Immunoisolation Device

HAIYAN WU,[a] EFSTATHIOS S. AVGOUSTINIATOS,[a] LARRY SWETTE,[b] SUSAN BONNER-WEIR,[c] GORDON C.WEIR,[c] AND CLARK K. COLTON[a,d]

[a]*Department of Chemical Engineering, Massachusetts Institute of Technology, Cambridge, Massachusetts 02139-4307, USA*

[b]*Giner, Inc., 14 Spring Street, Waltham, Massachusetts 02451, USA*

[c]*Section of Islet Transplantation and Cell Biology, Joslin Diabetes Center, Boston, Massachusetts 02215, USA*

**ABSTRACT: The viability and function of transplanted tissue encapsulated in immunobarrier devices is subject to oxygen transport limitation. In this study, we have designed and used an *in situ* electrochemical oxygen generator which decomposes water electrolyticaly to provide oxygen to the adjacent planer immunobarrier diffusion chamber. The rate of oxygen generation, which increases linearly with electrical current, was accurately controlled. A theoretical model of oxygen diffusion was also developed and was used to calculate the oxygen profiles in some of the experimental systems. *In vitro* culture experiments were carried out with βTC3 cells encapsulated in titanium ring devices. The growth and viability of cells with or without *in situ* oxygen generation was studied. We found that under otherwise similar culturing conditions, the thickness of the cell layer and the viability of cells was the highest in devices cultured in stirred media with oxygen generation, even though the thickness had not reached the theoretically predicted value, and lowest in those unstirred and without oxygen generation.**

## INTRODUCTION

Extravascular immunobarrier devices in the form of spherical capsules,[1,2] tubes,[3–8] or planar diffusion chambers[9–18] may be useful for protecting tissue from transplant rejection and autoimmunity. However, the process of immunoisolation removes the tissue from its normal blood supply, and the viability and function of the tissue depends on the supply of oxygen and nutrients from, and the removal of wastes to, the blood vessels nearest to the implanted device.[19,20] These transport limitations may be especially severe with planar diffusion chambers,[9,12,14,22] in part because of the formation of an avascular fibrotic tissue layer on a flat surface.[20] This problem is partially ameliorated by use of outer vascularizing membranes which induce neovascularization at the host tissue-membrane interface by virtue of their membrane microarchitecture.[22,24] However, when isogeneic islets in a planar diffusion chamber are implanted into diabetic mice,[25,26] substantial losses of viable tissue

[d]Author for correspondence: Room 66-452, Department of Chemical Engineering, Massachusetts Institute of Technology, 77 Massachusets Avenue, Cambridge, MA 02139-4307; 617-253-4585 (voice); 617-252-1651 (fax); ckcolton@mit.edu (e-mail).

are sustained in some devices, thereby suggesting that there are still oxygen supply limitations despite the presence of vascularizing membranes. Because the neovascularization process requires several days to begin and 10–14 days for completion,[24] the local hypoxic state following implantation likely results in the death of substantial tissue, as has been observed in the first few days following naked transplantation of islets under the kidney capsule.[27] One approach under study to prevent this early tissue death is to prevascularize the device, i.e., to substantially increase the local blood supply prior to placement of tissue in the device by infusion of an angiogenic factor through the membranes into the surrounding tissue.[28]

In this paper, we describe a new method for increasing oxygen supply to tissue implanted in an immunobarrier device involving *in situ* oxygen generation immediately adjacent to the device. For oxygen generation, we employ electrolytic decomposition of water into oxygen and hydrogen. The electrolyzer, in the form of a thin, multilayer sheet, is enclosed in silicone rubber membranes permeable to gas and water vapor but impermeable to liquids and dissolved materials. The anode side of the electrolyzer sheet is placed in contact with one face of a planar immunobarrier device in the form of a thin disk (in which the transplanted tissue is contained) which is sealed externally with titanium rings (henceforth referred to as the titanium ring device). The opposite face of the immunobarrier device is in contact with host tissue. The cathode side of the electrolyzer is also in contact with host tissue. In this arrangement, water vapor diffusing into the electrolyzer from both sides is decomposed at the anode; the oxygen generated at the anode diffuses back through the adjacent silicone rubber membrane to the implanted tissue, and the hydrogen generated at the cathode diffuses into the host tissue. This design provides a continuous supply of reactant water from the surrounding tissues, continuous diffusion of generated gases out of the electrolyzer disk, exclusion of biological components that would otherwise contaminate the electrolyzer, and requires only an input of electricity. Oxygen is supplied to the implanted tissue from two sides, one side being the electrolyzer, the other the adjacent blood supply from the host. Transport of nutrients in, and wastes and secreted products out, occurs only at the interface with the host.

The objectives of this study were to design and fabricate an electrolyzer of the type described above, to mate it with the titanium ring device, and to carry out initial *in vitro* experiments with cells cultured in the device to evaluate the feasibility of the concept. These initial experiments were carried out with the device suspended in well-oxygenated medium so that comparison could be made between supply of oxygen from the medium alone and supply from both the medium and the electrolyzer. In addition, a mathematical analysis of the oxygen transport in the device was developed in order to provide perspective on how it functions and to provide a basis for guiding further experimentation.

## EXPERIMENTAL MATERIALS AND METHODS

### *Planar Immunobarrier Device*

The planar diffusion chamber we employed has been previously described in detail.[25,26] Briefly, the device is a titanium ring chamber in which tissue was placed between two pieces of disk-shaped membrane (8.2 mm in diameter) which were held together by a titanium housing ring and a titanium sealing ring. The membrane consisted of three layers: (a) a hydrophilic polytetrafluoroethylene (PTFE) inner membrane with nominal pore size of 0.45 μm and thickness of 25–35 μm (Biopore Millipore Corp, Bedford, MA), which retained cells and would function *in vivo* as an immunobarrier layer; (b) a hydrophobic PTFE outer membrane with nominal pore size of 5 mm and thickness of approximately 15 μm (W.L. Gore and Associates, Elkton, MD), which would function *in vivo* as the vascularizing layer; and (c) a highly open outer meshwork about 125 μm thick of polyester fibers (about 50 μm in diameter) to provide support. The space between the two pieces of membrane was defined by a silicone rubber washer (inner diameter 6.6 mm, cross-sectional thickness 100 μm after the device is compressed during assembly).

### *Cells*

Experiments were carried out with βTC3 cells, a cell line derived from an insulinoma in a transgenic β6DZF1 mouse carrying a hybrid insulin-promoted SV40 T-antigen gene, which is among those β-cell lines being investigated with genetic engineering techniques for cell therapy of diabetes.[29,30] Cells were cultured in Dulbecco's Modification of Eagle's Medium (DMEM, Mediatech, Herndon, VA) with 400 mg/dl glucose, supplemented by 10% (v/v) fetal bovine serum (FBS, HyClone, Logan, UT), 100 IU penicillin, and 100 mg/ml streptomycin (Mediatech). Prior to loading the device, cells were detached from T-flasks using trypsin-EDTA solution (Mediatech) and washed three times by centrifugation, removal of the supernatant, and resuspension in culture medium. After the first wash, cells were suspended in 20 ml culture medium, and four aliquots of 200 ml each were taken, and counted in a hemocytometer with Trypan Blue staining. The average of these four counts was used to calculate the total cell numbers in the original cell suspension. Only batches with viability greater than 95% were used for loading. After the final wash, a thin Pasteur pipette (made by pulling a regular Pasteur pipette over flame) was used to remove as much supernatant as possible without removing cells, and the cells were resuspended in either phosphate buffered saline (PBS) or 1.7% (w/w) alginate solution to achieve the desired cell concentration. The suspension was carefully mixed without forming any air bubbles. A laminated membrane was placed inside the titanium housing ring with the hydrophilic side up and the silicone rubber washer was placed on top of the membrane. A volume of 3.5 ml of cell suspension was drawn into a 20 ml pipette tip and discharged at once on the center of the membrane. The other piece of membrane, with the hydrophilic side down, followed by the titanium sealing ring, were then placed on top of the cell suspension, and the whole device was pressed together with a hand press. When alginate was used, the assembled device was immersed in 10 mM BaCl2 solution for 30 seconds to crosslink the alginate. After three washes by immersion and shaking for 10 sec in $Ca^{2+}$ and $Mg^{2+}$-free PBS, the loaded device was ready to be cultured *in vitro*. Prior to loading, sterilization was achieved by autoclaving the titanium rings and washers, placing the electrolyzer in boiling water for at least 15 min, and immersing the membranes in 95% ethanol, 80% ethanol, and three times in PBS for at least 5 min in each. Sterilization was maintained by assembling the device in a laminar flow hood.

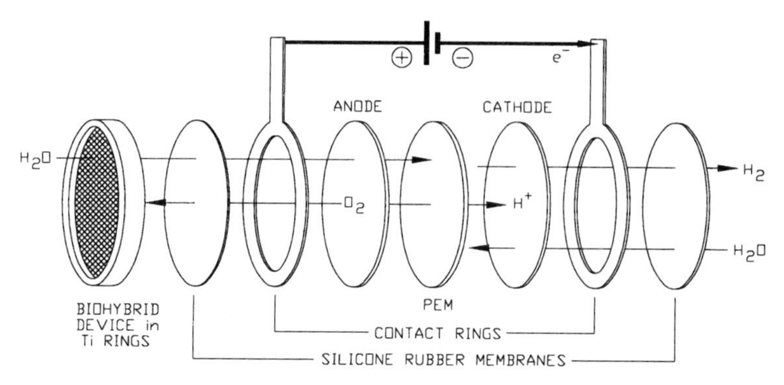


**FIGURE 1.** Exploded schematic diagram of *in situ* electrochemical oxygen generator (electrolyzer). PEM is the proton exchange membrane.

### *Electrochemical Oxygen Generation*

FIGURE 1 is an exploded schematic diagram of the components of the *in situ* electrochemical oxygen generator (electrolyzer) that carries out electrolysis of water.[31] The catalytic electrodes are separated by a solid polymer electrolyte proton exchange membrane (PEM)[32] which allows passage of hydrated $H^+$ but has much lower permeability to gases such as $O_2$ and $H_2$. As a consequence, the half-cell reactions at each electrode are compartmentalized. For normal acid electrolysis, the reactions are

| | | | |
|---|---|---|---|
| Anode | $2\,H_2O$ | $\longrightarrow$ | $O_2 + 4\,H^+ + 4\,e^-$ |
| Cathode | $4\,H^+ + 4\,e^-$ | $\longrightarrow$ | $2\,H_2$ |
| Net Reaction | $2\,H_2O$ | $\longrightarrow$ | $O_2 + 2\,H_2$ |

$O_2$ is formed at the anode. The $H^+$, which is also formed at the anode, is transported through the PEM under the influence of the potential gradient imposed by a constant current controller in the external circuit. The hydrogen ions arriving at the cathode recombine with electrons passed through the external circuit from the anode so as to form molecular hydrogen. Because of the permeability properties of the PEM, virtually all of the $O_2$ diffuses into the tissue contained in the titanium ring chamber, whereas the $H_2$ diffuses into the host tissue. $H_2$ is biologically inert in mammals under normal atmosphere condition and is not oxidized by mammalian tissues even under hyperbaric conditions.[33] Therefore, it should eventually reach the lungs from where it is exhaled. The quantity of hydrogen generated is expected to be less than the stoichiometric 2:1 ratio relative to oxygen for normal electrolysis because oxygen diffusing into the cathode side of the electrolyzer from the host tissue is preferentially reduced as compared to $H^+$. With oxygen present at the cathode, the reaction $O_2 + 4\,H^+ + 4e^- \rightarrow 2\,H_2O$ competes with $4\,H^+ + 4\,e^- \rightarrow 2H_2$, thereby decreasing the net hydrogen production. Both electrodes are covered by silicone rubber mem-

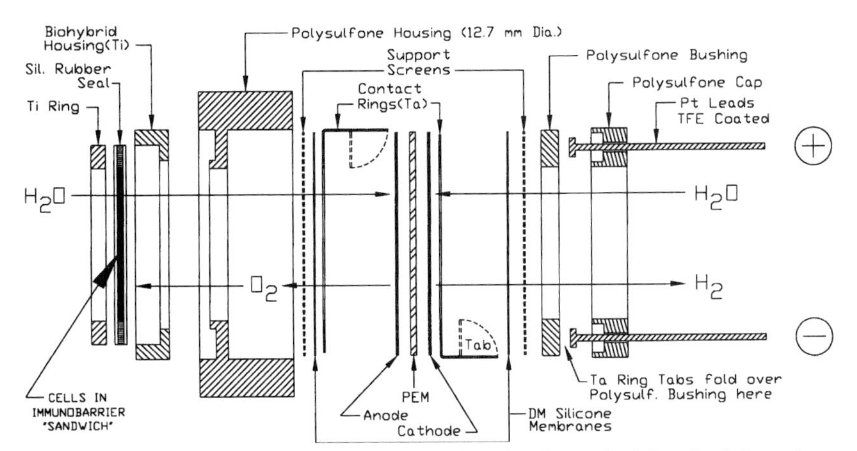


**FIGURE 2.** Schematic diagram of titanium ring chamber and miniaturized electrolyzer assembly. PEM is the proton exchange membrane.

branes, so that water enters the electrolyzer only in its vapor form and the electrolyzer interior is kept free of all other components of biological fluids.

The complete electrolyzer assembly is illustrated in FIGURE 2. The active components of the electrolyzer are the catalytic electrodes and the PEM. The PEM is Nafion 117 (1100 equivalent weight, about 1250 µm thick hydrated, DuPont Co., Wilmington, DE) which has $O_2$ and $H_2$ permeabilities more than two orders of magnitude less than silicone rubber. The Nafion membrane is received in the $Na^+$ form and is exchanged in acid to convert it to the proton form. The electrodes are placed in intimate contact with the PEM, one on each side, to form a membrane-electrode assembly (MEA). The substrate for the electrode was a very fine Pt screen (150 mesh with 43-mm diameter wire). The cathode catalyst is platinum (25 $m^2/g$), and the anode catalyst is platinum-iridium oxide (100 $m^2/g$). These high surface area particles are mixed with PTFE particles and pressed onto a fine-mesh substrate screen which in turn is pressed onto the PEM. To make electrical contact with the electrodes on the MEA disk, an annulus of tantalum foil, provided with a tab, is resistance welded to the edge of the electrodes before bonding to the PEM. The silicone rubber membranes are then hot pressed on either side of this MEA/Ta structure to complete the encapsulated electrolyzer assembly. To support the silicone rubber membrane, a disk of fine mesh titanium screen is added over the outside on both sides of the assembly. The entire thickness of the electrolyzer assembly, including the outer support screens, is about 0.75 mm. The encapsulated electrolyzer assembly was enclosed in a three-part polysulfone housing incorporating Pt wire leads for connection to the power supply and current control circuit. The titanium ring device was pressed into the polysulfone housing. The final assembly contained a gap between the outer surface of the silicone rubber membrane on the electrolyzer assembly and the outer membrane of the titanium ring device. The gap had a depth of about 0.75 mm and a diameter of 6.35 mm. The latter dimension defined an area of 0.317 $cm^2$, across which the generated oxygen diffused.

A power supply and a means for maintaining a constant current was necessary in order to maintain a constant rate of oxygen generation in the presence of resistance variations in the electrolyzer and declining battery voltage (when a battery is used). The constant current control was implemented with a Howland circuit,[34] a voltage-controlled current source which utilizes positive and negative feedback to provide precise current control. This circuit was powered by an AC–DC converter or by a single battery. The instrument which used this circuit incorporated meters for voltage and current measurement and a potentiometer to adjust current from 0 to 200 μA.

### In Vitro *Culture Experiments*

For oxygen generation experiments with *in vitro* culture, 50 ml Erlenmeyer flasks were filled with 40 ml of culture medium and prewarmed (37°C, 5% $CO_2$, 95% air in a humidified incubator, $P_{O_2}$ = 142 mm Hg). Each flask had a cylindrical magnetic stirring bar (2.6 cm long and 0.8 cm in diameter) on the bottom and a vented cap (taken from a 75 $cm^2$ T-flask) on the top. After the loaded immunobarrier device was mated with the oxygen electrolyzer in the polysulfone housing, the entire assembly was suspended in the flask below the level of the medium. The wires from the electrolyzer exited from under the cap and connected to an outside cable which was in turn connected to the current control device. Within the flask, the titanium ring device faced upward, and the electrolyzer was at the bottom so that oxygen was generated at the bottom of the device. The culture experiment started when the magnetic stirrer inside the incubator was turned on (150 rev/min). Culture medium was changed every 2 days.

Two types of experiments were carried out to examine the differences in cell growth and viability between 1) oxygen supplied only from the external medium (flask stirred without oxygen generation) and 2) oxygen supplied from both the external medium and the electrolyzer (flask stirred with oxygen generation). In addition, static unstirred control experiments were carried out with immunobarrier devices cultured in 6 cm petri dishes with a medium depth of 6 mm and with no electrolyzer attached and no stirring.

Each experiment within a given run was started with devices loaded with the same number of cells. After prescribed periods of time, one device with oxygen generation, together with the static control and/or a device exposed to stirred medium with no oxygen generation, were removed from culture. Culturing times from 0 to 9 days were examined.

### *Histology*

After removal from the culture flask, the immunobarrier device was first separated from the oxygen electrolyzer on a press made specifically for this purpose. The entire device was then immersed in fixative (Histochoice, Amresco, Solon, OH) for 2 hours. After fixation, the device was disassembled by separating the sealing ring from the housing ring using the same press employed for assembly. The silicone rubber washer was removed without disturbing the tissue inside, and the membrane-tissue sandwich was embedded in 7% agar gel. This was done by first dissolving the agar in 70°C water, placing a large drop of the solution on a glass slide, then placing the membrane-tissue sandwich in the middle, and finally placing another large drop of agar solution on top to cover it. After it solidified, the embedded sandwich was placed in a tissue cassette between biopsy sponges and was processed for paraffin embedding. Care was taken so that the original orientation of the device with respect to the side facing the electrolyzer remained identified. Serial sections 5–7 μm in thickness were cut perpendicular to the membrane surface. Only the longest sections which were nearest the center of the device were used. These sections, which numbered as many as 30, were then stained with hematoxylin and observed with light microscope (Olympus BH-2). Images selected for detailed examination were captured by a color video camera (DXC-960MD, Sony Corp., Japan) and a frame grabber (LG-3, Scion Corp., Frederick, MD) on a PowerMac as previously described.[25]

For use in numerical calculations with the theoretical model, the tissue volume fraction, $1-\varepsilon$, i.e., the volume fraction of a section occupied by cells, was estimated from a print of the part of the section being analyzed using the relation[35]

$$1-\varepsilon = \frac{n_n V_c}{A_{sec}(h+d_n)} \quad \textbf{(1)}$$

where $n_n$ is the number of stained nuclei identified in the section of surface area $A_{sec}$, $V_c = \pi d_c^3/6$ is the volume of one cell, $d_c$ is the cell diameter, $d_n$ is the nucleus diameter, and $h$ is the section thickness. $d_n$ was estimated to be about $10 \pm 1$ μm by measuring the diameters of the largest nuclei in prints of representative sections. $d_c$ was estimated to be $12 \pm 1$ μm by examination of cultured cells in suspension with light microscopy using a calibrated reticule.

## THEORY OF OPERATION

### *Oxygen Generation*

The oxygen generation rate M (mol/s) of the electrolyzer is related to the applied current $I$ (A) by

$$I = nFM, \quad \textbf{(2)}$$

where $n = 4$ is the number of electrons required to make one molecule of oxygen, and $F$ is Faraday's constant (96,500 A·s/equivalent). The imposed flux of oxygen $N_e$ from the electrolyzer into the planar diffusion chamber (mol/cm$^2$·s) is

$$N_e = \frac{M}{A_e}, \quad \textbf{(3)}$$

where $A_e = 0.317$ cm$^2$ is the cross-sectional area of the gap between the electrolyzer and the diffusion chamber. Equation **(2)** can thus be written as

$$i = nFN_e, \quad \textbf{(4)}$$

where $i = I/A_e$ is the effective current density at the electrodes.

### *Oxygen Diffusion and Consumption*

We present in this section the equations from which the important dependent parameters in our experiments can be estimated. These provide a useful framework for understanding oxygen diffusion and consumption in our experimental system. The derivation of those equations is an extension of analyses we have presented previously,[21,22] and is presented in full elsewhere.[35]

We consider one-dimensional oxygen diffusion, perpendicular to the membranes in Cartesian coordinates. Oxygen consumption is assumed to follow Michaelis-Menten kinetics with the local rate per unit volume $V$ given by $V = Vmax \cdot (1-\varepsilon) \cdot P/(Km + P)$ for $P > P_C$, where $P$ is the local oxygen partial pressure, $V$max is the maximum oxygen consumption rate per unit volume of tissue, $1-\varepsilon$ is the live tissue volume fraction in the tissue layer, $Km$ is the Michaelis–Menten constant, and $P_C$ is the critical value of $P$ below which loss of tissue viability occurs due to hypoxia, and oxygen consumption ceases. We present here the analytical solution to the oxygen diffusion-reaction equation using zero-order kinetics ($Km$ set equal to 0, $V = Vmax$ $(1-\varepsilon)$ = constant) and then examine the small difference that results from the solution obtained with numerical methods using the nonlinear Michaelis-Menten kinetics.

Assuming that all the tissue layer within the immunobarrier device is exposed to $P > P_C$, the solution for the local oxygen partial pressure is given by

$$P(x) = \frac{P_{Se} + P_{Sm}}{2} + (P_{Se} - P_{Sm})\frac{x}{L} - \frac{V}{2D\alpha}\left[\left(\frac{L}{2}\right)^2 - x^2\right] \quad \textbf{(5)}$$

where $x$ is the distance from the center plane of the tissue slab having a thickness $L$, considered positive in the direction towards the electrolyzer, $P_{Se}$ and $P_{Sm}$ are the values of $P$ at the tissue-membrane interfaces at the electrolyzer and medium side, respectively, $D$ is the effective diffusion coefficient of oxygen in tissue, and a is the Bunsen solubility of oxygen in tissue. $P_{Se}$ and $P_{Sm}$ are not known *a priori* but can be calculated in terms of the known quantities $N_e$ (the imposed oxygen flux from the electrolyzer) and $P_{med}$ (the oxygen partial pressure in the medium bulk):

$$P_{Sm} = P_{med} + (N_e - VL)R_{ext} \quad \textbf{(6)}$$

and

$$P_{Se} = P_{med} + (N_e - V_L)\left(\frac{L}{D\alpha} + R_{ext}\right) + \frac{VL^2}{2D\alpha} \quad \textbf{(7)}$$

where $R_{ext}$ is the sum of the diffusion resistances in series external to the tissue, i.e. those imposed by the membrane laminate and boundary layer, given by

$$R_{ext} = \frac{1}{k_c \alpha_{med}} + \left(\frac{L}{D\alpha}\right)_{M_2} + \left(\frac{L}{D\alpha}\right)_{M_1} \quad \textbf{(8)}$$

$M_1$ and $M_2$ refer to the cell retentive and vascularizing membranes, respectively, $k_c = D_{med}/\delta_c$ is the boundary layer mass transfer coefficient between the stirred medium and the vascularizing membrane $M_2$, and $\delta_c$ is the concentration boundary layer thickness (including the outermost polyester mesh).

The maximum thickness of viable tissue $L_{max}$ that can be supported in the device is

$$L_{max} = L_e + L_m \quad \textbf{(9)}$$

where $L_e$ and $L_m$ are the maximum tissue thicknesses that can be supported by the imposed oxygen flux and by oxygen diffusion from the bulk medium, respectively. $L_e$ can be calculated by making a mass balance around the tissue layer

$$N_m = N_e - VL \quad \textbf{(10)}$$

and setting the oxygen flux at the tissue-membrane interface at the medium side $N_m$ equal to 0:

$$L_e = \frac{N_e}{V} \quad \textbf{(11)}$$

$L_m$, equal to the distance from the tissue-membrane interface at the medium side ($x_C = -L/2$ ) to the point where the oxygen flux equals 0 and $P = P_C$, is given by

$$L_m = -D\alpha R_{ext} + \left[(D\alpha R_{ext})^2 + \frac{2D\alpha}{V}(P_{med} - P_C)\right]^{1/2}. \quad \textbf{(12)}$$

When the tissue thickness is not large enough for $P$ to fall to $P_C$, the minimum value of oxygen partial pressure $P_{min}$ can be calculated in a similar way, by replacing $P_C$ by $P_{min}$ and $L_m$ by $L - L_e$ to yield

$$P_{min} = P_{med} - V(L - L_e)R_{ext} - \frac{V}{2D\alpha}(L - L_e)^2. \quad \textbf{(13)}$$

This minimum occurs at distance $x_{min} = L/2 - L_e$ from the tissue-membrane interface at the electrolyzer side, provided that $L_e \leq L$.

For purposes of illustration, we calculated the oxygen partial pressure profiles in immunoisolated tissue supported on one face by an imposed oxygen flux from an electrolyzer for the case that $L \geq L_e$ so that $P$ decreases to $P_C$ in the interior of the device. Transport from the medium was not included. For zero-order kinetics, Equations **(5)** and **(11)** were used to calculate the maximum supportable thickness $L_e$, the local partial pressure $P(z)$ where $z = L/2 - x$, and the surface partial pressure $P_{Se}$. Calculation of the same dependent variables using Michaelis-Menten kinetics was carried out numerically.[35] Parameter values selected for these calculations were $1 - \varepsilon = 0.75$, $Vmax = 2.76 \times 10^{-8}$ mol/cm$^3$·s ,[36] $D\alpha = 1.70 \times 10^{-14}$ mol/cm·mm Hg·s,[22] $P_c$ = 0.1 mm Hg,[37–39] and $Km = 0.44$ mm Hg.[40]

Oxygen partial pressures are plotted as a function of distance from the interface in FIGURE 3 for values of imposed oxygen flux $N_e$ ranging from 1 to $6 \times 10^{-10}$ mol/cm$^2$·s. These values of $N_e$ correspond to current densities $i$ calculated from Equation **(4)** of 39 to 232 μA/cm$^2$ and to applied currents $I$ of 12 to 73 μA (with $A_e$ =

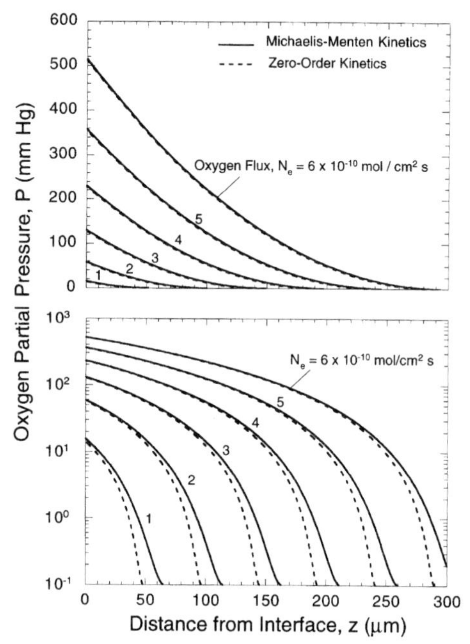


**FIGURE 3.** Oxygen partial pressure P as a function of the distance z from the electrolyzer-side tissue-membrane interface ($z = L/2 - x$) for different values of the oxygen flux $N_e$ generated by the electrolyzer. $P_{min} = P_C = 0.1$ mm Hg, $Km = 0.44$ mm Hg, $1 - \varepsilon = 0.75$, $Vmax \cdot (1 - \varepsilon) = 2.07 \times 10^{-8}$ mol/cm³·s, $D\alpha = 1.70 \times 10^{-14}$ mol/cm·mm Hg·s.

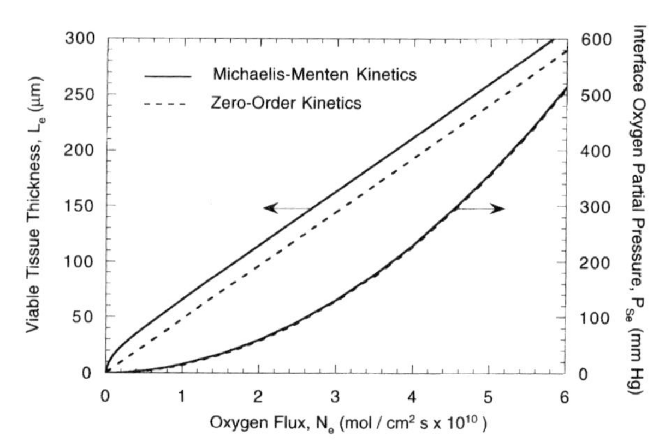


**FIGURE 4.** Viable tissue thickness $L_e$ supported by the electrolyzer and oxygen partial pressure $P_{Se}$ at the electrolyzer-side tissue-membrane interface as a function of the oxygen flux $N_e$ generated by the electrolyzer. Parameter values are the same as in FIGURE 3.

0.317 cm² in our system). With increasing oxygen flux, both the interface partial pressure and the maximum thickness increase. The underprediction of $P(z)$ by zero order as compared to Michaelis-Menten kinetics is hardly noticeable on the linear plot but is apparent on the semi-logarithmic plot (lower panel). At low partial pressures, the relative, but not the absolute, difference in $P(z)$ can be large.

FIGURE 4 is a plot of the interface oxygen partial pressure $P_{Se}$ and the maximum viable tissue thickness supported by the electrolyzer $L_e$ as a function of the imposed oxygen flux $N_e$. At the highest oxygen flux investigated, $L_e$ is about 300 µm, and $P_{Se}$ is about 500 mm Hg. Oxygen toxicity[41] at these $P_{Se}$ levels may be of concern with some cells and tissues, thereby setting a maximum limit on the imposed oxygen flux.

There is virtually no difference in FIGURE 4 between the two predictions for $P_{Se}$, but the zero-order model underpredicts $L_e$ by nearly 20 µm, except at very low $N_e$, as a consequence of the difference in profiles that develops at very low $P(z)$ (FIG. 3). Because the error in estimating oxygen partial pressure profiles is negligible and the error in $L_e$ relatively small, the zero-order kinetic model is used in the remainder of this paper.

## RESULTS AND DISCUSSION

In this initial feasibility study, we carried out five runs comprised of 18 sets of *in vitro* experiments. In each run, the imposed oxygen flux (or a specified pattern of changes with time) and the number of cells intended to be added to the device (from a single cell suspension) were held constant. Within a single run, each set of experiments included devices cultured for a specific time period. A single set included experiments with and without oxygen generation with stirred medium. In some cases, controls were also carried out with neither oxygen generation nor stirring. Some sets of experiments were carried out with alginate in the device, some without. Digital images taken from 5 mm paraffin sections through the device are presented here for three of the five runs. In runs 1 (FIG. 5) and 2 (FIG. 6), $I = 45$ µA, $N_e = 3.7 \times 10^{-10}$ mol/cm$^2$·s, and 2.3 or $2.5 \times 10^6$ cells were intended to be added to the device, respectively. In run 3 (FIG. 7), fewer cells were intended to be added ($0.35 \times 10^6$), and the low initial value of $I = 4.3$ µA ($N_e = 0.35 \times 10^{-10}$ mol/cm$^2$·s) was increased by a factor of $\sqrt{2}$ every 24 hours so as to parallel the doubling time of about 2 days we have observed with βTC3 cells in culture.

In runs 1 and 3, three devices were processed for histology immediately after being loaded in order to examine the initial cell distribution. In all devices, cells were usually distributed continuously within a region centered roughly around the center of the device, with a diameter of about 2 to 3.5 mm. In run 1, the cell layer ranged from one to four cells (about 10 to 40 mm) thick and was usually thinnest at the periphery and thickest close to the center. FIGURE 5a is a representative section of the layers observed. Thickness measurements were made with a calibrated reticule as a function of radial position, averaged, integrated radially, and then used to roughly estimate total cell volume by assuming that these results were constant circumferentially. The calculated volume was about 0.1–0.15 µl for run 1 and 0.05 – 0.1 µl for run 3. In contrast, the total volumes of 2.3 and $0.35 \times 10^6$ cells having a diameter of 12 µm are 2.1 and 0.32 µl, respectively. Thus, most of the cells intended for the device were lost during the cell suspension preparation or loading procedure. The exact source of the cell loss is unknown and now under study. These findings suggest that, although comparisons between sections from experiments in one run can be made

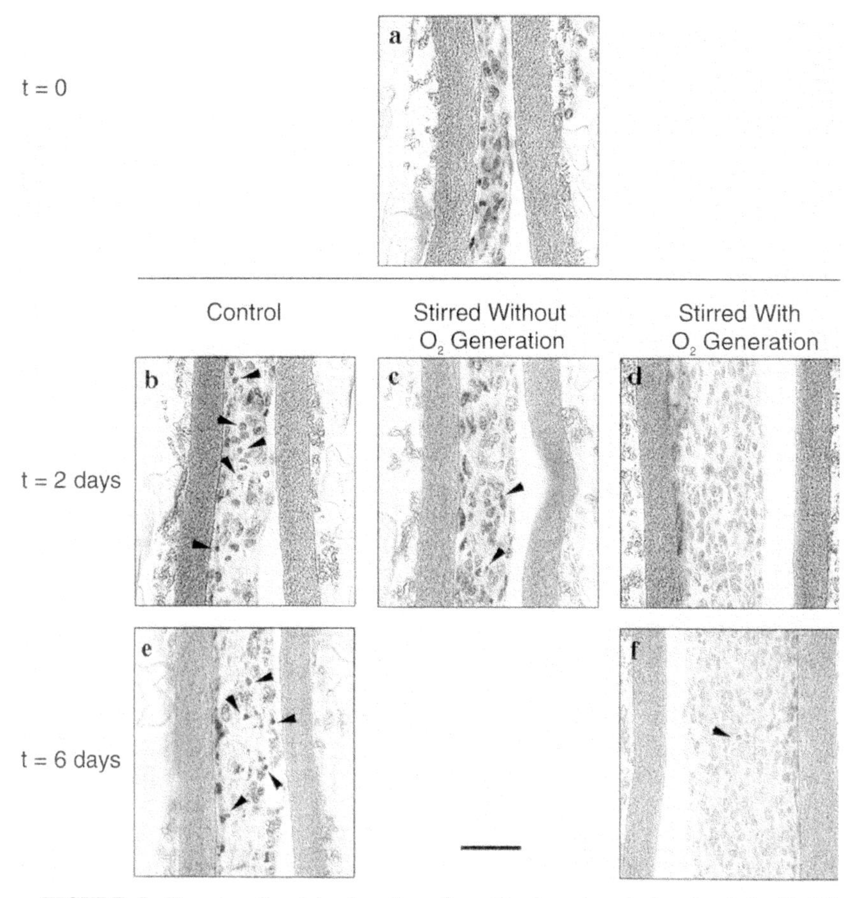


**FIGURE 5.** Hematoxylin stained sections from titanium ring devices loaded with 2.3 million βTC3 cells with alginate (Run 1). (**a**) $t$ = 0; (**b**) $t$ = 2 days; control (**c**) $t$ = 2 days, stirred without $O_2$ generation; (**d**) $t$ = 2 days, stirred with $O_2$ generation; (**e**) $t$ = 6 days, control; (**f**) $t$ = 6 days, stirred with $O_2$ generation. Arrows point to nuclei of apoptotic cells. Bar denotes 50 μm. In all stirred experiments, the membrane on the right faces the electrolyzer. In (**d**) and (**f**), $I$ = 45 μA, and $N_e = 3.7 \times 10^{-10}$ mol/cm$^2$·s.

with caution, comparison between sections from different runs may not be valid because of potentially large differences in number of cells loaded.

Histological section from devices that underwent culture for time $t$ = 1 to 9 days displayed cell layer thickness patterns qualitatively similar to those at $t$ = 0. The sections selected for presentation here met the criteria of being in focus, having no sectioning artifacts, and being representative of the thickest cell layer observed in the device.

In run 1 (FIG. 5), initial ($t$ = 0) tissue thickness $L$ was about 40 μm, and all cells were alive. After 2 days of culture, $L \approx 45$ μm in the control device, with many condensed nuclei characteristic of apoptotic cells. In the stirred experiments without and

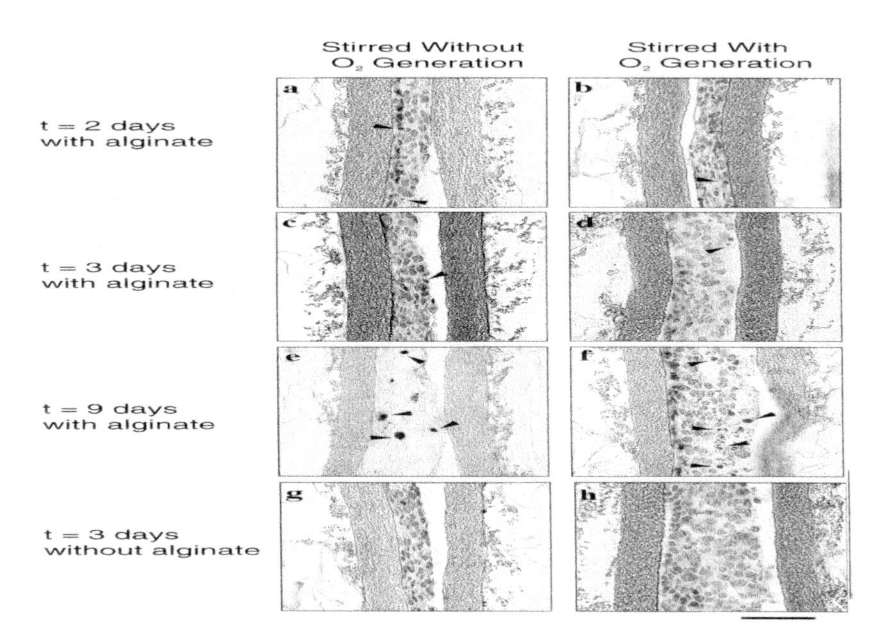


**FIGURE 6.** Hematoxylin stained sections from titanium ring devices loaded with 2.5 million βTC3 cells with alginate (Run 2). (**a**) $t$ = 1 day, control; (**b**) $t$ = 1 day, stirred with $O_2$ generation; (**c**) $t$ = 2 days, control; (**d**) $t$ = 2 days, stirred without $O_2$ generation; (**e**) $t$ = 2 days, stirred with $O_2$ generation. Arrows point to nuclei of apoptotic cells. Bar denotes 50 mm. In all stirred experiments, the membrane on the right faces the electrolyzer. In (**b**) and (**e**), $I$ = 45 μA, and $N_e = 3.7 \times 10^{-10}$ mol/cm²·s.

with $O_2$ generation, $L \approx 50$ and 70 μm, respectively. Cell viability was better with $O_2$ generation than without. After 6 days, $L$ increased only to about 50 μm in the control device, and there was substantial evidence of cell death. With stirring and $O_2$ generation at 6 days, $L$ increased to 100 μm and virtually all cells were viable.

Results from run 2 are summarized in FIGURE 6. After 1 day of culture, the control device had a tissue thickness of 20 μm, with substantial loss of cell viability, whereas with stirring and $O_2$ generation $L \approx 45$ mm with much fewer dead cells. After 2 days in the control device, $L \approx 45$ mm, but both the volume fraction and viability of cells were very low. With stirring and without $O_2$ generation, $L \approx 65$ μm, but there were many apoptotic cells indicative of low cell viability. With $O_2$ generation, $L \approx 60$ mm, and virtually all cells were viable.

FIGURE 7 shows the results from stirred experiments in run 3, in which cell loading and initial oxygen flux were much lower than in runs 1 and 2. At $t = 2$ days, tissue thickness ($L \approx 30$ μm) and viability were similar with or without $O_2$ generation. At 3 days, $L$ was still 25 μm without $O_2$ generation, while it increased to 50 μm with $O_2$ generation. At 9 days, most of cells in the experiment without $O_2$ generation were dead. With $O_2$ generation, $L \approx 70$ μm, but there were apoptotic cells and cell debris near the membrane adjacent to the electrolyzer where the oxygen partial pressure was highest. By 9 days and four doublings, $N_e$ had increased to the relatively high value of $5.6 \times 10^{-10}$ mol/cm²·s, thereby suggesting the possibility of oxygen toxicity

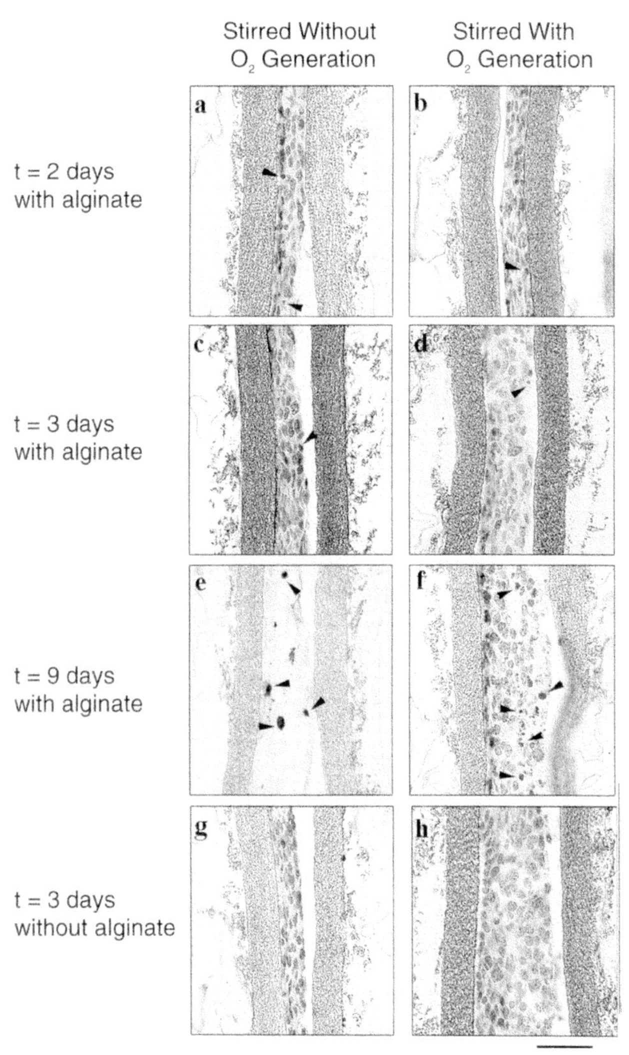


**FIGURE 7.** Hematoxylin stained sections from titanium ring devices loaded with 0.35 million βTC3 cells (Run 3). (**a**) $t = 2$ days, with alginate, stirred without $O_2$ generation; (**b**) $t = 2$ days, with alginate, stirred with $O_2$ generation, $N_e = 0.50 \times 10^{-10}$ mol/cm$^2$·s; (**c**) $t = 3$ days, with alginate, stirred without $O_2$ generation; (**d**) $t = 3$ days, with alginate, stirred with $O_2$ generation, $N_e = 0.70 \times 10^{-10}$ mol/cm$^2$·s; (**e**) $t = 9$ days, with alginate, stirred without $O_2$ generation; (**f**) $t = 9$ days, with alginate, stirred with $O_2$, $N_e = 5.6 \times 10^{-10}$ mol/cm$^2$·s; (**g**) $t = 3$ days, without alginate, stirred without $O_2$ generation; (**h**) $t = 3$ days, without alginate, stirred with $O_2$ generation, $N_e = 0.70 \times 10^{-10}$ mol/cm$^2$·s. Arrows point to nuclei of apoptotic cells. Bar denotes 50 mm. In all stirred experiments, the membrane on the right faces the electrolyzer. In (**b**), (**d**), (**f**), and (**h**), $I = 4.3$ µA, and $N_e = 0.35 \times 10^{-10}$ mol/cm$^2$·s initially. $I$ and $N_e$ were increased by a factor of $\sqrt{2}$ every day.

**TABLE 1.** Values of important parameters in analyzed experiments

| Parameters | Experiments | | | | | | | | |
|---|---|---|---|---|---|---|---|---|---|
| Figure number | 5a | 5a | 5c | 5d | 5f | 7a | 7b | 7g | 7h |
| Culture time, $t$ (d) | 0 | 0 | 2 | 2 | 6 | 2 | 2 | 3 | 3 |
| Oxygen flux, $N_e$ (mol/cm$^2$·s × 10$^{10}$) | 0[a] | 3.7[a] | 0 | 3.7 | 3.7 | 0 | 0.50 | 0 | 0.70 |
| Tissue thickness, $L$ (μm) | 40 | 40 | 50 | 70 | 100 | 30 | 25 | 25 | 75 |
| Tissue volume fraction, $1 - \varepsilon$ | 0.52 | 0.52 | 0.53 | 0.69 | 0.60 | 0.74 | 0.78 | 0.76 | 0.70 |
| Oxygen consumption rate, $V$ (mol/cm$^3$·s × 10$^8$) | 1.4 | 1.4 | 1.5 | 1.9 | 1.7 | 2.0 | 2.1 | 2.1 | 1.9 |
| Oxygen permeability, $D\alpha$ (mol/cm·mmHg·s × 10$^{14}$) | 2.2 | 2.2 | 2.1 | 1.8 | 2.0 | 1.7 | 1.6 | 1.7 | 1.8 |
| Tissue thickness supportable from electrolyzer, $L_e$ (μm) | 0 | 250 | 0 | 190 | 220 | 0 | 23 | 0 | 37 |
| Tissue thickness supportable from medium, $L_m$ (μm) | 140 | 140 | 140 | 110 | 130 | 110 | 100 | 100 | 110 |
| Interface $P$ at $x = -L/2$, $P_{Se}$ (mmHg) | 116 | 313 | 108 | 340 | 356 | 115 | 144 | 120 | 115 |
| Interface $P$ at $x = -L/2$, $P_{Sm}$ (mmHg) | 122 | 250 | 116 | 224 | 212 | 121 | 141[b] | 124 | 116 |
| Minimum $P$, $P_{min}$ (mmHg) | — | — | — | — | — | — | 141[b] | — | 108 |

For all examples, $P_m = 142$ mm Hg, $R_{ext} = 3.5 \times 10^{11}$ mm Hg/(mol/cm$^2$·s), $\delta = 50$, $L_{M_2} = 15$, and $L_{M_1} = 30$ μm, $(D\alpha)_{med} = 3.5$, $(D\alpha)_{M_2} = 2.8$, and $(D\alpha)_{M_1} = 2.0 \times 10^{-14}$ mol/cm·mmHg·s, $D_{med} = 2.8 \times 10^{-5}$ cm$^2$/s, $\alpha_{med} = 1.3 \times 10^{-9}$ mol/cm$^3$·mmHg, $Vmax = 2.76 \times 10^{-8}$ mol/cm$^3$·s, $P_C = 0.1$ mm Hg, and $Km = 0.44$ mm Hg.

Calculations were carried out with three or more digits, but all parameter results, except for partial pressures, were rounded to two.

[a]The results at $t = 0$ correspond to the hypothetical oxygen profiles in the absence and presence of an imposed oxygen flux, respectively.

[b]$P_{Sm} - P_{min} \ll 0.5$ mm Hg.

to the cells nearest the electrolyzer in this experiment. Up to this point, all of the experiments presented were carried out with alginate. FIGURES 7g and 7h show results from experiments without alginate. Without $O_2$ generation, thickness was similar to that with alginate ($L \approx 25$ μm) after 3 days (FIG. 7c). With $O_2$ generation, $L \approx 75$ μm, higher than with alginate (FIG. 7d). It is possible that cross-linked alginate posed a restriction on cell growth.

In all of these experiments, the thickness of the cell layer (and thus the growth rate of the cells), and their viability was highest in the stirred experiments with $O_2$ generation and lowest in the unstirred static controls (in which oxygen transport was most limited). These results verify the hypothesis that oxygen transport limitations can limit the growth and viability of cells in immunobarrier devices. Furthermore, they demonstrate that *in situ* oxygen generation leading to an imposed oxygen flux into the tissue compartment can have a beneficial effect on cell growth and viability.

The theoretical model developed earlier was used to analyze oxygen transport in nine of the experiments. Estimated values of parameters used in the calculations are summarized in TABLE 1, and additional details are provided elsewhere.[22] Each experiment is designated by its figure number. *Vmax* was based upon the value of 1.5 $\mu$mol/min$\cdot 10^9$ cells for a monolayer of $\beta$TC3 cells[33] and converted to a volume basis for cells with $d_c = 12$ $\mu$m to yield $2.76 \times 10^{-8}$ mol/cm$^3\cdot$s. Permeability of the cells was assumed to be the same as for islet tissue, $1.24 \times 10^{-14}$ mol/cm$\cdot$mm Hg$\cdot$s.[32] The values of $V$ and $D\alpha$ varied between experiments because of variation in the tissue volume fraction $1 - \varepsilon$ and were estimated as described elsewhere.[22] TABLE 1 also contains estimates of the dependent variables $L_e$, $L_m$, $P_{Se}$, $P_{Sm}$, and $P_{min}$ which were calculated from Equations **(11)**, **(12)**, **(7)**, **(6)**, and **(13)**, respectively.

The experiments analyzed represent three groups: 1) those with high imposed oxygen flux (experiments 5a, 5d, and 5f), 2) those with low oxygen flux (7b and 7h), and, 3) those without oxygen flux (5a, 5c, 7a, and 7g). In the first group, $L_e > L$, and there is an efflux of unconsumed oxygen from the device, described by Equation **(10)**. In the second group, $L_e < L$, and there is an influx of oxygen into the device from both sides, hence, a minimum in the $P$ profile develops. In the third group, oxygen is supplied only from the medium, so the maximum value of $P$ occurs at $y = 0$ and $P_{min}$ occurs at $z = 0$.

These trends are also shown graphically in FIGURE 8, where the predicted oxygen partial pressure profiles through the boundary layer, membrane, and tissue layers are plotted as a function of $y = L/2 + x$ for five of the nine experiments analyzed. Profiles for group 1), experiments 5d and 5f, group 2), experiment 7h, and group 3), experiments 5c and 7g are in panels a, b, and c, respectively. Changes in $N_e$ can have a dramatic effect on the profiles, even when tissue thickness and properties are similar, and can be best understood in terms of Equations **(6)**, **(7)**, and **(10)**. For example, experiments 5d and 7h have similar values of $L$ and $1 - \varepsilon$, but the partial pressure profiles are vastly different. In 5d, $N_e$ and $N_m$ are 3.7 and $2.4 \times 10^{-10}$ mol/cm$^2\cdot$s, respectively, so that 65% of the imposed flux exits the tissue at $y = 0$. This large value of $N_m$ leads to large partial pressure drops associated with diffusion across the external layers and across the tissue, amounting to 82 and 90 mm Hg, respectively, as compared to only 26 mm Hg resulting from oxygen consumption. In 7h, by contrast, $N_e$ and $N_m$ are 0.70 and $-0.74 \times 10^{-10}$ mol/cm$^2\cdot$s. In this case, $L_e < L$, $N_e$ is too small to support the full thickness of tissue, there are small, roughly equal values of oxygen influx on both sides of the tissue layer, and there is a nearly symmetrical oxygen partial pressure profile with a minimum very close to the center.

The precise values of the profiles plotted in FIGURE 8 depend upon the parameter value estimates in TABLE 1, some of which may be significantly in error. However, a sensitivity analysis using reasonable estimates of possible errors in the parameters indicates that the changes in profiles would not be large and would not affect the findings of this study. The largest uncertainty is in the boundary layer mass transfer coefficient $k_c$, which we estimated by setting $\delta_c = 50$ $\mu$m. Because there is an outer mesh about 125 $\mu$m thick containing large fibers, it is possible that $\delta_c$ should be much larger. If we set $\delta_c = 200$ $\mu$m, we find for experiment 5d that $L_m$ decreases from about 110 to 75 $\mu$m, and $P_{Sm}$ increases by 100 mm Hg, as do all values of $P(z)$. For

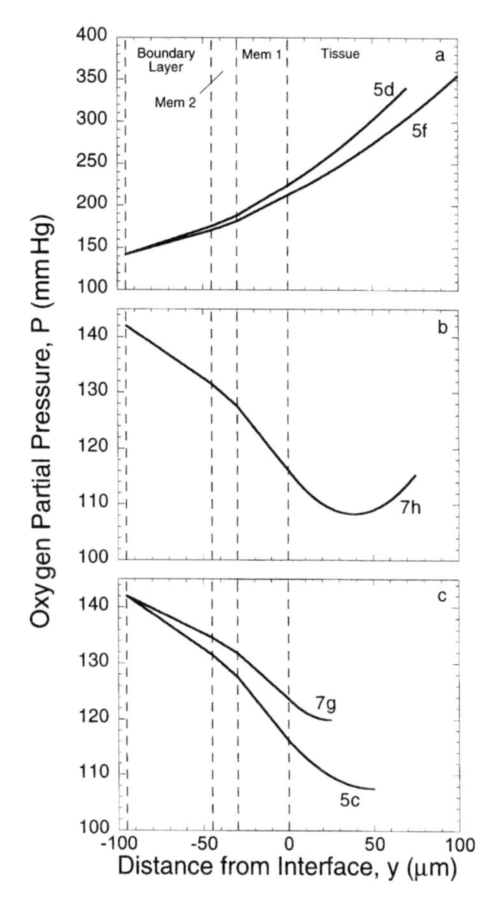


**FIGURE 8.** Predicted oxygen partial pressure $P$ as a function of the distance $y$ from the medium-side tissue-membrane interface ($y = L/2 + x$) corresponding to selected experiments. The distance coordinate is plotted to scale through the external resistances. The experiment to which each curve applies is designated by its associated figure number. (**a**) Experiments with relatively high imposed oxygen flux, FIGURES 5d and 5f, $N_e = 3.7 \times 10^{-10}$ mol/cm$^2$·s; (**b**) Experiments with low imposed oxygen flux, FIGURE 7h, $N_e = 0.7 \times 10^{-10}$ mol/cm$^2$·s; (**c**) Experiments with no imposed oxygen flux, FIGURES 5c and 7g. In all cases, $P_{med} = 142$ mm Hg.

experiment 5c, $L_m$ decreases from about 140 to 100 μm, and $P_{Sm}$ (and all values of $P(z)$) decrease by 31 mm Hg, so that the lowest value, $P_{Se}$, is about 77 mm Hg.

In none of the experiments was the observed cell layer thickness greater than about 100 μm, even in the high oxygen flux experiments where the estimated maximum thickness supportable form both sides was 300 μm or more. A likely explanation is that in no case did the cells have enough time to proliferate to their maximum thickness because the initial load of cells placed in the devices was far lower than intended. As a consequence, none of these experiments provided a test of the maximum thickness of tissue that could be supported in the device. Furthermore, the estimated minimum partial pressure in the stirred experiments never came close to the hypoxic limit and, for the analyzed cases (TABLE 1), never fell below 100 mm Hg. Nonetheless, the use of oxygen generation and exposure of the cells to higher oxygen partial pressure led to clearly identifiable improvements in cell layer thickness and viability. This conclusion leads to the notion that the higher partial pressure directly provided benefits through increased proliferation rates and improved maintenance of cell viability.

Although the bench-top current controller used in our *in vitro* experiments is large because it provides displays and controls, we have also constructed a miniaturized controller (6.5 × 3.5 × 5.4 cm) that can be worn by a rat. Furthermore, microelectronic technology can be used to make a miniaturized implantable device with a size suitable for implantation. The current can be preset or controlled by telemetry. We have calculated that an oxygen generation rate sufficient to support a biohybrid artificial pancreas in a human could be powered by a an implantable battery with 3000 mAh capacity which would require recharging every four weeks. Recharging could be achieved with a transcutaneous energy transfer (TET) system of the type developed to power implantable devices such as artificial hearts, defibrillators, and electrical stimulators.[42] The power transmission requirements for biohybrid artificial pancreas is many orders of magnitude smaller than the capacity of currently available TET systems. Therefore, we do not believe that the power supply would be a major obstacle for human implantation of our electrolyzer-backed immunobarrier device.

## SUMMARY

We have designed and fabricated a thin, multilayered sheet electrolyzer for in situ electrochemical oxygen generation by electrolysis of water which can be placed in contact with one face of a planar immunobarrier diffusion chamber. *In vitro* feasibility experiments with βTC3 cells loaded into the chamber showed that growth and viability are improved with oxygen generation. A theoretical model was developed to describe oxygen diffusion and consumption in the system. Application of the model to analysis of selected experiments revealed that oxygen partial pressures were relatively high and that substantial increases in the thickness of the cell layer supported in these devices should be attainable.

## ACKNOWLEDGMENTS

The titanium ring chamber was kindly supplied by Baxter Healthcare Corp. We thank Dr. Klearchos K. Papas (Novartis Pharmaceuticals Corporation) for helpful discussions.

This work was supported in part by grants from the National Institutes of Health (1R43DK51909-01 to L.S. and DK-35449 and DK-50657 to G.C.W.) and from the juvenile Diabetes Foundation International (File No. 198300 to C.K.C. and through the the JDFI Center for Islet Transplantation at Harvard Medical School to G.C.W. and C.K.C.).

## REFERENCES

1. DE VOS, P., B. DE HAAN, J. PATER & R. VAN SCHILFGAARDE. 1996. Association between capsule diameter, adequacy of encapsulation, and survival of macroencapsulated rat islet allografts. Transplantation **62:** 893–899.
2. SUN, Y., X. MA, D. ZHOU, I. VACEK & A.M. SUN. 1996. Normalization of diabetes in spontaneously diabetic cynomolous monkeys by xenograft of microencapsulated porcine islets without immunosuppression. J. Clin. Invest. **98:** 1417–1422.
3. ALTMAN, J.J., A. PENFORNIS, J. BOILLOT & M. MALETTI. 1988. Bioartificial pancreas: long-term function of discordant islet xenografts in streptozotocin diabetic rats. Trans. Am. Soc. Artif. Int. Organs **34:** 247–249.
4. LACY, P.E., O.D. HEGRE, A. GERASIMIDI-VEZEOU, F.T. GENTILE & K.E. DIONNE. 1991. Maintenance of normoglycemia in diabetic mice by subcutaneous xenograft of encapsulated islets. Science **254:** 1782–1784.
5. LANZA, R.P., K.M. BORLAND, J.E. STARUK, M.C. APPEL & W.L. CHICK. 1992. Transplantation of encapsulated canine islets into spontaneously diabetic BB/Wor rats without immunosuppression. Endocrinology **131:** 637–642.
6. LANZA, R.P., K.M. BORLAND, P. LODGE, M. CARRETTA, S.J. SULLIVAN, T.E. MULLER, B.A. SOLOMON, T. MAKI, A.P. MONACO & W.L. CHICK. 1992. Treatment of severely diabetic pancreatectomized dogs using a diffusion-based hybrid pancreas. Diabetes **41:** 886–888.
7. LANZA, R.P., K.M. BORLAND, J.E. STARUK & W.L. CHICK. 1993. Bioartificial pancreas: long term function of discordant islet xenografts in streptozotocin diabetic rats. Transplantation **56:** 1067–1072.
8. SCHARP, D.W., C.J. SWANSON, B.J. OLACK, P.P. LATTA, O.D. HEGRE, E.J. DOHERTY, F.T. GENTILE, K.S. FLAVIN, M.F. ANSARA & P.E. LACY. 1994. Protection of encapsulated human islets implanted without immunosupression in patients with type I or II diabetes and in nondiabetic control subjects. Diabetes **43:** 1167–1170.
9. BRAUKER, J., L.A. MARTINSON, T. LOUDOVARIS, R.S. HILL, V. CARR-BRENDEL, R. HODGSON, S. YOUNG, T.E. MANDEL, B. CHARLTON & R.C. JOHNSON. 1992. Immunoisolation with large pore membranes: allografts are protected under conditions that result in destruction of xenografts. Cell Transplant. **1:** 16.
10. HILL, R.S., S.K. YOUNG, S.A. JACOBS, L.A. MARTINSON & R.C. JOHNSON. 1992. Membrane encapsulated islets implanted in epididymal fat pads corrects diabetes in rats. Cell Transplant. **1:** 168.
11. MARTINSON, L., R. PAULEY, J. BRAUKER, D. BOGGS, D. MARYANOV, S. STERNBERG & R.C. JOHNSON. 1995. Protection of xenografts with immunoisolation membranes. Cell Transplant. **3:** 249.
12. BRAUKER, J., L. MARTINSON, S.K. YOUNG & R.C. JOHNSON. 1996. Local inflammatory response around diffusion chambers containing xenografts. Transplantation **61:** 1671–1677.
13. LOUDOVARIS, T., T. E. MANDEL & B. CHARLTON. 1996. $CD4^+$ T cell mediated destruction of xenografts within cell-impermeable membranes in the absence of $CD8^+$ T cells and B cells. Transplantation **61:** 1678-1684.
14. CARR-BRENDEL, V.E., R.L. GELLER, T.J. THOMAS, D.R. BOGGS, S.K. YOUNG, J. CRUDELE, L.A. MARTINSON, D.A. MARYANOV, R.C. JOHNSON & J.H. BRAUKER. 1997. Transplantation of cells in an immunoisolation device for gene therapy. *In* Methods in Molecular Biology: Expression and Detection of Recombinant Genes. R. Tuan, Ed. **63:** 373–387. Humana. Totowa, NJ.
15. GELLER, R.L., T. LOUDOVARIS, S. NEUENFELDT, R.C. JOHNSON & J.H. BRAUKER. 1997. Use of an immunoisolation device for cell transplantation and tumor immunotherapy. Ann. N.Y. Acad. Sci. **831:** 438–451.

16. BRAUKER, J. G.H. GROST, V. DWARKI, T. NIJJAAR, R. CHIN, V. CARR-BRENDEL, C. JASUNS, D. HODGETT, W. STONE, L.K. COHEN & R.C. JOHNSON. 1998. Sustained expression of high levels of human factor IX from human cells implanted within an immunoisolation device into athymic rodents. Human Gene Therapy. **9:** 879–888.
17. LOUDOVARIS, T, S. JACOBS, S. YOUNG, D. MARYANOV, J. BRAUKER & R.C. JOHNSON. 1999. Correction of diabetic nod mice with insulinomas implanted within Baxter immunoisolation devices. J. Mol. Med. **77:** 219–223.
18. JOSEPHS, S.F., T. LOUDOVARIS, A. DIXIT, S.K. YOUNG & R.C. JOHNSON. 1999. In vivo delivery of recombinant human growth hormone from genetically engineered human fibroblasts implanted within Baxter immunoisolation devices. J. Mol. Med. In press.
19. COLTON, C.K. & E.S. AVGOUSTINIATOS. 1991. Bioengineering in development of the hybrid artificial pancreas. J. Biomech. Eng. **113:** 152-170.
20. COLTON, C.K. 1995. Implantable biohybrid artificial organs. Cell Transplant. **4:** 415–436.
21. AVGOUSTINIATOS, E.S. & C.K. COLTON. 1997. Design considerations in immunoisolation. *In* Principles of Tissue Engineering, R.P. Lanza, R. Langer & W.L. Chick, Eds. :333–346. R.G. Landes, Austin, TX.
22. AVGOUSTINIATOS, E.S. & C.K. COLTON. 1997. Effect of external oxygen mass transfer resistances on viability of immunoisolated tissue. Ann. N.Y. Acad. Sci. **831:** 145–167.
23. BRAUKER, J.H., V.E. CARR-BRENDEL, L.A. MARTINSON, J. CRUDELE, W.D. JOHNSTON & R.C. JOHNSON. 1995. Neovascularization of synthetic membranes directed by membrane microarchitecture. J. Biomed. Mat. Res. **29:** 1517–1524.
24. PADERA, R.F. & C.K. COLTON. 1996. Time course of membrane microarchitecture-driven neovascularization. Biomaterials **17:** 277–284.
25. SUZUKI, K., S. BONNER-WEIR, J. HOLLISTER-LOCK, C.K. COLTON & G.C. WEIR. 1998. Number and volume of islets transplanted in immunobarrier devices. Cell Transplant. **7:** 47–52.
26. SUZUKI, K., S. BONNER-WEIR, N. TRIVEDI, K.-H. YOON, J. HOLLISTER-LOCK, C.K. COLTON & G.C. WEIR. 1998. Function and survival of macroencapsulated syngeneic islets transplanted into streptozotocin-diabetic mice. Transplantation **66:** 21–28.
27. DAVALLI, A., L. SCAGLIA, D. ZANGEN, J. HOLLISTER, S. BONNER-WEIR & G.C. WEIR. 1996. Vulnerability of islets in the immediate posttransplantation period—dynamic changes in structure and function. Diabetes **45:** 1161–1167.
28. TRIVEDI, N., G.M. STEIL, C.K. COLTON, S. BONNER-WEIR & G.C. WEIR. Improved vascularization of planar diffusion membrane devices following continuous infusion of vascular endothelial growth factor. Am. J. Physiol. Submitted.
29. EFRAT, S. 1996. Genetic engineering of β-cells for cell therapy of diabetes: cell growth, function, and immunogenicity. Diabetes Rev. **4:** 224–234.
30. POITOUT, V., L.K. OLSON & R.P. ROBERTSON. 1996. Insulin-secreting cell lines: classification, characteristics and potential applications. Diabetes & Metab. **22:** 7–14.
31. ERICKSON, A.C. & J.H. RUSSELL. 1977. Development status of a preprototype water electrolysis system. Presented at the Intersociety Conference on Environmental Systems, San Francisco, CA, July 11–14, 1977. 77-ENAs-34.
32. LACONTI, A.B., A.R. FRAGALA & J.R. BOYARK. 1977. Solid polymer electrolyte electrochemical cells: electrode and other materials considerations. Proceedings of the Symposium on Electrode Materials and Processes for Energy Conversion and Storage. **77-6:** 354–374.
33. KAYAR, S.R., M.J. AXLEY, L.D. HOMER & A.L. HARABIN. 1994. Hydrogen gas is not oxidized by mammalian tissues under hyperbaric conditions. Undersea & Hyperbaric Med. **21:** 265–275.
34. JUNG, W.G. 1981. IC Op-Amp Cookbook, 2nd Edition. :192–194. Howard W. Sams Pub.
35. AVGOUSTINIATOS, E.S. 1999. Oxygen transfer limitations in the bioartificial pancreas. Ph.D. Thesis. Massachusetts Institute of Technology, Cambridge, MA.

36. MUKUNDAN, N.E., P.C. FLANDERS, I. CONSTANTINIDIS, K.K. PAPAS & A. SAMBANIS. 1995. Oxygen consumption rates of free and alginate-entrapped βTC3 mouse insulinoma cells. Biochem. Biophys. Res. Commun. **210:** 113–118.
37. CHANCE, B., B. OSHINO, T. SUGANO & A. MAYEVSKY. 1973. Basic principles of tissue oxygen determination from mitochondrial signals. *In* Oxygen Transport to Tissue. Instrumentation, Methods, and Physiology. H.I. Bicher & D.F. Bruley, Eds. **37A:** 277–292. Plenum Press. New York.
38. SILVER, I.A. 1973. Brain oxygen tension and cellular activity. *In* Oxygen Supply; Theoretical and Practical Aspects of Oxygen Supply and Microcirculation of Tissue. M. Kessler, D.F. Bruley, L.C. Clark, D.W. Lübbers, I.A. Silver & J. Strauss, Eds. : 186–188. University Park Press. Baltimore, MD.
39. ANUNDI, I. & H. DE GROOT. 1989. Hypoxic liver cell death: critical $Po_2$ and dependence of viability on glycolysis. Am. J. Physiol. **257:** G58–G64.
40. DIONNE, K.E. 1990. Effect of hypoxia on insulin secretion and viability of pancreatic tissue. Ph.D. Thesis. Massachusetts Institute of Technology, Cambridge, MA.
41. JENKINSON, S.G. 1993. Oxygen toxicity. New Horiz. **1:** 504–511.
42. MUSSIVAND, T., J.A. MILLER, P.J. SANTERRE, G. BELANGER, K.C. RAJAGOPALAN, P.J. HENDRY, R.G. MASTERS, K.S. HOLMES, R. ROBICHAUD, M. KEANEY, V.M. WALLEY & W.J. KEON. 1993. Transcutaneous energy transfer system performance evaluation. Artif. Organs **17:** 940–947.

# Conformal Coating of Small Particles and Cell Aggregates at a Liquid-Liquid Interface

MICHAEL H. MAY[a] AND MICHAEL V. SEFTON[b]

*Department of Chemical Engineering and Applied Chemistry, University of Toronto, 200 College Street, Toronto, Ontario, Canada M5S 3E5*

**ABSTRACT: Polymer encapsulation of allogeneic or xenogeneic tissue is under active investigation as a means of isolating transplanted cells, such as pancreatic islets, from the immune system. We report here a method for coating small particles and cell aggregates with a very thin water insoluble hydroxyethyl methacrylate-methyl methacrylate (HEMA-MMA) membrane that conforms to the shape of the aggregate, and minimizes the polymer's contribution to the total transplant volume. Cell aggregates were coated at a liquid-liquid interface of a discontinuous density gradient composed of both aqueous and organic liquids. By increasing the viscosity difference and decreasing the density difference between the two liquids of the coating interface, coatings from approximately 1 to 15 μm thick were formed. Aggregates of HepG2 cells and pancreatic islets were coated and remained viable.**

## INTRODUCTION

Under hypoxic conditions, pancreatic islets have been shown to exhibit reduced insulin secretion.[1] Encapsulation of the tissue in a polymer designed to exclude the elements of the immune system contributes additional resistance to the diffusion of nutrients and cellular products, further decreasing the steady-state production rate of the cells, as well as increasing their response time to chemical stimuli.[2,3] Furthermore, the volume added by the membrane produces unrealistic total transplant volumes,[4–6] a problem which is appreciated more fully by the likely need to transplant $> 5 \times 10^5$ islets to control glycemia.[5]

Using smaller and thinner capsules should alleviate the aforementioned implications of immunoisolation; however, conventional microencapsulation processes rely on forming a droplet of cell suspension. Minimizing capsule size, therefore, depends on the ability to make small drops, and the fragility of mammalian cells appears to limit droplet formation to not less than 300–400 μm in diameter in most cases. In contrast, the final size of the capsules produced by the mechanism reported here depends directly on the size of the cell aggregate to be coated.

[a]Current address: Rimon Therapeutics. Ltd., 200 College St., Toronto, Ontario, Canada M5S 3E5; 416-978-3088 (voice); 416-978-8605 (fax); maymi@chem-eng.utoronto.ca (e-mail).

[b]Author to whom correspondence should be addressed: 416-978-3088 (voice); 416-978-8605 (fax); sefton@chem-eng.utoronto.ca (e-mail).

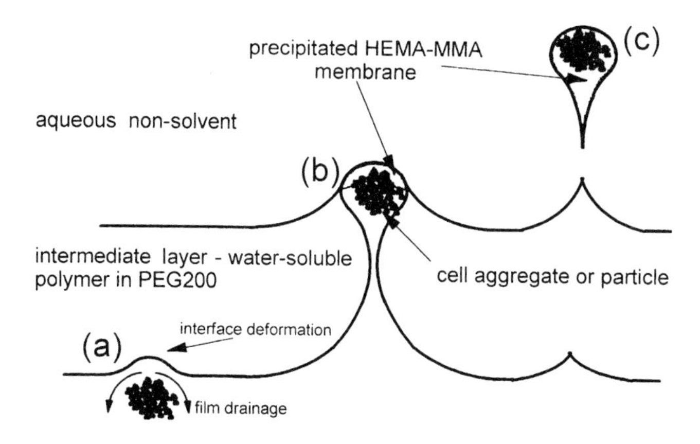


**FIGURE 1.** Schematic representation of the conformal coating mechanism: **(a)** approach of a particle to a liquid-liquid interface resulting in large interface deformation and entrainment of HEMA-MMA solution into the intermediate layer; **(b)** passage of the particle plus entrained HEMA-MMA solution into an aqueous non-solvent layer, where the thin film of polymer solution precipitates; **(c)** precipitation of the coating, detachment of the "tail" and recovery of the interfaces.

## CONFORMAL COATING AT A LIQUID-LIQUID INTERFACE

In its simplest form, the coating apparatus consists of three liquid layers: a polymer (HEMA-MMA) solution layer, an aqueous non-solvent layer, and an intermediate layer to prevent premature contact between the other two layers. Entrainment of polymer solution around small particles and cell aggregates occurred as they approached the interface between the HEMA-MMA solution and the intermediate layer during centrifugation as shown in FIGURE 1. Entrainment of HEMA-MMA solution depended on the balance between two processes: large deformation of the liquid-liquid interface by the approaching particles, and slow drainage of the thin film between the particles and the interface (FIG. 1a).[7–10] If the interfacial tension and specific gravity difference between the two liquids was relatively low, and the viscosity of the HEMA-MMA solution was much greater than the intermediate layer, interface deformation in the direction of the particle motion was extensive and drainage of the thin film between the particle and the interface was slow. If the particle plus entrained polymer solution reached the non-solvent layer (phosphate-buffered saline (PBS) in our case) before the HEMA-MMA solution drained from around the particle (FIG. 1b), then a membrane precipitated around the particle in the non-solvent layer (FIG. 1c). The volume of HEMA-MMA solution entrained depended on the "average" specific gravity of the particle plus entrained HEMA-MMA solution, which could not be greater than the specific gravity of the intermediate layer. Similarly, the coated bead would not pass into the precipitation layer, unless the "average" specific gravity of the coated particle was less than that of the aqueous non-solvent. Thus, the maximum possible coating thickness depended on the specif-

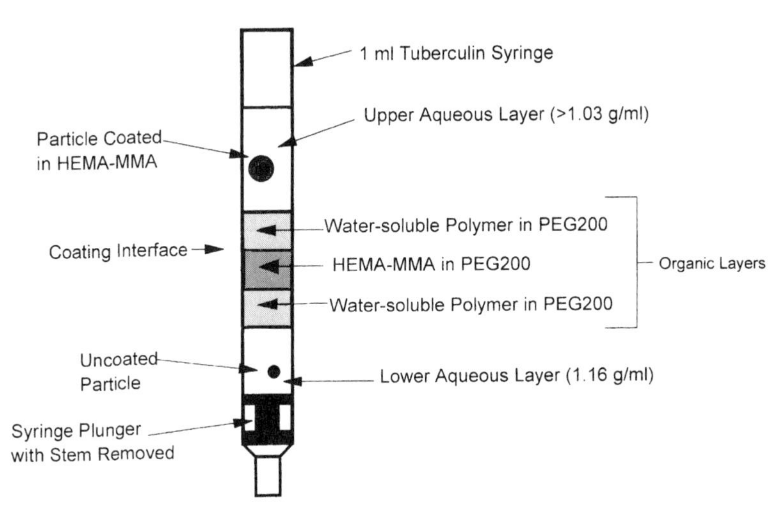


**FIGURE 2.** Schematic diagram of the conformal coating discontinuous density gradient. Representative specific gravities are shown for the upper and lower layers, which are aqueous solutions of glycerol in PBS. The middle layer is a solution of 5–20% (w/w) HEMA-MMA in PEG200. The other two intermediate layers are solutions of water-soluble polymers (e.g., PVP or PAA) in PEG200.

ic gravity of the precipitation layer; however, achieving this maximum thickness required slow drainage of the polymer solution.

The more complex coating apparatus needed to coat cell aggregates consisted of a discontinuous density gradient (ranging from 1.16 to 1.08 g/ml) composed of three organic layers surrounded by two aqueous layers (FIG. 2). Having aqueous layers at both ends of the gradient minimized cell exposure to the organic layers. Interface deformation by small particles with specific gravity near unity required that the interfacial tensions throughout the apparatus,[7] and especially at the coating interface,[9] were extremely low ($< 10^{-2}$–$10^{-3}$ dynes/cm), and that the gradient was centrifuged at greater than $100 \times g$. The former was achieved by using the same solvent, polyethylene glycol 200 (PEG200), for all three organic layers; PEG200 is a solvent for HEMA-MMA that can be tolerated by cells, at least to a limited extent, despite its non-aqueous nature.[11] The two organic layers between the HEMA-MMA layer and the aqueous layers were composed of solutions of polymers other than HEMA-MMA, which are soluble in water in addition to PEG200. Mixing of the organic layers was minimized, despite the low interfacial tensions, because the polymers tended to demix in the same way that multiphase aqueous systems are formed for biological separations.[12] In addition, changing polymer concentrations varied the specific gravities and viscosities of the layers; viscosity was also varied by using different polymer molecular weights. A silicone glycol copolymer DC193 from Dow Corning®, poly(vinyl pyrrolidone) (PVP) and poly(acrylic acid) (PAA) were suitable polymers for the intermediate organic layers.

## METHODS AND MATERIALS

Liquids were layered carefully in a 1.0 cc tuberculin syringe (Becton Dickinson, NJ) with a plunger, but with the stem removed. With cell aggregates in the top layer or polystyrene beads suspended in the bottom layer, the gradient was centrifuged at 100–500×*g* for 5 to 10 minutes. Coated beads or cell aggregates were removed from the gradient with a pasteur pipette into PBS or cell medium for further curing and subsequent analysis. The syringe was capped and then cut with centrifuge tube cutters to expose the bottom layer so that the coated cell aggregates could be removed.

Polystyrene beads (Polysciences, Warrington, PA) were coated using 3 of the 5 layers shown in FIGURE 2: approximately 200 beads (~120 μm in diameter and 1.04 g/ml) were suspended in 0.05 ml 15% (w/w) HEMA-MMA in PEG200 (BDH Chemicals, Toronto, Ontario), on top of which was layered 0.05 ml of 25% (w/w) PVP (Polysciences) (MW 2.5 kD) and 0.05 ml 40% (w/w) aqueous glycerol (BDH Chemicals) solution for thick coatings or 5% (w/w) PVP (360 kD) and 0.2 ml 30% (w/w) aqueous glycerol (BDH Chemicals) solution for thin coatings. Coated beads were viewed with a Zeiss (Zeiss, Oberkochen, Germany) inverted light microscope or freeze-dried and gold-coated prior to viewing with a Hitachi S520 scanning electron microscope (SEM).

HepG2 cells were cultured in suspension in 10 cm polystyrene petri dishes for 3–5 days and spontaneously formed 50–400 μm spheroids. For cell aggregate coating, the gradient was formed in a 1.0 cc tuberculin syringe and consisted of (from bottom to top): 0.3 ml of an aqueous solution consisting of 60% (w/w) glycerol, 0.05 ml 35% (w/w) PVP (MW 2.5 kD), 0.05 ml 10% (w/w) HEMA-MMA in PEG200, 0.05 ml pure PEG200, 0.2 ml α-MEM + antibiotics + 10% fetal bovine serum (prepared at the Tissue Culture Preparation Facility, University of Toronto, Toronto, Ontario) and 200–300 HepG2 cell aggregates (ATCC, Rockland, MD). Coated aggregates were fixed in 3.5% glutaraldehyde in 2% tannic acid in 0.1M Sorenson's phosphate buffer, freeze-dried, gold-coated, and examined under SEM.

Confocal scanning laser images were obtained by staining coated cells with 0.05 μg/ml ethidium homodimer and 0.25 μg/ml of calcein AM (both from Molecular Probes, Eugene, OR) for 30 minutes in cell medium and then rinsing twice with PBS. Images represent an optical cross-section through the center of the coated cell aggregates and were obtained using an MRC-600 confocal scanning laser microscope.

## RESULTS AND DISCUSSION

FIGURE 3a shows a thin HEMA-MMA coating around an approximately 300 μm diameter polystyrene bead (specific gravity ~1.05 g/ml). A small viscosity ratio ($\lambda$ ~ 6) and a relatively large density difference of 0. 02 g/ml at the coating interface resulted in a coating that was approximately 0.5 % the diameter of the bead (1.5 μm). The presence of a "tail" is an artifact of the entrainment/interface deformation mechanism and for the smallest particles or cell aggregates that we coated (20 μm), the tail was often the only indicator of the presence of a coating.

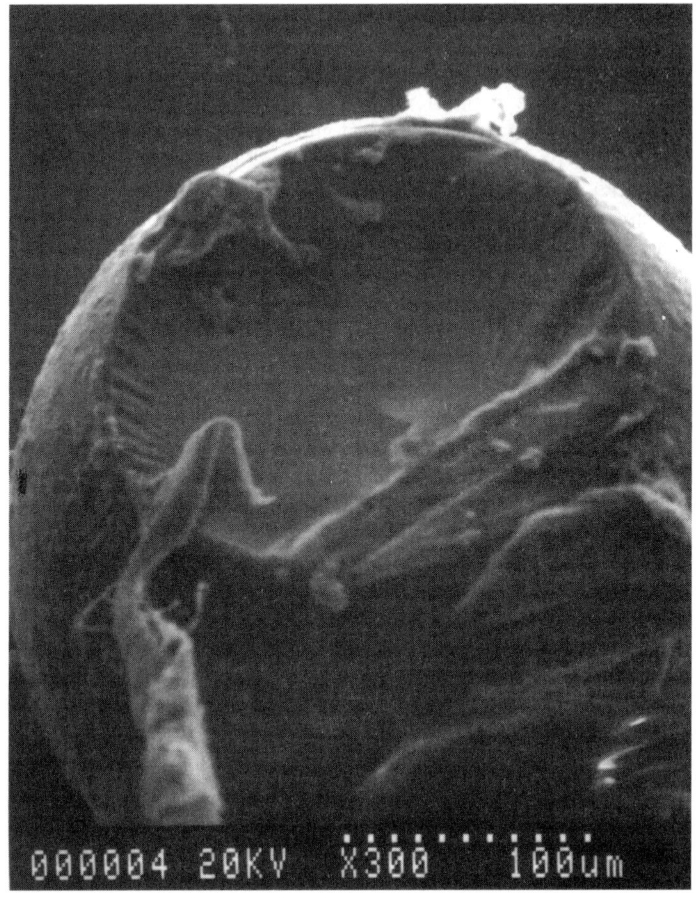


**FIGURE 3.** Conformally coated polystyrene beads as model cell aggregates: **(a)** (above) scanning electron micrograph of a ~300 μm diameter polystyrene bead coated with a ~1.5 μm conformal coating of HEMA-MMA using a 3-layer gradient; **(b)** a light micrograph showing a ~120 (m polystyrene bead with a ~15 μm thick coating.

FIGURE 3b shows a ~120 μm polystyrene bead with a much thicker coating of HEMA-MMA, ~15 % of the diameter of the uncoated bead, produced by increasing λ to ~30, decreasing the density difference at the coating interface 1 to 0.004 g/ml, and increasing the specific gravity of the precipitation layer.

FIGURE 4 shows two spherical HepG2 cell aggregates conformally coated in a single HEMA-MMA membrane. Individual cells of the aggregates are visible through a defect in the coating. FIGURE 5a shows the presence of a thin HEMA-MMA coating around viable HepG2 cell aggregates shortly after passage through the density gradient and exposure to the organic components. Coated rat islets (FIG. 5b) also appeared viable and secreted insulin afterwards (data not shown). Green fluorescence indicated the presence of metabolizing cells; red fluorescence revealed dead cells and indicated the presence of a HEMA-MMA coating.

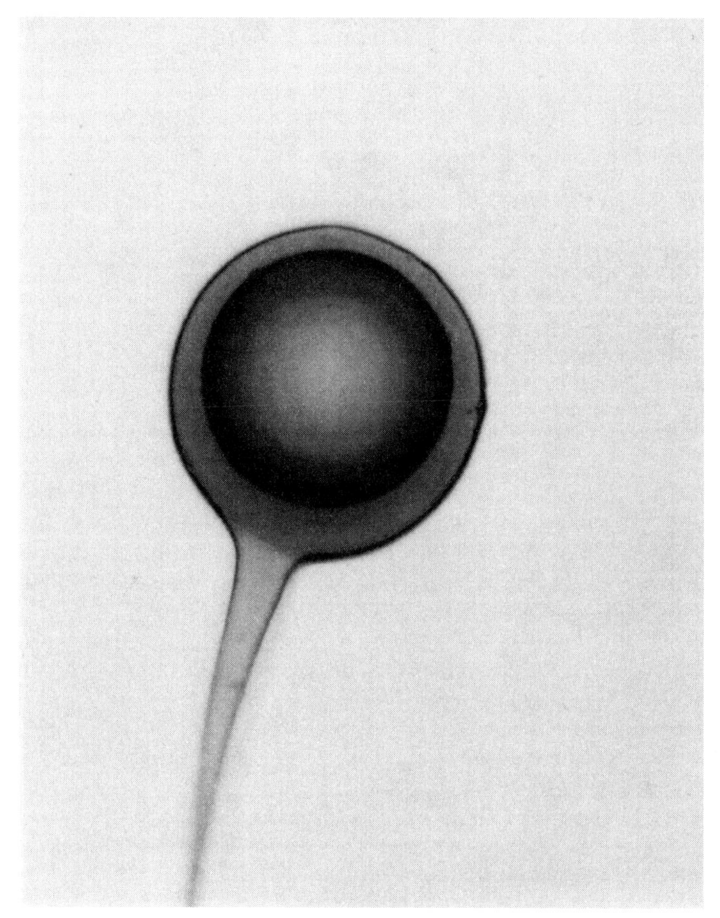

**FIGURE 3b.**

The gradient was modified to coat cells because their specific gravity increased (to > 1.18 g/ml) from exposure to PEG200. Consequently, cell aggregates were coated as they passed from the top of the gradient to the bottom, and the coating interface became the interface between HEMA-MMA solution and the lower intermediate layer. The increase in cell aggregate specific gravity indicated that the PEG200 solvent dehydrated the cell aggregates. The long-term effects on viability and function of this dehydration, as well as the rehydration that occurs in the precipitation layer, are being investigated.

HepG2 spheroids cultured for coating were relatively dense and tightly packed. The coating process, however, did not appear limited by minor differences in size, shape, or packing of the HepG2 cell aggregates or in the size of the islets that were coated; the process depended fundamentally on the presence of a "particle" to deform the coating interface. Tightly packed aggregates might resist dehydration be-

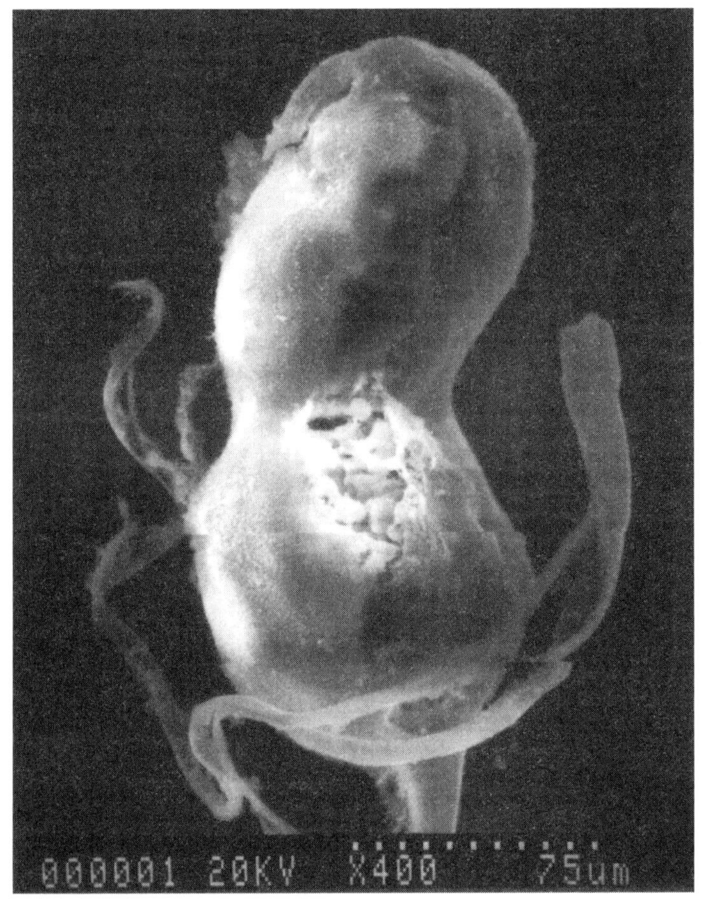


**FIGURE 4.** Scanning electron microscope image of a thin conformal coating around HepG2 cell aggregates.

yond the periphery of the aggregate more readily than less densely packed aggregates. As a consequence, exposure times to the organic layers of the gradient may have to be optimized for different cell types.

Sawhney *et al.*[13] developed a conformal coating process whereby multifunctional PEG-based macromers are photopolymerized outward from the surface of islets of Langerhans to any desired thickness. Zekorn *et al.*[6] reported on a method to coat islets in alginate using an aqueous discontinuous density gradient. Although the mechanism was not described, the presence of liquid-liquid interfaces in the Zekorn system, and tails on 30% of their coated islets, suggests that the islets were coated via the mechanism described here. Using alginate avoided the complexities of dealing with organic solvents in their gradient; however, as a natural polymer, alginate may be less stable *in vivo* and may have biocompatibility limitations.[14,15]

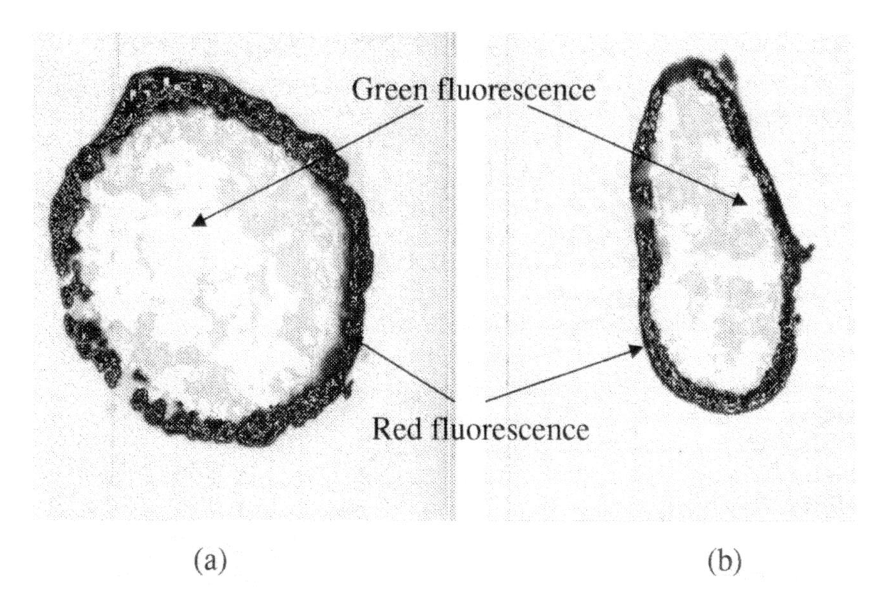


**FIGURE 5.** Confocal scanning laser microscope images of conformally coated (**a**) a HepG2 cell aggregate and (**b**) a rat islet, respectively, indicating that the cell aggregates are viable after being coated. Original colored image was digitized and converted to a grey-scale to permit publication.

It is not expected that the presence of tails on most of the coatings will affect the delivery of therapeutic biomolecules from the cells; it is possible, however, that the tails might reduce the biocompatibility of the coated tissue, or make implantation more difficult. In fact, coated cell aggregates or beads often clumped together after membrane precipitation owing to tail entanglement. It may be possible to minimize tailing by optimizing the interfacial tensions of the liquids of the gradient. A larger interfacial tension between the HEMA-MMA solution and the adjacent intermediate layer would induce "pinching" of the tail and drive the coating towards a spherical shape before precipitation.

Conformal coating at a liquid-liquid interface shows promise as a method to produce ultra-thin conformal coatings of synthetic polymers around small particles and cell aggregates, as well as bubbles and drops. Whether the membrane has the necessary permselectivity to isolate cells from the immune system or whether the coated cells maintain their functional attributes *in vivo* are under investigation.

## ACKNOWLEDGMENTS

We would like to thank Dr. Xijia Gu of the Ontario Laser and Lightwave Research Centre for his assistance with the confocal microscopy and Dr. Peter Zucker of the Islet Transplant Facility, University Hospital, London, Ontario, for supplying us with rat islets.

## REFERENCES

1. DIONNE, K., C. COLTON & M. YARMUSH. 1993. Effect of Hypoxia on insulin secretion by isolated rat and canine islets of Langerhans. Diabetes **42:** 12–21.
2. TZIAMPAZIS, E. & A. SAMBANIS. 1995. Tissue engineering of a bioartificial pancreas: modeling the cell environment and device function. Biotechnol. Prog. **11:** 115–126.
3. MAY, M. H. 1998. Conformal Coating of Mammalian Cells at a Liquid-Liquid Interface. Ph.D. Dissertation, University of Toronto.
4. CHICHEPORTICHE, D. & G. REACH. 1993. In vitro kinetics of insulin release by microencapsulated rat islets: effect of the size of the microcapsules. Diabetologia **31:** 54–57.
5. COLTON, C.K. & E.S. AVGOUSTINIATOS. 1993. Bioengineering in the development of the hybrid artificial pancreas. Trans. ASME **113:** 152–170.
6. ZEKORN, T., U. SEIBERS, A. HORCHER *et al.* 1992. Alginate coating of islets of Langerhans: in vitro studies on a new method for microencapsulation for immuno-isolated transplantation. Acta Diabetologia **29:** 41–45.
7. MARU, H.C., D.T. WASAN & R.C. KINTNER. 1971. Behaviour of a rigid sphere at a liquid-liquid interface. Chem. Eng. Sci. **26:** 1615-28.
8. HARTLAND, S. 1967. The approach of a rigid sphere to a deformable liquid/liquid interface. J. Colloid Interface Sci. **26:** 383–394.
9. GELLER, A.S., S. H. LEE & L.G. LEAL. 1986. The creeping motion of a spherical particle normal to a deformable interface. J. Fluid Mech. **169:** 27–69.
10. MANGA, M. & H.A. STONE. 1995. Low Reynolds number motion of bubbles, drops, and rigid spheres through fluid-fluid interfaces. J. Fluid Mech. **287:** 270–298.
11. CROOKS, C.A., J.A. DOUGLAS, R.L. BROUGHTON & M.V. SEFTON. 1990. Microencapsulation of mammalian cells in a HEMA-MMA copolymer: effects on capsule morphology and permeability. J. Biomed. Res. **24:** 1241–.
12. ALBERTSSON, P. 1986. Partition of cell particles and macromolecules. New York. John Wiley and Sons.
13. SAWHNEY, A.S., P.P. CHANDRASHEKHAR & J.A. HUBBELL. 1994. Modification of islet of Langerhans surfaces with immunoprotective poly(ethylene glycol) coatings via interfacial photopolymerization. Biotechnol. Bioeng. **44:** 383–386.
14. DE VOS, P., G.H.J. WOLTERS, W.M. FRITSCHY & R.V. VAN SCHILFGAARDE. 1993. Obstacles in the application of microencapsulation in islet transplantation. Int. J. Artif. Organs **16:** 205–212.
15. O'SHEA, G.M. & A.M. SUN. 1986. Encapsulation of rat islets of Langerhans prolongs xenograft survival in diabetic mice. Diabetes **35:** 943–946.

# New Multicomponent Capsules for Immunoisolation

ARTUR BARTKOWIAK,[a] LAURENCE CANAPLE,[b] ION CEAUSOGLU,[a] NATHALIE NURDIN,[a] ANDREAS RENKEN,[a] LORENZ RINDISBACHER,[a] CHRISTINE WANDREY,[a] BÉATRICE DESVERGNE,[b] AND DAVID HUNKELER[a,c]

[a]*Laboratory of Polymers and Biomaterials, Swiss Federal Institute of Technology, CH-1015 Lausanne, Switzerland*

[b]*Institut de Biologie Animale, Bâtiment de Biologie, University of Lausanne, CH-1015 Lausanne, Switzerland*

**ABSTRACT: A new generation of microcapsules based on the use of oligomers which participate in polyelectrolyte complexation reactions has been developed. These freeze-thaw stable capsules have been applied as a bioartificial pancreas and have resulted in normoglycemia for periods of six months in concordant xenotransplantations. The new chemistry permits the control of permeability and mechanical properties over a wide range and can be adapted both to microcapsule and hollow fiber geometries rendering it a robust tool for encapsulation in general. Methods, and metrics, for the characterization of the mechanical properties and permeability of microcapsules are presented.**

## INTRODUCTION

Bioartificial organ research has been targeted at several hormone deficiencies and neurodegenerative conditions such as Parkinson's disease, Alzheimer's disease and Huntington's chorea as well as in the control of chronic pain and human growth factors. The encapsulation of hepatocytes for the production of a bioartificial liver and the development of artificial skin are other emerging applications. However, bone marrow transplantation is the only cellular transplantation technique that is currently clinically practiced, although limited clinical trials have been performed with a bioartificial pancreas.

A bioartificial organ involves the immunoisolation of mammalian cells[d] in order to provide a steric selectivity to the ingress and egress of various molecules. Semipermeable polymeric membranes have been developed with the aim of permitting the transplantation of xenogenic cells from species with a large phylogenic separation from humans, thus removing the need for immunosuppression therapy. Although several biologically active species have been encapsulated or immobilized, and the techniques generally have potential for the treatment of diseases requiring enzyme or endocrine replacement, this chapter will focus on the microencapsulation. of non-dividing mammalian cells. In particular, the immunoisolation of pancreatic islets for the treatment of diabetes mellitus will be discussed. In general, microcap-

[c]Corresponding author. The names of the first 7 authors are in alphabetic order.

[d]An exception to this categorization is "bioartificial" skin, though the seeding of cells on a polymer construct is more appropriately termed "tissue engineering."

sules avoid the problems of coagulation and vascular anastomoses associated with hollow fiber (macroencapsulation) devices[1] owing to a lack of blood contact.

### *The Bioartificial Pancreas Problem*

Steady state normoglycemia cannot be achieved through daily treatments with extracorporeal insulin. Therefore, the development of a bioartificial pancreas, over the past two decades, has been centered on the belief that tightly regulated glucose homeostasis can only be achieved by transplantation of Langerhans islets. It may ultimately be that genetically engineered cell lines present alternatives to massive islet isolation and banking. However, this, at present, is not a viable solution. Ethical and political considerations are also likely to hinder the implementation of devices based on genetically modified cells.

A permselective polymeric membrane must permit the diffusion of oxygen (hypoxia leads to a reduction in the metabolic effectiveness of islets) and glucose to the islet as well as the exodiffusion of the insulin hexamer, with a nominal molar mass of 36 kD. Additionally, the barrier must sterically exclude larger molecules such as immunoglobulins. To achieve glucose homeostasis requires rapid insulin delivery (< 15 minutes)[2] in response to a glucose challenge. Evidently the polymers that contact the islets must be noncytotoxic, while the polymers contacting the physiological fluid should be 'biocompatible'. The latter definition is site specific and still a matter of debate. For example, immunoprivileged sites with blood-tissue barriers, such as the eye, brain and testes, also exist. The possibility of providing a local immunomodulation via cell co-culture and coencapsulation, for example with growth factors, is under investigation. Furthermore, the partial pressure of oxygen differs at various locations within the body (~40 mmHg intraperitoneally versus ~100 mmHg intravascularly),[2] influencing the long-term functioning of transplants. Zekorn *et al.*[3] have suggested that there are three components to consider in the biocompatibility of a microencapsulated islet: i) the reaction of the entrapped islets to the polymer and method of encapsulation, ii) the reaction of the recipient to the device (the so-called foreign body reaction), and iii) the reaction of the recipient against the encapsulated islets. Certainly, immunoisolation is less problematic, and the encapsulation more viable, if allogenic tissue is used in place of xenogenic cells. However, allogenic tissue sources are limited, particularly for diabetes where the demand is high.

Unfortunately, humans have high levels of IgM and IgB antibodies that could be directed against expressed xenoantigens found in likely tissue donors (porcine, bovine).[4] Cytotoxic events may occur if specific antibodies pass through the membrane. However, the chemical structure and purity of the polymer employed, as well as the encapsulation process itself, also contribute to cytotoxicity. Therefore, the cytotoxic response observed *in vivo*, can be the result of variables controlled during the encapsulation process, including the reagent quality and toxicity of residual solvents. Additionally, the viability of microencapsulated islets depends on the host, even in the absence of active rejection mechanisms. The polymeric membrane is also sensitive to the surrounding media, which influence capsules swelling, shrinking and integrity through the osmotic pressure. Furthermore, larger capsule diameters, and larger volumes of encapsulated tissue, are suspected to enhance the necrosis that can occur at the center of the capsule due to reduced oxygen mass transfer. Therefore, the development of a bioartificial pancreas comprises multidimensional problems concerning biocompatibility, permselectivity and specific mechanical requirements. Since most biocompatible materials, such as poly(ethylene oxide), have very poor mechanical properties, blending is likely required in order to obtain the threshold of 0.5 Newtons that Dautzenberg *et al.* have proposed for the safe handling of capsules.[5]

### *Polymeric Biomaterials*

A recent review has evaluated the types of material and encapsulation technologies employed in the development of the bioartificial pancreas.[6] Other than some innovative chemistries introduced by Sefton[7] and Dautzenberg,[8] who respectively employ phase inversion and complex coacervation to form the capsular membranes, the overwhelming majority of the literature over the past two decades has utilized the alginate/poly-L-lysine system. While Sun, who pioneered this chemistry,[9] was successful, originally in rodents and more recently in larger animal discordant xenografts, many authors have failed to repeat his results. This is likely due to the batch-to-batch variabilities in the molar mass, viscosity and chemical composition of the alginates employed. Indeed, there is a strong debate as to whether the alginate purity or mannuronic/guluronic acid ratio controls the immunogenecity of the capsule.

From a clinical perspective, three critical problems remain unresolved: i) the lack of a reproducible means for islet, or encapsulated islet, banking,[e] ii) the lack of an off-the-shelf technology for cellular encapsulation, and iii) the batch-to-batch irreproducibility of polysaccharides utilized as biomaterials. In parallel, clinicians require proven systems (capsules and biological materials) so that issues such as the volume of site of the implant and number of islets transplanted can be statistically evaluated. While xenotransplantation using the alginate/poly-L-lysine capsule may provide an alternative, first to auto- and allografts and ultimately in xenotransplantation, the medical risk is large if a single material chemistry is retained. Patients are likely to develop responses to any foreign material over the five decades they typically contract diabetes, and alternative implant chemistries would be desirable for various patients. For these reasons a large-scale screening of polyelectrolyte complexation was carried out with the aim of identifying alternative systems to the alginate/poly-L-lysine chemistry which offered equal or improved mechanical properties, sterilizability, lack of islet/cell cytotoxicity and biocompatibility.[12]

The screening study revealed that a variety of naturally occurring polymers, including carboxymethylcellulose, carrageenans, cellulose sulfate, gellan and xanthan were suitable for islet contacting applications. Furthermore, of the 1235 polyelectrolyte pairs investigated (35 polyanions and 40 polycations), 47 were found to provide mechanically stable microcapsules. While this list provided a promising number of alternatives to Sun's classical system, the combination of two high molar mass polymers continued to present a tradeoff between permeability and mechanical properties. Prokop *et al.*[13] subsequently developed a multicomponent microcapsule comprised of two inner polyanions, cellulose sulfate to provide a network structure, and alginate to control the droplet rheology. In addition to simple electrolytes (sodi-

[e]Although Rajotte[10] and Sun[11] developed methods to freeze and thaw islets while maintaining yields as high as 97%, their technique has not been successfully reproduced by others.

um and calcium chloride), which influence permeability and gelation respectively, an oligomeric cation was used to form a thick membrane (on the order of 100 μm) which acted as an immunoisolation barrier. This capsule has been shown, using rat xenografts, to reverse diabetes in both chemically induced and spontaneously diabetic mice for periods of 120 and 180 days, respectively. Although the permeability of the multicomponent capsule can be controlled,[14] the range of manipulation is somewhat limited. There is additional concern as to the ultimate cytotoxicity of cellulose sulfate and the leaching out of the oligocation, poly(methylene-co-guanidine), which may induce a specific foreign body reaction.

The various polymers employed in the multicomponent capsule act as rheology modifiers and to produce the capsule network, with mechanical properties optimized by appropriately blending the components. Recently the authors of this paper have shown that a simple two component capsule can be used based on a high molar mass polyelectrolyte and an oligomer of the opposite charge.[17] By appropriately degrading the oligomer to a controlled molar mass,[15] capsules can be produced with optimum mechanical properties and a molar mass cutoff (MMCO) variable between 0.5 and 300 kD. The properties of this capsule, relative to the multicomponent system, is the topic of this chapter. A discussion of metrics for the mechanical characterization and permeability of microcapsules will also be presented.

## EXPERIMENTAL

### *Materials*

Alginate (Keltone HV, Kelco/NutraSweet, San Diego, CA, USA), iota-carrageenan (Fluka, Buchs, Switzerland) and cellulose sulfate (CS: Across Organics, Geel, Belgium) were purified by ultrafiltration with hollow-fibers with a MMCO of 30 kDa. Poly(methylene-co-guanidine) hydrochloride (PMCG: 35% aqueous solution) was purchased from Scientific Polymer Products. Inc. (Ontario, NY, USA) and used without any further purification. Polycation solutions contained 1.2% PMCG dissolved in an aqueous solution containing 1.0 % $CaCl_2$ and 0.9% NaCl. The polyanion solution consisted of 0.5% alginate mixed with either 0.5% of cellulose sulfate in 0.9% NaCl or iota-carrageenan in deionized water (Millipore, MILLI-Qplus, Model PF). Samples of oligochitosan with different molar masses were obtained in controlled radical degradation of chitosan by hydrogen peroxide.[15]

### *Capsule Preparation*

Multicomponent capsules of various diameters were formed by dropping an aqueous polyanion solution into a polycation receiving bath. The standard reaction time was 3 minutes, for capsules on the order of 2 mm, though this was varied as part of the experimental design. Following the reaction, capsules were isolated from polycation solution on the stainless steel screen grid and washed several times with a 0.9% NaCl solution. Calcium removal, and core liquefaction, with a 0.05 M sodium citrate solution were carried out for 15 minutes prior to a final washing with the 0.9% NaCl. All experiments were performed at room temperature. FIGURE 1 shows a photo of an islet within a multicomponent capsule based on alginate/cellulose sul-

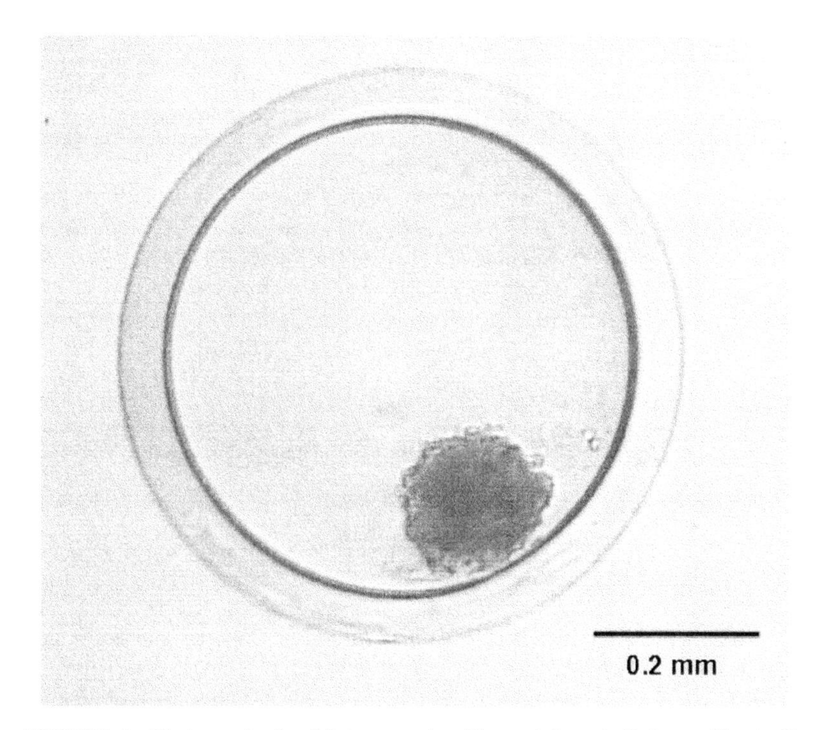


**FIGURE 1.** Photograph of an islet encapsulated in an alginate/cellulose sulfate/sodium chloride/calcium chloride/poly(methylene-co-guanidine) capsule. The capsule diameter is 650 μm.

fate/poly(methylene-co-guanidine). In order to vary the membrane thickness of the multicomponent capsules, a procedure outlined in TABLE 1 was followed. Sodium chloride was added to all solutions to minimize the osmotic stress during capsule formation.

The novel oligocapsules were prepared by polyelectrolyte complexation.[17] Capsules were formed from a pair of oppositely charged polyelectrolytes, where a 1% aqueous sodium alginate solution, in deionized water, was added dropwise to the complexation bath containing 1% of an oligochitosan in water (molar mass varied between 1–40 kD). The reaction time was adjusted from few minutes up to 1 hour to control permeability. For the mechanical strength optimization the capsules were collected after a reaction time of 30 minutes. Further details are available on polymer degradation[15] and capsule preparation.[17]

### *Permeability Measurements*

Two mL of empty capsules were placed in a 10 mL recipient bath. Two mL of a 0.1% polymer standard, in 0.9% NaCl, was added under agitation. Aliquots were withdrawn at various times and injected into a liquid chromatograph equipped with a Shodex SB-803 HQ column and a Shodex SB-G guard column. The eluent was

**TABLE 1.** Summary of multicomponent capsule reaction conditions and preparation procedures

| Condition/Procedure | Specifications |
|---|---|
| Anionic Polymer Blend | 0.6% Alginate (Keltone HV: Kelco Chemical Company, UK)<br>0.6% Cellulose Sulfate, Batch A006986201<br>(Acros Organics, Geel, Belgium) |
| Receiving Bath | Solution 1: 1.0% $CaCl_2$ + 0.9% NaCl<br>Solution 2: 1.2% PMCG + 0.9% NaCl<br>The pH was adjusted to 7.0 using 0.1 M NaOH. |
| Atomization | Syringe G 27¾, bevel tip<br>(Becton Dickinson, Drogheda, Ireland) |
| Washing Steps | 2 washing steps with 0.9% NaCl solution prior to Sodium Citrate treatment and 3 times at the end of the procedure |
| Citrate Treatment | 15 min. in 0.05 M Sodium Citrate |
| Procedure | Atomization of polyanion blend into solution 1 during 30 s.<br>Reaction in solution 1 for 5 min<br>Various reaction times (1–7 min) in solution 2, washing steps<br>Citrate treatment for 15 min, washing steps |

0.9% NaCl applied at a flow rate of 0.5 mL/min. The polymer concentration was proportional to the height of the detected chromatographic peak. The radii of gyration Rg were calculated from molar masses (MM) according to the formulae:

Rg = 0.015 MM0.495 for dextran [14]
Rg = 0.026 MM0.550 for pullulan[14]
Rg = 0.0255 MM0.56 for polyacrylamide[22]

Molar mass cutoffs were also estimated by gel electrophoresis. Fifty µL of a mixture containing protein standards were suspended in 500 mL of 0.6% alginate/0.6% cellulose sulfate solution in PBS and capsules were formed as described in TABLE 1. The capsules were placed in 400 mL of 0.9% NaCl solution. Fifty mL of the medium were collected at different times and heated in 1 × SDS gel loading buffer. The samples were then separated on 8% SDS polyacrylamide in Tris-glycine buffer. Gels were then stained with Coomassie Brilliant Blue R-250. The radius of gyration Rg of the proteins was calculated according to the following formula[14]: $Rg = 0.051\ MM^{0.378}$.

### *Mechanical Characterization*

Capsules were tested on a Texture Analyzer (TA-2xi, Stable Micro Systems, Godalming, UK). The apparatus consists in a mobile probe moving vertically, up or down, at a constant velocity. The capsules were placed in a 0.9% NaCl solution and the test speed was 0.1 mm/s. The capsules had an average size of 1.9 mm diameter and were compressed until bursting occurred. The force exerted by the probe on the capsule was recorded as a function of the displacement (compression distance), therefore leading to a force vs. strain curve. Thirty capsules per batch were analyzed in order to obtain statistically relevant data.

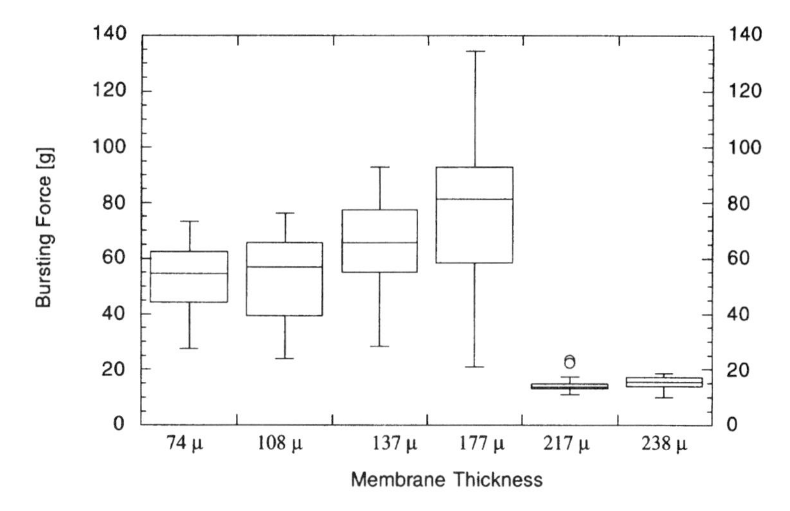


**FIGURE 2.** Box plot for the comparison of bursting forces of capsules with differing wall thicknesses. The average capsule size was 1.9 mm.

## RESULTS AND DISCUSSION

### *Mechanical Properties*

The mechanical properties of the multicomponent microcapsules have been found to be independent of capsule diameter, at least for capsules above 1 mm (data not shown). The bursting force was however determined to be quite sensitive to the membrane thickness as is shown in FIGURE 2, with thicker membranes improving the mechanical resistance, as would be expected. The data in FIGURE 2 are represented by a box plot. The horizontal lines within the boxes represent the median values of the specific observation and the limits of the box are given by the upper and lower quartiles. The box, therefore, represents 50% of the data. The bars are delimited by the maximum and minimum values whereas the circles represent extremes. The multicomponent capsules had a high impact resistance while maintaining their elasticity. They are "soft" in their behavior, deforming rather than rupturing following an applied force. This is contrary to the alginate/poly-L-lysine capsules, which tend to rupture catastrophically above a critical load that is lower than the bursting force of the multicomponent system described herein.

Above a maximum membrane thickness (in this case $d_m > 177$ μm) capsule mechanical resistance drops dramatically, a situation that is rather unexpected. The origin of this phenomenon cannot yet be explained, although a thermodynamic cause may be postulated. Indeed, component demixing may occur at longer reaction times due to the inhomogeneity of the original alginate/CS bead. In the absence of alginate, cellulose sulfate reacts with PMCG to form a white precipitate. The alginate chains provide a network, spacing the CS chains and avoiding precipitation. However, due to the formation of inhomogeneous beads with higher network density on

**TABLE 2.** Capsule permeability as measured by the ingress of the polymer standards and egress of protein standards from alginate/cellulose sulfate/ poly(methylene-co-guanidine)/ $cacl_2$ capsules

| Polymers | Molar Mass (kDa) | Rg (nm) | % of Diffusion (Ingress) into Capsules after 3 h |
|---|---|---|---|
| Dextran | 15 | 3.0 | 28 |
| | 70 | 6.5 | 24 |
| | 110 | 8.3 | 0 |
| Pullulans | 22.9 | 3.7 | 30 |
| | 95.3 | 8.2 | 12 |
| Polyethyleneoxide | 25 | — | 14 |
| | 92 | — | 4 |
| Polyacrylamide | 21.9 | 6.9 | 34 |
| | 79.0 | 14.0 | 21 |
| **Proteins** | **Molar Mass (kDa)** | **Rg (nm)** | **Diffusion (Egress) from the Capsules after 3 h** |
| Ovalbumin | 45.0 | 2.9 | Yes |
| Bovine Serum Albumin | 66.2 | 3.4 | Yes |
| Rabbit Muscle Phosphorylase B | 97.4 | 3.9 | Yes |
| β-galactosidase | 116.25 | 4.2 | Yes |
| Rabbit Muscle Myosin | 200.00 | 5.1 | No |

the bead surface, the spacing of CS chains in the center of the particle may be insufficient to prevent the precipitation reaction with PMCG. This would explain the precipitate-like structure observed in thick walled capsules, the higher opacity of the capsules and the increase in the observed wall thickness without further mechanical improvements. The weakening of the capsules could be explained by a thermodynamic demixing of the wall forming polymers which lowers the elasticity, though this requires further investigation.

### *Permeability*

TABLE 2 summarizes the permeability measurements on the multicomponent alginate/cellulose sulfate/poly(methylene-co-guanidine) capsules. Clearly, with a variety of synthetic and naturally occurring probes of different molar masses and radii of gyration, a true molar mass cutoff is observed at 90 kD. That is to say that for polyacrylamide, polyethyleneoxide, dextran and pullulan of the same molar mass, but different coil sizes, the membrane appeared to offer the same permeability characteristics. The gel electrophoresis tests with globular proteins revealed a slightly higher MMCO than observed by chromatography. In this case the sphericity of the proteins certainly facilitated their pore passage. The results illustrate that the permeability of capsules can be accurately determined by using both polymer influx and efflux of encapsulated biologically relevant molecules. The authors believe that both

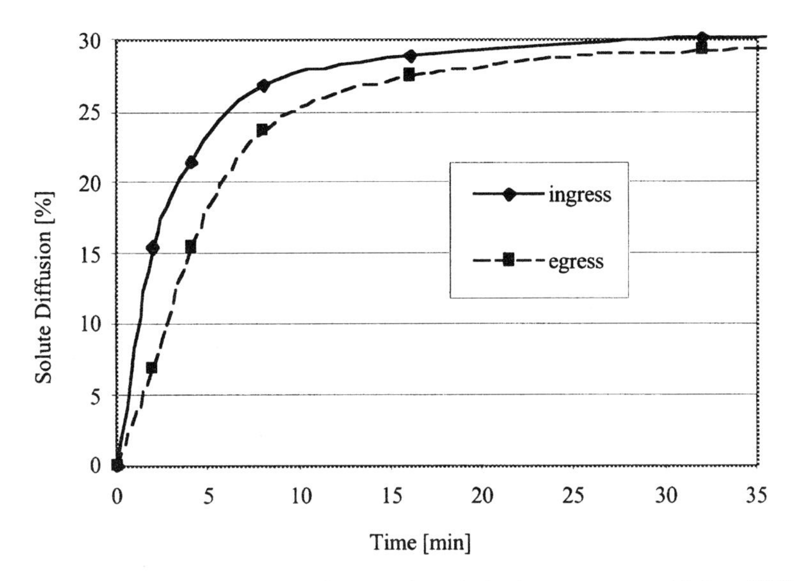


**FIGURE 3.** Glucose ingress and egress through the iota-carrageenan/alginate/PMCG capsule membrane. The capsules were prepared with a reaction time of 3 minutes.

the chromatography and gel electrophoresis methods provide reasonable metrics which can, and will be, correlated with *in vivo* performance and survival of a xenograft.

### *Novel Capsule Chemistries*

The standard multicomponent capsule chemistry based on an alginate/cellulose sulfate blend[16] has been modified through the replacement of the structure forming polyanion with iota-carrageenan. Carrageenans tend to create gels in the presence of mono- and divalent metal cations due to a coil-to-double-helix transition. Therefore, in order to control the osmotic pressure during the capsule formation process, a small molecule such as mannitol is recommended. FIGURE 3 illustrates that, using glucose as a probe, the ingress and egress are not the same for the carrageenan-based multicomponent capsule, with the initial diffusion kinetics (ingress) approximately two times faster, likely due to a larger external surface area. More significantly, the permeability of these capsules is quite sensitive to the reaction time[f] (FIG. 4), with longer reactions providing a more dense network and a lower molar mass cut-off.

A binary alginate-oligochitosan system has also been developed[17] based on polyelectrolyte complexation. An advantage of the use of oligochitosan, relative to other patents in the literature[19–21] is the fact that membrane formation can occur over more physiological pH ranges (up to pH of 7.6). In comparison, higher molar mass chito-

[f]The permeability of carrageenan-based multicomponent capsules is more sensitive to reaction parameters then for those derived from alginate.

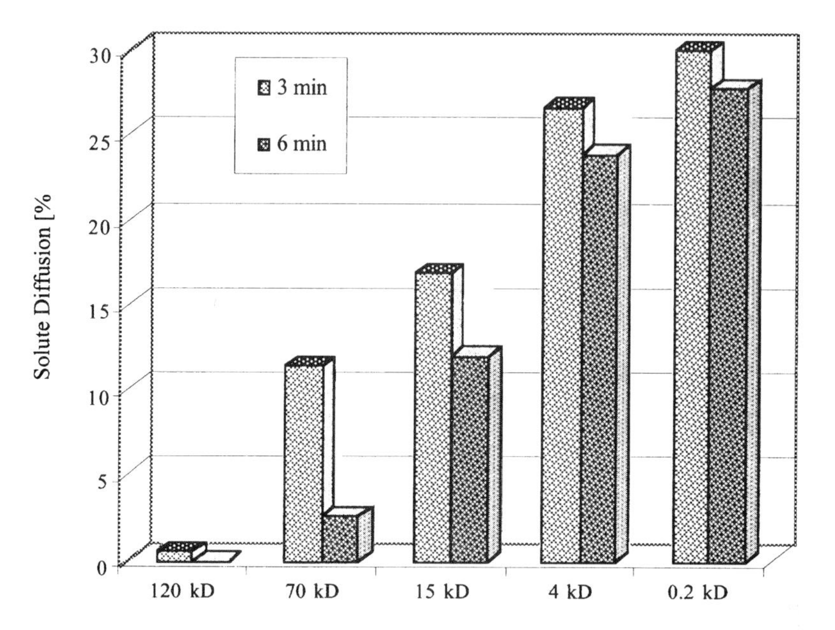


**FIGURE 4.** Diffusion of glucose and dextrans of different molar mass through the iota-carrageenan/alginate/PMCG capsule membrane. The ingress was measured after a contact time of 32 minutes.

san is insoluble at pH's above 6.6, limiting the application for certain bioartificial organs as well as some biotechnology applications. Figure 1 from Bartkowiak and Hunkeler (p. 39 of this volume) illustrates that the mechanical behavior of such capsules are optimized at a molar mass of approximately 2000 daltons, far below the region typically employed for microencapsulation. The *in vivo* testing of these binary capsules is presently in progress.

## CONCLUSIONS

A new capsule chemistry based on polyelectrolyte complexation with an oligomeric component permits the decoupling of mechanical properties from permeability. These freeze-thaw stable microcapsules (data not shown) have been applied in islet immunoisolation to provide normoglycemia for periods of up to six months in concordant xenografts. The simultaneous control of permeability and mechanical properties provides a robust, non-toxic sterilizable material for encapsulation of various cell types including genetically modified cell lines. The chemistry is unique in that it can be applied both in spherical microcapsules or in hollow fibers.

Future developments in the bioartificial pancreas are likely to be derived from advances in biology and materials interface. Clinical auto- and allografts of encapsulated islets will almost certainly precede cellular xenotransplantation. In order to evaluate the efficacy of such transplants the development of valid *in vitro* metrics which correlate with *in vivo* performance will be required. Ultimately the optimal transplantation site as well as the role of vascularization will have to be evaluated in light of the risks involved in major surgery and the desire for implant recoverability.

## REFERENCES

1. SEFTON, M.V. & L. KHARLIP. 1994. *In* Pancreatic Islet Transplatation III: Immunoisolation of Pancreatic Islets. R.P. Lanza & W.L. Crick, Eds.: 107–117. R.G. Landes Co.
2. COLTON, C. 1996. Trends Biotechnol. **14:** 158.
3. ZEKORN, T.D.C., *et al.* 1996. Int. J. Artif. Organs **19:** 251.
4. MORRIS, P.J. 1996. Trends Biotechnol. **14:** 163.
5. DAUTZENBERG, H., B. LUKANOFF, U. ECKERt, B. TIERSCH & U. SCHULDT. 1996. Ber. Bunsenges. Phys. Chem. **100:** 1045.
6. HUNKELER, D. 1997. Trends Polym. Sci. **5:** 286.
7. SEFTON, M.V. 1989. Can. J. Chem. Eng. **67:** 705.
8. DAUTZENBERG, H., F. LOTH, K. POMMERENING, K.-J. LINOW & D. BARTSCH. 1984. UK Patent 2 135 954 A.
9. LIM, F. & A.M. SUN. 1980. Science **210:** 908.
10. RAJOTTE, R.V., Z. AO, G.S. KORBUTT, J.R.T. LAKEY, M. FLASHNER, C.B. COLBY & G.L. WARNOCK. 1995. Transplant. Proc. **27:** 6.
11. INABA, K., D. ZHOU, B. YANG, I. VACEK & A.M. SUN. 1996. Transplantation **61:** 175.
12. PROKOP, A., D. HUNKELER, S. DIMARI, D. HARALSON & T. WANG. 1998. Adv. Polym. Sci. **136:** 1.
13. PROKOP, A., M. HUNKELER, A.C. POWERS, R.R. WHITESELL & T. WANG. 1998. Adv. Polym. Sci. **136:** 53.
14. BRISSOVA, M., M. PETRO, I. LACIK, A.C. POWERS & T. WANG. 1996. Analytical Biochem. **242:** 104–111.
15. BARTKOWIAK, A., CH. WANDREY & D. HUNKELER. Second International Symposium on Polyelectrolytes, Inuyama, Japan, 31 May–3 June, 1998.
16. WANG, T., I LACIK, M. BRISSOVA, A. ANILKUMAR, A. PROKOP, D. HUNKELER, R. GREEN, K. SHAHROKHI & A.C. POWERS. 1997. Nature Biotechnol. **15:** 358.
17. BARTKOWIAK, A. & D. HUNKELER. 1998. UK Patent Application no. GB-A-9814619.4.
18. WANG, T.G. 1988. Artif. Organs **22**(1)**:** 68–74.
19. DAUTZENBERG, H., F. LOTH, J. POMMERENING, K.-J. LINOW & D. BARTSCH. 1984. UK Patent Application no. 2 135 954 A.
20. RHA, C., & D. RODRIGEZ-SANCHEZ. 1988. US Patent no. 4,744,933.
21. DALY, M.M., R.KEOWN & D.W. KNORR. 1989. US Patent no. 4,808,707.
22. GRIEBEL, T. & W.M. KULICKE. 1992. Makromol. Chem. **193:** 811.

# Encapsulation for Somatic Gene Therapy

PATRICIA L. CHANG[a]

*Departments of Biology and Pediatrics, McMaster University, Hamilton, Ontario, Canada*

**ABSTRACT: With the human genome project approaching its completion date of 2005, gene-based technology will play an increasingly important role in health-care delivery. Non-autologous somatic gene therapy is a novel application in which non-autologous cell lines engineered to secrete a recombinant protein are enclosed within immunoisolation devices and implanted into all patients requiring the same product for therapy. The development of this technology requires a multi-disciplinary effort towards optimization of the biomaterial used to manufacture the implantable devices and selection of the appropriate cell lines for enclosure. The efficacy of this technology is illustrated in the treatment of dwarfism and lysosomal storage disease in murine models. The potential of a safe and cost-effective gene-based delivery method should have wide applications in treating both classical genetic disorders and non-Mendelian diseases.**

## INTRODUCTION

Since the first human gene therapy clinical trial took place in 1990,[1] the number of patients enrolled and trials approved have increased exponentially. There are over 3000 patients enrolled world-wide and almost 300 human clinical trials have been approved.[2] Such activities attest to the momentum of this new direction in health-care towards a gene-based technology.

According to the FDA, human gene therapy is defined as a medical intervention based on the alteration of genetic material of living cells in humans. Currently, there are primarily two approaches to altering cells genetically in humans: *in vivo* and *ex vivo*.[3] Through the *in vivo* method, favored in 60% of the clinical trials, new genetic material in the form of viral vectors or plasmid DNA encoding the desirable genes is introduced directly into the patient's tissue *in situ*. Subsequent uptake of the genetic material into tissues such as liver or muscle may result in expression of the recombinant product. The advantage of this method is that it is usually a benign procedure and simple to administer. However, some of the earlier problems of transient and low level expression are still to be resolved, and there is also a relative lack of understanding of the cellular and molecular controls underlying such events.

The second approach to introducing genetic material is by way of *ex vivo* routes. Cells (e.g., lymphocytes, bone marrow cells, fibroblasts), are explanted from the patient, expanded in culture, and genetically modified *in vitro* before implantation back to the patients. The advantage of this approach is that cells are optimally modified

[a]Address for correspondence: Department of Pediatrics, Health Sciences Centre Room 3N18, McMaster University, 1200 Main Street West, Hamilton, Ontario L8N 3Z5 Canada; 905-521-2100 ext. 3716 (voice); 905-521-1703 (fax); changp@fhs.mcmaster.ca

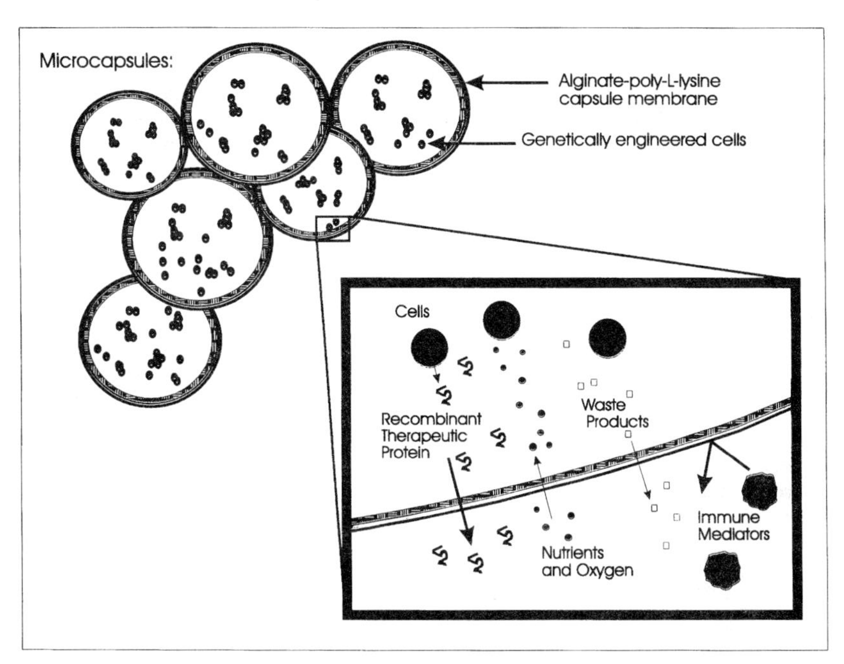


**FIGURE 1.** Immune isolation in gene therapy. Genetically engineered recombinant cells are enclosed in immuno-protective alginate microcapsules whose permeability permits exit of recombinant proteins and exchange of nutrients and wastes, but excludes immune mediators from the host. (From Stockley & Chang,[10] reproduced with permission.)

and characterized *ex vivo* before implantation, but problems in the lack of sustained and high level expression, and the labor-intensive nature of the manipulation are significant. This approach accounts for about 40% of all the current human clinical trials.

In our laboratory, we have developed a third approach to gene therapy. Our "nonautologous somatic gene therapy" approach relies on the implantation of "universal" recombinant cell lines protected in immunoisolation devices to deliver a therapeutic gene product.[4] Cell lines genetically engineered to secrete a desired gene product are enclosed in immunoprotective devices, thus allowing such nonautologous cells to be implanted into any host to deliver the desired gene product without triggering graft rejection. The primary requirement is that such devices must have a permeability threshold that allows transit of nutrients and recombinant products, while prohibiting entry of the host's immune mediators, such as the complement system and lymphocytes, owing to their larger molecular sizes (FIG. 1).

The advantages of this nonautologous method of gene delivery are: 1) it does not require chemical purification of the gene product, an often daunting task in terms of labor and cost; 2) it does not require modification of the host's genome, thus providing additional measures of safety and cost-saving; and 3) it provides ample material for quality assessment before implantation, a safety feature not available to most other forms of delivery.

**TABLE 1.** Delivery of heterologous recombinant product with various types of biomaterial implants

| Immunoisolation Device | Protein Delivered | Encapsulated Cell Type | Implanted Animal | Targeted Disease | Ref. |
|---|---|---|---|---|---|
| Alginate-Poly-L-lysine-alginate microcapsules | β-glucuronidase | murine fibroblast | mucopolysaccharidosis VII mice | lysosomal storage diseases | 39 |
| | factor IX(h) | murine myoblasts | C57BL/6 mice | hemophilia | 28 |
| | growth hormone(m) | murine myoblasts | dwarf mice | hypopituitarism | 29 |
| | growth hormone(h) | canine myoblasts | dogs | hypopituitarism | 41 |
| | urease(k) | *E. coli* DH5α | uremic Wistar rats | kidney failure | 42 |
| Barium-alginate capsules | growth hormone(h) | canine myoblasts | dogs | hypopituitarism | 41 |
| Barium-Poly-L-lysine-alginate capsules | growth hormone(h) | canine myoblasts | dogs | hypopituitarism | 41 |
| PAN/PVC hollow fiber | nerve growth factor(h) | rat fibroblasts | Lesioned Sprague Dawley rats | neurodegenerative disorders | 9 |
| Polyethersulfone(PES) hollow fiber | ciliary neurotrophic factor(h) | baby hamster kidney cells | humans | Amyotrophic lateral sclerosis | 43 |
| | erythropoietin(h) | murine myoblasts | DBA/2J mice fisher rats | anemia | 44 |
| | nerve growth factor(h) | baby hamster kidney cells | Rhesus monkeys | Alzheimer | 45 |

NOTATION: h = human, m = murine, k = K. aerogens. (Reproduced from Chang *et al.*,[46] 1999, with permission.)

## SCIENTIFIC ISSUES

### *Biomaterial*

The basic requirements of the immunoisolation device are that it must be biocompatible, mechanically stable, and able to provide a suitable environment for the recombinant cells to survive and secrete a therapeutic product.[6,7] While numerous biomaterials have been studied for the purpose of immunoisolation, e.g., alginate,[8] acrylic hollow fibers,[9] hydroxyethyl methacrylate-methyl methacrylate,[7] polyphosphazene,[11] agarose,[12] etc., none has been shown to be totally ideal. Different geometrical configurations have been constructed from these materials, including spherical microcapsules, diffusion chambers and hollow fibers. Microcapsules offer advantages in their ease of implantation and effective geometry for fluid exchange, whereas diffusion chambers and hollow fibers permit easy manipulation and device containment once implanted. Among the microcapsules, alginate is the most widely used material since it is well-characterized,[13] easy to fabricate into microcapsules,[14] and biocompatible. However, because alginate is a naturally occurring polysaccharide composed of alternating blocks of D-mannuronic acid and α-L-guluronic acid,[15] the varying proportion of these residues among different samples can alter its properties. Alginate with a high guluronic acid content is mechanically more stable with greater affinity to divalent cations.[16,17] Some studies have shown that mannuronic acid elicit an immune reaction,[18,19] whereas other studies have concluded that the response is due to impurities[20] and that microcapsules made with a high guluronic acid content may actually predispose those capsules to fibrotic reaction.[21,22] Nevertheless, a variety of immunoisolation devices fabricated from various polymers, including alginate, have been explored as vehicles to deliver transgene products secreted from genetically engineered cells (TABLE 1).

### *Recombinant Cells*

For cells to be useful for the delivery of therapeutic recombinant gene products within immunoisolation devices, they should have several important properties: robust proliferative potential necessary for gene transfection and expansion *in vitro*, capability to produce and secrete the transgene product, and the ability to exhibit stable transgene expression after encapsulation. While also dependent on the vector constructed to encode the transgene, many established cell lines do fulfill these requirements. However, a more difficult condition to meet is that these cells should also be able to differentiate terminally. Withdrawing from the cell cycle would prevent continued proliferation and over-crowding of cells within the capsular space. Otherwise this would lead to nutrient depletion and apoptosis. An added advantage of using cells which terminally differentiate is safety. The risk of a proliferative cell line becoming tumorigenic is significantly reduced when cells do not undergo further mitosis.[5]

Although early studies on the delivery of recombinant products with fibroblasts were successful in demonstrating the feasibility of this approach with immunoisolation devices, e.g., delivery of human growth hormone,[6,23,24] adenosine deaminase,[25] insulin,[26] coagulation factor IX,[27]and neural growth factor,[9] these cells clearly were not ideal for long-term survival as they cannot exit the cell cycle in order to differentiate. In contrast, myoblasts are proliferative cells that do possess this important property. They can be transfected *in vitro*, and express and secrete transgene products, but are also capable of differentiating terminally into myotubes, circumventing the problem of continued proliferation and overcrowding of cells within immunoisolation devices.[4] This differentiation capability allows for long-term viability of the encapsulated cells[28] without the problem of continued proliferation and overcrowding within the capsular space, as evident with microencapsulated fibroblasts.[23] Even though the biology of myoblast differentiation within implantable devices has not been well elucidated,[5] microencapsulated recombinant myoblasts have successfully delivered transgene products including growth hormone,[29,30] human factor IX,[28] and ciliary neurotrophic factor.[31]

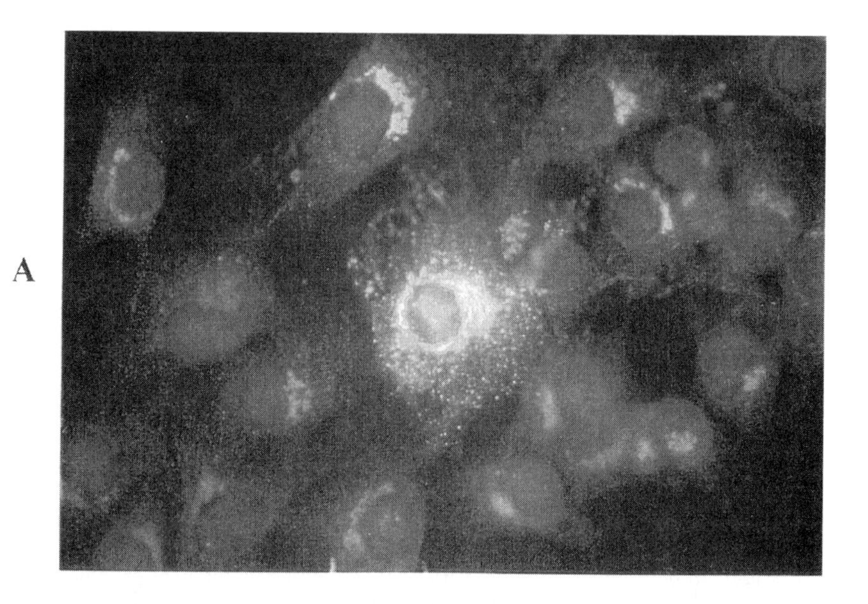


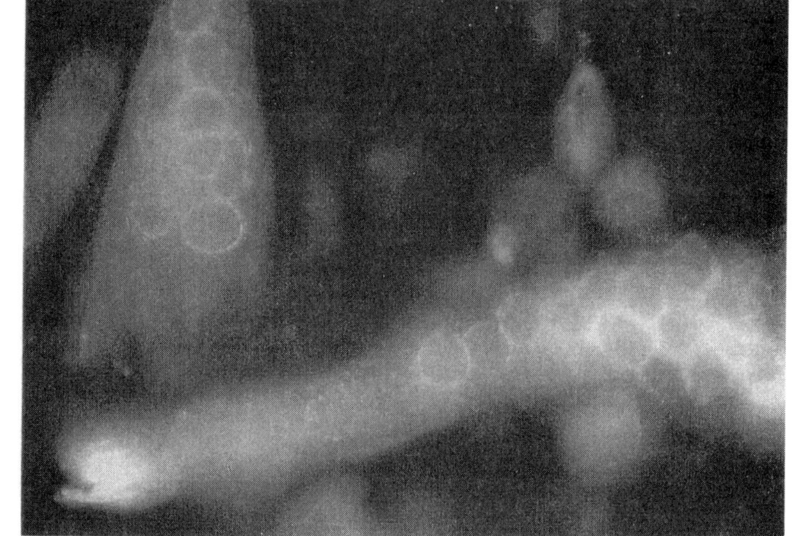


**FIGURE 2.** Differentiation of recombinant myoblasts into myotubes. Mouse C2C12 myoblasts (**A**) expressing the transgene product, human growth hormone, localized with fluorescent immuno-staining, are clearly distinguishable from the fused myotubes (**B**) showing the multi-nucleated syncytium. Magnification: 630×. (From Chang & Bowie,[5] reproduced with permission.)

The differentiation of murine C2C12 myoblasts (engineered to secrete human growth hormone) on a morphogenic level, from mononucleate myoblasts to a multi-

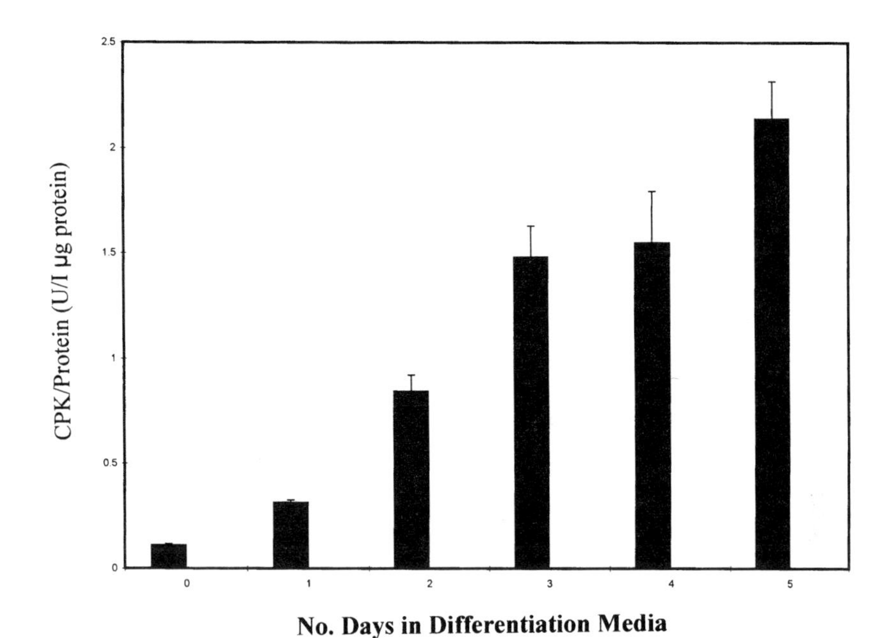


**FIGURE 3.** Up-regulation of creatine phosphokinase activity during differentiation of myoblasts into myotubes. Mouse C2C12 myoblasts were cultured in differentiation-inducing media. Creatine phosphokinase activity was assayed on various days following the exposure. (From Chang & Bowie, [5] reproduced with permission.)

nucleate myotube upon cell fusion, is illustrated in FIGURE 2. This differentiation event is accompanied by marked increase in the production of various differentiation-specific enzymes. Examples of enzyme systems which change dramatically during the course of differentiation include phosphoglycerokinase, glycogen synthetase, glycogen phosphorylase, and creatine phosphokinase (CPK), although none of these is produced exclusively in muscle tissue.[32] The rapid increase in CPK activity in differentiating transfected C2C12 myoblasts upon exposure to differentiation-inducing media is often taken to be a marker of differentiation (FIG. 3). CPK is a good indicator of myoblast differentiation and fusion as its activity is up-regulated tremendously in myotubes, whereas in non-committed myoblasts, it is expressed at a very low basal level similar to that seen in non-muscle tissues.

In addition to the enzymes, genes encoding structural and contractile proteins, such as desmin, actin, myosin, troponin and tropomyosin, are transcriptionally activated during muscle differentiation. FIGURE 4 depicts the pattern of up-regulation in some of these muscle-specific genes during the differentiation of transfected C2C12 myoblasts. The rise in muscle-specific regulatory gene expression (e.g., myogenin) as well as genes encoding structural and/or contractile proteins (e.g., Troponin I slow) is evident. The differentiation of mammalian myoblasts into mature myotubes depends upon the up-regulation of various muscle-specific genes, enzymatic systems and extensive changes in cell morphology.[33] It is important to note that throughout such differentiation-specific changes, the expression of the transgene

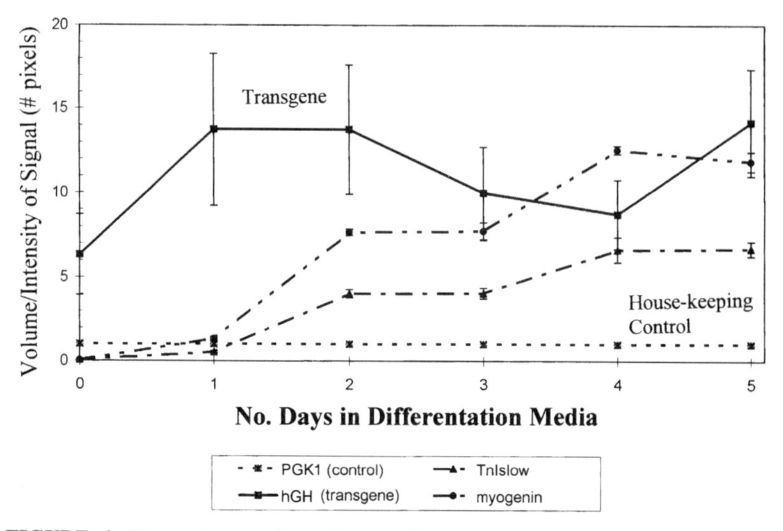


**FIGURE 4.** Up-regulation of muscle-specific transcripts during differentiation of myoblasts into myotubes. Mouse C2C12 myoblasts transfected to express the transgene, human growth hormone, were exposed to differentiation-inducing media. On various days after the exposure, total RNA was extracted, probed for the various transcripts with dot blotting, and quantified with phosphoimaging. The transgene and the house-keeping control (phosphokinase I) transcripts were expressed at a constitutive level throughout but the differentiation-specific transcripts (myogenin and troponin I slow) were clearly elevated during differentiation. (From Chang & Bowie,[5] reproduced with permission.)

(human growth hormone) remained constitutive and persistent. This is clearly an important attribute if such a myoblast-myotube "organoid" is to be useful for gene product delivery.

### *Preclinical Studies*

The most obvious therapeutic application of nonautologous somatic gene therapy is to treat well-characterized classical Mendelian disorders caused by deficiency of single gene products. The first "proof of principle" of the clinical efficacy of this technology was obtained by treating growth retardation in the Snell dwarf mice. These mutant mice suffer from an autosomal recessive form of dwarfism due to a mutation of the *pit-1* transcription factor,[34] which down regulates the secretion of various pituitary hormones including growth hormone. As a result, the body size of the dwarf mutant is only about 30% of that of the unaffected litter mate (FIG. 5, Al-Hendy and Chang, unpublished data). After implantation of microcapsules containing myoblasts engineered to secrete mouse growth hormone, the treated animals showed increased growth of all the appropriate target organs, including most of the internal organs, muscle mass, and bone growth plate. By 35 days post-implantation, both the length and body weight were increased by >20%, a visually detectable difference from the sham-treated litter mates.[29] This work demonstrated not only the clinical efficacy of this technology, but also the ability of intraperitoneally delivered

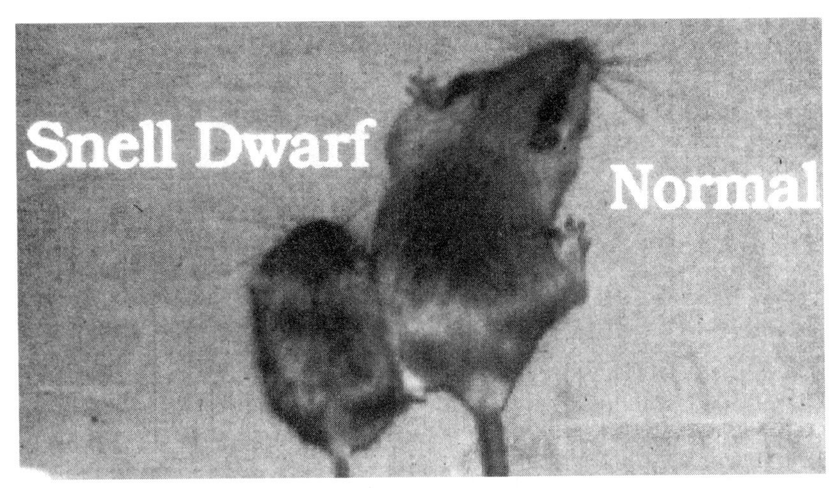


**FIGURE 5.** The Snell dwarf mouse. The Snell dwarf mouse (*left*) suffers from an autosomal recessive mutation causing deficient growth hormone secretion. Its body size is hence reduced to about 30% of that of its normal littermate (*right*).

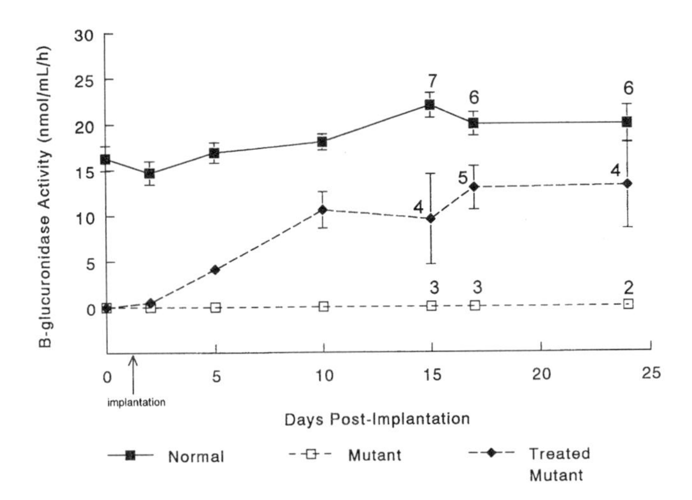


**FIGURE 6.** Delivery of a lysosomal enzyme, β-glucuronidase, from microencapsulated cells to the plasma. Alginate microcapsules enclosing mouse fibroblasts secreting mouse β-glucuronidase were implanted intraperitoneally into the mutant Gus/Gus mice suffering from the enzyme deficiency. At various days post-implantation, plasma from the normal and mutant controls and treated mutants was assayed for the enzyme activity. The dramatic increase in the enzyme activity to about 50% of normal activity provided a level of correction consistent with that of heterozygous carriers which are clinically normal. (From Bastedo *et al.*,[47] reproduced with permission.)

heterologous proteins to effect changes in target organs distant from the implantation site. It proves that product transfer from the microcapsules through the systemic cir-

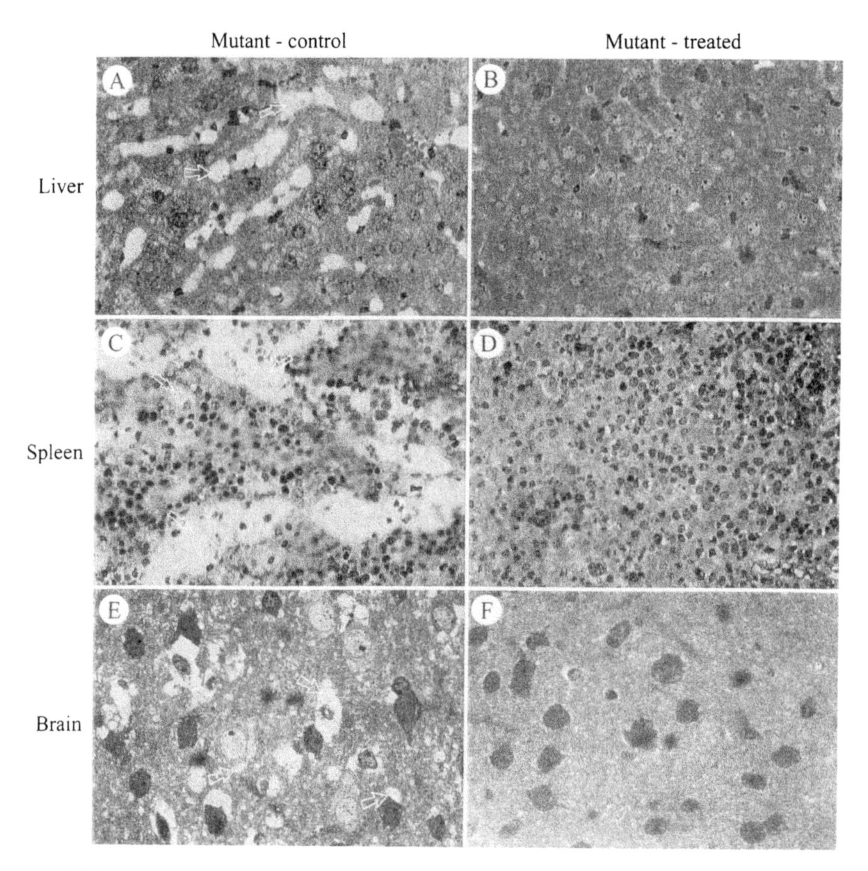


**FIGURE 7.** Correction of the pathological lysosomal inclusions in tissues of the mutant mice. After intraperitoneal (**B** and **D**) or intraventricular (**F**) implantation of microcapsules enclosing cells secreting β-glucuronidase, the pathognomonic lysosomal inclusions containing undegraded glycosaminoglycans (*open arrows*) in the mutant mice largely disappeared from the various organs. Tissues were processed for resin embedding and toluidine-blue staining. Original magnification of **A–D** is 160× and of **E–F** is 1000×. (From Ross & Chang,[39] reproduced with permission.)

culation is a realistic goal. The results are particularly remarkable, considering the half-life of growth hormone in circulation is only in the order of minutes. The transfer must have occurred efficiently and rapidly after the hormone was released from the microcapsules to elicit such dramatic response.

There are genetic disorders with more devastating consequences, however, that are in great need of therapy. An example is the lysosomal storage diseases. These are heritable genetic disorders due to the deficiency of any one of the >30 lysosomal enzymes.[35] In the more severe forms, patients suffer from total neurodegeneration resulting in a vegetative state and early death. Unfortunately, there is no general treatment available, and gene therapy is being considered as the treatment with the most potential.[36] The efficacy of the microencapsulation technology has now been shown in the treatment of one of these forms of lysosomal storage disease in a murine model. The $gus^{mps}/gus^{mps}$ mice provide a model of human mucopolysaccharidosis type VII.[37] This disease is a subgroup of hereditary lysosomal storage disorders resulting from an inability to degrade glycosaminoglycans due to failure in producing the lysosomal enzyme, β-glucuronidase. The glycosaminoglycans accumulate in the lysosomes of various organs, including the liver, heart and brain.[38] After the implantation of microencapsulated cells engineered to secrete the missing enzyme, correction at both the biochemical (FIG. 6) and pathological (FIG. 7) levels was observed in the peripheral organs. The plasma level of the enzyme was increased to normal range and the lysosomal storage granules were largely cleared from the peripheral organs. Even more exciting, our laboratory has shown that implantation of these microcapsules into the lateral ventricles of affected mice to bypass the blood brain barrier leads to a clearing of lysosomal accumulations even in the brain (FIG. 7). More importantly, this treatment was able to correct the abnormal circadian rhythms characteristic of the mutant mice, thus showing promise that behavioral and cognitive deficits can be reversed in this very severe neurodegenerative disease (see review by Ross and Chang[39]).

## CONCLUSIONS

As the Human Genome Project may be completed even ahead of the previously projected date of 2005, a new era of gene-based technologies is evolving. The concept of using genes as templates, and immunoisolated cells as microreactors to produce heterologous recombinant products has now been proven in practice.[46] The therapeutic areas in which this technology can be applied have yet to be explored fully. In addition to classical Mendelian genetic disorders, non-Mendelian conditions such as cancer or cardiovascular and systemic diseases are also potential targets. Microencapsulation of recombinant cells provides a platform technology for a wide variety of therapeutic applications, and such cost-effective means of gene product delivery will help to realize some of the potentials of biotechnology in the coming decades.

## ACKNOWLEDGMENTS

The development of this program has been supported by the following agencies: Medical Research Council of Canada, NSERC, Canadian Red Cross, Canadian Hemophilia Society, and Ontario Mental Health Foundation. The author is particularly indebted to the many graduate and post-doctoral trainees and colleagues who have helped to make this development possible and their contributions have been acknowledged in our related publications.

## REFERENCES

1. BLAESE, R.M., K.W. CULVER, A.D. MILLER, *et al.* 1995. T lymphocyte-directed gene therapy for ADA$^-$ SCID: initial trial results after 4 years. Science **270:** 475–480.

2. MARCEL, T. & J.D. GRAUSZ. 1997. The TMC Worldwide Gene Therapy Enrollment Report, End 1996. Hum. Gene Ther. **8:** 775–800.
3. POTTER, M.A. & P. L. CHANG. 1998. Gene Therapy in Pediatrics—Executive Summary. Drug News & Perspectives. Drugs of Today **34:** 759–766.
4. CHANG, P. L. 1995. Non-autologous somatic gene therapy. *In* Somatic Gene Therapy. P.L. Chang, Ed.: 203–224. CRC Press, Inc. Boca Raton, FL.
5. CHANG, P.L. & K.M. BOWIE. 1998. Development of engineered cells for implantation in gene therapy *In* Advanced Drug Delivery Reviews—Special Issue on Tissue Engineering, W. M. Saltzman & J. A. Hubbell, Eds. Elsevier Ltd. Ireland. **33:** 31–43..
6. CHANG, P.L., G. HORTELANO, M. TSE & D.E. AWREY. 1994. Growth of recombinant fibroblasts in alginate microcapsules. Biotechnol. Bioeng. **43:** 925–933.
7. TSE, M., H. ULUDAG, M.V. SEFTON & P.L. CHANG. 1993. Secretion of recombinant proteins from hydroxyethyl methacrylate-methyl methacrylate capsules. Biotechnol. Bioeng. **51:** 271–280.
8. O'SHEA, G., M. GOOSEN & A. SUN. 1984. Prolonged survival of transplanted islets of Langerhans encapsulated in a biocompatible membrane. Biochim. Biophys. Acta **804:** 133–136.
9. HOFFMAN, D., X.O. BREAKEFIELD, M.P. SHORT & P. AEBISCHER. 1993. Transplantation of a polymer-encapsulated cell line genetically engineered to release NGF. Exp. Neurol. **122:** 100–106.
10. STOCKLEY, T.L. & P.L. CHANG. 1997. Nonautologous somatic gene therapy: a novel approach to drug delivery. Drug News & Perspectives **10:** 331–340.
11. CARMEN BANO, M., S. CHEN, K.B. VISSCHER, H.R. ALLCOCK & R. LANGER. 1991. A novel synthetic method for hybridoma cell encapsulation. Biotechnology **9**(5): 468–471.
12. AOMATSU, Y., H. IWATA, T. TAKAGI, Y. AMEMIYA, H. KANEHIRO, M. HISANAGA, T. FUKUOKA & H. NAKANO. 1992. Microencapsulated Islets in agarose gel as bioartificial pancreas for discordant xenotransplantation. Transplant. Proc. **24**(6): 2922–2923.
13. SMIDSROD, O., & G. SKJAK-BRAEK. 1990. Alginate as immobilization matrix for cells. Trends Biotechnol. **8**(3): 71–78.
14. SUN, A. 1988. Microencapsulation of pancreatic islet cells: a bioartificial endocrine pancreas. Meth. Enzym. **137:** 575–579.
15. MARTINSEN, A. 1990. Alginates as Immobilization Materials—A Study of Some Molecular and Functional Properties. Ph.D. thesis, Trondheim Institute for Biotechnology. Trondhein, Norway.
16. MARTINSEN, A., G. SKJAK-BRAEK & O. SMIDSROD. 1989. Alginate as immobilization material: I. Correlation between chemical and physical properties of alginate gel beads. Biotechnol. Bioeng. **33:** 79–89.
17. THU, B.J. 1996. Alginate Polycation Microcapsules: A Study of Some Molecular and Functional Properties Relevant to Their Use as a Bioartificial Pancreas. Ph.D. Thesis, Department of Biotechnology, Norwegian University of Science and Technology.
18. SOON-SHIONG, P., M. OTTERLIE, G. SKJAK-BRAEK, O. SMIDSROD, R. HEINTZ, R.P. LANZA & T. ESPEVIK. 1991. An immunologic basis for the fibrotic reaction to implanted microcapsules. Transplant. Proc. **23**(1): 758–759.
19. OTTERLEI, M., K. OSTGAARD, G. SKJAK-BRAEK, O. SMIDSROD, P. SOON-SHIONG & T. ESPEVIK. 1991. Induction of cytokine production from human monocytes stimulated with alginate. J. Immunotherapy **10:** 286–291.
20. KLOCK, G., A. PFEFFERMAN, C. RYSER, P. GROHN, B. KUTTLER, H.J. HAHN & U. ZIMMERmann. 1997. Biocompatibility of mannuronic acid-rich alginates. Biomaterials **18**(10): 707–713.
21. ZIMMERMANN, U., G. KLOCK, K. FEDERLIN, K. HANNIG, M. KOWALSKI, R.G. BRETZEL, A. HORCHER, H. ENTENMANN, U. SIEBER & T. ZEKORN. 1992. Production of mirogen-contamination free alginates with variable ratios of mannuronic acid to guluronic acid by free flow electrophoresis. Electrophoresis **13**(5): 269–274.

22. De Vos, P, B. De Haan & R. Van Schilfgaarde. 1997. Effect of the alginate composition on the biocompatability of alginate-polylysine microcapsules. Biomaterials **18**(3): 273–278.
23. Chang, P.L., N. Shen & A.J. Westcott. 1993. Delivery of recombinant gene products with microencapsulated cells in vivo. Hum. Gene Ther. **4:** 433–440.
24. Tai, I.T. & A.M. Sun. 1993. Microencapsulation of recombinant cells: a new delivery system for gene therapy. FASEB **7:** 1061–1069.
25. Hughes, M., A. Vassilakos, D.W. Andrews, G. Hortelano, J.W. Belmont & P.L. Chang. 1994. Delivery of a secretable adenosine deaminase through microcapsules —A Nov
26. Taniguchi, H., K. Fufao & H. Nakauchi. 1997. Constant delivery of proinsulin by encapsulation of transfected cells. Surg. Res. **70:** 41–45.
27. Liu, H.W., F.A. Ofosu, & P.L. Chang. 1993. Expression of human factor IX by microencapsulated recombinant fibroblasts. Hum. Gene Ther. **4:** 291–301.
28. Hortelano, G., A. Al-Hendy, F. A. Ofosu & P. L. Chang. 1996. Delivery of human factor IX in mice by encapsulated recombinant myoblasts: a novel approach towards allogeneic gene. Blood **87:** 5095–5103.
29. Al-Hendy, A., G. Hortelano, G. S. Tannenbaum & P. L. Chang. 1995. Correction of the growth defect in dwarf mice with nonautologous microencapsulated myoblasts—an alternative approach to somatic gene therapy. Hum. Gene Ther. **6:** 165–175.
30. Al-Hendy A, G. Hortelano, G.S. Tannenbaum & P.L. Chang. 1996. Growth retardation—an unexpected outcome from growth hormone gene therapy in normal mice with microencapsulated myoblasts. Hum. Gene Ther. **7:** 61–70
31. Delgon, N., B. Heyd, S.A. Tan, J.M. Joseph, A.D. Zurn & P. Aebisher. 1996. Central nervous system delivery of recombinant ciliary neurotrophic factor by polymer encapsulated differentiated C2C12 myoblasts. Hum. Gene Ther.**7:** 2135–2146.
32. Shainberg, A., G. Yagil & D. Yaffe. 1971. Alterations of enzymatic activities during muscle differentiation *in vitro*. Develop. Biol. **25:** 1–29.
33. Mangan, M.E. & J.B. Olmsted. 1996. A muscle-specific variant of microtubule-associated protein 4 (MAP4) is required in myogenesis. Development **122:** 771–781.
34. Lin, C., S.-C.Lin, C.-P. Chang & M. Rosenfeld. 1992. Pit-1-dependent expression of the receptor for growth hormone releasing factor mediates pituitary cell growth. Nature **360:** 765–768.
35. Gieselmann, V. 1995. Lysosomal storage diseases. Biochim. Biophys. Acta Mol. Basis Dis.**1270:** 103–136.
36. Beutler, E. 1993. Gaucher disease as a paradigm of current issues regarding single gene mutations of humans. Proc. Natl. Acad. Sci. USA **90:** 5384--390.
37. Birkenmeier, E.H., M.T. Davisson W.G. Beamer, R.E. Ganschow, C.A. Vogler, B. Gwynn, K.A. Lyford, L.M. Maltais & C.J. Wawrzyniak. 1989. Murine mucopolysaccharidosis type VII—characterization of a mouse with β-glucuronidase deficiency. J. Clin. Invest. **83:** 1258–1266.
38. Sly, W.S., B.A. Quinton, W.H. McAlister & D.L. Rimoin. 1973. β-glucuronidase deficiency: report clinical, radiologic, and biochemical features of a new mucopolysaccharidosis. J. Pediatr. **82:** 249–257.
39. Ross, C.J.D. & P.L. Chang. 1999. Microencapsulation—a novel gene therapy for lysosomal storage diseases. *In* Handbook of Cell Encapsulation and Therapeutics. Springer-Verlag. In press.
40. Chang, P. L. 1997. Microcapsules as bio-organs for somatic gene therapy. Ann. N.Y. Acad. Sci. **831:** 461–473.
41. Peirone, M., K. Delaney, J. Kwiecin, A. Fletch & P.L. Chang. 1998. Delivery of recombinant gene product to canines with nonautologous microencapsulated cells. Hum. Gene Ther. **9:** 195–206.
42. Prakash, S., & T.M.S. Chang. 1996. Microencapsulated genetically engineered live *E. coli* DH5 (cells admininstered orally to maintain normal plasma urea level in uremic rats. Nat. Med. **2:** 883–889

43. Aebischer, P., M. Schluep, N. Deglon, J.-M. Joseph, L. Hirt, B. Heyd, M. Goddard J.P. Hammang, A.D. Zurn, A.C. Kato, F. Regli & E.E. Baetge. 1996. Intrathecal delivery of CNTF using encapsulated genetically modified xenogeneic cells in amyotrophic lateral sclerosis patients. Nat. Med. **2**(6)**:** 696–699.
44. Rinsch, C., E. Regulier, N. Deglon, B. Dalle, Y. Beuzard & P. Aebischer. 1997. A gene therapy approach to regulated delivery of erythropoietin as a function of oxygen tension. Hum. Gene Ther. **8:** 1881–1889.
45. Kordower, J.H., S.R. Winn, Y-T. Liu, E.J. Mufson, J.R. Sladek, J.P. Hammang, E.E. Baetge & D.F. Emerich. 1994. The aged monkey forebrain: rescue and sprouting of axotomized basal forebrain neurons after grafts of encapsulated cells secreting human nerve growth factor. Proc. Natl. Acad. Sci. USA **91:** 10898–10902.
46. Chang, P.L., J.M. Van Raamsdonk, G. Hortelano, S.C. Barsoum, N.C. MacDonald & T.L. Stockley. 1999. The in vivo delivery of heterologous proteins by microencapsulated cells. TIBECH **17:** 78–84.
47. Bastedo, L., M.S. Sands, B. Hortelano, A. Al-Hendy & P.L. Chang. 1994. Partial correction of murine mucopolysaccharidosis VII with micro-encapsulated nonautologous recombinant fibroblasts. Am. J. Hum. Genet. **55:** A211.

# Review—The Use of Immunosuppressive Agents to Prevent Neutralizing Antibodies Against a Transgene Product

MURRAY A. POTTER[a] AND PATRICIA L. CHANG[b–d]

[a]*The Departments of Medical Biochemistry,* [b]*Biology , and* [c]*Pediatrics, McMaster University, Hamilton, Ontario L8N 3Z5 Canada*

**ABSTRACT: A potential obstacle to successful gene therapy for some patients is the *in vivo* production of neutralizing antibodies against the recombinant therapeutic product delivered. This is a problem inherent to all gene therapy methods, regardless of the vector used to deliver the protein. This clinical situation can be mimicked in animal models by delivering a foreign protein (i.e., a human protein) to the animal to provoke anti-human protein antibody production. The efficacy of different immunosuppressive treatments to inhibit the development of neutralizing antibodies can then be investigated. The immunosuppressive agents examined here include drugs (e.g., cyclophosphamide, FK506), cytokines (e.g., interferon-γ, interleukin-12), and monoclonal antibodies (e.g., anti-CD4, anti-gp39, CTLA4-Ig). It has been found that a high level of antibody suppression is necessary to allow prolonged delivery of a foreign protein. Immunosuppressive agents capable of this high level of suppression will be important adjuncts to prevent treatment failures in situations where patients are at risk of developing neutralizing antibodies.**

## INTRODUCTION

Many genetic diseases, which are caused by the absence of a functional protein, are potentially amenable to treatment by gene therapy protocols. However, protein replacement therapy for some of these disorders has revealed that neutralizing antibodies can form against the therapeutic product. Approximately 10–15% of hemophilia A[1] and 2% of hemophilia B[2] chronic transfusion patients develop antibodies to factor VIII or IX, respectively, which inhibit clotting functions and decrease the efficacy of the replacement therapy. Similarly 13% of patients[3,4] with Gaucher disease, one of the more than 30 lysosomal storage disorders, developed antibodies against the enzyme glucocerebrosidase used for replacement therapy. Even in animal models of many lysosomal storage disorders, development of antibodies against the therapeutic product is common. For example, in the mucopolysaccharidosis (MPS) type I dog deficient in α-iduronidase[5] and the MPSVII mouse deficient in β-glucuronidase,[6] the development of antibodies to the replacement protein has been well documented. In addition to loss of efficacy, anaphylaxis during subsequent treatments is a potential clinical complication. Unfortunately, it appears that the more se-

[d]Corresponding author: Department of Pediatrics, Health Sciences Centre Room, 3N18 McMaster University, 1200 Main Street West, Hamilton, Ontario L8N 3Z5 Canada; 905-521-2100 ext. 3716 (voice); 905-521-1703 (fax);changp@fhs.McMaster.CA (e-mail).

verely affected the patients, the greater tendency for them to become sensitized against the replacement protein as a result of their cross-reacting-material-negative phenotype. Thus, for patients who need the therapy most may have a higher risk of becoming resistant to the treatment.

Other sources causing immunological response from the host include the viral vectors used in gene therapy. The vector, usually a recombinant virus or plasmid, is genetically engineered to contain the gene of interest, along with various regulatory sequences, such as promoters, enhancers, and genes used to select for transfected cells (e.g., antibiotic-resistance factors or cell surface markers). The most common vectors used are retroviruses, followed by plasmids, adenoviruses, pox-viruses, and adeno-associated viruses. Vectors which elicit a host inflammatory or immune response are less likely to be able to sustain delivery of the trans-gene product. Viruses have numerous proteins which can stimulate the immune system. Adenoviruses are strong activators of host inflammatory and immune responses (cellular and humoral) leading to loss of transgene delivery.[7] Newer adenoviral constructs with fewer viral proteins have been shown to decrease T-cell response. The most recent development is adenoviral vectors with no viral proteins at all,[8] or with co-expression of anti-inflammatory cytokine to avoid inflammatory and immune responses.[9] A commonly used retrovirus is the Moloney murine leukemia virus (MLV), which has the advantage that it does not elicit a host inflammatory/immune response.

Non-viral methods usually use recombinant plasmid DNA to deliver the target gene to the host cell. Compared to viral transduction, these methods generally have poor efficiency. However, depending on the delivery method, the host inflammatory response can be avoided. In our approach, a nonautologous universal cell line (mouse C2C12 myoblasts) containing a plasmid engineered to produce human growth hormone (hGH) was placed in immuno-protective alginate-poly-L-lysine-alginate microcapsules. The microcapsules were protected from immune rejection after intraperitoneal implantation into the allogeneic hosts, C57Bl/6 mice, thus allowing a continuous delivery of hGH *in vivo* by the encapsulated cells.[10] Owing to the size exclusion property of the microcapsule membrane, the larger immune mediators, likely including complement and lymphocytes, are excluded from entry, while passage remains unimpeded for the smaller molecules such as nutrients, metabolic waste products and the transgene product, with molecular weights below the cut-off threshold.[11] While immunoisolation protected the encapsulated cells from rejection, the immune system was fully capable of reacting to the recombinant protein secreted from the encapsulated cells.[12] This method of gene product delivery provides a useful model to mimic the clinical complication of neutralizing antibodies in gene therapy and to develop strategies to suppress such immune response.

## PRINCIPLE OF IMMUNOSUPPRESSION

Stimulation of T-cell dependent antibody production is a complex process (FIG. 1). Antigen-presenting cells (APC) such as macrophages, dendritic cells, and B-cells internalize foreign antigens and then present them on their cell surface in association with the major histocompatibility complex (MHC) class II. This complex is recognized by the CD4–T-cell receptor (TCR) on T-helper cells, but a second signal is re-

Step 1: helper T-cell activation

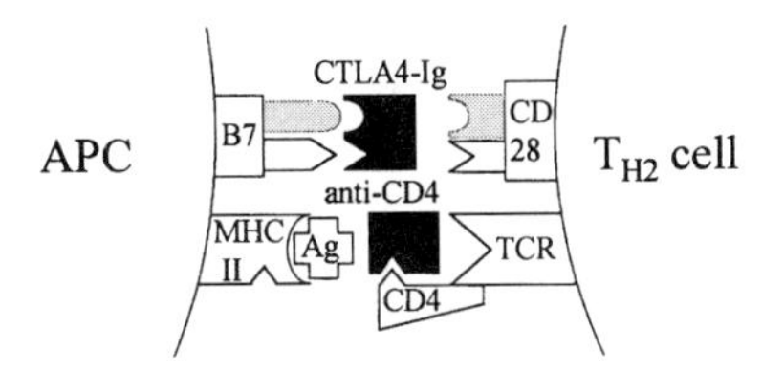


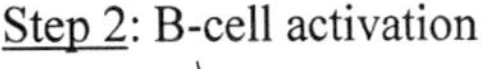


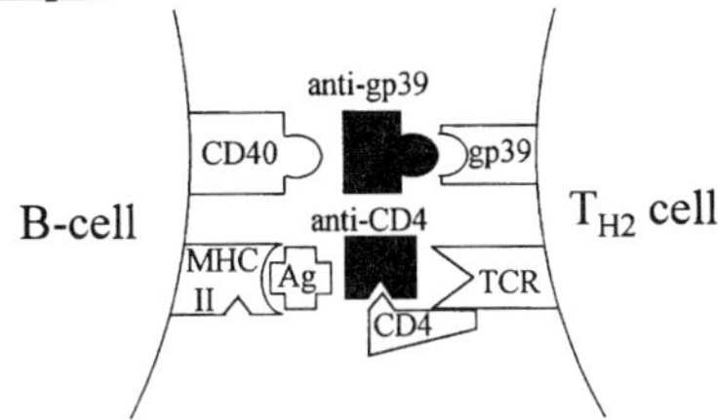


**FIGURE 1.** Immune signaling for antibody production and then immune suppressive agents. ***Step 1***: Antigen presenting cells (APC) present foreign antigens (Ag) along with the major histocompatibility complex type II (MHC-II) to T-helper cells. This signal is recognized by the T-cell receptor (TCR) and CD4 molecule on the T-helper cell. Activation of the T-helper cell also requires a second signal, the B7–CD28 interaction. If the APC secretes IL-12 (e.g., if it is a macrophage), the activated T-helper cells preferentially differentiate into IL-2, IFN-γ, and tumor necrosis factor (TNF) β–secreting $T_{H1}$, cells instead of the $T_{H2}$ cells which are more important in antibody production. The immunosuppressive agents which act during this step are FK506, CTLA4-Ig, anti-CD4 antibodies, IL-12 and IFN-γ (see TABLE 1 for details). ***Step 2***: The activated $T_{H2}$ cell then activates B-cells via the MHC-II restricted recognition of the antigen, also requiring a second signal, the gp39–CD40 interaction. The $T_{H2}$ cells secrete IL-4, -5, -6, -10, and -13 to stimulate B-cell proliferation and differentiation into antibody-producing plasma cells. The immunosuppressive agents which act during this step are cyclophosphamide and anti-gp39 (see TABLE 1 for details).

quired for activation of the T-cell. A potent costimulator is the B7 molecule on the APC, which binds to the CD28 molecule on the T cell, stimulating T-cell proliferation. These activated T-helper cells can then stimulated resting B-cells by MHC-II restricted antigen interaction with the CD4-TCR on the T-helper cell. A costimulatory interaction between CD40 on the B-cell and gp39 (CD40 ligand) on the T-cell ensures B-cell activation. Activated B-cells are then stimulated into clonal proliferation and to differentiate into immunoglobulin producing plasma cells.[13]

Several methods of immune suppression may be potentially useful in attenuating the formation of neutralizing antibodies. They include the use of general immunosuppressive drugs or specific immune modulators that block the various pathways leading from antigen presentation to T- and B-cell activation (TABLE 1). The immunosuppressive agents examined here include the immunosuppressive or cytotoxic drugs cyclophosphamide and FK506 (group I). As well, immune signal blocking

**TABLE 1.** Immunosuppressive agents and their possible mechanisms of action

| Agent | Mechanism | Reference |
|---|---|---|
| Group I: Immunosyppressive drugs | | |
| cyclophosphamide | prevents clonal expansion of B cells and antibody expression | Dai *et al.*, 1995[14] |
| FK506 | interferes with T-cell differentiation and proliferation | Lochmuller *et al.*, 1996[15] |
| Group II: Antibodies | | |
| CTLA4-Ig | competitive inhibitor of CD28 | Abbas *et al.*, 1994[17] |
| anti-gp39 | blocks the interaction between the gp39 protein and the CD40 B-cell receptor | Foy *et al.*, 1993[20] |
| anti-CD4 | transiently depletes CD4 cells | Yang *et al.*, 1996[21] |
| Group III: Cytokines | | |
| interleukin-12 | induction of $T_{H1}$clones | Paul and Seder, 1994[24] |
| interferon-γ | inhibits proliferation of $T_{H2}$ clones | Paul and Seder, 1994[24] |

monoclonal antibodies such as anti-CD4, anti-gp39, CTLA4-Ig (group II) and immune mediators such as the cytokines interferon-γ and interleukin-12 (group III) are also examined.

## EXPERIMENTAL METHODS

### *Recombinant Cells for Encapsulation*

A mouse C2C12 myoblast cell line (C41) was transfected with the plasmid pNMG3. The pNMG3 plasmid coded for the *hGH* gene driven by the mouse metallothionein-1 promoter and the *NeoR* gene conferring resistance to G418. Prior to encapsulation, cells were maintained in Dulbecco's medium supplemented with 10% fetal bovine serum (FBS) and Penicillin (100 units/mL), streptomycin (100 μg/mL) and G418 (400 μg/mL). Immediately following encapsulation and washing, the cells were maintained in SkBM low-serum medium (Clonetics, San Diego, CA) until implantation.

### *Encapsulation*

The cells were encapsulated in alginate-poly-L-lysine-alginate microcapsules. Briefly, cells harvested with trypsin were resuspended in 1.5% potassium alginate (Improved Kelmar, Lot 17703A, Kelco, San Diego, CA) at $2 \times 10^6$ cells/mL, extruded with a 27G blunt end needle as droplets into 1.1% $CaCl_2$ to form gelled beads, coated with poly-L-lysine and alginate to form the outer membrane, and the core solubilized with sodium citrate to form microcapsules enclosing the recombinant cells. The microcapsules were kept in SkBM low serum medium until implantation.

### *Animals*

Male C57Bl/6 mice (3–4 week old, ~15 g body weight) were housed in pathogen-free housing with micro-isolator hooded cages. All procedures were performed under a laminar flow hood with sterile techniques and in accordance with Canadian Institutional Animal Care Guidelines.

### *Capsule Implantation*

The animals were briefly anesthetized with a small-animal anesthetic machine providing a controlled amount of isofluorane and oxygen. Approximately 3 mL of washed microcapsules were implanted into the peritoneal cavity of each mouse with a 16G catheter. Baseline blood sampling and body weight measurement were performed immediately before the implantation. The procedure took 10–15 min and the animals were soon freely mobile in their cages.

### *Blood Collection*

Retro-orbital bleeds were conducted on anesthetized mice on days 0, 2, 7, 14, 21, and 28 post-implantation. Approximate 100 μL of whole blood was collected with a heparinized capillary tube and plasma stored at –20°C until assayed. On day 28, one mouse from each group was sacrificed via terminal cardiac bleed for retrieval of microcapsules.

### *Capsule Retrieval*

A full midline incision of the abdominal skin and a 0.75 cm incision through the abdominal wall were made to retrieve the capsules from the peritoneal cavity. They were washed three times with ice-cold PBS and then with supplemented Dulbecco's medium. The capsules were maintained in this medium under the usual culture conditions

### *Clearance Study*

Three animals from a treatment group (CTLA4-Ig) sensitized to hGH, owing to microcapsules implanted 22 weeks previously, and four naïve mice of similar weight and sex were each injected into the tail vein with 6 μg of purified hGH (gift from Eli Lilly Inc., Indianapolis, IN). Blood was sampled by retro-orbital bleeds at 1, 3, 5, 10, 15 and 30 min after the injection. The mice were sacrificed after the final blood sample.

### *Reagents and Treatment Protocols*

Four mice were used for each treatment. Two mice died on day 1 following implantation (one each from the FK506 and IFN-γ treatments).

*Controls*[e]

- Negative control: received only microcapsules but no immune suppressive treatments.
- L6 (a miscellaneous fusion protein as a matched negative control for CTLA4-Ig, Bristol-Myers Squibb Pharmaceutical Research Institute, Seattle, WA): 200 μg IP (1 mg/mL saline) q2d × 5 doses starting on day 0 of implantation (total dose 1000 μg/mouse).

*Group I: Immunosuppressive Drugs*

- Cyclophosphamide (Carter-Horner, Mississauga, Ont., Canada): 250 mg/kg injected IP (20 mg/mL), one dose on day –1 prior to implantation.
- FK506 (Fujisawa USA, Inc., Deerfield, IL, USA): 5 mg/kg SC (0.5 mg/mL saline) daily starting at day –2 prior to implantation.

*Group II: Monoclonal Antibodies*

- CTLA4-Ig (Bristol-Myers Squibb, Pharmaceutical Research Institute, Seattle, WA): 200 μg IP (1 mg/mL saline) q2d × 5 doses starting on day 0 of implantation (total dose 1000 μg/mouse).
- Anti-gp39 (Pharmingen Canada, Ontario, Canada): 250 μg IP q2d × 3 doses starting on day 0 of implantation (total dose 750 mg/mouse).
- Anti-CD4 (Pharmingen Canada, Ontario, Canada): 250 mg IP q3d × 3 doses starting on day –3 prior to implantation (total dose 750 μg/mouse).

*Group III: Cytokines*

- Interferon-γ (Pharmingen Canada, Ontario, Canada): 2 μg IP (10 μg/mL PBS) on day 0 and day 1 post-implantation (total dose 4 μg/mouse).
- Interleukin-12 (Hoffmann-LaRoche, Nutley, NJ): 2 μg IP (1 mg/mL PBS) on day 0 and 1 post-implantation (total dose 4 μg/mouse).

### *Human Growth Hormone Assay*

An ELISA kit (UBI-Magiwel hGH kit, United Biotech, CA) was used according to the supplier's instructions. The rate of hGH secretion from capsules was determined by sampling aliquots of the media at 0, 1, 2, and 4 hours. Mouse plasma levels were determined at 1:3 dilutions. The limit of detection for the assay was 0.2 ng/mL, which gave a limit of detection of 4 ng/mL for the rate of secretion assay and 0.6 ng/mL for the plasma assay.

### *Human Growth Hormone Antibody Assay*

Antibodies to hGH were assayed with an ELISA protocol as follows, washing 3 times with PBS/Tween (10 mM $Na_2HPO_4$, 150 mM NaCl, 0.05% Tween 20, pH 7.4)

[e]Abbreviations: q2d–every two days; q3d–every three days; OD–once daily; IP–intraperitoneal; SC–subcutaneous.

between steps. Each well was coated with 200 ng pure hGH (Humatrope, supplied by Eli Lilly Inc. Indianapolis, IN) for 2 h at 37°C, blocked with 5% skim milk powder in PBS/Tween for 2 h at 37°C, treated with 100 μL plasma sample diluted 1:300 in 5% skim milk powder in PBS/Tween at 37°C for 1 h, incubated with goat anti-mouse antibody conjugated to alkaline phosphatase (Promega, Madison, WI) at 37°C for 1 hr, and then detected with Sigma 104 Phosphatase substrate. A standard curve was constructed by making serial dilutions serum from a positive control mouse that was immunized with pure hGH. All sample antibody titers were expressed as the equivalent dilution of the positive control serum to contain the same amount of anti-hGH antibodies.

### *Statistical Analysis*

ANOVA was carried out to detect significant differences between the groups at each time point. When a significant difference was detected ($p < 0.05$), a Scheffe test was performed to identify the significant groups.

## SUPPRESSION OF IMMUNE RESPONSE IN A MODEL OF GENE THERAPY

Using the murine model for nonautologous gene therapy, we delivered hGH to mice by intraperitoneal implantation of microencapsulated recombinant cells. Plasma hGH levels and the antibody response to hGH in control mice were then compared to those in mice treated with one of the immunosuppressive agents. In the control mice, the circulating hGH was clearly detectable by day 2 post-implantation, reaching a peak level of ~2 ng of hGH/mL plasma on day 7, but declining to background level by day 14 (FIG. 2A, left panel). As expected, the xenogeneic hGH, being a foreign antigen, provoked an immunological response, leading to a corresponding rise in anti-hGH antibodies, which were first detectable by day 14 and continued to increase until day 28 (FIG. 2A, right panel). When the implanted mice were treated with the three groups of immunosuppressive agents, their responses were highly variable, depending on the protocol used (TABLE 2).

### *Group I*

These mice were treated with one of the two immunosuppressive drugs, cyclophosphamide or FK506. The delivery pattern was similar to that of the controls, peaking on day 7 at 2.0 ng/mL and 0.9 ng/mL plasma, respectively, before subsiding to background level by day 14 (FIG. 2B, left panel). However, both drugs in this group were able to down regulate the antibody response to hGH when compared to the untreated controls. The cyclophosphamide-treated mice showed only a low titer response beginning on day 14, while FK506 did not show any antibody response until day 21 (FIG. 2B, right panel). Cyclophosphamide is used primarily as an anti-cancer drug while FK506 (Tacrolimus, Prograf™) is a newer drug that has been used as an anti-rejection agent in organ transplants as well as in somatic gene therapy models to suppress host antibody response. Treatment with cyclophosphamide prevents clonal expansion of B cells and antibody expression[14] whereas FK506 is an antibi-

**TABLE 2.** Treatment groups and growth of encapsulated cells retrieved on day 28 post-implantation[a]

| Treatment | Protocol | % Cell Viability | No. Viable Cells/Capsule |
|---|---|---|---|
| *In Vitro* | | | |
| Day 0 | N/A | 94 ± 5 | 231 ± 64 |
| Day 7 | N/A | 93 ± 1 | 185 ± 1 |
| Day 14 | N/A | 83 ± 2 | 425 ± 158 |
| Day 28 | N/A | 80 ± 7 | 302 ± 91 |
| *In Vivo* | | | |
| Controls: | | | |
| Negative control (N = 4) | no treatment | 87 ± 1 | 999 ± 370 |
| L6 (N = 4) | 200 μg IP q2d on days 0 to 8 | 69 ± 11 | 1230 ± 617 |
| Group I: Immunosuppressive drugs | | | |
| Cyclophosphamide (N=4) | 250 mg/kg IP on day –1 | 89 ± 5 | 1430 ± 551 |
| FK506 (N = 3) | 5 mg/kg SC daily | 94 ± 2 | 2360 ± 465 |
| Group II: Antibodies | | | |
| Anti-gp39 (N = 4) | 250 μg IP q2d on days 0 to 4 | 84 ± 3 | 1390 ± 383 |
| Anti-CD4 (N = 4) | 250 μg IP q3d on days –3 to 3 | 83 ± 5 | 1150 ± 141 |
| CTLA4-Ig (N = 4) | 200 μg IP q2d on days 0 to 8 | 84 ± 4 | 1870 ± 845 |
| Group III: Cytokines | | | |
| IFN-γ (N = 3) | 2 μg IP on days 0 and 1 | 88 ± 4 | 1420 ± 171 |
| IL-12 (N = 4) | 2 μg IP on days 0 and 1 | 83 ± 12 | 2500 ± 351 |

[a]Encapsulated hGH-secreting cells were either kept *in vitro* for 28 days or implanted intraperitoneally into mice treated with various immunosuppressive reagents according to the different protocols. On day 28 post-implantation, the microcapsules were retrieved with intraperitoneal lavage to determine the viability and number of encapsulated cells. The data are means ± standard error. Abbreviations: IP–intraperitoneal; SC–subcutaneous; q2d–every second day, q3d–every third day. (From Potter *et al.* 1998,[26] reprinted with permission.)

otic produced by *Streptomyces tsukubaenis* that interferes with T-cell differentiation and proliferation.[15] They both showed good suppression of antibody response (11 ± 3% and 6 ± 5% of the control, FIG. 2). In other experiments, cyclophosphamide had been used successfully at a dose of 300 mg/kg to prevent the formation of anti-adenovirus–neutralizing antibody in C57Bl/6 mice,[16] thus allowing a repeat administration of human factor IX via an adeno-viral vector. We were not able to achieve total antibody suppression at a dose of 250 mg/kg cyclophosphamide, and a dose of 300 mg/kg cyclophosphamide was poorly tolerated in a pilot study (unpublished data). Similarly, FK506 had been used to suppress antibody response to dystrophin and an adenovirus vector, allowing dystrophin transgene expression for more than 2 months.[15] In our study, FK506 was an effective agent in suppressing the anti-hGH antibody response (FIG. 3), thus verifying the effectiveness of this drug treatment.

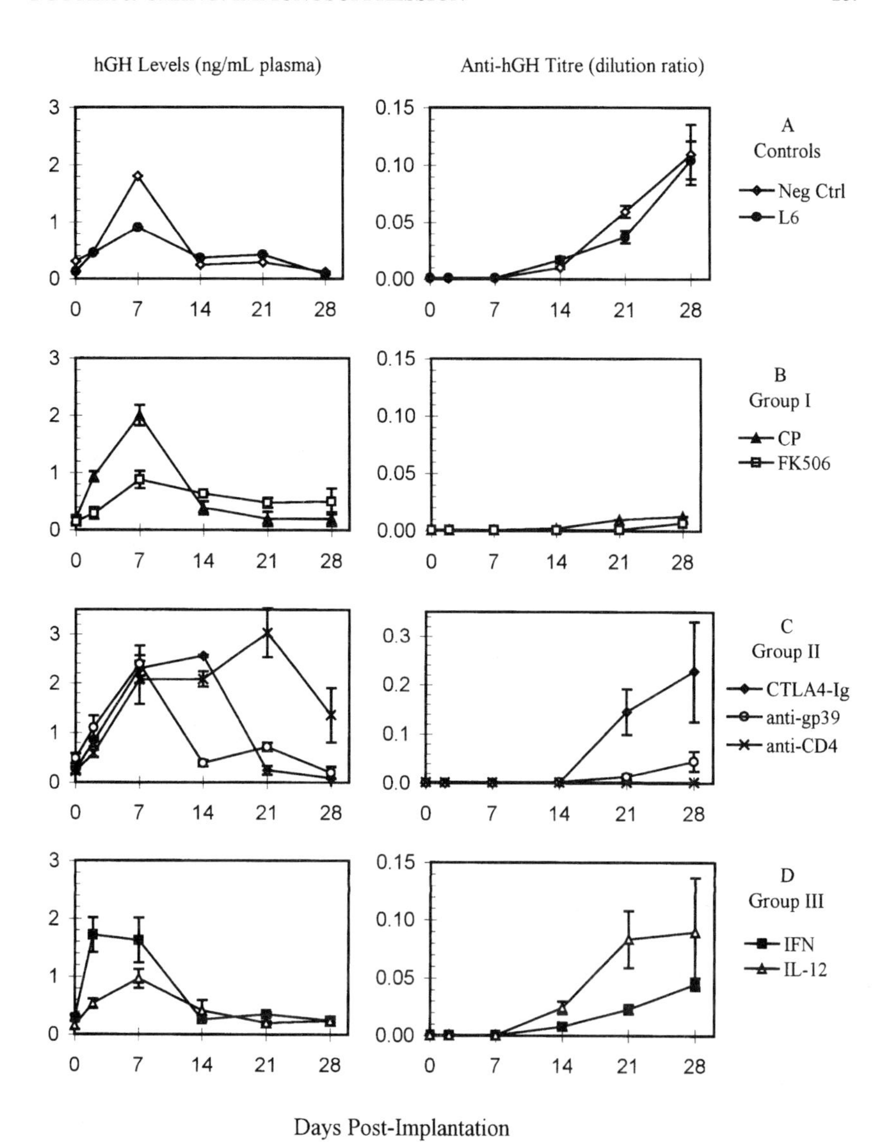


**FIGURE 2.** *In vivo* comparison of plasma hGH and anti-hGH antibody levels. Each animal was implanted with encapsulated hGH-secreting myoblasts on day 0 and treated with one of the immunosuppressive agents. The control groups included the negative control group, which were implanted with encapsulated hGH-secreting cells but received no immunosuppression, and the L6 group, which was similarly implanted but was treated with an irrelevant fusion protein. Group I included the immunosuppressive drug treatments (CP: cyclophosphamide; FK506), Group II the anti-T-cell receptor antibody treatments (CTLA4-Ig; anti-gp39; antiCD4) and Group III the cytokine treatments (IFN: interferon-γ; IL-12: interleukin 12). On various days post-implantation, the levels of hGH (ng/mL plasma) and titers of anti-hGH antibodies were determined. The anti-hGH antibody titer was ex-

### *Group II*

These mice were treated with antibodies directed against various T-cell receptors. Their responses were highly variable depending on the antibody used (FIG. 2C, left panel). The CTLA4-Ig treated mice had a peak level of hGH on day 14 with 2.5 ng/mL before declining to near zero on day 28. CTLA4-Ig is a fusion protein that acts as a competitive inhibitor of CD28. It prevents stimulation of T cells by blocking the T-cell CD28 receptor from interacting with ligands on antigen presenting cells.[17, 18] In experimental systems, its administration results in suppression of the inflammatory response with the inhibition of $T_{H1}$ cytokines (IL-2 and IFN-$\gamma$) but not $T_{H2}$ cytokines (IL-4, IL-10 and IL-13).[19] The elevation in anti-hGH antibody titer to twice that of its control L6, an irrelevant fusion protein (FIG. 2C), indicates that the $T_{H2}$ response to hGH was probably more important than the $T_{H1}$ response to mediate B-cell expansion and antibody production. Similarly, the anti-gp39–treated mice showed a peak delivery of hGH at 2.4 ng/mL on day 7, which declined to background level by day 28, a pattern that was almost identical to the controls. In contrast, the anti-CD4–treated mice had a much more sustained delivery, rising to the same level as the controls on day 7 (~2 ng/mL) but continuing to increase to 3 ng/mL by day 21 before declining by day 28 to 1.4 ng/mL (a level that was still statistically greater than the controls, $p < 0.05$).

The immune response to hGH was also highly variable in this group (FIG. 2C, right panel). The CTLA4-Ig–treated mice had a delayed but exaggerated antibody response, the titer rising sharply only on day 21 and continuing to escalate until day 28 to a level about 200% of its controls, which were implanted mice treated with an irrelevant antibody L6 (FIG. 2A, right panel). In contrast, the anti-gp39–treated animals showed a moderate suppression compared to the controls with a slight rise in titer by day 14 which then escalated during the remaining 14 days to about 35% of the control level. The anti-gp39 antibodies are thought to block the interaction between the gp39 protein and the CD40 receptor expressed on all mature B-cells. Blockage of CD40 and gp39 interactions via antibodies to gp39 is thought to prevent initiation of B-cell proliferation and antibody class switching. It has been shown to reduce both primary and secondary humoral immune response in mice when administered with soluble protein antigens, achieving >90% antibody suppression.[20] However, in our current protocol, anti-gp39 treatment only modestly lowered the anti-hGH antibody titer (42 ± 19% of control, FIG. 3), and was insufficient to influence hGH delivery *in vivo* (FIG. 2C). The anti-CD4 group showed the most effective suppression of anti-hGH response. Throughout the 28 days of the experiment, there was very little detectable titer of anti-hGH antibodies beyond background (FIG. 2C, right panel). The anti-CD4 antibody has been used to transiently deplete CD4 cells (T-helper cells) to prevent neutralizing antibody formation in recombinant gene therapy.[21] This treatment almost completely suppressed antibody response to hGH (1.2 ± 0.6% of the control, FIG. 3), and also allowed sustained circulation of hGH even up

---

pressed as the dilution of a positive control plasma (mice specifically immunized with purified hGH) to contain an equivalent amount of anti-hGH antibodies. All data are expressed as the mean ± standard error (N = 4 per treatment except for FK506 and IFN-$\gamma$ where N = 3). (From Potter *et al.* 1998,[26] reprinted with permission.)

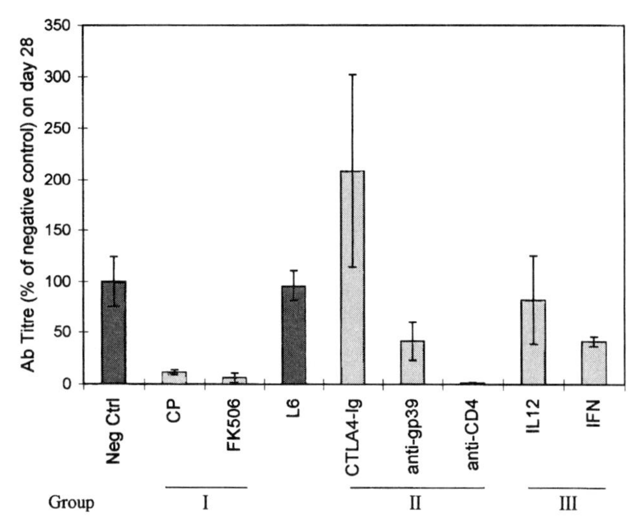


**FIGURE 3.** Comparison of antibody titers on day 28 post-implantation. Day 28 antibody titers against hGH were measured in plasma from animals treated with the seven immunosuppressive protocols (as described in FIG. 2) and the group mean expressed as a percent of the negative control group ± standard error. (From Potter *et al.* 1998,[26] reprinted with permission.)

to day 28 at levels of 1 ng/mL of plasma. This result agreed with those obtained by Yang,[21, 22] who used anti-CD4 antibodies to suppress adenovirus vector–neutralizing antibodies and to improve transgene delivery. Therapeutic approaches using anti-CD4 antibodies have already been designed in humans for the treatment of transplant rejection and autoimmune diseases,[23] suggesting that anti-CD4 treatment may be a promising agent for use in human gene therapy protocols.

### *Group III*

These mice were treated with the cytokines IL-12 or IFN-γ. Their circulating levels of hGH were similar to that of the control group at 1.0 and 1.6 ng/mL on day 7, respectively (FIG. 2D, left panel). Although they both showed an antibody response by day 14, IFN-γ appeared partially successful in suppressing the anti-hGH response, with titers rising to less than half of the control levels (41%) by day 28, whereas the IL-12 treated mice had a similar level of response as the controls with an even earlier peak at day 21 (FIG. 2D, right panel). IL-12 is a cytokine that activates $T_{H1}$ cells at the expense of $T_{H2}$ activation, which are thought to be more important in broader antibody responses, inhibiting the production of antibodies.[24] IL-12 is expected to suppress the anti-hGH IgG response better than CTLA4-Ig, since CTLA4-Ig only blocks the $T_{H2}$ response by inhibiting the second signal required for $T_{H2}$ cell stimulation. Although this was indeed observed (FIGS. 2C and 2D), the suppression by IL-12 was not low enough to reduce it from those of the controls (FIG. 2A). IL-12 has been successfully used to reduce neutralizing (IgA) antibodies and improve transgene delivery, but these therapies had no effect on IgG levels in lung tissue.[22]

In another experiment targeting liver cells, IL-12 achieved only a partial reduction in neutralizing antibody levels insufficient to improve transgene expression.[21] Hence, it is likely that both $T_{H1}$ and $T_{H2}$ response were important in the mounting of antibody response against hGH delivered continuously by implanted cells. Suppression of either one alone was thus ineffective. Interferon-γ is another cytokine secreted by activated macrophages and T-helper cells. It is thought to mediate the effect of IL-12 and thus achieves the same immune suppression[24] of antibody production by activating $T_{H1}$ cells to promote cytotoxic lymphocyte and $IgG_{2A}$ antibody response. However, although IL-12 treatment had little effect on antibody titer (82 ± 43% of control), IFN-γ actually achieved a modest suppression of the antibody response, at 41 ± 5% of the control (FIG. 3), thus indicating the complexity of the immune response.

Hence, the efficacy of the different treatment protocols in suppressing the antibody response to a foreign protein appeared to be highly variable. While the differences between most of the groups were not statistically significant by ANOVA, there was a trend of decreasing suppression in the order: anti-CD4 > FK506 > cyclophosphamide > anti-gp39 = IFN-γ, while IL-12 and CTLA4-Ig were not effective (FIG. 3). In particular, the suppression by anti-CD4 was almost 100% with little detectable antibody to hGH while that of FK506 and cyclophosphamide was ≥ 90% compared to the controls.

## LOSS OF GENE PRODUCT DELIVERY

With the exception of the anti-CD4–treated animals, all other groups showed a loss of hGH by day 28 post-implantation. In general, this loss was accompanied by a corresponding rise in antibody titer. It was postulated that the lack of detectable circulating hGH was either due to clearance of hGH from the plasma by anti-hGH antibodies[12] or the loss of microcapsule function after implantation. To investigate the first possibility, we injected 6 mg of purified hGH into each of three mice from a group previously implanted with microcapsules and hence sensitized to hGH (CTLA4-Ig–treated mice). No hGH could be detected in the plasma of any of these implanted mice, even at 1 minute after the hGH injection (FIG. 4). However, when four naïve mice which had not received any prior microcapsule implantations were similarly treated, they showed a high level of hGH immediately after the injection, which continued to be measurable at a level of 75 ng hGH/mL plasma at 30 minutes after the injection (FIG. 4). Since the level of hGH expression at implantation was 83 ± 24 ng/$10^6$ cells/h and $1.26 \pm 0.36 \times 10^6$ cells were implanted, the maximal amount of hGH delivered *in vivo* was expected to be 104 ng/h. Because the half-life of hGH in mice is only 2.2 ± 0.5 min,[25] such a level of delivery would have been readily cleared from the circulation by the sensitized mice, thus accounting for the loss of detectable hGH.

To verify that the loss of detectable hGH was not due to breakdown of microcapsules or loss of transgene expression, representative animals from all groups were sacrificed on day 28 to recover the microcapsules. The microcapsules appeared intact and free within the abdominal cavity. When compared to the encapsulated cells kept *in vitro*, the viability of those retrieved after IP implantation was quite similar,

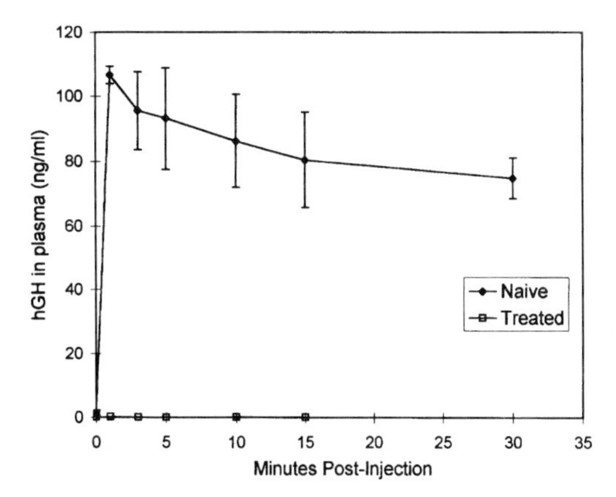


**FIGURE 4.** Clearance of hGH by naïve vs. treated mice. Naïve mice never exposed to hGH (N = 4) and treated mice that had been implanted with microcapsules secreting hGH two months prior to the clearance study (N = 3) were each injected with 6 μg hGH IV at time 0. Blood was sampled at the times shown post-injection and assayed for hGH in the plasma. Data are expressed as the mean ± standard error. (From Potter *et al.* 1998,[26] reprinted with permission.)

ranging from a low of 69% for the L6 control mice to a high of 94% for the FK506 treated mice, with an average viability for all retrieved capsules of 83% (TABLE 2). There was no statistically significant difference in cell viability among the different treatment groups. However, compared to the microcapsules kept *in vitro*, those retrieved after 28 days of implantation showed a vastly increased cell density. As shown in TABLE 2, the retrieved capsules had cell numbers ranging from approximately 1000/capsule for the negative control mice to about 2500/capsule for the IL-12 treated mice, with an average of around 1600/capsule for all the retrieved capsules. This represented an increase of fivefold in cell density compared to the capsules kept *in vitro* (approximately 300 cells/capsule) for the same duration.

Secretion rates of hGH from the capsules after retrieval on day 28 were similar to those of capsules kept *in vitro* until day 28 (FIG. 5), i.e., no significant difference between groups by ANOVA. The average hGH secretion from recovered capsules for the nine treatment and control groups was 44 ng/$10^6$ cells/h, which represented an overall decrease in secretion from the pre-implantation level of 83 ± 24 ng/$10^6$ cells/h, possibly owing to the removal of G418-selection pressure *in vivo*.

## CONCLUSION

The responses of the recipients to the various treatments can be classified into three categories. The first category, shown by treatment with CTLA4-Ig or interleukin-12, was similar to the untreated controls: no suppression of anti-hGH antibodies and no significant improvement in delivery of hGH. The second category of response observed in four treatment protocols (cyclophosphamide, FK506, anti-gp39 and interferon-γ), was suppression of antibodies but no improvement in sustaining delivery

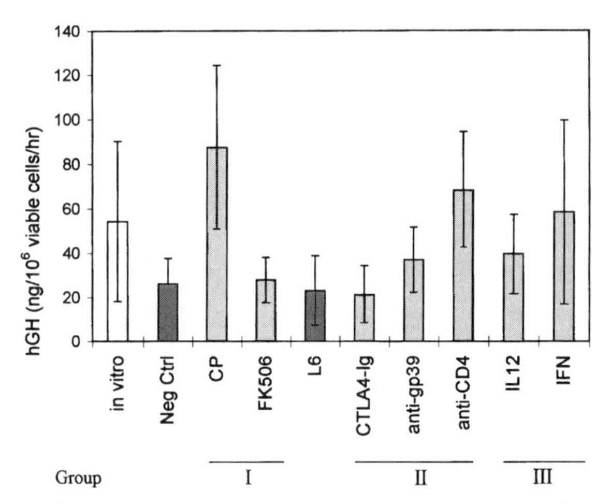


**FIGURE 5.** hGH secretion from retrieved capsules after day 28 of implantation. On day 28 post-implantation, microcapsules were retrieved from the intraperitoneal cavity by lavage, washed, and kept under the usual tissue culture conditions to determine the rate of hGH secretion (see METHODS). The microcapsules were then ruptured to determine the viable cell number. The data represented mean secretion ± S.D. The *in vitro* group refers to non-implanted microcapsules kept *in vitro* for 28 days under the usual tissue culture conditions (see FIG. 2 for remainder of legend). (From Potter *et al.* 1998,[26] reprinted with permission.)

of transgene product (FIG. 2). It is clear that while these treatments are more effective in antibody suppression than CTLA4-Ig and IL-12, they were unable to exert sufficient suppression of the humoral response to permit a sustained level of circulating recombinant hGH produced by the encapsulated cells. The last category of response was seen in the group of mice receiving anti-CD4: strong antibody suppression and the most sustained hormone delivery.

In conclusion, of the seven immune suppressive reagents, the use of anti-CD4 that interferes with T-helper cell response and B-cell activation appears most promising. It allowed prolonged delivery of a foreign protein and suppression of antibody response to a recombinant gene product. Hence, its role as adjunct treatment for appropriate patients at risk for developing inhibitors merits further consideration.

## REFERENCES

1. ALLAIN, J. 1984. Transfusion support for hemophiliacs. Clinics Haematol. **13:** 99–117.
2. ROBERTS, H.R. & M.E. EBERST. 1993. Current management of hemophilia B. Hematol./Oncol. Clinics N. Am. **7:** 1269–1279.
3. GRABOWSKI, G.A., N.W. BARTON, G. PASTORES, J.M. DAMBROSIA, T.K. BANERJEE, M.A. MCKEE, C. PARKER, R. SCHIFFMANN, S.C. HILL & R.O. BRADY. 1995. Enzyme therapy in type 1 Gaucher disease: comparative efficacy of mannose-terminated glucocerebrosidase from natural and recombinant sources. Ann. Intern. Med. **122:** 33–39.

4. RICHARDS S.M., T.A. OLSON & J.M. MCPHERSON. 1993. Antibody response in patients with Gaucher disease after repeated infusion with macrophage-targeted glucocerebrosidase. Blood **82:** 1402–1409.
5. SHULL, R., X. LU, I. DUBE, C. LUTZKO, S. KRUTH, A. ABRAMS-OGG, H.P. KIEM, S. GOEHLE, F. SCUENING, C. MILLAN, C. & R. CARTER. 1996. Humoral immune response limits gene therapy in canine MPS I. Blood **88:** 377–379.
6. SANDS, M.S., C. VOLGER, J.W. KYLE, J.H. GRUBB, B. LEVY, N. GALVIN, W.S. SLY & E.H. BIRKENMEIER. 1994. Enzyme replacement therapy for murine mucopolysaccharidosis Type VII. J. Clin. Invest. **93:** 2324–2331.
7. KAY, M.A., C.N. LANDEN, S.R. ROTHENBERG, L.A. TAYLOR, F. LELAND, S.WIEHLE, B. FANG, D. BELLINGER, M. FINEGOLD, A.R. THOMPSON, M. READ, K.M. BRINKHOUS & S.L.C. WOO. 1994. In vivo hepatic gene therapy: complete albeit transient correction of factor IX deficiency in hemophilia B dogs. Proc. Natl. Acad. Sci. USA **91:** 2353–2357.
8. SCHIEDNER, G., N. MORRAL, R.J. PARKS, *et al.* 1998. Genomic DNA transfer with a high-capacity adenovirus vector results in improved in vivo gene expression and decreased toxicity. Nature Genetics **18:** 180–183.
9. FISHER, K.J., K. CHOI, J. BURDA, *et al.* 1996. Recombinant adenovirus deleted of all viral genes for gene therapy of cystic fibrosis. Virology **217:** 11–22.
10. CHANG, P.L., N. SHEN & A.J. WESTCOTT. 1993. Delivery of recombinant gene products with microencapsulated cells in vivo. Hum. Gene Ther. **4:** 433–440.
11. CHANG, P.L. 1995. Nonautologous somatic gene therapy. *In* Somatic Gene Therapy. P.L. Chang, Ed. : 203–223. CRC Press Inc. Boca Raton, FL.
12. HORTELANO, G., A. AL-HENDY, F.A. OFOSU & P.L. CHANG. 1996 Delivery of human factor IX in mice by encapsulated recombinant myoblasts: a novel approach towards allogeneic gene therapy of hemophilia B. Blood **87:** 5095–5103
13. ROITT, I.M. 1997. Roitt's essential immunology, 9th edition. : 168–177. Blackwell Science Ltd. Oxford.
14. DAI, Y., E.M. SCHWARZ, D. GU, W.W. ZHANG, N. SARVETNICK & I.M. VERMA. 1995. Cellular and humoral immune responses to adenoviral vectors containing factor IX gene: tolerization of factor IX and vector antigens allows for long term expression. Proc. Natl. Acad. Sci. USA **92:**1401–1405.
15. LOCHMULLER, H., B.J. PETROF, G. PARI, N. LAROCHELLE, V. DODELET, Q. WANG, C. ALLEN, S. PRESCOTT, B. MASSIE, J. NALBANTOGLU & G. KARPATI. 1996. Transient immunosuppression by FK506 permits a sustained high-level dystrophin expression after adenovirus-mediated dystrophin minigene transfer to skeletal muscles of adult dystrophic (mdx) mice. Gene Ther. **3:** 706–716.
16. SMITH, T.A., B.D. WHITE, J.M. GARDNER, M. KALEKO & A. MCCLELLAND. 1996. Transient immunosuppression permits successful repetitive intravenous administration of an adenovirus vector. Gene Ther. **3:** 496–502.
17. ABBAS, A.K., A.H. LICHTMAN & J.S. POBER. 1994. Cellular and Molecular Immunology. W.B. Saunders & Co, Philadelphia.
18. LENSCHOW, D.J., Y. ZENG, J.R. THISTLEWAITE, A. MONTAG, W. BRADY, M.G. GIBSON, P.S. LINSLEY & J.A. BLUESTONE. 1992. Long-term survival of xenogeneic pancreatic islet grafts induced by CTLA4Ig. Science **257:** 789–792.
19. KHOURY, S.J., E. AKALIN, A. CHANDRAKER, L.A. TURKA, P.S. LINSLEY, M.H. SAYEGH & W.W. HANCOCK. 1995. CD28-B7 costimulatory blockade by CTLA4Ig prevents actively induced experimental autoimmune encephalomyelitis and inhibits TH1 but spares TH2 cytokines in the central nervous system. J. Immunol. **155:** 4521–4524.
20. FOY, T.M., D.M. SHEPHERD, F.H. DURIE, A. ARUFFO, J.A .LEDBETTER & R.J. NOELLE. 1993. In vivo CD40-gp39 interactions are essential for thymus dependent humoral immunity: prolonged suppression of the humoral immune response by an antibody to the ligand for CD40, gp39.J. Exp. Med. **178:** 1567–1575.
21. YANG, Y., K. GREENOUGH & J.M. WILSON. 1996. Transient immune blockade prevents formation of neutralizing antibody to recombinant adenovirus and allows repeated gene transfer to mouse liver. Gene Ther. **3:** 412–420.

22. YANG, Y., G. TRINCHIERI & J.M. WILSON. 1995. Recombinant IL-12 prevents formation of blocking IgA antibodies to recombinant adenovirus and allows repeated gene therapy to mouse lung. Nat. Med. **1:** 890–893.
23. RUIZ, P.J., H. ZINGER & E. MOZES. 1996. Effect of injection of anti- CD4 and anti-CD8 monoclonal antibodies on the development of experimental systemic lupus erythematosus in mice. Cell. Immunol. **167:** 30–37.
24. PAUL, W.E. & R.A. SEDER. 1994. Lymphocyte responses and cytokines. Cell **76:** 241–251.
25. TURYN, D. & BARTKE.1993. Pharmacokinetics of radioiodinated human and bovine growth hormones in mice expressing bovine growth hormone. Transgenic Rev. **2:** 219–226.
26. POTTER, M.A., S. HYMUS, T. STOCKLEY & P.L. CHANG. 1998. Suppression of immunological response against a transgene product delivered from microencapsulated cells. Hum. Gene Ther. **9:** 1275–1282.

# Potential Application of Neonatal Porcine Islets as Treatment for Type 1 Diabetes: A Review

GINA R. RAYAT, RAY V. RAJOTTE, AND GREGORY S. KORBUTT[a]

*Department of Surgery, Surgical-Medical Research Institute, University of Alberta, Edmonton, Canada*

**ABSTRACT: Islet transplantation has been shown to be a viable option for treating patients with type 1 diabetes. However, widespread clinical application of this treatment will necessitate an alternative source of insulin-producing tissue. Porcine pancreata may be a potential source of islets since pigs are inexpensive, readily available, and exhibit morphological and physiological characteristics comparable to humans. Recently, we developed a simple, standardized procedure for isolating large numbers of neonatal porcine islets with a reproducible and defined cellular composition. Following nine days of *in vitro* culture, tissue from one neonatal pig pancreas yielded approximately 50,000 islet cell aggregates, consisting of primarily epithelial cells (57%) and pancreatic endocrine cells (35%). In addition, neonatal porcine islets were responsive to glucose challenge *in vitro* and were capable of correcting hyperglycemia in alloxan-induced diabetic nude mice. Although neonatal porcine islets constitute an attractive alternative source of insulin-producing tissue for clinical transplantation, many aspects such as the immunological responses to these tissue and the latent period (2 to 8 weeks) between transplantation of these islets and the reversal of hyperglycemia need further investigation. This article discusses these issues and presents possible solutions to problems that may hinder the potential application of neonatal porcine islets for transplantation into patients with type 1 diabetes.**

## INTRODUCTION

The discovery of insulin at the University of Toronto in 1922 was one of the most dramatic events in the history of the treatment of type 1 diabetes.[1] Insulin therapy has improved the quality of life and extended the life expectancy of patients with diabetes; however, this current mode of treatment does not protect diabetic patients from episodes of abnormally high blood glucose levels, which can lead to chronic complications unless intensive insulin therapy is used. The main focus of diabetes research has been to develop better methods of treatment which can prevent the long-term complications of this disease. Endocrine replacement by islet transplantation is an attractive alternative treatment because it offers a physiological means for precise restoration of euglycemia in patients with type 1 diabetes.

Over the past 16 years, significant advances have been made in the number and purity of islets that can be harvested from the human pancreas.[2–7] Reports of both

[a]Author for correspondence: Surgical-Medical Research Institute, 1074 Dentistry/Pharmacy Building, University of Alberta, Edmonton, Alberta T6G 2N8 Canada; 780-492-4657 (voice); 780-492-1627 (fax); korbutt@gpu.srv.ualberta.ca (e-mail).

short-term and long-term insulin independence following human islet allotransplantation has encouraged many centers in the world to continue clinical trials of islet transplantation in patients with type 1 diabetes.[8–14] However, if islet transplantation is to become a widespread treatment for type 1 diabetes the supply of donors will become a major limitation. The shortage of available allogeneic organs and tissues for clinical transplantation has resulted in considering other sources of insulin-producing tissue which includes: porcine[15–19] and bovine[20] islets, fish Brockman bodies,[21] genetically engineered insulin-secreting cell lines,[22–24] and *in vitro* production of human fetal[25] or adult cells.[26] Porcine islets represent the most likely practical alternative source of insulin-producing tissue, since pigs are inexpensive, readily available, and they exhibit physiological and morphological characteristics comparable to humans. Porcine insulin is also structurally similar to human insulin and has been used safely for treating patients with type 1 diabetes for many years.

Adult pigs are often employed as tissue sources; however, adult porcine islets are difficult to isolate and they exhibit poor growth potential.[27] Recently, we have developed a simple, standardized procedure for isolating large numbers of neonatal porcine islets with a reproducible and defined cellular composition.[28] After nine days culture, approximately 50,000 islets/pancreas can be recovered and these islets were shown to consist primarily of 35% fully differentiated endocrine and 57% endocrine precursor cells. *In vitro* viability assessment of the cultured islets demonstrated that in the presence of 20 mM glucose, the islets were capable of releasing 7-fold more insulin than at 2.8 mM glucose. When these islets were exposed to 20 mM glucose in combination with 10 mM theophylline, the stimulation index increased to 30-fold as compared to basal release. When 2000 neonatal porcine islets were transplanted into alloxan diabetic nude mice ($n = 10$), 100% of the recipients became normoglycemic within 6–8 weeks post-transplantation and remained euglycemic until the graft-bearing kidney was removed at 100 days follow-up, after which all recipients returned to a hyperglycemic state. Examination of the grafts derived from normalized mice revealed that they were largely composed of insulin-positive cells, and their cellular insulin content was 5- to 20-fold higher than at the day of transplantation. Weber *et al.*[29] has also demonstrated that neonatal porcine islet cells secrete insulin *in vitro* after microencapsulation and biopsies of these grafts at ≥100 days following transplantation to streptozotocin-diabetic NOD-Scid mice revealed increased numbers of intensely insulin-positive islet cells in most cell aggregates. These results also suggest that neonatal porcine islets differentiate and divide during the transplant period.

## IMMUNOLOGICAL RESPONSES TO NEONATAL PORCINE ISLETS

### *Humoral-mediated Immune Responses*

A major barrier to discordant (e.g., pig-to-human) xenotransplantation of whole organs is hyperacute rejection (HAR), a process believed to be initiated when naturally occurring xenoreactive antibodies in the recipient's sera binds to antigens present on the surface of endothelial (and other) cells within the xenograft. Antibody binding in turn activates complement, which rapidly destroys the transplanted organ or tissue.[30–34] The most important target for these antibodies has been identified as the terminal carbohydrate galactose α(1,3)-galactose or Galα(1,3)Gal (αGal).[35–37] Pigs and most mammals express α 1-3 galactosyltransferase, which places αGal on glycoconjugates while humans and Old World monkeys lack this enzyme. Humans presumably developed antibodies against αGal from exposure to αGal antigen on bacteria present in the gut. More than 2% of total human IgM and IgG in the circulation represents αGal antibody.[38]

The αGal carbohydrate residue is present in high concentrations on all porcine endothelial cells[37, 39, 40] and has been detected on fetal porcine islet cells.[41,42] It is generally believed that the only component of fully differentiated adult porcine islets that expresses αGal is the small number of contaminating vascular endothelial cells present immediately after isolation and which can be eliminated through tissue culture. However, we and others have demonstrated that natural xenoreactive antibodies bind to fetal,[43] neonatal,[44] and adult[45, 46] porcine islet cells, and exposure to human sera containing active complement *in vitro* results in rapid destruction of these tissues.[44–46] We have also recently shown *in vitro* that following fluorescence-activated cell sorter analysis with a Gal-specific lectin (IB4-FITC), 30% of the neonatal porcine islet cells expressed the Gal epitope and 70% did not.[47] Histological assessment of those cells expressing αGal revealed that 55% stained positive for either insulin or glucagon and 69% of the αGal-negative cells stained positive for these same pancreatic hormones. Incubation of either αGal-positive or -negative cells with human AB serum plus rabbit complement for 1.5 hours resulted in the lysis of >90% of the cells. This study demonstrates that neonatal porcine islets are composed of cells expressing αGal and that expression of this epitope is not restricted to non-endocrine cells. Furthermore, both αGal-positive and -negative cells are susceptible to human antibody/complement–mediated lysis, which suggests the presence of other xenoantigens recognized by human antibodies and that this form of immunological destruction may be a problem if the cells are implanted in humans. In agreement with this finding, recent studies by McKenzie *et al.*[48] showed that pig islet xenografts are susceptible to “anti-pig” but not Galα(1,3)Gal antibody plus complement in Gal o/o mice.

Several strategies are being developed to block serum antibody/complement–mediated destruction of xenografts. One approach involves circulating human blood plasma over αGal immunoadsorbent columns to remove anti-αGal antibodies.[49] However, the benefit of this procedure is transient since anti-αGal antibody levels quickly return to normal in the blood.[50] Another method is to inhibit triggering of the complement cascade by treatment with excess amounts of a soluble form of complement receptor.[51–54] A third strategy is to generate transgenic pigs that over express a fucosyltransferase that competes with the substrate for αGal attachment so that a fucose group, representing a natural human blood group antigen, is substituted for αGal.[50,55–57] A fourth approach is to knock out the pig gene that encodes α 1-3 galactosyltransferase.[58,59] This would presumably eliminate the main cause of hyperacute rejection, but the technology for porcine knockouts is not yet available.[50] At present, it is not possible to generate pigs lacking the αGal epitope because porcine pluripotent cells, which are essential for gene inactivation, are not yet available.[58] The fifth strategy is to generate transgenic pigs that express human complement-regulatory proteins.[60–65] These proteins, CD55 (decay accelerating factor, DAF), CD46 (membrane cofactor protein, MCP-1) and CD59 (protectin) do not prevent anti-αGal antibody binding to endothelial cells to trigger the classical pathway of complement activation; rather they inhibit downstream steps in the complement cascade so that cell lysis may be prevented.[50] Several transgenic pig herds have been developed that express one or more of the human genes encoding CD55, CD46 and CD59.[60]

### *T-Cell–mediated Immune Responses*

It is generally accepted that two signals are needed for T-cell activation, engagement of the antigen-specific T-cell receptor and a second non-antigen–specific inductive stimulus, or costimulator, provided by a metabolically active antigen-presenting cell (APC). Two pathways of graft antigen presentation would fulfill this two-signal requirement for T cell activation: 1) direct pathway, where host T cells recognize antigen on the surface of donor APC that are capable of costimulatory activity (donor APC-dependent), and 2) indirect pathway, whereby host T cells recognize graft antigens which are processed and presented by host APC (host APC-dependent). In allorejection, both pathways are believed to play a role although the direct pathway is perhaps most crucial initially, whereas, during xenorejection the indirect pathway is thought to be dominant. Gill *et al.*[66,67] has demonstrated that elimination of donor APC from mouse islet allografts led to indefinite survival, while similar treatment of concordant (rat-to-mouse) islet xenografts had little benefit for survival. Furthermore, rejection of the islet xenografts showed a specific dependence on $CD4^+$ T cells, and not on the presence of donor APC and host $CD8^+$ cells.[67] It has also been shown that marked prolongation of islet xenografts can be achieved in adult pig-to-mouse model by the administration of anti-CD4 antibody.[68] Islet xenograft rejection may therefore occur predominantly through the processing and presentation of xenogeneic antigens in association with class II MHC molecules of host APC, leading to a CD4-dependent inflammatory response—where other cells (i.e., macrophages and NK cells) recruited by this response, may also contribute to rejection. It has also been shown in skin xenograft model that removal of mouse $CD4^+$ T cells with anti-CD4 antibody can prolong monkey or rabbit skin xenograft survival even after whole MHC-disparate allogeneic mouse skin had been rejected.[69] Other studies also showed that islet allografts from transgenic mice that are deficient in class I MHC expression survived long-term as allografts but are acutely rejected as xenografts.[70,71] The role of direct antigen presentation in xenografts appears to be minor, however, one must not neglect the possibility that direct recognition may also contribute to cell-mediated destruction of xenogeneic cells. Work by Murray *et al.*[72] has demonstrated that human T cells can recognize porcine endothelial cells directly and Yamada *et al.*[73] recently observed that human T cells that recognize porcine class II MHC antigens through the direct pathway can discriminate among swine leukocyte antigens in a manner that allows for xenospecific responses. Whether xenoantigens are presented directly or indirectly by APC, a requirement for a costimulatory signal exists in both pathways. Thus, one current immunosuppressive strategy invokes blocking this signal by treatment with the soluble protein CTLA4Ig. This approach has been successful in preventing islet xenograft survival in rodents.[29,74]

Transplantation of islets into abdominal testis has also been shown to protect islets from immune destruction without the requirement of systemic immunosuppression.[75–79] Sertoli cells are thought to confer immune privilege to the testis, possibly by producing factors that act locally to inhibit immune responses. Expression of Fas (CD95) ligand in the testes [80,81] has been shown to be responsible in part for maintaining the immunoprivileged status of this site. Fas receptor (FasR) and its ligand (FasL) are components of the immune system that play a role in killing activated T cells. Binding of FasL to FasR-bearing activated T cells leads to apoptosis of these cells.[82–84] More recently, it has been shown that allografts consisting of purified Sertoli cells alone can survive long-term in immune-competent mice.[80] We have also demonstrated that long-term graft survival of allogeneic rat islets without systemic immunosuppression can be achieved by cotransplantation of allogeneic islets with allogeneic testicular cell aggregates.[85] Transplantation of a sufficient quantity of testicular aggregates (containing $11 \times 10^6$ cells, 75% Sertoli cells), together with 2000 purified Lewis rat islets, reversed the diabetic state for >95 days in 100% of the streptozotocin-diabetic Wistar-Furth recipients. Similar grafts consisting of islets alone or islets plus 50% fewer testicular cell aggregates survived for only 10 days. Functioning composite allografts harvested from normoglycemic animals at approximately 100 days showed healthy cells in close association with Fas ligand-expressing Sertoli cells.

The effect of cotransplantation of neonatal porcine Sertoli cells on the survival of neonatal porcine islet xenografts is not known and still under investigation. Preliminary results in our laboratory however, indicate that neonatal porcine Sertoli cells can survive under the kidney capsule in Balb/c mice for periods of 6 weeks without immunosuppression. Sertoli cells are not only responsible for the synthesis of a wide variety of proteins and hormones required for the orderly differentiation of sperm cells, they also secrete a number of immunosuppressive agents[80,86] such as clusterin. This is a heterodimeric glycoprotein found in a wide variety of tissues under a number of different names such as sulfated glycoprotein-2 (SGP-2), SP-40, 40, Apo J, and gpIII.[87] This 70–80 kD protein is the most abundant protein synthesized by Sertoli cells and its exact function is not known. However, clusterin has been identified as a component of circulating cytolytically inactive terminal complement complex and appears to associate with C5b67 and C8 and C9 to form clusterin-C5b-9, which is analogous to SC5b-9.[88] This protein was shown to inhibit complement-mediated cell lysis.[89] Clusterin has also recently been shown to accelerate the formation of immune complexes *in vitro,* which suggests that the protein has a binding site for immunoglobulins.[90] From these findings, it has been speculated that clusterin may protect sperm from complement-mediated attack. In addition to clusterin, Sertoli cells also secrete cytokines such as transforming-growth factor (TGF) which is a multi-regulatory molecule that can stimulate or inhibit aspects of cellular growth and differentiation.[91] TGF also antagonizes many responses of lymphocytes by counteracting the effects of pro-inflammatory cytokines which may be beneficial to the protection of neonatal porcine islet xenografts from T-cell–mediated destruction. With this idea in mind, cotransplantation of neonatal porcine islets with neonatal porcine Sertoli cells may therefore prevent both antibody/complement and T-cell–mediated destruction of islet xenografts.

## GROWTH AND PROLIFERATION OF NEONATAL PORCINE ISLETS

Although neonatal porcine islets constitute an attractive source of xenogeneic insulin-producing tissue for clinical transplantation, many aspects of the model need further investigation. Since we have previously demonstrated that neonatal porcine islets have inherent ability for growth both *in vitro* and *in vivo*, one approach to more rapidly correct diabetes is to enhance the growth and proliferation of new cells *in vitro* prior to transplantation so that the islets contain a majority of endocrine cells. There is clearly a latent period (2–8 weeks) between transplantation of neonatal porcine islets and the reversal of hyperglycemia, albeit somewhat shorter than that observed for fetal porcine islet grafts (>2 months).[92] This delay presumably reflects the differentiation and growth of the grafted tissue after implantation and before diabetes can be corrected. To enhance this process, much attention has focused on factors that might regulate the differentiation and replication of cells *in vitro* and *in vivo*. Particular interest has been given to the possibility of influencing these variables *in vitro* before transplantation in order to promote an adequate graft function *in vivo*. In contrast to the extensive literature available on rodent fetal and adult islet growth and the growth factors involved in such a process,[93] information concerning porcine cell growth is limited. On the other hand, growth of fetal and to some extent adult human pancreatic cells, has been successfully accomplished by culturing with nicotinamide,[94] sodium-butyrate,[95] hepatocyte growth factor/scatter factor,[96–98] and by providing an extracellular matrix *in vitro*.[96,98,99] Extracellular matrices have also played a significant role in inducing neonatal rat islet cell growth *in vitro*,[100] and it has been shown that the cellular environment, including collagen and extracellular matrix components, can modulate cellular differentiation *in vitro*.[101] Furthermore, mature epithelia that normally lack expression of mesenchymal genes can be induced to express them by suspension of collagen gels *in vitro*,[102] and mammary epithelial cells, which tend to normally flatten and lose their differentiated phenotype when attached to plastic dishes, become round, polarized, secrete milk proteins, and accumulate a continuous basement membrane when the collagen gel is allowed to contract.[103] In addition to its role in cellular growth and differentiation, extracellular matrix has been recognized as a regulator of cell survival.[104] Disruption of the cell-to-matrix leads to apoptosis,[105,106] morphological changes,[107] and rapid dissolution of basement membrane can result in cell death.[108] It therefore appears likely that a cell-to-matrix and/or cell-to-cell interrelationships may play an essential role in islet cell survival and differentiation during *in vitro* tissue culture. Moreover, identification of the critical matrix and media constituents (i.e., growth factors), may potentially provide a means for enhancing *in vitro* proliferation of neonatal porcine cells, which is not only important for transplantation purposes, it may also identify mechanisms and growth factors that control islet neogenesis *in vivo*. Preliminary results from our laboratory indicated that microencapsulation and culture in the presence of autologous serum (i.e., provision of matrix and growth factors, respectively) allows for the growth and maturation of neonatal porcine islets *in vitro* and *in vivo*. When eight-day cultured neonatal porcine islets were microencapsulated with purified alginate, then re-cultured for 8 days in the presence of 5% (v/v) non–heat-inactivated autologous serum, the amount of insulin recovered increased by 89%. When transplants were then carried out in diabetic nude mice, all mice implanted intraperitoneally with 2000 encapsulated islets cultured with serum became normoglycemic within 14 days post-transplantation. These results suggest that microencapsulation and culture in the presence of serum enhance the functional maturation of neonatal porcine islets.

## XENOSIS

While progress has been made on the immunological problems of xenotransplantation, the risk of infectious disease transmission from graft to recipient, and conceivably on to the new host population, remains a topic of lively debate but relatively little research.[27] The risks can be reduced or eliminated by using specific-pathogen–free animal colonies, but this approach will not work for the porcine endogenous retrovirus (PERV) because the genome of these viruses is in the germline of every pig.[109] Multiple copies of PERV are integrated in the pig genome, which suggests that breeding "clean" pigs will be extremely difficult.[110] PERV particles are released spontaneously by cell lines originating from pig kidney, lymph node, testis, and fallopian tube.[110–112] PERV have approximately 60% sequence homology to the gibbon ape leukemia and murine leukemia C-type retrovirus.[112–115] Retroviruses result in lifelong infection[116] and reports that PERV from cell lines and porcine lymphocytes can infect human cells *in vitro*,[112, 114] have prompted the US Food and Drug Administration to put porcine xenograft trials on hold until previously exposed patients are assessed for PERV infection and until prospective monitoring of xenograft recipients is established. More recent studies[109, 117] in xenotransplantation had addressed these issues and promising results have been reported. Having established that the nested PCRs could detect single molecules of target sequence, Patience *et al.*,[117] had analyzed DNA isolated from patients' peripheral blood mononuclear cells and found no evidence of pig or PERV DNA in two renal dialysis patients whose circulation had been linked extracorporeally to pig kidneys. In addition, they found no seroconversion for PERV-specific antibodies. Similarly, Heneine *et al.*[109] were unable to detect markers of PERV infection in 10 diabetic patients who had received porcine fetal islets despite the evidence for extended exposure to pig cells and despite concomitant immunosuppressive therapy. These studies are important because they suggest the absence of PERV infection in patients which received pig tissue as well as established useful methods for detection of possible PERV infection in patients given pig xenografts.

## CONCLUSION

The finding that islet cell grafts can achieve and maintain long-term glucose homeostasis in human subjects has proven that islet transplantation can be a therapeutic option for management of type 1 diabetes. However, the shortage of human organ donors and the use of immunosuppressive drugs to prevent rejection of islet grafts, are one of the limiting factors for the application of islet transplantation in patients with type 1 diabetes. The potential of neonatal pigs as a source of unlimited supply of insulin-producing tissue for clinical transplantation is promising and protocols on how to avoid the need for continuous use of immunosuppression in patients with type 1 diabetes must be thoroughly examined. The safety and regulatory issues encompassing the use of animal tissue for clinical transplantation is a growing area of concern, and whether any of the identified PERVs would pose a hazard for humans is not known. Research intended to define and quantify infectious risks must be further developed so progress in the development of xenotransplantation can be achieved with enhanced safety.

## ACKNOWLEDGMENTS

This work was funded by the Medical Research Council of Canada, the Edmonton Civic Employees Charitable Assistance Fund, and the MacLachlan Fund of the University Hospitals Foundation. Miss Rayat is supported by a 75th Anniversary Faculty of Medicine Graduate Student Award and Dr. Korbutt is a recipient of a scholarship from the Canadian Diabetes Association and the Alberta Heritage Foundation for Medical Research.

## REFERENCES

1. Bliss, M. 1982. The discovery of insulin. McLelland & Stewart Inc. Toronto, p. 11.
2. Lacy, P.E. 1995. Islet cell transplantation for insulin-dependent diabetes. Hospital Practice **30:** 41–45.
3. Brandhorst, D., H. Brandhorst, B.J. Hering, K. Federlin & R.G Bretzel. 1995. Islet isolation from the pancreas of large mammals and humans: 10 years of experience. Exp. Clin. Endocrinol. **103:** 3–14.
4. Brandhorst, H., D. Brandhorst, B.J. Hering, K. Federlin & R.G. Bretzel. 1995. Body mass index of pancreatic donors: a decisive factor for human islet isolation. Exp. Clin. Endocrinol. **103:** 23–26.
5. Bretzel, R.G., B.J. Hering & K.F. Federlin. 1995. Islet cell transplantation in diabetes mellitus—from bench to bedside. Exp. Clin. Endocrinol. **103:** 143–159.
6. Calafiore, R. 1997. Perspectives in pancreatic and islet cell transplantation for the therapy of IDDM. Diabetes Care **20:** 889–896.
7. Slover, R.H. & G.S Eisenbarth. 1997. Prevention of type I diabetes and recurrence of β-cell destruction of transplanted islets. Endocrine Rev. **18:** 241–258.
8. Scharp, D.W., P.E. Lacy, J.V. Santiago, C.S. McCullough, L.G. Weide, L. Falqui, P. Marchetti, R.L. Gingerich, A.S. Jaffe, P.E. Cryer, C.B. Anderson & M.W. Flye. 1990. Insulin independence after islet transplantation into type 1 diabetic patient. Diabetes **39:** 515–518.
9. Warnock, G.L., N.M. Kneteman, E. Ryan, R.E. Seelis, A. Rabinovitch & R.V. Rajotte. 1991. Normoglycemia after transplantation of freshly isolated and cryopreserved pancreatic islets in type 1 (insulin-dependent) diabetes mellitus. Diabetologia **34:** 55–58.
10. Socci, C., L. Falqui, A.M. Davalli, C. Ricordi, S. Braghi, F. Bertuzzi, P. Maffi, A. Secci, F. Gavazzi, M. Freschi, P. Magistretti, S. Socci, A. Vignali, V. Di Carlo & G. Pozza. 1991. Fresh human islet transplantation to replace pancreatic endocrine function in type 1 diabetic patients: report of six cases. Acta Diabetol. **128:** 151–157.
11. Warnock, G.L., N.M. Kneteman, E.A. Ryan, A. Rabinovitch & R.V. Rajotte. 1992. Long-term follow-up after transplantation of insulin-producing pancreatic islets into patients with type 1 (insulin-dependent) diabetes mellitus. Diabetologia **35:** 89–95.

12. RICORDI, C., A.G. TZAKIS, P.B. CARROLL, Y.J. ZENG, H.L. RILO, R. ALEJANDRO, A. SHAPIRO, J.J. FUNG, A.J. DEMETRIS, D.H. MINTZ & T.E. STARZL. 1992. Human islet isolation and allotransplantation in 22 consecutive cases. Transplantation **53:** 407–414.
13. GORES, P.F., J.S. NAJARIAN, E. STEPHANIAN, J.J. LLOVERAS, S.L. KELLEY & D.E. SUTHERLAND. 1993. Insulin independence in type 1 diabetes after transplantation of unpurified islets from single donor with 15-deoxyspergualin. Lancet **341:** 19–21.
14. ALEJANDRO R., R. LEHMANN, C. RICORDI, N.S. KENYON, M.C. ANGELICO, G. BURKE, V. ESQUENAZI, J. NERY, A.E. BETANCOURT, S.S. KONG, J. MILLER & D.H. MINTZ. 1997. Long-term function (6 years) of islet allografts in type 1 diabetes. Diabetes **46:** 1983–1989.
15. RICORDI, C., C. SOCCI, C. DAVALLI, C. STAUDACHER, P. BARO, A. VERTOVA, I. SASSI, F. GAVAZZI, G. POZZA & V. DICARLO. 1989. Isolation of the elusive pig islet. Surgery **107:** 688–694.
16. KORSGREN, O., L. JANSSON, D. EIZIRIK & A. ANDERSSON. 1991. Functional and morphological differentiation of fetal porcine islet-like clusters after transplantation into nude mice. Diabetologia **34:** 379–386.
17. LUI X., K.F. FEDERLIN, R.G. BRETZEL, B.J. HERING & M.D. BRENDAI. 1991. Persistent reversal of diabetes by transplantation of fetal pig proislets into nude mice. Diabetes **40:** 858–866.
18. GROTH, C.G., O KORSGREN, A. TIBELL, J. TOLLFMAR, E. MOLLER, J. BOLINDER, J. OSTMAN, F.R. REINHOLD, C. HELLERSTROM & A. ANDERSSON. 1994. Transplantation of porcine fetal pancreas to diabetic patients. Lancet **344:** 1402– 1404.
19. DAVALLI, A.M., Y. OGAWA, L. SCALIA, Y-J. WU, J. HOLLISTER, S. BONNER-WEIR & G.C. WEIR. 1995. Function, mass and replication of porcine and rat islets transplanted into diabetic nude mice. Diabetes **44:** 104–111.
20. MARCHETTI, P., R. GIANNARELLI, S. COSMI, P. MASIELLO, A. COPPELLI, P. VIACAVA & R. NAVALESI. 1995. Massive isolation, morphological and functional characterization, and xenotransplantation of bovine pancreatic islets. Diabetes **44:** 375– 381.
21. WRIGHT, J.R., S. POLVI & S. MACLEAN. 1992. Experimental transplantation with principal islets of teleost fish (Brockman bodies). Long-term function of tilapia islet tissue in diabetic nude mice. Diabetes **41:** 1528–1532.
22. FERBER S., H. BELTRANDELRIO, J.H. JOHNSON, R.J. NOEL, L.E. CASSIDY, S. CLARK, T.C. BECKER, S.D. HUGHES & C.B. NEWGARD. 1994. GLUT-2 gene transfer into insulinoma cells confers both low and high affinity glucose-stimulated insulin release. J. Biol. Chem. **269:** 11523–11529.
23. KNAACK, D., D.M. FIORE, M. SURANA, M. LEISER, M. LAURANCE, D. FUSCO-DEMANE, O. D. HEGRE, N. FLEISCER & S. EFRAT. 1994. Clonal insulinoma cell line that stably maintains correct glucose responsiveness. Diabetes **43:** 1413–1417.
24. EFRAT, S., D. FUSCO-DEMANE, H. LEMBERG, O. EMRAN & X. WANG. 1995. Conditional transformation of a pancreatic beta-cell line derived from transgenic mice expressing a tetracycline-regulated oncogene. Proc. Natl. Acad. Sci. USA **92:** 3576– 3580.
25. KOVER K. & W. V. MOORE. 1989. Development of a method for isolation of islets from human fetal pancreas. Diabetes **38:** 917–924.
26. HAYEK, A., G. M. BEATTIE, V. CIRULLI, A. D. LOPEZ, C. RICORDI & J.S. RUBIN. 1995. Growth factor/matrix-induced proliferation of human adult β-cells. Diabetes **44:** 1458–1460.
27. SMITH, R. M. & T. E. MANDEL. 1998. Transplantation treatment for diabetes. Immunol. Today **19:** 444–447.
28. KORBUTT, G.S., J.F. ELLIOTT, Z. AO, D.K. SMITH, G.L. WARNOCK & R.V. RAJOTTE. 1996. Large scale isolation, growth, and function of porcine neonatal islet cells. J. Clin. Invest. **97:** 2119–2129.
29. WEBER, C.J., M.K. HAGLER, J.T. CHRYSSOCHOOS, J.A. KAPP, G.S. KORBUTT, R.V. RAJOTTE & P.S. LINSLEY. 1997. CTLA4-Ig prolongs survival of microencapsulated neonatal porcine islet xenografts in diabetic NOD mice. Cell Transplant. **6:** 505–508.

30. Schilling, A., W. Land, E. Pratschke, K. Pielsticker & W. Brendel. 1976. Dominant role of complement in the hyperacute xenograft rejection reaction. Surgery, Gynecol. & Obst. **142:** 29–32.
31. Auchincloss, H., Jr. 1988. Xenogeneic transplantation. A review. Transplantation **46:** 1–20.
32. Platt, J.L., G.M. Vercellotti, A.P. Dalmasso, A.J. Matas, R.M. Bolman, J.S. Najarian & F.H. Bach. 1990. Transplantation of discordant xenografts: A review of progress. Immunol. Today **11:** 450–456
33. Platt, J.L. & F.H. Bach. 1991. The barrier to xenotransplantation. Transplantation **52:** 937–947.
34. Baldwin, W.M. III, S.K. Pruitt, R.B. Brauer, M.R. Daha & F. Sanfilippo. 1995. Complement in organ transplantation—contributions to inflammation, injury and rejection. Transplantation **59:** 797–808.
35. Galili, U., E.A. Rachmilewitz, A. Peleg & I. Flechner. 1984. A unique natural human IgG antibody with anti-galactosyl specificity. J. Exp. Med. **160:** 1519–1531.
36. Galili, U. 1993. Interaction of natural anti-Gal antibody with galactosyl epitopes: a major obstacle for xenotransplantation in humans. Immunol. Today **14:** 480–482.
37. Sandrin, M.S., H.A. Vaughan, P.L. Dabkowski & I.F.C. McKenzie. 1993. Anti-pig IgM antibodies in human serum react predominantly with Galα(1,3)Gal epitopes. Proc. Natl. Acad. Sci. USA **90:** 11391–11395.
38. McMorrow, I., C. Comrack, D. Sachs & H. Dersimonian. 1997. Transplantation **64:** 501–510.
39. Oriol, R., Y. Ye, E. Koren & D.K.C. Cooper. 1993. Carbohydrate antigens of pig tissues reacting with human natural antibodies as potential targets for hyperacute vascular rejection in pig-to-man organ xenotransplantation. Transplantation **56:** 1433– 1442.
40. McKenzie, I.F.C., P.X. Xing, H.A. Vaughan, J. Prenzoska, P.L. Dabkowski & M.S. Sandrin. 1994. Distribution of the major xenoantigen (galα(1-3)gal) for pig to human xenografts. Transplant. Immunol. **2:** 81–86.
41. Rydberg, L., C.G. Groth, E. Moller, A. Tibell & B.E. Samuelsson: 1995. Is the Galα(1,3)Gal epitopes a major target for xenoantibodies on pig fetal islet cells? Xenotransplantation **2:** 148–153.
42. McKenzie, I.F.C., M. Koulmanda, T.E. Mandel, P.X. Xing & M.S. Sandrin. 1995. Pig-to-human xenotransplantation. The expression of Galα(1,3)Gal epitopes on pig islet cells. Xenotransplantation **2:** 1–7.
43. Satake, M., M. Kumagai-Braesch, O. Korsgren, A. Andersson & E. Moller. 1993. Characterization of humoral human anti-porcine xenoreactivity. Clin. Transplant. **7:** 281–288.
44. Korbutt, G.S., L. Aspeslet, R.V. Rajotte, G.L Warnock, Z. Ao, J. Ezekowitz, A.J. Malcolm, A. Koshal & R.W. Yatscoff. 1996. Natural human antibody-mediated destruction of porcine neonatal islet cell grafts. Xenotransplantation **3:** 207–216.
45. Schaapherder, A.F.M., M.R. Daha, F.J. Van Der Woude, J.A. Bruijn & H.G. Gooszen. 1993. IgM, IgG, and IgA antibodies in human sera directed against porcine islets of Langerhans. Transplantation **58:** 1576–1578.
46. Schaapherder, A.F.M., M.C.J. Wolvekamp, M.T.J.W. Te Bulte, E. Bouwman, H.G. Gooszen & M.R. Daha. 1996. Porcine islets of Langerhans are destroyed by human complement and not by antibody-dependent cell-mediated mechanisms. Transplantation **62:** 29–33.
47. Rayat, G.R., R.V. Rajotte, J.F. Elliott & G.S. Korbutt. 1998. Expression of Galα(1,3)Gal on neonatal porcine islet β-cells and susceptibility to human antibody/complement lysis. Diabetes **47:** 1406–1411.
48. McKenzie, I.F., M. Koulmanda, T.E. Mandel & M.S. Sandrin. 1998. Pig islet xenografts are susceptible to anti-pig but not to Galα(1,3)Gal antibody plus complement in Gal o/o mice. J. Immunol. **161:** 5116–5119.
49. Azimzadeh, A., I. Anegon, K. Thibaudeau, B. Charreau, P. Zibolt, J. Cinqualbre & J.P. Soulillou. 1997. Removal of anti-Galα(1,3)Gal antibodies diminishes

the cytotoxic effect of primate xenoreactive antibodies on rat endothelial cells. Transplant. Proc. **29:** 2337.
50. WEISS, R. A. Transgenic pigs and virus adaptation. 1998. Nature **39:** 327–328.
51. PRUITT, S.K., W.M. BALDWIN III, H.C. MARSH JR., S.S. LIN, C.G. YEH & R.R. BOLLINGER. 1991. The effect of soluble complement receptor type 1 on hyperacute xenograft rejection. Transplantation **52:** 868–873.
52. XIA, W., D.T. FEARON & R.L. KIRKMAN. 1993. Effect of repetitive doses of soluble human complement receptor type 1 on survival of discordant cardiac xenografts. Transplant. Proc. **25:** 410–411.
53. PRUITT, S.K., A.D. KIRK, R.R. BOLLINGER, H.C. MARSH JR., B.H. COLLINS, J.L. LEVIN, J.R. MAULT, J.S. HEINLE, S. IBRAHIM, A.R. RUDOLPH, W.M. BALDWIN III & F. SANFILIPPO. 1994. The effect of soluble complement receptor type 1 on hyperacute rejection of porcine xenografts. Transplantation **57:** 363–370.
54. CANDINAS, D., B.-A. LESNIKOSKI, S.C. ROBSON, T. MIYATAKE, S.M. SCESNEY, H.C. MARSH JR., U.S. RYAN, A.P. DALMASSO, W.W. HANCOCK & F.H. BACH. 1996. Effect of repetitive high-dose treatment with soluble complement receptor type 1 and cobra venom factor on discordant xenograft survival. Transplantation **62:** 336–342.
55. CHEN, C.-G., N. FISICARO, T.A. SHINKEL, V. AITKEN, M. KETERELOS, B.J.W. VAN DENDEREN, M.J. TANGE, R.J. CRAWFORD, A.J. ROBINS, M.J. PEARSE & A.J.F. D'APICE. 1996. Reduction in Gal-α1,3-Gal epitope expression in transgenic mice expressing human H-transferase. Xenotransplantation **3:** 69–75.
56. SANDRIN, M.S., W.L. FODOR, S. COHNEY, E. MOUHTOURIS, N. OSMAN, S.A. ROLLINS, S.P. SQUINTO & I.F.C. MCKENZIE. 1996. Reduction of the major porcine xenoantigen Gal(1,3)Gal by expression of α(1,2)fucosyltransferase. Xenotransplantation **3:** 134–140.
57. KOIKE, C., R. KANNAGI, Y. TAKUMA, F. AKUTSU, S. HAYASHI, N. HIRAIWA, K. KAOMATSU, T. MURAMATSU, H. YAMAKAWA, T. NAGAI, S. KOBAYASHI, H. OKADA, I. NAKASHIMA, K. UCHIDA, I. YOKOYAMA & H. TAKAGI. 1996. Introduction of α(1,2)-fucosyltransferase and its effect on α-Gal epitopes in transgenic pig. Xenotransplantation **3:** 81–86.
58. TEARLE, R.G., M.J. TANGE, Z.L. ZANNETTINO, M. KATERELOS, T.A. SHINKEL, B.J.W. VAN DENDEREN, A.J. LONIE, I. LYONS, M.B. NOTTLE, T. COX, C. BECKER, A.M. PEURA, P.L. WIGLEY, R.J. CRAWFORD, A.J. ROBINS, M.J. PEARSE & A.J.F. D'APICE. 1996. The α-1,3-Galactosyltransferase knockout mouse. Transplantation **61:** 13–19.
59. TANGE, M.J., E. SALVARIS, M. ROMANELLA, A. AMINIAN, M. KATERELOS, C. SOMERVILLE, R.G. TEARLE, M.J. PEARSE & A.J.F. D'APICE. 1997. Additive effects of CD59 expression in Gal knockout mice in vitro but not in an ex vivo model. Xenotransplantation **4:** 25–33.
60. MCCURRY, K.R., D.L. KOOYMAN, C.G. ALVARADO, A.H. COTTERELL, M.J. MARTIN, J.S. LOGAN & J.L. PLATT. 1995. Human complement regulatory proteins protect swine-to-primate cardiac xenografts from humoral injury. Nature Med. **1:** 423–427.
61. COZZI, E. & D.J.G. WHITE. 1995. The generation of transgenic pigs as potential organ donors for humans. Nature Med. **1:** 964–966.
62. CARY, N., J. MOODY, N. YANNOUTSOS, J. WALLWORK & D. WHITE. 1993. Tissue expression of human decay accelerating factor, a regulator of complement activation expressed in mice: A potential approach to inhibition of hyperacute xenograft rejection. Transplant. Proc. **25:** 400–401.
63. DIAMOND, L., E.R. OLDHAM, J. L. PLATT, H. WALDMANN, M. TONE, L.A. WALSH & J.S. LOGAN. 1994. Cell and tissue specific expression of a human CD59 minigene in transgenic mice. Transplant. Proc. **26:** 1239.
64. ROSENGARD, A.M., N.R. CARY, G.A. LANGFORD, A.W. TUCKER, J. WALLWORK & D.J. WHITE. 1995. Tissue expression of human complement inhibitor, decay-accelerating factor, in transgenic pigs—a potential approach for preventing xenograft rejection. Transplantation **59:** 1325–1333.

65. LANGFORD, G.A., N. YANNOUTSOS, E. COZZI, R. LANCASTER, K. ELSOME, P. CHEN, A. RICHARDS & D.J. WHITE. 1995. Production of pigs transgenic for human decay accelerating factor. Transplant. Proc. **26:** 1400–1401.
66. GILL, R. G., L. WOLF & M. COULOMBE. 1994. CD4+ T cells are both necessary and sufficient for islet xenograft rejection. Transplant. Proc. **26:** 1203.
67. WOLF, L. A., M. COULOMBE & R.G. GILL. 1995. Donor antigen-presenting cell-independent rejection of islet xenografts. Transplantation **60:** 1164–1170.
68. MARCHETTI, P., D.W. SCHARP, E.H. FINKE, C.J. SWANSON, B.J. OLEK, D. GERASIMIDI-VAZEOU, R. GIANNARELLI, R. NAVALESI & P.E. LACY. 1996. Prolonged survival of discordant porcine islet xenografts. Transplantation **61:** 1100–1102.
69. PIERSON, R. N. III, H.J. WINN, P.S. RUSSELL & H. AUCHINCLOSS JR. 1989. Xenogeneic skin graft rejection is especially dependent on CD4+ T cells. J. Exp. Med. **170:** 991–996.
70. DESAI, N.M., H. BASSIRI, J.S. ODORICO, B.H. KOLLER, O. SMITHIES, A. NAJI, C.F. BARKER & J.F. MARKMANN. 1993. Pancreatic islet allograft and xenograft survival in CD8+ T-lymphocyte-deficient recipients. Transplant. Proc. **25:** 961.
71. OSORIO, R.W., N.L. ASCHER & P.G STOCK. 1994. Prolongation of in vivo mouse islet allograft survival by modulation of MHC class I antigen. Transplantation **57:** 783–788.
72. MURRAY, A.G., M.M. KHODADOUST, J.S. POBER & A.L. BOTHWELL. 1994. Porcine aortic endothelial cells activate human T cells: direct presentation of MHC antigens and costimulation by ligands for human CD2 and CD28. Immunity **1:** 57–63.
73. YAMADA, K., D.H. SACHS & H. DERSIMONIAN. 1995. Human anti-porcine xenogeneic T cell response. Evidence for allelic specificity of mixed leukocyte reaction and for both direct and indirect pathways of recognition. J. Immunol. **155:** 5249–5256.
74. LENSCHOW, D. J., Y. ZENG, J.R. THISTLETHWAITE, A. MONTAG, W. BRADY, M.G. GIBSON, P.S. LINSLEY & J.A. BLUESTONE. 1992. Long-term survival of xenogeneic pancreatic islet grafts induced by CTLA4Ig. Science **257:** 789– 792.
75. SELAWRY, H.P., K.B. WHITTINGTON & D. BELLGRAU. 1989. Abdominal intratesticular islet xenograft survival in rats. Diabetes **38:** 220–223.
76. BAKER, C.F. & R.E. BILLINGHAM. 1977. Immunologically privileged sites. Adv. Immunol **25:** 1–54.
77. BOBZIEN, B., Y. YASUNAMI, M. MAJERCIK, P.E. LACY & J.M. DAVIE. 1983. Intratesticular transplants of islet xenografts (rat to mouse). Diabetes **32:** 213–216.
78. SELAWRY, H. & K. WHITTINGTON. 1984. Extended survival of islets grafted into the intra-abdominally placed testis. Diabetes **33:** 405–406.
79. WHITMORE III, W.F., L. KARSH & R.F. GITTES. 1985. The role of germinal epithelium and spermatogenesis in the privileged survival of intratesticular grafts. J. Urol. **134:** 782–786.
80. BELLGRAU, D., D. GOLD, H. SELAWRY, J. MOORE, A. FRANZUSOFF & R.C. DUKE. 1995. A role of CD95 ligand in preventing graft rejection. Nature **377:** 630–632.
81. STREILEIN, J.W. 1995. Unraveling immune privilege. Science **270:** 1158–1159.
82. NAGATA, S. & P. GOLSTEIN. 1995. The Fas death factor. Science **267:** 1449–1456.
83. ALDERSON, M.R., T.W. ROUGH, T. DAVIS-SMITH, S. BRADDY, B. FALK, K.A. SCHOOLEY, R.G. GOODWIN, C.A. SMITH, F. RAMSDELL & D.H. LYNCH. 1995. Fas ligand mediates activation-induced cell death in human T lymphocytes. J. Exp. Med. **181:** 71–77.
84. LYNCH, D.H., F. RAMSDELL & M.R. ALDERSON. 1995. Fas and Fas l in the homeostatic regulation of immune responses. Immunol. Today **16:** 569–574.
85. KORBUTT, G.S., J.F. ELLIOTT & R.V. RAJOTTE. 1997. Cotransplantation of allogeneic islets with testicular cell aggregates allows long-term graft survival without systemic immunosuppression. Diabetes **46:** 317–322.
86. SKINNER, M.K. 1991. Cell-cell interactions in the testis. Endocrin. Rev. **12:** 45–77.
87. CLARK, A. M. & M.D. GRISWOLD. 1997. Expression of clusterin/sulfated glycoprotein-2 under conditions of heat stress in rat sertoli cells and a mouse sertoli cell line. J. Androl. **18:** 257–263.
88. MURPHY, B.F., I.D. WALKER, L. KIRSZBAUM & A.J.F. D'APICE. 1988. SP-40-40-a newly identified normal human serum protein found in the SC5b-9 complex of

complement and in the immune deposits in glomerulonephritis. J. Clin. Invest. **81:** 1858–1864.
89. MURPHY, B.F., J.R. SAUNDERS, M.K. O'BRYAN, L. KIRSZBAUM, I.D. WALKER & A.J.F. D'APICE. 1989. SP-40-40 is an inhibitor of C5b-6 initiated hemolysis. Int. J. Immunol. **1:** 551–554.
90. WILSON, M.R., P.J. ROETH & S.B. EASTERBROOK-SMITH. 1991. Clusterin enhances the formation of insoluble immune complexes. Biochem. Biophys. Res. Commun. **177:** 985–990.
91. ROBERTS, A.B. & M.B. SPORN. 1988. Transforming growth factor beta. Adv. Can. Res. **51:** 107–145.
92. KORSGREN, O., L. JANSSON, D. EIZIRIK & A. ANDERSSON. 1991. Functional and morphological differentiation of fetal porcine islet-like clusters after transplantation into nude mice. Diabetologia **34:** 379–386.
93. BONNER-WEIR, S. & F.E. SMITH. 1994. Islet cell growth and the growth factors involved. Trends Endocrin. Metab. **5:** 60–64.
94. OTONKOSKI, T., G.M. BEATTIE, M.I. MALLY, C. RICORDI & A. HAYEK. 1993. Nicotinamide is a potent inducer of endocrine differentiation in cultured human fetal pancreatic cells. J. Clin. Invest. **92:** 1459–1466.
95. OTONKOSKI, T., J. USTINOV, M.A. HUOTARI, E. KALLIO & P. HAYRY. 1996. Nicotinamide and sodium butyrate potent synergistic effects on fetal porcine β cell differentiation. Diabetologia **39** (Suppl. 1)**:** 232A.
96. HAYEK, A., G.M. BEATTIE, V. CIRULLI, A.D. LOPEZ, C. RICORDI & J.S. RUBIN. 1995. Growth factor/matrix-induced proliferation of human adult b-cells. Diabetes **44:** 1458–1460.
97. OTONKOSKI, T., G.M. BEATTIE, J.S. RUBIN, A.D. LOPEZ, A. BAIRD & A. HAYEK. 1994. Hepatocyte growth factor/scatter factor has insulitropic activity in human fetal pancreatic cells. Diabetes **43:** 947–953.
98. BEATTIE, G.M., J.S. RUBIN, M.I. MALLY, T. OTONKOSKI & A. HAYEK. 1996. Regulation of proliferation and differentiation of human fetal pancreatic islet cells by extracellular matrix, hepatocyte growth factor, and cell-cell contact. Diabetes **45:** 1223–1228.
99. KERR-CONTE, J., F. PATTOU, M. LECOMTE-HOUCKE, X.J. XIA, B. BOILLY, C. PROYE & J. LEFEBVRE. 1996. Ductal cyst formation in collagen-embedded adult human islet preparations. Diabetes **45:** 1108–1114.
100. MONTESANO, R., P. MOURN, M. AMHERDT & L. ORCI. 1983. Collagen matrix promotes reorganization of pancreatic endocrine cell monolayers into islet-like organoids. J. Cell Biol. **97:** 935–939.
101. GOSPODAROWICZ, D., G. GREENBURG & C.R. BIRDWELL. 1978. Determination of cellular shape by the extracellular matrix and its correlation with the control of cellular growth. Cancer Res. **38:** 4155–4171.
102. HAY, E.D. 1993. Extracellular matrix alters epithelial differentiation. Curr. Opin. Cell Biol. **5:** 1029–1035.
103. EMERAN, J.T. & D.R. PITELKA. 1977. Maintenance and induction of morphological differentiation in dissociated mammary epithelium on floating collagen membranes. In Vitro **13:** 316–328.
104. BATES, R.C., L.F. LINCZ & G.F. BURNS. 1995. Involvement of integrins in cell survival. Cancer Metastasis Rev. **14:** 191–203.
105. FRISCH, S.M. & H. FRANCIS. 1994. Disruption of epithelial cell-matrix interaction induces apoptosis. J. Cell Biol. **124:** 619–126.
106. SCHWARTZ, S M. & M.R. BENNETT. 1995. Death by any other name. Am. J. Pathol. **147:** 229–234.
107. KERR, J.F.R., A.H. WYLLIE & A.R. CURRIE. 1972. Apoptosis: a basic biological phenomenon with wide-ranging implications in tissue kinetics. Br. J. Cancer **26:** 239–257.
108. BEN ZE'EV, A., S.R. FARMER & S. PENMAN. 1980. Protein synthesis requires cell-surface contact while nuclear events respond to cell shape in anchorage-dependent fibroblasts. Cell **21:** 365–372.

109. HENEINE, W., A. TIBELL, W.M. SWITZER, P. SANDSTROM, G. VASQUEZ ROSALES, A. MATHEWS, O. KORSGREN, L.E. CHAPMAN, T.M. FOLKS & C.G. GROTH. 1998. No evidence of infection with porcine endogenous retrovirus in recipients of porcine islet-cell xenografts. Lancet **352:** 695–699.
110. EIBER, M.M., C.J. SHERR, R.E. BENVENSISTE & G.J. TODARO. 1975. Biologic and immunologic properties of porcine type C viruses. Virology **66:** 616–619.
111. UZUKA, I., N. SHIMIZU, K. SEKIGUCHI, H. HOSHINO, M. KODAMA & K. SHIMOTOHNO. 1986. Molecular cloning of unintegrated closed circular DNA of porcine retrovirus. FEBA **198:** 339–343.
112. PATIENCE, C., Y. TAKEUCHI & R.A. WEISS. 1997. Infection of human cells by an endogenous retrovirus of pigs. Nat. Med. **3:** 282–286.
113. LE TESSIER, P., J. P. STOYE, Y. YASUHIRO, C. PATIENCE & R. A. WEISS. 1997. Two sets of human-tropic pig retrovirus. Nature **389:** 681–682.
114. WILSON, C.A., S. WONG, J. MULLER, C.E. DAVIDSON, T.M. ROSE & P. BURD.1998. Type C retrovirus released from porcine primary peripheral blood mononuclear cells infects human cells. J. Virol. **72:** 3082–3087.
115. AKIYOSI, D.E., M. DENARO, H. ZHU, J.L. GREENSTEIN, P. BANERJEE & J.A. FISHMAN. 1998. Identification of a full length cDNA for an endogenous retrovirus of miniature swine. J. Virol. **72:** 4503–4507.
116. COFFIN, J.M. 1990. Retroviridae and their replication. *In* Fields Virology, 2nd edition. B.N. Fields, D.M. Knipe, R.M. Chanock, *et al.*, Eds.: 1437–1500. Raven Press. New York.
117. PATIENCE, C., G.S. PATTON, Y. TAKEUCHI, R.A. WEISS, M.O. MCCLURE, L. RYDBERG & M.E. BREIMER. 1998. No evidence of pig DNA or retroviral infection in patients with short-term extracorporeal connection to pig kidneys. Lancet **352:** 699–701.

# Clinical Islet Transplantation: A Review

JOSÉ OBERHOLZER,[a] FRÉDÉRIC TRIPONEZ, JINNING LOU, AND PHILIPPE MOREL

*Division of Surgical Research, Department of Surgery, University Hospital, Rue Micheli-du-Crest 24, 1211 Geneva 14, Switzerland*

**ABSTRACT: For decades, the inability of insulin therapy to physiologically control glycemia in type I diabetic patients has motivated the search for insulin-delivering grafts. Islet autotransplantation is such a therapeutic approach to prevent diabetes mellitus following a major pancreatectomy, whereas allotransplantation is generally prescribed for type I diabetic patients with a functional solid organ graft, or for patients awaiting one. As of today, over 150 patients have been autotransplanted world-wide, following total or subtotal pancreatectomy, permitting an insulin-independence in nearly 40% of patients. Furthermore, more than 350 islet allotransplantations have been performed. Recent results show improved metabolic control in over 50% of cases and insulin-independence in approximately 20%. This chapter presents a literature review including preliminary human islet transplantation data from the University of Geneva.**

## INTRODUCTION

Islet transplantation may be the most emotionally charged area in diabetes research since its availability would provide the equivalent of a cure, bringing not only freedom from the burdens of injections, glucose testing, dietary restriction, and even more importantly, protection from the dreaded complications of the disease.[1] Since the discovery of insulin in 1921 by Banting and Best, insulin therapy has permitted diabetic patients to survive. Nevertheless, chronic complications evolving years after the onset of diabetes, including blindness and renal failure, damage the quality of life and represent a multi-billion dollar annual burden on the health care systems of industrialized countries.[2] These figures can be appreciated in light of kidney transplant expenses, which, in Switzerland, are billed to insurance at a rate of approximately $50,000 per operation. It is estimated that the prevalence of type II diabetes in Western countries is as much as 5% and of insulin-dependent type I diabetes approximately 0.4%, with the highest incidence of 42 cases per 100,000 per year in Finland.[3] Approximately 50% of diabetics will develop chronic diabetic complications.[4]

Several clinical trials have demonstrated that strict glycemic control can prevent or even stop the progression of diabetic complications.[5,6] Unfortunately, intensive insulin therapy increases by a factor of three the incidence of hypoglycemic episodes and is only suitable for selected patients.[7] Therefore, pancreas transplantation is the only therapeutic modality which can prevent the progression of diabetic complica-

[a]Corresponding author: Division of Surgical Research, Department of Surgery, University Hospital, Rue Micheli-du-Crest 24, 1211 Genève 14, Switzerland; (41) 22 372 33 11 (voice); (41) 22 372 77 55 (fax); celtrans@cmu.unige.ch (e-mail).

tions without increasing the incidence of hypoglycemic events.[8] Unfortunately, this procedure, which is usually performed simultaneously with a kidney transplant, has a high morbidity and a significant mortality rate.[9] Evidently, pancreas transplantation, in spite of an important impact on the quality of life in successful cases,[10] will be restricted to a small group of highly selected patients. In this context, islet transplantation appears to be the ideal solution, allowing a normalization of glucose metabolism without the risk of hypoglycemia[11] and avoiding the potentially life-threatening complications of whole pancreas grafts:

> On December 20th (1893) my surgical colleague, Mr. Harsant, placed the patient under chloroform, while I extracted the pancreas with strict aseptic precautions from a freshly-slaughtered sheep, so that by the time the patient was anaesthesied the pancreas was at hand, and three pieces each of the size of a brazil nut had been grafted into the subcutaneous tissues of the breast and abdomen, and the operation completed within twenty minutes of the death of the sheep.[12]

Although the first "islet transplantation" was performed more than 100 years ago, only in the last 20 years has light shone on this endeavor. While the islet transplantation concept is simple, its wide-spread clinical applicability is hampered by technical and biological obstacles. This chapter presents a review of clinical islet auto- and allotransplantation.

## ISLET ISOLATION

During the 1970s pioneering work by Lacy involving the development of islet isolation[13] and islet transplantation in rats[14] was rapidly applied in large animal models[15,16] and consequently in humans.[17,18] While in the small animal model, two mice (total body weight 50 g) can be transplanted with islets from one rat (body weight 300 g), a clinical therapy will demand more efficient islet usage. Specifically, the serious human organ shortage demands more efficient islet isolation procedures permitting a transplant for one person from each donor. Such statistics are not presently attainable in clinical practice. Indeed, some centers have reported to use as much as 6 to 9 pancreata for one islet transplantation.[19] Nonetheless, most centers tend to use, if possible, an islet graft from one excellent isolation procedure (e.g., the Universities of Miami and Giessen, personal communications from C. Ricordi and M. Brendel). Under optimal conditions, every third to fifth islet isolation can deliver a single pancreas islet graft. Furthermore, the enormous variability of donor factors and organ procurement–related variables reduces the potential number of clinical islet transplants.[20] Factors affecting the success of islet isolation have been extensively studied.[21] While donor factors are largely fixed and can be influenced only by adequate donor selection (donor > 20 years, high body mass index, no cardiac arrest, no severe hypotension, no or low vasoactive medication, short intensive-care stay), the procurement technique has a major impact on the outcome of islet isolation and a short (< 20 min) secondary ischemia time is of crucial importance.[22]

The development of an automated digestion and purification procedure for islet isolation by C. Ricordi[23] was a breakthrough in this field and allowed reproducible clinical application. Nonetheless, the large variability in collagenase activity added another uncertainty to the isolation procedure.[24] Purified enzyme blends such as Liberase® (Boehringer-Mannheim) are, therefore, promising.[25] However, in spite of initial convincing results and a less aggressive digestion allowing the isolation of more intact islets, lots with low enzymatic activity still remain a problem.

The purification process of the digest has been the focus of intense research.[26–31] Although, a large variety of continous and discontinous density gradients have been tested, the tradeoff between purity and islet loss remains unresolved owing to the limiting factor of density gradients, namely, the minimal difference of density between islets and exocrine tissue. The purification of islets by magnetic beads linked to islet specific antibodies is an interesting concept; however, it has not gained acceptence for large scale purification of human islets.[32]

Evidently, as long as the islet-isolation procedure remains unreliable, thereby rendering islet yields irreproducible among the different reporting laboratories, clinical islet transplantation will be restricted to some experienced centers. In the last 10 years, research in the field of islet-isolation techniques has not made any important advances and has lost some attractiveness as documented by the lack of any recent "landmark article" in this field. However, the islet isolation technique is of fundamental importance, as good islet isolation is the *conditio sine qua non* of successful islet transplantation. It is probable that the actual isolation technique with the available enzymes and the purification by density gradients has reached a plateau (5–10,000 islet equivalent per g pancreatic tissue) and that for further improvement a completely different approach will be required. While in the intraductal collagenase technique used in the Ricordi procedure, the islets are isolated by partial destruction of the connective tissue and subsequent separation from exocrine tissue by slightly different densities, another approach would be the selective destruction of the exocrine tissue allowing a more elegant direct isolation of intact islets. Methods for selective destruction of exocrine tissue could be developed by using antibody-mediated radiosensitization, induction of gene transfer–mediated apoptosis or destruction.

## ISLET AUTOTRANSPLANTATION

In the absence of endogenous insulin delivery and lack of counter-regulatory hormones, e.g., glucagon, postpancreatectomy diabetes tends to be particularly difficult to treat, with frequent hypoglycemic events. In addition, the underlying alcohol and narcotics abuse in chronic pancreatitis patients complicates the diabetic treatment after extensive pancreatectomy by non-compliance and malnutrition. The fact that, in most of these patients, the endocrine function prior to surgery is sufficient to maintain insulin-independence has led to the concept of islet autotransplantation. Prevention of diabetes by islet autotransplantation has an important impact on the quality of life of pancreatectomized patients. To date, over 150 patients have been autotransplanted world-wide after total or subtotal pancreatectomy with persisting insulin-independence in 37% and 58%, respectively.[33]

The main indication for total or subtotal pancreatectomy is actually chronic, small duct pancreatitis with disabling chronic pain. Reported results for this indication are rather encouraging,[34–36] and the clinical application should gain more acceptance in the future.

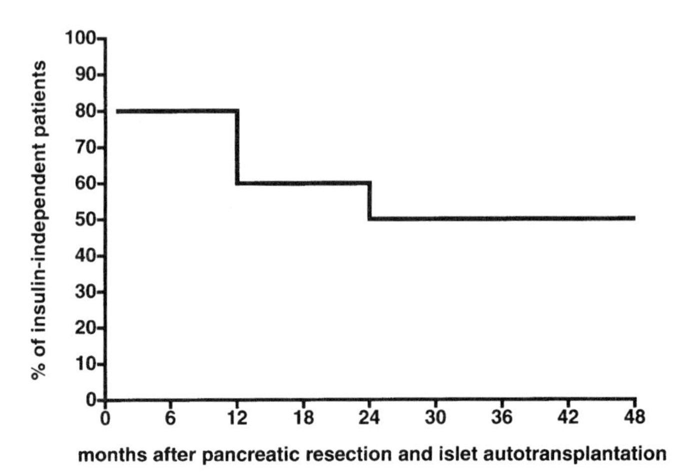


**FIGURE 1.** Actuarial insulin-independence after islet autotransplantation following extensive to total pancreatectomy in 10 patients.

Our group has extended the indication for islet autotransplantation to extensive (> 80%) pancreatectomy for benign tumors of the pancreas.[37] From 1992 to 1998 thirteen islet autotransplantations have been performed at our institution. The rate of insulin-independence in ten patients with a follow up of more than one year is summarized in FIGURE 1. Approximately 50% of our patients remained insulin-independent for more than two years (FIG. 1). Two patients were still insulin-independent 5 years after total and subtotal pancreatectomy. The main cause of immediate graft failure was an insufficient islet mass by preexisting glucose intolerance (3 out of 13). Recurrence of alcohol abuse was responsible for late islet failure in another two patients.

Autotransplantation may be restricted to a small group of patients undergoing extensive pancreatectomy for benign disease, nonetheless its clinical application has not only prevented postoperative diabetes in some patients, but has additionally brought to light the pathophysiology of ectopic, endogenous insulin production by intrahepatic islets. The short-term results of clinical trials of islet autotransplantation with some primary failures, indicate that actual islet isolation procedures inevitably decrease islet mass. Moreover, in spite of having to deal with neither allo- nor autoimmunity, long-term data suggest that islets transplanted into the portal circulation are exposed to deleterious factors (nutritional toxins, high postprandial glucose levels and endotoxins from intestinal bacteria) which, in some patients, leads to gradual graft loss. The mechanisms that ultimately decrease the islet mass in some patients remain, thus far, unkown. In spite of these unanswered questions, the authors believe that there is sufficient clinical evidence to validate the islet transplantation concept.

## ISLET ALLOTRANSPLANTATION

Allotransplantation is prescribed for type I diabetic patients with a functional solid organ graft, or for patients on the waiting list.[38] Following islet isolation, purifi-

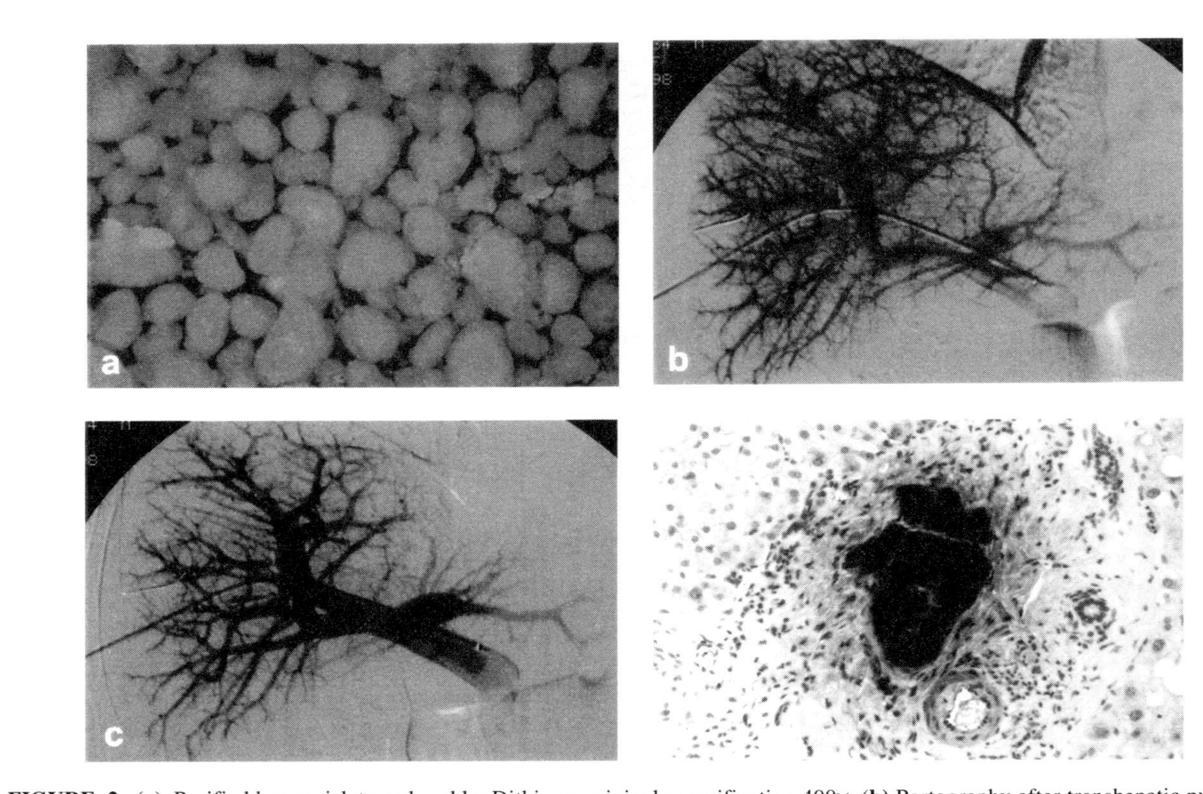


**FIGURE 2.** **(a)** Purified human islets, colored by Dithizon, original magnification 400×. **(b)** Portography after transhepatic puncture of the portal vein (courtesy of Dr. C. Becker and Dr. P. A. Schneider, Division of Radiology, Geneva University Hospital) prior to and **(c)** after islet transplantation. **(d)** Islet in a portal vein, 1 year after transplantation, positive insulin-staining, original magnification 400×.

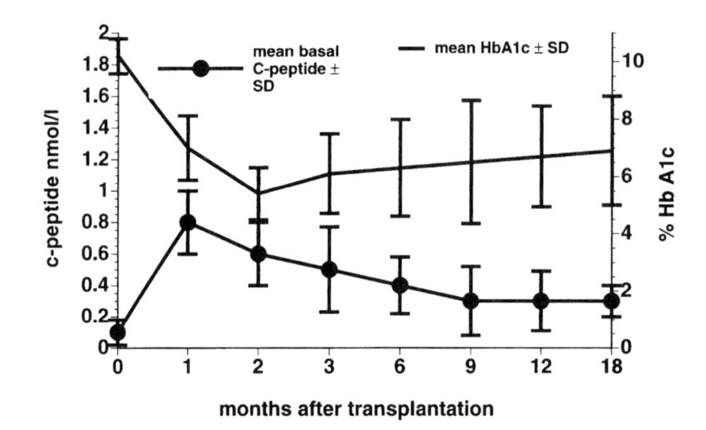


**FIGURE 3.** Summary of the evolution of c-peptide and HbA1c in 7 islet allotransplantations with a follow up of more than 1 year at the Geneva University Hospital. Endogenous insulin production permits a clear decrease in HbA1c.

cation and culture for 24 to 72 hours, the islets are transplanted by a transhepatic puncture of the portal vein and embolized in small portal veins (FIG. 2). More than 350 islet allotransplantations have been performed to date. Recent results show improved metabolic control in over 50% of cases and insulin-independence in approximately 20% (results presented by the International Islet Transplant Registry ITR in July 1998 at the World Congress of the Transplantation Society in Montreal). These data have been confirmed by our group.[39]

While our short-term results of islet allotransplantation in patients with type I diabetes are excellent, with 100% graft function within the first months, middle- and long-term data are less encouraging, with graft loss in 3 out of 10 patients after 3 to 6 months and a decrease in c-peptide production in an other 3 patients (FIG. 3). Nevertheless, one patient has been completely off insulin and presents normal metabolic tests for more than 2.5 years (FIG. 4), confirming that islet allotransplantation has the potential to cure diabetes.

The majority of the allotransplantations have been performed in type I diabetic patients with end stage renal disease—a clinical situation exposing the graft not only to allo- but also to automimmunity. However, fifteen patients with extensive abdominal surgery for abdominal tumors requiring total hepatectomy and pancretectomy have been transplanted with alloislets.[40–42] In this small group, nine patients (60%) became insulin-independant, indicating that the co-transplanted liver might modulate alloreactivity and suggesting that autoimmunity plays a crucial role in the islet loss in type I diabetic patients. The clinical data presented recently by Giessen's group, demonstrated a significantly increased incidence of graft loss in patients testing positive for anti-GAD 65 and anti-islets antibodies.[43,44] A high recurrence rate of diabetes after partial pancreas transplantation between identical twins and its very low incidence in unrelated allografts[45] underscore the implication of autoimmunity in the chronic loss of endogenous insulin production.[46]

In whole organ transplantation, the conventional immunosuppression prevents recurrence of autoimmunity in the vast majority of cases. To date, there is no convinc-

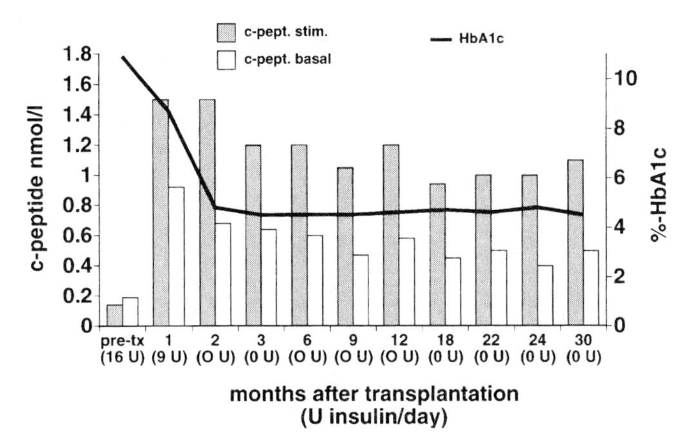


**FIGURE 4.** Metabolic follow up in a type I diabetic patient who became insulin-independent after islet allotransplantation.

ing explanation for why isolated islets with similar immunosuppression are more susceptible to autoimmune factors than islets embedded in the whole pancreas.

## FUTURE PERSPECTIVES

The limited availability of human tissue has motivated research in the field of islet xenotransplantation. Apart from concerns about infectious diseases, the major obstacle to xenotransplantation is the inevitable rejection. Thus, research in this field has mainly focused on new immunotherapeutic modalities. The various proposed approaches can be grossly divided into immunosuppression, immunomodulation, and immunoisolation. Among others techniques, immunomodulation was attempted with different culture conditions, antibodies[47] and using UVB irradiation;[48] in spite of promising and excellent experimental reports in small animals, immunomodulation has not gained clinically successful applicability.

A number of immunoisolation systems have been developed over the past decades. Three major types of immunoisolation have been studied by different groups: perfusion shunt devices anastomosed to the vascular system,[49] diffusion chambers or macrocapsules, and microcapsules. However, the clinical application of these devices is hindered, in many cases, by problems such as fragility, limited surface area, and, in the case of perfused vascular devices, the surgery required for implantation. Shunt connection, with risks of hemorrhage, thrombosis, embolism and infection, and the relatively high diffusion resistance inherent in the plastic membrane[50] are additional concerns. Immunoisolation barriers, such as microcaspules, bypass these problems and provide additional options for the method and site of implantation. Specifically, Sun, in 1980 provided the first evidence that encapsulated islets could regulate blood glucose in rats.[51] By isolating rat islets and encapsulating these in water soluble polymeric capsules with a semipermeable membrane, the ingress of nutrients and egress of cellular debris could be controlled, while protecting the graft (an islet cluster containing insulin-secreting β-cells) from the host's immune system. These capsules, based on naturally occurring polysaccharides and polyaminoacids have been shown to regulate the blood glucose for periods exceeding six months.[52] The results have recently been extended to spontaneously diabetic cynomogulus monkeys providing the first "large" animal (Sun's monkeys weigh 2–3 kg) evidence of discordant xenograft function.[53]

In light of the recent fear of transmission of zoonosis by xenotransplantation,[54] reproduction of human tissue by genetic engineering appears to be an attractive alternative. In fact, new HIV-derived viruses developed by D. Trono[55] infect non-dividing cells and potentially could incorporate oncogenes into the genom of the target cell and Ph. Halban's group has developed a large-scale method for isolating human β-cells by a targeted expression of green fluorescent protein.[56] These two tools inaugurate a new area in the field of islet transplantation. The future will show whether the surgical approach of xenotransplantation or the more sophisticated, molecular biology method of mass reproduction of human islets or β-cells will lead to a cure for established diabetes mellitus. To date, while the bioartificial pancreas has remained a promising therapy, with the exception of one reported case,[57] there have been no systematic demonstrations of clinical efficacy of the combined use of islet or β-cell transplantation (allograft) and immunoisolaton (e.g., microencapsulation).

In summary, the clinical data obtained thus far, and the results of basic research suggest, that islet transplantation is a valid concept and that immunoisolation may be a straightforward way to long-term clinical success. The authors recommend that research in clinical islet transplantation continue to focus auto- and allotransplantation, providing a limited number of worst-case patients the chance to alleviate the burdens of an unstable diabetes, or even cure an onset diabetes, while accumulating data sufficient to scale up the technology to a larger population. Specifically, the bioartificial pancreas community needs to enhance the investigations in xenotransplantation, genetically modified cell lines, and biomaterials to lay the framework for a second generation of devices which can treat type I diabetics in a non-obtrusive manner.

## ACKNOWLEDGMENTS

We thank Corinne Sinigaglia, Raymond Mage, David Matthey and Elisabeth Bernoulli for their technical assistance. Without the initial and continuous efforts of Léo Bühler, Shaopping Deng, Elisabeth Andereggen, Béatrice Fournier, and Nathalie Cretin our series of 24 clinical islet transplantations would not have been possible. We also thank the Division of Diabetology (Jacques Philippe, Aileen Caulfield and Tatjana Daneva) for their precious help in the clinical follow up of transplanted patients and David Hunkeler from EPFL for his suggestions in the field of encapsulation.

This work was supported by grant No. 32-50865.97 from the Swiss National Science Foundation (to Ph. Morel, J. Philippe, and J. Lou).

## REFERENCES

1. WEIR, G.C. & S. BONNER-WEIR. 1997. Scientific and political impediments to successful islet transplantation. Diabetes **46:** 1247–1256.
2. 1997. National Diabetes Fact Sheet: National Estimates and General Information on Diabetes in the United States. Department of Health and Human Services, Centers for Disease Control and Prevention. Atlanta, GA, USA
3. GREEN, A., E.A. GALE & C.C. PATTERSON. 1992. Incidence of childhood-onset insulin-dependent diabetes mellitus: the EURODIAB ACE Study. Lancet **339:** 905–909.
4. HASSLACHER, C., E. RITZ, P. WAHL, *et al.* 1989. Similar risks of nephropathy in patients with type I or type II diabetes mellitus. Nephrol. Dial. Transplant. **4:** 859–863.
5. THE DIABETES CONTROL AND COMPLICATIONS TRIAL RESEARCH GROUP. 1993. The effect of intensive treatment of diabetes on the development and progression of long-term complications in insulin-dependent diabetes mellitus. N. Engl. J. Med. **329:** 977–986.
6. WANG, P.H., J. LAU & T.C. CHALMERS. 1993. Meta-analysis of effects of intensive blood-glucose control on late complications of type I diabetes. Lancet **341:** 1306–1309.
7. GAUTIER, J.F., J.P. BERESSI, H. LEBLANC, *et al.* 1996. Are the implications of the Diabetes Control and Complications Trial (DCCT) feasible in daily clinical practice? Diabetes Metab. **22:** 415–419.
8. MOREL, P., C. CHAU, K. BRAYMAN, *et al.* 1992. Quality of metabolic control at 2 to 12 years after a pancreas transplant. Transplant. Proc. **24:** 835–838.
9. GRUESSNER, A.C., D.E. SUTHERLAND & R.W. GRUESSNER. 1998. Report of the International Pancreas Transplant Registry. Transplan. Proc. **30:** 242–243.
10. LANDGRAF, R. 1996. Impact of pancreas transplantation on diabetic secondary complications and quality of life. Diabetologia **39:** 1415–1424.
11. MEYER, C., B.J. HERING, R. GROSSMANN, *et al.* 1998. Improved glucose counterregulation and autonomic symptoms after intraportal islet transplants alone in patients with long-standing type I diabetes mellitus. Transplantation **66:** 233–240.
12. WILLIAMS, P.W. 1894. Notes on diabetes treated with grafts of sheep's pancreas. Br. Med. J. **2:** 1303.
13. LACY, P.E. & M. KOSTIANOVSKY. 1967. Method for the isolation of intact islets of Langerhans from the rat pancreas. Diabetes **16:** 35–39.
14. BALLINGER, W.F. & P.E. LACY. 1972. Transplantation of intact pancreatic islets in rats. Surgery **72:** 175–186.
15. MIRKOVITCH, V. & M. CAMPICHE. 1976. Successful intrasplenic autotransplantation of pancreatic tissue in totally pancreatectomised dogs. Transplantation **21:** 265–269.
16. LORENZ, D., R. REDING, J. PETERMANN, *et al.* 1976. Transplantation of isolated islets of Langerhans into the liver of diabetic dogs. Zentralbl. Chir. **101:** 1359–1368.
17. NAJARIAN, J.S., D.E. SUTHERLAND, A.J. MATAS, *et al.* 1977. Human islet transplantation: a preliminary report. Transplant. Proc. **9:** 233–236.
18. SUTHERLAND, D.E., A.J. MATAS, F.C. GOETZ, *et al.* 1980. Transplantation of dispersed pancreatic islet tissue in humans: autografts and allografts. Diabetes **29** (Suppl. 1)**:** 31–44.
19. KEYMEULEN, B., Z. LING, F. GORUS, *et al.* 1998. Implantation of standardized beta-cell grafts in a liver segment of IDDM patients: graft and recipient characteristics in two cases of insulin-independence under maintenance immunosuppression for prior kidney graft. Diabetologia **41:** 452–459.
20. BRANDHORST, D., H. BRANDHORST, M. BRENDEL, *et al.* 1998. Problems of islet isolation from the human and porcine pancreas for islet transplantation into men. Zentralbl. Chir. **123:** 814–822.
21. BENHAMOU, P.Y., P.C. WATT, Y. MULLEN, *et al.* 1994. Human islet isolation in 104 consecutive cases. Factors affecting isolation success. Transplantation **57:** 1804–1810.

22. BRANDHORST, D., H. BRANDHORST, B.J. HERING, *et al.* 1995. Islet isolation from the pancreas of large mammals and humans: 10 years of experience. Exp. Clin. Endocrinol. Diabetes **103** (Suppl. 2): 3–14.
23. RICORDI, C., P.E. LACY, E.H. FINKE, *et al.* 1988. Automated method for isolation of human pancreatic islets. Diabetes **37:** 413–420.
24. JOHNSON, P.R., S.A. WHITE & N.J. LONDON. 1996. Collagenase and human islet isolation. Cell Transplant. **5:** 437–452.
25. LINETSKY, E., R. BOTTINO, R. LEHMANN, *et al.* 1997. Improved human islet isolation using a new enzyme blend, liberase. Diabetes **46:** 1120–1123.
26. ALEJANDRO, R., S. STRASSER, P.F. ZUCKER, *et al.* 1990. Isolation of pancreatic islets from dogs. Semiautomated purification on albumin gradients. Transplantation **50:** 207–210.
27. BEHBOO, R., P.B. CARROLL, F. UKAH, *et al.* 1994. One-hour of hypothermic incubation in Euro-Collins improves islet purification. Transplant. Proc. **26:** 645.
28. SOON-SHIONG, P., R. HEINTZ, T. FUJIOKA, *et al.* 1990. Utilization of anti-acinar cell monoclonal antibodies in the purification of rat and canine islets. Horm. Metab. Res. **25** (Suppl.): 45–50.
29. SAMEJIMA, T., K. YAMAGUCHI, H. IWATA, *et al.* 1998. Gelatin density gradient for isolation of islets of Langerhans. Cell Transplant. **7:** 37–45.
30. LAKEY, J.R., T.J. CAVANAGH & M.A. ZIEGER. 1998. A prospective comparison of discontinuous EuroFicoll and EuroDextran gradients for islet purification. Cell Transplant. **7:** 479–487.
31. LONDON, N.J., S.M. SWIFT & H.A. CLAYTON. 1998. Isolation, culture and functional evaluation of islets of Langerhans. Diabetes Metab. **24:** 200–207.
32. NANDIGALA, P., T.H. CHEN, C. YANG, *et al.* 1997. Immunomagnetic isolation of islets from the rat pancreas. Biotechnol. Prog. **13:** 844–848.
33. ROBERTSON, G.S., A.R. DENNISON, P.R. JOHNSON, *et al.* 1998. A review of pancreatic islet autotransplantation. Hepatogastroenterology **45:** 226–235.
34. WAHOFF, D.C., B.E. PAPALOIS, J.S. NAJARIAN, *et al.* 1995. Autologous islet transplantation to prevent diabetes after pancreatic resection. Ann. Surg. **222:** 562–575.
35. TEUSCHER, A.U., D.M. KENDALL, Y.F. SMETS, *et al.* 1998. Successful islet autotransplantation in humans: functional insulin secretory reserve as an estimate of surviving islet cell mass. Diabetes **47:** 324–330.
36. FOURNIER, B., E. ANDEREGGEN, L. BUHLER, ***et al.*** 1998. Long term evaluation of 9 islet autotransplantations after pancreatic resection. Schweiz. Med. Wochenschr. **128:** 856–859.
37. FOURNIER, B., E. ANDEREGGEN, L. BUHLER, *et al.* 1997. Human islet autotransplantations: new indications. Transplant. Proc. **29:** 2420–2422.
38. OBERHOLZER, J., F. TRIPONEZ, A. CAULFIELD, *et al.* 1998. Islet transplantation: quo vadis? Méd. et Hyg. **56:** 1337–1341.
39. CRETIN, N., L. BUHLER, B. FOUMIER, *et al.* 1998. Results of human islet allotransplantation in cystic fibrosis and type I diabetic patients. Transplant. Proc. **30:** 315–316.
40. TZAKIS, A.G., C. RICORDI, R. ALEJANDRO, *et al.* 1990. Pancreatic islet transplantation after upper abdominal exenteration and liver replacement. Lancet **336:** 402–405.
41. CARROLL, P.B., H.L. RILO, R. ALEJANDRO, *et al.* 1995. Long-term (> 3-year) insulin independence in a patient with pancreatic islet cell transplantation following upper abdominal exenteration and liver replacement for fibrolamellar hepatocellular carcinoma. Transplantation **59:** 875–879.
42. 1995/96. International Islet Transplant Registry. Justus-Liebig-University of Giessen.
43. JAEGER, C., M.D. BRENDEL, B.J. HERING, *et al.* 1998. IA-2 antibodies are only positive in association with GAD 65 and islet cell antibodies in islet transplanted insulin-dependent diabetes mellitus patients. Transplant. Proc. **30:** 659–660.
44. JAEGER, C., M.D. BRENDEL, B.J. HERING, *et al.* 1997. Progressive islet graft failure occurs significantly earlier in autoantibody-positive than in autoantibody-negative IDDM recipients of intrahepatic islet allografts. Diabetes **46:** 1907–1910.

45. TYDEN, G., F.P. REINHOLT, G. SUNDKVIST, *et al.* 1996. Recurrence of autoimmune diabetes mellitus in recipients of cadaveric pancreatic grafts. N. Engl. J. Med. **335:** 860–863.
46. SUTHERLAND, D.E., F.C. GOETZ & R.K. SIBLEY. 1989. Recurrence of disease in pancreas transplants. Diabetes **38** (Suppl. 1)**:** 85–87.
47. LACY, P.E., J.M. DAVIE & E.H. FINKE. 1980. Prolongation of islet xenograft survival without continuous immunosuppression. Science **209:** 283–285.
48. LAU, H., K. REEMTSMA & M.A. HARDY. 1984. Prolongation of rat islet allograft survival by direct ultraviolet irradiation of the graft. Science **223:** 607–609.
49. PETRUZZO, P., L. PIBIRI, M.A. DE GIUDICI, *et al.* 1991. Xenotransplantation of microencapsulated pancreatic islets contained in a vascular prosthesis: preliminary results. Transplant. Int. **4:** 200–204.
50. LANZA, R.P. & W.L. CHICK. 1997. Experimental pancreatic islet cell xenotransplantation. *In* Xenotransplantation, D.K.C. Cooper, E. Kemp, J.L. Platt, *et al.*, Eds.: 534–544. Springer. Berlin.
51. LIM, F. & A.M. SUN. 1980. Microencapsulated islets as bioartificial endocrine pancreas. Science **210:** 908–910.
52. O'SHEA, G.M., M.F. GOOSEN & A.M. SUN. 1984. Prolonged survival of transplanted islets of Langerhans encapsulated in a biocompatible membrane. Biochim. Biophys. Acta **804:** 133–136.
53. SUN, Y., X. MA, D. ZHOU, *et al.* 1996. Normalization of diabetes in spontaneously diabetic cynomologus monkeys by xenografts of microencapsulated porcine islets without immunosuppression. J. Clin. Invest. **98:** 1417–1422.
54. BACH, F.H. & H.V. FINEBERG. 1998. Call for moratorium on xenotransplants. Nature **391:** 326.
55. NALDINI, L., U. BLOMER, P. GALLAY, *et al.* 1996. In vivo gene delivery and stable transduction of nondividing cells by a lentiviral vector. Science **272:** 263–267.
56. MEYER, K., J.C. IRMINGER, L.G. MOSS, *et al.* 1998. Sorting human beta-cells consequent to targeted expression of green fluorescent protein. Diabetes **47:** 1974–1977.
57. SOON-SHIONG, P., R.E. HEINTZ, N. MERIDETH, *et al.* 1994. Insulin independence in a type 1 diabetic patient after encapsulated islet transplantation. Lancet **343:** 950–951.

# Islet Cryopreservation Protocols

RAY V. RAJOTTE[a]

*Departments of Surgery and Medicine, Surgical-Medical Research Institute, University of Alberta, Edmonton, Alberta T6G 2N8 Canada*

**ABSTRACT: Low temperature banking of islets has facilitated ongoing clinical trials, allowing for the collection and long-term storage of islets during which viability and sterility assessment can be carried out. Islets from most species of animals have been cryopreserved using various freeze-thaw protocols; however, the best to date is slow cooling to −40°C and rapid thawing from −196°C. If one carefully follows the three distinct steps of freezing and thawing human islets can be successfully cryopreserved, allowing for the establishment of a low temperature bank with diverse HLA (Human Leukocyte Antigen) and ABO phenotypes. Using a combination of fresh and cryopreserved islets to transplant type I diabetic patients, long-term insulin independence has been obtained.**

## INTRODUCTION

The transplantation of isolated islets has been shown to induce long-term normoglycemia and insulin independence in type I insulin-dependent diabetic patients.[1–8] Evaluation of recent clinical islet transplants by the International Islet Transplant Registry identified several common characteristics in all patients achieving insulin independence following islet transplantation. One of these factors was the transplantation of an islet mass exceeding 6000 islet equivalents per kilogram body weight.[6] The limitation in the ability to isolate such large numbers of viable islets from one pancreas has made it necessary to pool islets from several donors to achieve this critical β-cell mass. Several methods have been proposed to store islets; however, cryopreservation is the most effective means of long-term storage of donor islets.[8] Once a low temperature bank of cryopreserved islets is established, supplementing freshly isolated islets with pretested, viable, microbiologically sterile, frozen-thawed tissue can be easily accomplished and has been shown to produce insulin independence long term in a number of type I diabetic patients.[1,9] Of the cases reported to the International Islet Transplant Registry, type I diabetic recipients transplanted with freshly isolated islets in combination with cryopreserved islets are insulin independent at 1 year in 18% of the cases.[6] This is higher than the 11% of the cases that are insulin independent when freshly isolated islets from a single cadaveric donor were transplanted. To date, the longest duration of insulin independence in a type I diabetic patient receiving an islet transplant simultaneously with a kidney transplant, received a combination of fresh and cryopreserved islets.[4,6]

[a]Address for correspondence:Surgical-Medical Research Institute, 1074 Dentistry/Pharmacy Building, University of Alberta, Edmonton, AB T6G 2N8 Canada; 780-492-3386 (voice); 780-492-1627 (fax); rrajotte@gpu.srv.ualberta.ca (e-mail).

## SMALL AND LARGE ANIMALS

Since 1977 much work has been carried out on islet cryopreservation when the present author first demonstrated that frozen-thawed islets were able to normalize diabetic rats posttransplant.[10] Using adult rat islets, a number of different freezing protocols have been proposed with viability demonstrated both *in vivo* and *in vitro.*[11,12] *In vivo* success with rodent islets has been with both slow and fast cooling rates.[10,13–18] Postcryopreservation tissue culture was found to improve insulin release from the islets,[10,11,19] while Sandler[20] has shown similar effects of culture when used before freezing. We have found, however, this not to be the case for syngeneic islets transplanted into rats[21] and for human islets isolated from pancreata with a short cold-storage period before the islet isolation process.[22] However, the use of a culture period before freezing was not found to be deleterious to *in vivo* function[22] and may in fact improve the postcryopreservation function if the islets are isolated from a pancreas that has had a prolonged cold-storage period before the islet isolation process (unpublished observations). It is also reasonable to consider using a preculture period if the islets suffer some damage during the isolation procedure thus allowing them time to recover prior to freeze-thaw stress.

We have found that slow cooling to –40°C with rapid thawing from –196°C gives a high percentage survival, with an identical clinical response regardless whether 3000 frozen-thawed or the same number of fresh islets were transplanted beneath the kidney capsule.[23] Using this cryopreservation protocol for mouse islets 80% of the islets were recovered post-thaw,[24] and, when variable numbers of syngeneic islets were transplanted after correcting for the freeze-thaw loss, an identical clinical response was observed with the insulin content of the graft (300 islets) at 100 days post transplant equivalent in both the freshly isolated and the frozen-thawed groups.[25] Over the years many studies have reported optimum cryopreservation of islets; however, comparison of various freezing protocols has been difficult because of the variation in the methods used for freezing and thawing. When our slow cooling protocol was compared with that of others that have been cited as optimum,[13,14,16–26] we found that slow cooling to –40°C in combination with rapid thawing from –196°C gave the best results as assessed by perifusion and transplantation.[27, 28] This has been confirmed by another group who, when comparing various protocols, found that slow cooling to –40°C and rapid thawing from –196°C resulted in the best *in vivo* survival following the freeze-thaw process.[29]

In addition, using this freezing procedure dog pancreatic microfragments can normalize carbohydrate metabolism when autografted into totally pancreatectomized dogs[17,30,31] and particularly pancreatectomized pigs.[32,33] Using a similar freeze-thaw protocol for purified dog islets, the same number of fresh or cryopreserved syngeneic islets induced normoglycemia[34] past 100 days. Some dogs were monitored long term with euglycemia maintained in both groups 5–7 years post islet autotransplant (unpublished observation).

When allografts were carried out an increased number of frozen-thawed islets were needed to induce normoglycemia in combination with cyclosporine immunosuppression.[35] This effect could not be attributed to rejection, since insulin secretion persisted in the splenic vein during an intravenous glucose tolerance 30 days posttransplant.[36] This problem was not observed in cryopreserved allografted mouse is-

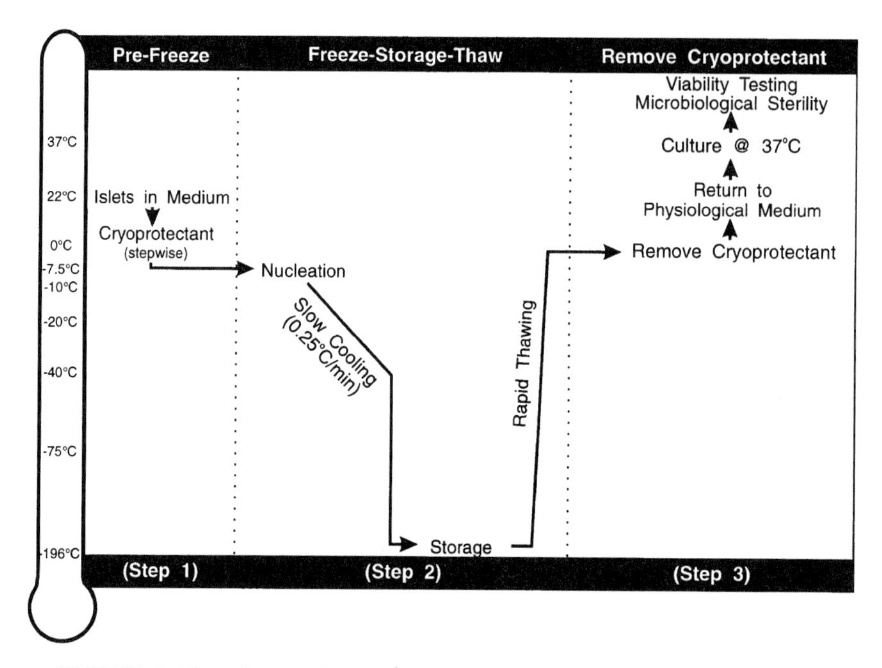


**FIGURE 1.** Flow diagram for cryopreservation of isolated islets using a three-step approach.

lets, which functioned as well as fresh islets when the same number were transplanted.[24,25] The cryopreserved allografts in this murine model did not appear to be less immunogenic, in contrast with cryopreserved xenografts,[37] although MHC (Major Histocompatibility Complex) Class I expression was reduced.[24]

## HUMAN

The ability to cryopreserve human islets with diverse HLA and ABO phenotypes has facilitated ongoing clinical islet transplantation trials.[8,9] Once frozen at −196°C, the storage of human islets is indefinite, transportation between centers is facilitated, and the ability to test viability and microbiological sterility improves the chances of success following clinical transplantation.

The methods used to cryopreserve human islets are based on our preclinical large animal canine model.[10,17,27] Using this freeze-thaw protocol human islets can respond to glucose *in vitro* and survive long term when transplanted beneath the kidney capsule of nude athymic rodents.[38] Using this cryopreservation protocol, it has been possible to produce insulin independence long term when a combination of fresh and cryopreserved islets were transplanted in patients with longstanding diabetes.[4,6,7]

## CRYOPRESERVATION PROTOCOL

During freezing and thawing there are three distinct steps (FIG. 1): 1) a prefreeze phase during which the islets are equilibrated with the cryoprotectant, 2) freezing, storage, and thawing, and 3) return of the islets to a physiological medium.[9,39]

### *Prefreezing Phase*

Following islet isolation 1000–2000 mouse and rat islets are suspended at 22°C in 0.2 mL of Medium 199 (Gibco, Burlington, ON) which is supplemented with 25 mM HEPES, 10% fetal calf serum (v/v), penicillin (100 U/mL), and streptomycin (100 μg/mL). For dog and human islets, 10–15,000 are suspended in 1 mL of the above medium with supplements. To these islets, DMSO is added in a stepwise fashion as previously described,[39] with time allowed between the steps for equilibration with the cryoprotectant to occur. All the test tubes are then transferred to the seeding bath of 95% ethanol (–7.5°C).

### *Freezing and Thawing*

Once in the seeding bath the test tubes are held at this temperature until they are supercooled to –7.5°C. The test tubes are then nucleated with an ice crystal and time is then allowed for release of the latent heat of fusion, which takes 10–15 minutes depending on the volume of liquid being frozen. They are then transferred to an evacuated freezing dewar which gives a controlled cooling rate of 0.25°C/min from –7.5°C to –40°C.[9] Once –40°C is reached, the test tubes are removed from the freezing dewar and plunged into liquid nitrogen. For low temperature storage, the test tubes are placed on freezing canes, which are then transferred to the liquid nitrogen storage vessel. One test tube from the preparation is kept separate and is used for viability and sterility assessment.[8]

Using this freezing procedure we have found that rapid thawing (150–200°C/min) from –196°C is needed to maximize islet recovery and viability. For thawing, the test tubes are agitated quickly in a 37°C water bath just until the last piece of ice disappears (0°C), at which point they are transferred to an ice slush (0°C) until all the test tubes are thawed.

### *Removal of the Cryoprotectant*

Once all the test tubes are thawed, they are centrifuged at 450×*g* and the 2M DMSO removed using a sucrose dilution.[39] One milliliter of 0.75M sucrose is added to the test tubes at 0°C and the test tubes kept in an ice slush for 30 minutes. The sucrose is then serially diluted with 5 minutes allowed between steps. All the test tubes are then centrifuged, the supernatant removed, and the islets transferred to isotonic medium and placed in tissue culture media for a period of 24–48 hours prior to *in vitro* testing or transplantation.

### *Viability Testing and Quality Control*

For human islets, it is important that both viability and microbiological testing is carried out before the islets are used for transplantation to diabetic recipients. Low temperature banking allows this flexibility before the islets are used clinically.[8] We measure the response of the islets to glucose challenge and the ability of the frozen-thawed islets to normalize a diabetic nude mouse. Before *in vitro* viability assessment the islets need to be cultured at 37°C for at least 24 hours to allow time for metabolic recovery following the freeze-thaw insult. For *in vivo* assessment, 2000 frozen-thawed islets are transplanted beneath the kidney capsule of experimentally induced diabetic nude mice. For comparison, nonfrozen islets from the same isolation are also tested *in vitro* and *in vivo*, which guarantees islet viability prior to cryopreservation. The thawed islet samples used for viability assessment are also used for confirmation of microbiological sterility. Islets that are nonresponsive to glucose or that are unable to normalize the diabetic nude mice are discarded and not used for our clinical trials.

## SUMMARY

There are several steps involved in the freeze and thaw protocol which must be carefully followed to ensure a high recovery of viable islets.[39] The time and temperature at which islets are equilibrated with the cryoprotectant are variables that require careful control to ensure full equilibration with the cryoprotectant while minimizing the toxic effect of the cryoprotectant. Furthermore, since cryoprotectants are very hypertonic, their addition and removal should be carried out in a stepwise fashion to minimize osmotic stress to the cells.

The freezing protocol developed for a permeating cryoprotectant is specific for that agent and, therefore, needs to be modified if a different cryoprotectant is used. For example, the permeating kinetics of glycol is different from DMSO and requires a longer equilibration time at a higher temperature.

The cooling rate used to freeze islets will be dictated by how the islets were treated before freezing—time and temperature of exposure and type of cryoprotectant. The cooling rate optimum for multicellular structures (i.e., islets, embryos, etc.) is usually slower than single cells when a permeating cryoprotectant (DMSO) is used as the cryoprotectant. Controlled cooling can be to different subzero temperatures; however, this will affect the thawing rate. Slow cooling to −40°C needs rapid thawing from −196°C, while slow cooling to −75°C needs a slow thawing rate. The reason thawing rate is different relates to the amount of intracellular ice and size of the ice crystals which can grow during rewarming.

A viability assessment is critical to ensure the tissue is capable of functioning in a normal physiologic manner. Such an assessment, immediately after thawing, usually provides a poor response in that the islets need some time in tissue culture to recover from a freeze-thaw insult. If islets are not optimally cryoprotected they may still respond to high glucose but lose their ability to turn off insulin secretion during low glucose. This damage is usually irreversible and cannot be corrected in tissue culture. The best test of viability is the ability to correct diabetes in a transplant model using the same number of islets as nonfrozen control. If this can be achieved then the cryoproectant protocol is optimum for that specific islet type.

## ACKNOWLEDGMENTS

This work was supported by funds from the Alberta Foundation for Diabetes Research, the Edmonton Civic Employees' Charitable Assistance Fund, and the Medical Research Council of Canada.

## REFERENCES

1. WARNOCK, G.L., N.M. KNETEMAN, E.A. RYAN, M.G. EVANS, R.E.A. SEELIS, P.F. HALLORAN, A. RABINOVITCH & R.V. RAJOTTE. 1989. Continued function of pancreatic islets after transplantation in type 1 diabetes. Lancet **2:** 570–572.
2. SCHARP, D.W., P.E. LACY, J.V. SANTIAGO, C.S. MCCULLOUGH, L.G. WEIDE, L. FALQUI, P. MARCHETTI, R.L. GINGERICH, A.S. JAFFE, P.E. CRYER, C.B. ANDERSON & M.W. FLYE. 1990. Insulin independence after islet transplantation into type I diabetic patient. Diabetes **39:** 515–518.
3. TZAKIS, A.G., C. RICORDI, R. ALEJANDRO, Y. ZENG, J.J. FUNG, S. TODO, A.J. DEMETRIS, D.H. MINTZ & T.E. STARZL. 1990. Pancreatic islet transplantation after upper abdominal exenteration and liver replacement. Lancet **336:** 402–405.
4. WARNOCK, G.L., N.M. KNETEMAN, E.A. RYAN, A. RABINOVITCH & R.V. RAJOTTE. 1992. Long-term follow-up after transplantation of insulin-producing pancreatic islets into patients with type 1 (insulin-dependent) diabetes mellitus. Diabetologia **35:** 89–95.
5. GORES, P.F., J.S. NAJARIAN, E. STEPHANIAN, J.J. LLOVERAS, S.L. KELLEY & D.E.R. SUTHERLAND. 1993. Insulin independence in type 1 diabetes after transplantation of unpurified islets from a single donor with 15-deoxyspergualin. Lancet **341:** 19–21.
6. HERING, B.J., C.C. BROWATZKI, A. SCHULTZ, R.G. BRETZEL & K.F. FEDERLIN. 1993. Clinical islet transplantation—Registry report, accomplishments in the past and future research needs. Cell Transplant. **2:** 269–282.
7. SOCCI, C., A.M. DAVALLI, P. MAFFI, L. FALQUI, A. SECCHI, F. BERTUZZI, A. VIGNALI, P. MAGISTRETTI, *et al.* 1993. Allotransplantation of fresh and cryopreserved islets in patients with type 1 diabetes: two-year experience. Transplant. Proc. **25:** 989–991.
8. WARNOCK, G.L., J.R.T. LAKEY, Z. AO & R.V. RAJOTTE. 1994. Tissue banking of cryopreserved islets for clinical islet transplantation. Transplant. Proc. **26:** 3438
9. RAJOTTE, R.V., J.R.T. LAKEY & G.L. WARNOCK. 1995. Adult islet cryopreservation. *In* Methods in Cell Transplantation. C. Ricordi, Ed.: 517–524. R.G. Landes Company. Austin, TX.
10. RAJOTTE, R.V., H.L. STEWART, W.A.G. VOSS, T.K. SHNITKA & J.B. DOSSETOR. 1977. Viability studies on frozen-thawed rat islets of Langerhans. Cryobiology **14:** 116–120.
11. SCHATZ, H. 1981. Section III: Cryopreservation and culture. *In* Islet Isolation, Culture and Cryopreservation. K. Federlin & R.G. Bretzel, Eds.: 124–128. Thieme-Stratton Inc. New York.
12. BANK, H.L. 1983. Cryobiology of isolated islets of Langerhans, circa 1982. Cryobiology **20:** 119–128.
13. BANK, H.L., R.F. DAVIS & D. EMERSON. 1979. Cryogenic preservations of isolated rat islets of Langerhans: effect of cooling and warming rates. Diabetologia **16:** 195–199.
14. BRETZEL, R.G., J. SCHNEIDER, J. DOBROSCHKE, K. SCHWEMMLE, E.F. PFEIFFER & K. FEDERLIN. 1980. Islet transplantation in experimental diabetes of the rat. VII. Cryopreservation of rat and human islets. Preliminary results. Horm. Metab. Res. **12:** 274–275.
15. RAJOTTE, R.V., D.W. SCHARP, R. DOWNING, R. PRESTON, G.D. MOLNAR, W.F. BALLINGER & M.H. GREIDER. 1981. Pancreatic islet banking: the transplantation of frozen-thawed rat islets transported between centers. Cryobiology **18:** 357–369.

16. ANDERSSON, A. & S. SANDLER. 1983. Viability tests of cryopreserved endocrine pancreatic cells. Cryobiology **20:** 161–168.
17. RAJOTTE, R.V., G.L. WARNOCK & N.M. KNETEMAN. 1984. Cryopreservation of insulin-producing tissue in rats and dogs. World J. Surg. **8:** 179–186.
18. RAJOTTE, R.V. & T.J. DEGROOT. 1986. Effects of warming rate on slowly cooled islets. Cryobiology **23:** 572.
19. FERGUSON, J., R.H. ALLSOPP, R.M.R. TAYLOR & I.D.A. JOHNSTON. 1976. Isolation and preservation of islets from the mouse, rat, guinea pig, and human pancreas. Br. J. Surg. **63:** 767–773.
20. SANDLER, S. & A. ANDERSSON. 1984. The significance of culture for successful cryopreservation of isolated pancreatic islets of Langerhans. Cryobiology **21:** 503–510.
21. WARNOCK, G.L. & R.V. RAJOTTE. 1989. Effects of precryopreservation culture on survival of rat islets transplanted after slow cooling and rapid thawing. Cryobiology **26:** 103–111.
22. LAKEY, J.R.T., G.L. WARNOCK, N.M. KNETEMAN, Z. AO & R.V. RAJOTTE. 1994. Effects of pre-cryopreservation culture on human islet recovery and in vitro function. Transplant. Proc. **26:** 820.
23. COULOMBE, M.G., G.L. WARNOCK & R.V. RAJOTTE. 1988. Reversal of diabetes by transplantation of cryopreserved rat islets of Langerhans to the renal subcapsular space. Diabetes Research **8:** 9–15.
24. CATTRAL, M.S., G.L. WARNOCK, N.M. KNETEMAN, P.F. HALLORAN & R.V. RAJOTTE. 1993. Effect of cryopreservation on the survival and MHC antigen expression of murine islet allografts. Transplantation **55:** 159–163.
25. CATTRAL, M.S., J.R.T. LAKEY, G.L. WARNOCK, N.M. KNETEMAN & R.V. RAJOTTE. 1998. Effect of cryopreservation on the survival and function of murine islet isografts and allografts. Cell Transplant. **7:** 373–379.
26. TAYLOR, M.J. & M.J. BENTON. 1987. Interaction of cooling rate, warming rate, and extent of permeation of cryoprotectant in determining survival of isolated rat islets of Langerhans during cryopreservation. Diabetes **36:** 59–65.
27. RAJOTTE, R.V., G.L. WARNOCK & L.E. MCGANN. 1988. Cryopreservation of islets of Langerhans for transplantation. *In* Low Temperature Biotechnology: Emerging Applications and Engineering Contributions. J.J. McGrath & K.R. Diller, Eds.: 25–45. The American Society of Mechanical Engineers.
28. RAJOTTE, R.V., G.L. WARNOCK, N.M. KNETEMAN, C. ERICKSON & D.K. ELLIS. 1989. Optimizing cryopreservation of isolated islets. Transplant. Proc. **21:** 2638–2640.
29. RICH, S.J., S. SWIFT, S.M. THIRDBOROUGH, G. RUMFORD, R.F.L. JAMES & N.J.M. LONDON. 1993. Cryopreservation of rat islets of Langerhans: a comparison of two techniques. Cryobiology **30:** 407–412.
30. RAJOTTE, R.V., G.L. WARNOCK, R.C. BRUCH & A.W. PROCYSHYN. 1983. Transplantation of cryopreserved and fresh rat islets and canine pancreatic fragments: comparison of cryopreservation protocols. Cryobiology **20:** 169–184.
31. KNETEMAN, N.M., R.V. RAJOTTE & G.L. WARNOCK. 1986. Long-term normoglycemia in pancreatectomized dogs transplanted with frozen/thawed pancreatic islets. Cryobiology **23:** 214–221.
32. WISE, M.H., A. YATES, C. GORDON & R.W.G. JOHNSON. 1983. Subzero preservation of mechanically prepared porcine islets of Langerhans: response to a glucose challenge in vitro. Cryobiology **20:** 211–218.
33. WISE, M.H., C. GORDON & R.W.G. JOHNSON. 1985. Intraportal autotransplantation of cryopreserved porcine islets of Langerhans. Cryobiology **22:** 359–366.
34. EVANS, M.G., G.L. WARNOCK, N.M. KNETEMAN & R.V. RAJOTTE. 1990. Reversal of diabetes in dogs by transplantation of pure cryopreserved islets. Transplantation **50:** 202–206.
35. CATTRAL, M.S., G.L. WARNOCK, M.G. EVANS & R.V. RAJOTTE. 1991. Transplantation of purified frozen/thawed canine pancreatic islet allografts with cyclosporine. Transplantation **52:** 457–461.
36. DAUDI, F.A., G.L. WARNOCK, M.S. CATTRAL, M.G. EVANS & R.V. RAJOTTE. 1990. Islet banking: transplantation of cryopreserved canine islet auto- and allografts. Can. J. Surg. **33:** 322.

37. COULOMBE, M.G., G.L. WARNOCK & R.V. RAJOTTE. 1987. Prolongation of islet xenograft survival by cryopreservation. Diabetes **36:** 1086–1088.
38. WARNOCK, G.L., D.W.R. GRAY & P.J. MORRIS. 1986. Transplantation of cryopreserved isolated adult human islets of Langerhans into nude rats. Surgical Forum **37:** 334–336.
39. RAJOTTE, R.V., G.L. WARNOCK & N.M. KNETEMAN. 1992. Methods of islet cryopreservation. *In* Pancreatic Islet Cell Transplantation. C. Ricordi, Ed. : 124–131. R.G. Landes Company. Austin, TX.

# Bioartificial Pancreas:

## Alternative Supply of Insulin-secreting Cells

DAOBIAO ZHOU, EKATERINA KINTSOURASHVILI, SALIM MAMUJEE, IVAN VACEK, AND ANTHONY M. SUN[a]

*Department of Physiology, Faculty of Medicine, University of Toronto, 1 King's College Circle, Toronto, Ontario M5S 1A8 Canada*

**ABSTRACT: In this study, insulin secretion function of INS-1 cells immunoisolated in microcapsules was evaluated. Following encapsulation, the immunoisolated INS-1 cells continued to propagate and flourish within the microcapsules during the entire two-month *in vitro* incubation period. The insulin secretion from encapsulated INS-1 cells following seven days of *in vitro* culture increased from 1.6 ± 0.2 ng/2h/$10^6$ cells in a glucose-free medium to 11.5 ± 2.1 ng/2h/$10^6$ cells at 16.7 mM glucose.**

***In vivo*, transplants of 1.2 × $10^7$ cells into each of six diabetic C57BL/6 mice resulted in the restoration of normoglycemia in all graft recipients for up to 60 days post transplantation. Most capsules recovered from two animals 30 days post transplantation were free of cell overgrowth and physically intact. Immunostaining for insulin of the cells within the recovered capsules clearly indicated the presence of insulin.**

**The presented data demonstrate the potential use of an immunoisolated β-cell line for the treatment of diabetes.**

## INTRODUCTION

The transplantation of pancreatic islet tissue, either as a whole pancreas or as isolated islets, has been pursued because the technique can provide normal blood glucose control and thus potentially prevent or reduce diabetic complications.[1–3] The concept of immunoisolation by microencapsulation advanced in this laboratory obviated the need for immunosuppression and demonstrated the potential for the use of allo- and xenotransplantation as therapeutic alternatives to exogenous insulin therapy in insulin-dependent diabetics.[4–8] Although there is little question that transplanted islets offer a potential alternative to exogenous insulin therapy, both large-scale islet isolation and cryopreservation are technically difficult and expensive. Insulin-secreting cell lines derived from β cells represent a potential alternative approach to pancreatic islet transplantation. These cells can be grown inexpensively, and in unlimited quantity. Several such lines were developed from the x-ray–induced transplantable rat insulinoma.[9–13] Although these cells have retained many characteristics of normal β cells, many of them have lost the capacity to secrete insulin in response to glucose[10,12] and to synthetize and store insulin.

[a]Author for correspondence: 416-978-8781 (voice); anthony.sun@utoronto.ca (e-mail).

In our past studies[14,15] we selected as a model an insulin-producing clonal line βTC6-F7, originally derived from insulinomas arising in transgenic mice expressing the SV40 T antigen gene under control of the insulin promoter.

Following microencapsulation, the βTC6-F7 cell mass expanded within the capsules, displaying a pattern of distribution that was substantially different from that of the free, unencapsulated cells. In monolayer culture, cells would grow to approximately 70% confluence, at which point the cells would quite rapidly start necrotizing. The encapsulated cells grew in a three-dimensional fashion, initially in a few aggregates that would later, in 4 to 6 weeks, expand and fill the entire capsule, visualized under light microscopy as a solid mass.

In our experiments, the glucose responsiveness of the encapsulated βTC6-F7 cells was subphysiological, shifted to the 2.8mM to 5.6mM range. Exposure of the encapsulated cells to 1 mM IBMX or 100 nM tGLP-1 resulted in a significantly higher insulin response compared to IBMX-free or tGLP-1–free media, regardless of the glucose concentration. In general, IBMX was found to be a more potent stimulator of insulin release than tGLP-1.

*In vitro*, the insulin secretion from microencapsulated βTC6-F7 cells showed little change over the first 20 days of culture while the cell density increased 35-fold. Most likely, the lag in insulin secretion may be attributed to the cell adaptation to growth in their new surroundings. While little or no change in insulin accumulation into the medium was observed over the first 21 days in culture, an approximately 5-fold increase occurred over the next 14 days. In our experiments, at 55 days when the cell numbers appeared to have stabilized, the insulin secretion was found to be about 10-fold greater than the secretion at 19 days.

The intraperitoneal implantation of a sufficient number of encapsulated βTC6-F7 cells into streptozotocin-diabetic mice and rats ($3 \times 10^6$ cells per mouse, $3 \times 10^7$ cells per rat) in most cases, resulted in normalization of blood glucose within 24 hours and was maintained for up to 60 days. Continuous insulin secretion with little glucose responsiveness often resulted in the hypoglycemic condition of the recipients. When capsules were recovered from graft recipients 30 and 60 days after the graft administration, they were found free of cell overgrowth and physically intact with enclosed clusters of cells clearly visible. Immunostaining of the cells within the capsules recovered from rats at 30 days post-transplantation indicated a strong presence of insulin.

The growth and secretory properties of βTC6-F7 cells within the microcapsule environment provide an excellent model for the eventual application of insulin-secreting cells as a means of providing endogenous insulin therapy. However, it is clear that while the cells are capable of reversing hyperglycemia in diabetic mice and rats for up to 60 days, their responsiveness to glucose is of crucial importance for the proper regulation of blood glucose concentrations of recipients. In addition, the fact that all of the current insulin-producing cell lines are potentially cancerogenic hinders the immediate clinical experimentation and application.

In 1991, Asfari *et al.*[16] reported on establishment of two stable insulin-secreting cell lines (INS-1, INS-2) whose morphology, insulin biosynthesis, and secretion are remarkably similar to those of the parent tumor propagated *in vivo*. Although INS-1 cells have retained capacity to secrete insulin in response to glucose during an acute challenge, this response is much reduced in comparison to perfused pancreas and islet preparations.[17] The cells do not secrete insulin when exposed to 1mM glucose and a 2.2-fold enhancement of insulin secretion was demonstrated at 10 mM glucose. In the presence of forskolin and 3-isobutyl-1-methylxanthine, increase of glucose concentration from 2.8–20 mM caused a 4-fold enhancement of the rate of insulin secretion. These cells were reported to have retained differentiated functions for more than two years.[18]

In a recent study, Frodin *et al.*[19] studied the signaling pathways whereby glucose and hormonal secretagogues regulate insulin-secretory function in INS-1 cells and showed that in these cells, major secretagogue-stimulated–signaling pathways converge to activate 44-kD mitogen-activated protein kinase.

In this study we have endeavored to evaluate the insulin secretion function of INS-1 cells immunoisolated in alginate-polylysine-alginate (APA) membranes *in vitro* and *in vivo*.

## MATERIALS AND METHODS

### *Cell Culture*

INS-1 cells (passage 72–86) were grown in RPMI 1640 medium supplemented with 10mM HEPES, 10% heat-inactivated fetal calf serum, 100 μ/ml penicillin, 100 μg/ml streptomycin, 1 mM sodium pyruvate and 50 μM 2-mercaptoethanol in a humidified atmosphere of 5% CO2 and 95% air at 37°C. The INS-1 cells were a kind gift from Dr. M. Asfari of the University of Geneva, Geneva, Switzerland.

### *Cell Encapsulation*

The encapsulation technique was a modification of Sun's method.[4] The modification involved the use of an electrostatic droplet generator,[5–8] which produces smaller and more uniform capsules. Briefly, the cells were suspended in 1.7% (w/v) sodium alginate (Kelco Gel LV. Kelco, San Diego, CA, USA) at a concentration of approximately $8 \times 10^6$ cells per ml. Spherical droplets were formed by the electrostatic field interaction coupled with syringe pump extrusion (Razel A 99 syringe pump, pump speed 55–65) and were collected in a 100 mM calcium lactate solution. To achieve this, the negative pole is attached to the loop which is submerged in the calcium lactate solution, and the positive pole is attached to the needle. The droplets were suspended in 0.05% poly-L-lysine (Sigma, MW 22,000 to 24,000 daltons) for five minutes and were then washed with 0.9% saline and reacted with 0.15% alginate for five minutes. After another wash with 0.9% saline, the capsules were allowed to react with 55 mM sodium citrate for five minutes and finally washed with 0.9% saline and with culture medium. The encapsulated cells were then ready to use for *in vivo* or *in vitro* studies. Overall, the sizes of the capsules were 0.25–0.35 mm in diameter and each capsule contained 150–200 cells.

### In Vitro *Study*

The growth of the INS-1 cells within the APA microcapsules and their insulin secretion in response to secretagogues were studied during a two-month observation period. The cell number inside the capsules was assessed once a week as previously described.[15] To evaluate insulin secretion, 100 cell-containing capsules were placed in each well of the multiwell plate (Flow Laboratories Inc., McLean, VA, USA). The cells were preincubated in glucose-free medium for one hour and then exposed to media containing different concentrations of glucose (0 mM, 2.8 mM, 5.6 mM, 11.1 mM, and 16.7 mM), or glucose (16.7 mM) plus 0.1 mM isobutylmethylxanthine (IBMX) for two hours. Samples of media were collected for insulin content determination using a rat insulin solid-phase $^{125}$I radioimmunoassay (Linco Research Inc., St. Louis, MO, USA). At the same time, the cell density within the capsules was determined.

### In Vivo *Study*

Male C57BL/6 mice(Charles River, St. Constant, Quebec, Canada) were used as graft recipients. Diabetes was induced in the animals by intravenous injection of streptozotocin (Sigma, St. Louis, MO, USA, 185 mg/kg body weight). The animals were considered suitable for transplantation after registering three consecutive, non-fasting blood glucose measurements above 20 mM. Six diabetic mice received intraperitoneal transplants of $1.2 \times 10^7$ microencapsulated cells (passage 72–86), contained in $7–8 \times 10^4$ capsules. Two control groups of animals, six mice per group, received either the same number of free, non-encapsulated cells, or empty capsules. The grafts were delivered using an 18-gauge catheter. Blood samples for glucose determination were obtained from the tail vein of the animals, daily during the first week post-transplantation, then every two days for a month, and every four days thereafter until the conclusion of the study. In this study, blood glucose levels below 10 mM are considered as normal, while the range of 10–16 mM is defined as partially normalized. To confirm that the grafts were responsible for the restoration of normoglycemia in the recipient animals, the capsules were recovered from two randomly selected animals, 30 days post transplantation, by peritoneal lavage using warm sterile 0.9% saline.

### *Statistical Analysis*

Data are presented as mean ± SE. The student *t*-test was used to evaluate the statistical significance of differences, as appropriate; $p < 0.05$ was considered statistically significant.

## RESULTS

### *Insulin Secretion*

The insulin secretion from encapsulated INS-1 cells following seven days of culture in response to glucose and IBMX is shown in TABLE 1. The insulin secretion rose from 1.6 ± 0.2 ng/2h/$10^6$ cells in glucose-free medium to 6.5 ± 0.5 ng/2h/$10^6$ cells at 2.8 mM glucose, to 8.0 ± 0.6 ng/2h/$10^6$ cells at 5.6 mM glucose, to 9.5 ± 1.0 ng/2h/$10^6$ cells at 11.1 mM glucose and to 11.5 ± 2.1 ng/2h/$10^6$ cells in the presence of 16.7 mM glucose. The exposure to 16.7 mM glucose plus 0.1 mM IBMX triggered a further increase in insulin secretion at 15.6 ± 1.6 ng/2h/$10^6$ cells. The corresponding values for the control, unencapsulated cells were 1.7 ± 0.2 (no glucose),

**TABLE 1.** *In vitro* challenge study

| Type of Stimulant | Insulin Secretion (ng/2hr/$10^6$cells) | |
|---|---|---|
| | Encap. ($n$ = 5) | Free ($n$ = 5) |
| Glucose 0 mM | 1.6 ± 0.2 | 1.7 ± 0.2 |
| Glucose 2.8 mM | 6.5 ± 0.5 | 7.4 ± 0.8 |
| Glucose 5.6 mM | 8.0 ± 0.6 | 8.5 ± 0.5 |
| Glucose 11.1 mM | 9.5 ± 1.0 | 10.9 ± 1.2 |
| Glucose 16.7 mM | 11.5 ± 2.1 | 12.0 ± 1.8 |
| Glucose 16.7 mM + 0.1mM IBMX | 15.6 ± 1.6 | 16.7 ± 1.9 |

7.4 ± 0.8 (2.8 mM glucose), 8.5 ± 0.5 (5.6 mM glucose), 10.9 ± 1.2 (11.1 mM glucose), 12.0 ± 1.8 (16.7 mM), and 16.7 ± 1.9 ng/2h/$10^6$ cells (16.7 mM glucose plus 0.1 mM IBMX). While after one week of culture, the insulin secretion at 11.1 mM glucose was determined at 9.5 ± 1.0 ng/2h/$10^6$ cells, three weeks later it was measured at 11.7 ± 1.5 ng/2h/$10^6$ cells ($n = 5$, $p > 0.05$ compared to first week).

### *Cell Growth within Microcapsules*

As shown in FIGURE 1, the encapsulated INS-1 cells continued to propagate and flourish during the entire two-month incubation period. The cell density within the microcapsule increased from the initial number of 150 to 200 cells per capsule,

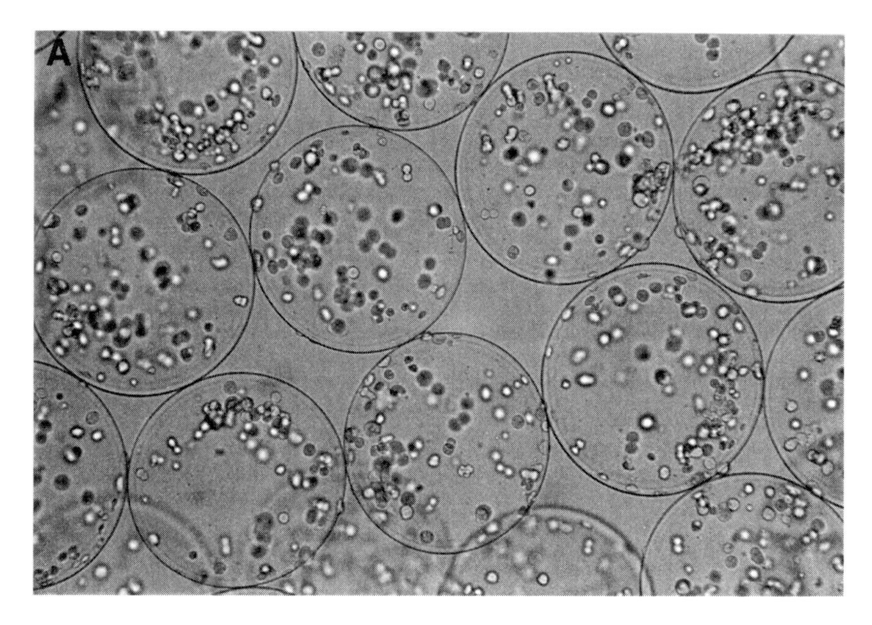


**FIGURE 1.** Micrographs of encapsulated INS-1 cells (×130) **A**: freshly encapsulated; **B**: cultured for half a month; **C**: cultured for two months.

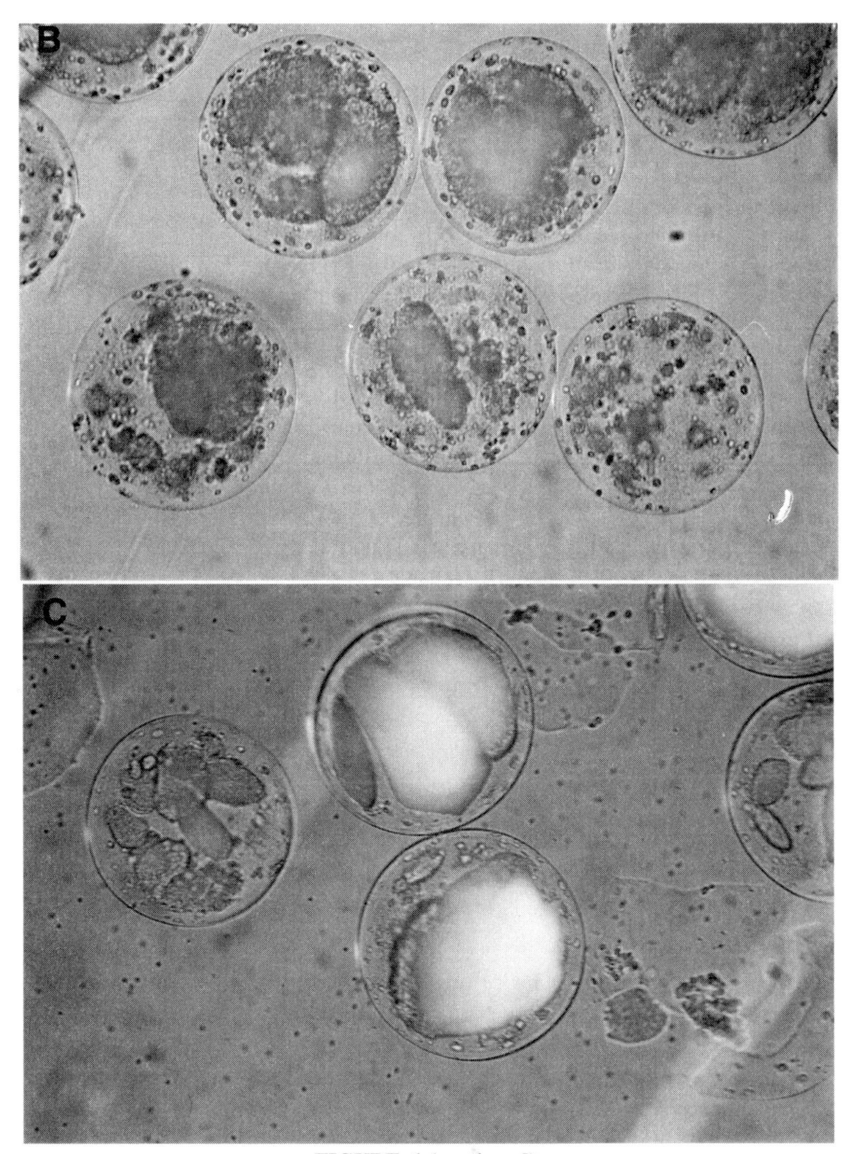


FIGURE 1 (continued).

reaching a plateau at about 2100 cells/per capsule in one month. Two weeks following encapsulation, the cells started to form aggregates. During the next thirty days these aggregates became progressively bigger until they formed islet-like clumps. A trypan blue exclusion test performed on the cells after 1.5 months indicated that more than 90% of cells were viable.

**TABLE 2.** Restoration of normoglycemia in streptozotocin-diabetic mice transplanted with microencapsulated INS-1 cells

| Type of Graft | Normoglycemia | Partially Normoglycemic | Hyperglycemia | Total |
|---|---|---|---|---|
| $1.2 \times 10^7$ Encapsulated cells | 6 | 0 | 0 | 6 |
| $1.2 \times 10^7$ Free cells | 0 | 0 | 6 | 6 |
| Empty capsules | 0 | 0 | 6 | 6 |

### *Transplantation of Microencapsulated INS-1 Cells*

The results of the intraperitoneal transplantation of microencapsulated INS cells into diabetic mice are shown in TABLE 2 and FIGURE 2. All of the recipients in $1.2 \times 10^7$ cells group became normoglycemic (8–10 mM). While the recipients of free, unencapsulated cells showed only a slight decrease in their hyperglycemic blood glucose levels (to $17.6 \pm 1.5$ mM) for the duration of 48 hours, no change was registered in the recipients of empty capsules. Of the normoglycemic recipients, two animals maintained normoglycemia for 60 days after transplantation, while in the rest of the graft recipients the duration of normoglycemia varied between 30 and 45 days. The serum insulin concentrations in the diabetic mice prior to the graft administration were determined at $0.3 \pm 0.1$ ng/ml, while thirty days after the transplantation they increased to $1.8 \pm 1.2$ ng/ml ($n = 6$, $p < 0.05$, compared to the pre-transplant concentration; normal control:$1.9 \pm 0.5$ ng/ml). The body weights of the recipients increased with the diabetic improvement, increasing from the pretransplant level of $18.4 \pm 0.3$ grams to $20.6 \pm 0.6$ thirty days after the graft administration.

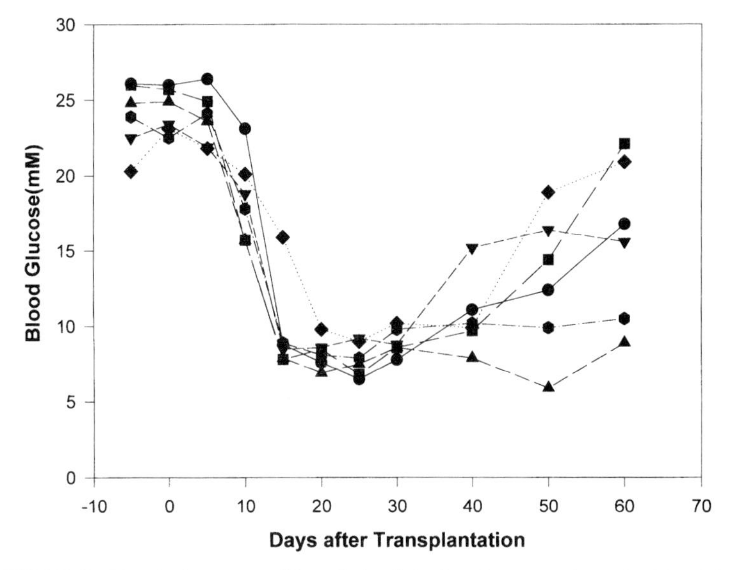


**FIGURE 2.** Blood glucose profiles of six diabetic mice transplanted with with $1.2 \times 10^7$ microencapsulated INS-1 cells.

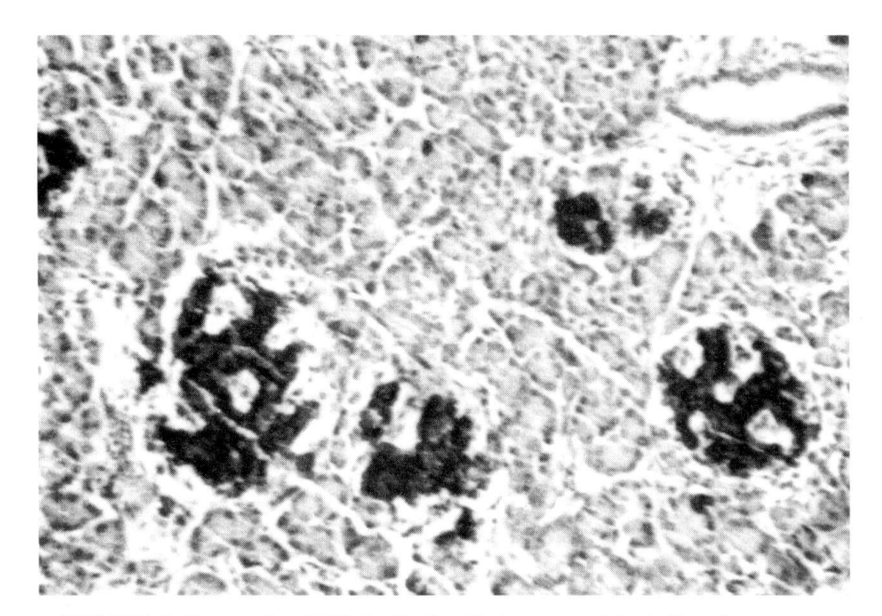

**FIGURE 3.** Encapsulated INS-1 cells (insulin immunostaining): Capsules were recovered from a diabetic mouse at 1.5 months; picture shows typical insulin stain of the cells inside the capsule.

### *Capsule Recovery*

Thirty days post transplantation, the grafted capsules were recovered from two randomly chosen animals in which normoglycemia had been established. As a result, the blood glucose concentration increased from 9.8 ± 0.63 mM to 20.3 ± 0.9 mM two days later, thus indicating that the graft was responsible for the restoration of normoglycemia. Most of the recovered capsules were free of cell overgrowth and physically intact. The enclosed cell clusters were clearly visible. When compared with the *in vitro* cultured capsules, a similar cell growth pattern was detected. The recovered encapsulated cells were shown to respond to glucose challenge by an increase in insulin secretion (0.9 ± 0.2 ng/2h/$10^6$ cells at 0 mM glucose vs 5.6 ± 0.7 ng/2h/$10^6$ cells at 16.7 mM glucose). Immunostaining for insulin of the cells within the capsules recovered from a diabetic mouse at one month post transplantation clearly indicated the presence of insulin (FIG. 3).

## DISCUSSION

The use of insulin-secreting pancreatic β-cell lines commands increasing interest as a potential alternative to pancreatic islets for insulin replacement therapy in diabetes mellitus. A number of such lines generated either from insulinomas or from hyperplastic islets displayed insulin secretion characteristics similar to those observed in intact adult islets; however, their phenotypic instability constitutes a serious problem. The data reported by Asfari *et al.*[16–18] indicate that their INS-1 cells remained stable for more than two years and that they retained a high degree of differentiation, which should make them a suitable model to study various aspects of β-cell function.

In the current study, the microencapsulation of the INS-1 cells within the alginate-polylysine-alginate membrane constitutes the most significant departure from the pioneering work of Asfari.[16,17]

Microencapsulation of the cells results in a radical change in the cell environment, from monolayer growth on flat-surfaced petri dish to radial, three dimensional growth within hydrogel inside a capsule. This would result in a pattern of distribution substantially different from that of free, unencapsulated cells. Similar to our earlier studies using microencapsulated insulin producing βTC6-F7 cells,[14,15] the cells growing in a three-dimensional pattern—both *in vitro* and *in vivo*—would start forming aggregates which would eventually expand and fill virtually the entire capsule, visualized under light microscopy as a solid mass (FIG. 1C).

In this study, the rate of insulin secretion in the *in vitro* glucose challenge experiments showed very little difference between microencapsulated and free cells, thus indicating that the capsule membrane does not impede the passage of glucose or insulin. While the previously studied βTC6-F7 cells showed a rather limited and clearly subphysiological insulin secretion response to glucose,[14,15] the INS-1 cells were shown to have secreted glucose in a distinctly more physiological pattern. In particular, in comparison to the βTC6-F7 cells, the INS-1 cells showed improved sensitivity in the 11.1 to 16.7 mM glucose range. The phosphodiesterase inhibitor 3-isobutyl-1-methylxanthine potentiated further the response to glucose, similar to βTC6-F7 cells.

Although the response to glucose is markedly reduced in comparison to islet preparations, in our experiments the magnitude of the response in the 0–11.1 mM glucose range was distinctly greater in comparison to data reported by Asfari.[16] While in his experiment a 75% increase was detected in the above range, a six-fold increase was measured in the current study followed by a further small increase at 16.7 mM glucose. This compares with a slight decrease in insulin secretion reported by Asfari at 16.7 mM glucose as compared to 11.2 mM.

The graft of 12 million microencapsulated INS-1 cells clearly resulted in the reversal of the diabetic hyperglycemia for up to sixty days, the duration of the entire observation period. In comparison to our previous *in vivo* studies using βTC6-F7 cells,[14] in which about three million of these cells were grafted into each diabetic mouse, no instances of post-transplantation hypoglycemia were noted, with the normalized blood glucose levels in our INS-1 cell graft recipients higher than in the βTC6-F7 cell–transplanted animals. This undoubtedly reflects the fact that the insulin secretion responsiveness of the INS-1 cells tends to be distinctly more physiological compared to the βTC6-F7 cells in which the insulin release appears to be continuous, with the cells not responding to the dynamics of serum glucose concentrations.

The graft size of $1.2 \times 10^7$ microencapsulated cells employed in the current study was chosen arbitrarily; however the relatively long time necessary for the graft to establish normoglycemia may suggests that a larger graft may be needed to result in a more prompt reversal of the diabetic hyperglycemia. In comparison, a much smaller graft of three million βTC6-F7 cells per diabetic mouse was sufficient to bring the recipients blood glucose levels promptly to levels significantly lower[14] than was the case in the current study.

One can only speculate as to the factors responsible for the return of diabetic hyperglycemia in the recipient animals and the failure of the graft following the normoglycemic period. It may have been caused by a decrease in insulin secretion or by an eventual death of the transplanted cells.

Also, the capsule construction is of a critical importance in this respect since the capsules strength determines the duration of the graft function. Similarly, imperfectly constructed capsules may limit the duration of the graft function because of surficial cell overgrowth. Following the graft failure, the absolute majority of recovered capsules were found intact, with some of them displaying varying degrees of cell overgrowth. In these initial experiments the reported periods of normoglycemia were shorter than those we had previously reported for transplants of pancreatic islets, possibly indicating a limited life span of the implanted cells. Future studies will be directed at prolonging graft survival and at enhancing the glucose responsivity of the cells.

## REFERENCES


1. THE DIABETES CONTROL AND COMPLICATIONS TRIAL RESEARCH GROUP. 1993. The effect of intensive treatment of diabetes on the development and progression of long term complications in insulin-dependent diabetes mellitus. N. Engl. J. Med. **329:** 977.
2. REICHARD, P., B.Y. NILSSON & U. ROSENQUIST. 1993. The effect of long-term intensified insulin treatment on the development of microvascular complications of diabetes mellitus. N. Engl. J. Med. **329:** 304.
3. WANG, P.H., J. LAU & T.C. CHALMERS. 1990. Meta-analysis of effects of intensive blood glucose control on late complications of Type I diabetes. Lancet **341:** 1306.
4. FAN, M.Y., Z. LUM, X. FU, L. LEVESQUE, I.T. TAI & A.M. SUN. 1990. Reversal of diabetes in BB rats by transplantation of encapsulated rat islets. Diabetes **39:** 519.
5. LUM, Z.P., M. KRESTOW, J. NORTON, I. VACEK & A.M. SUN. 1991. Prolonged reversal of the diabetic stateIn NOD mice by xenografts of microencapsulated rat islets. Diabetes **40:** 1511.
6. LUM, Z.P., M. KRESTOW, I.T. TAI & A.M. SUN. 1992. Xenografts of rat islets into diabetic mice. Transplantation **53:** 1180.
7. KRESTOW, M., Z.P. LUM, I. TAI & A.M. SUN. 1991. Xenotransplantation of microencapsulated fetal rat islets. Transplantation **51:** 651–655.
8. SUN, Y., X. MA, D. ZHOU, I. VACEK & A.M. SUN. 1996. Normalization of diabetes in spontaneously diabetic monkeys by xenografts of microencapsulated porcine islets without immunosuppression. J. Clin. Invest. **98:** 1417.
9. GAZDAR, A.F., W.L. CHICK, H.K. OIE, H.L. SIMS, D.L. KING, G.C. WEIR & V. LAURIS. 1980. Continuous clonal insulin and somatostatin secreting cell line established from a transplantable rat islet cell tumor. Proc. Natl. Acad. Sci. USA **77:** 3519–3523.
10. PRAZ, G.A., P.A. HALBAN, C.B. WOLLHEIM, B. BLONDEL, A.J. STRAUSS & A.E. RENOLD. 1983. Regulation of immunoreactive insulin release from a rat cell line (RINm5F). Biochem. J. **210**: 345–352.
11. CARRINGTON, C.A., E.D. RUBERY, E.C. PEARSON & C.N. HALES. 1986. Five new insulin-producing cell lines with differing secretory properties. J. Endocrinol. **109:** 193–200.
12. TRAUTMANN, M.E, B. BLONDEL, A. GJINOVACI & C.B. WOLLHEIM. 1990. Inverse relationship between glucose metabolism and glucose-induced insulin secretion in rat insulinoma cells. Horm. Res. **34:** 75–82.

13. CHICK, W.L., S. WARREN, R.N. CHUTE, A.A. LIKE, V. LAURIS & K.C. KITCHEN. 1977. A transplantable insulinoma in the rat. Proc. Natl. Acad. Sci. USA **74:** 628–632.
14. ZHOU, D., A.M. SUN, X. LI, S.N. MAMUJEE, I. VACEK, J. GEORGIOU & M.B. WHEELER. 1998. In vitro and in vivo evaluation of insulin producing βTC6-F7 cells in microcapsules. Am. J. Physiol. **274** (Cell Physiol.**43**)**:** C1356–C1362.
15. MAMUJEE, S.N., D. ZDOU, M. WHEELER, I. VACEK & A. SUN. 1997. Evaluation of immunoisolated insulin-secreting βTC6-F6 cells as a bioartificial pancreas. Ann. Transplant. **2:** 27–32.
16. ASFARI, M., D. JANJIC, P. MEDA, G. LI, P.A. HALBAN & C.B. WOLLHEIM. 1982. Establishment of 2- mercaptoethanol-dependent differentiated insulin secreting cell-lines. Endocrinology **130:** 167–178.
17. ASFARI, M., W. DE, M. NOEL, P.E. HOLTHUIZEN & P. CZERNICHOW. 1995. Insulin-like growth factor-II gene expression in a rat insulin-producing beta-cell line (INS-1) is regulated by glucose. Diabetologia **38:** 927–935.
18. JANJIC, D. & M. ASFARI. 1992. Effects of cytokines on rat insulinoma INS-1 cells. J. Endocrinol. **132:** 67–76.
19. FRODIN, M., N. SEKINE, E. ROCHE, C. FILLOUX, M. PRENTKI, C.B. WOLLHEIM & E. VAN OBBERGHEN. 1995. Glucose, other secretagogues, and nerve growth factor stimulate mitogen-activated protein kinase in the insulin-secreting beta cell line, INS-1. J. Biol. Chem. **270:** 7882–7889.

# Transplantation of Pancreatic Islets Contained in Minimal Volume Microcapsules in Diabetic High Mammalians

RICCARDO CALAFIORE,[a,d] GIUSEPPE BASTA,[a] GIOVANNI LUCA,[a] CARLO BOSELLI,[b] ANDREA BUFALARI,[b] ANTONELLO BUFALARI,[c] MARIA PAOLA CASSARANI,[c] GIAN MARIO GIUSTOZZI,[b] AND PAOLO BRUNETTI[a]

[a]*Departments of Internal Medicine and Endocrine and Metabolic Sciences (DIMISEM),* [b]*Surgery and Surgical Emergencies, and* [c]*Veterinary Surgery, University of Perugia, Perugia, Italy*

**ABSTRACT: To minimize technical problems relating to excessive size (600–800μ in diameter) of standard alginate microcapsules (CSM) for pancreatic islet graft immunoisolation, we have developed two novel minimal volume, chemically identical, capsule prototypes (MVC): 1) coherent microcapsules (CM), and 2) medium-size microcapsules (300–400μ, MSM). CM, which envelop each individual islet within a thin alginate hydrogel cast, are prepared by emulsification, whereas MSM are made by atomizing the islet-alginate suspension through a special microdroplet generator. Upon graft into diabetic rodents, CM have shown to immunoprotect both allo- and xenogeneic nondiscordant islets, and restored normoglycemia. In higher mammals, at subtherapeutic doses, CM fully immunoprotected islet allografts (pig→pig), but only temporarily xenografts (dog→pig). We then used MSM to immunoisolate canine islet allografts in the peritoneal cavity of dogs with spontaneous insulin-dependent diabetes. Of three grafted dogs, two showed full remission of hyperglycemia with insulin withdrawal. MSM could represent an intermediate solution between CSM and CM for peritoneal immunoisolated islet transplants.**

## INTRODUCTION

In spite of almost two decades of steady technical progress and promising data, immunoisolation of pancreatic islet grafts within highly biocompatible and immunoselective microcapsules, usually but not solely formulated with alginic acid and polyaminoacidic derivatives, has not been yet associated with uniform and susbstantial success. Although there is general consensus about the fact that transplantation of microencapsulated islets may consistently reverse hyperglycemia in streptozotocin (STZ)-induced diabetic rodents, profound controversy has emerged between different laboratories about the possibility of restoring normoglycemia in rodent animal models (such as NOD mice and BB rats) of spontaneous autoimmune, insulin-dependent diabetes mellitus (IDDM). The latter goal has been fully accomplished, with simple use of microcapsules and no other immune intervention, only by a very few

[d]Author for correspondence: DIMISEM, University of Perugia, Via E. Dal Pozzo, 06126 Perugia, Italy; +39-075-578-3682 (voice); +39-075-573-0855 (fax); islet@unipg.it (e-mail).

laboratories,[1,2] while the majority of researchers experienced unsurmountable obstacles in achieving remission of IDDM in these recipients.[3,4] Whether discrepancies in results between spontaneously vs. STZ-induced diabetic rodents may depend either on the former's higher stringency in immune responsiveness, or rather on non-specific, toxic agents which accelerate intracapsular islet cell death, or finally, on higher propensity of the microcapsules' constituent polymers to degrade faster in the autoimmune animals, remains, at this juncture, unclear.

A major pitfall associated with the microencapsulation system may consist of poor standardization in selecting chemically suitable and endotoxin-free polymers to engineer the microcapsule's membrane. Other significant differences occur in regard to the microencapsulation methodology. Therefore, it is possible that results achieved in some laboratories are not comparable with those obtained in others. These problems become even more stringent when microcapsules are applied to islet transplant into diabetic higher mammalians. With the single exception of a brilliant trial of encapsulated porcine islet xenografts in spontaneously diabetic primates, which resulted in full and prolonged reversal of hyperglycemia in these nonimmunosuppressed recipients,[5] all other attempts to re-establish normal blood glucose levels in diabetic large-size mammals have been associated with only partial and transient success. In particular, as far as diabetic dogs are concerned, time-limited remission of hyperglycemia was accomplished only when the recipients underwent a course of general immunosuppression with cyclosporin. Similar results were described, by the same group, in a IDDM patient who had previously undergone a kidney transplant.[6] However, use of immunosuppressants does not seem to help understand whether microcapsules may represent, per se, an effective immunobarrier to weather the host's immune attack under various circumstances. Furthermore, in the specific instance of IDDM, the immune response comprises both, immune rejection and autoimmune recurrence of the disease on the implanted tissue.[7] Therefore, another major challenge of microencapsulation consists of preventing autoimmunity, which remains a formidable, still unanswered issue, also in IDDM-patients receiving unencapsulated human islet allografts, who undertake conventional, general immunosuppression. Finally, it has been rightfully speculated that if microcapsules might successfully circumvent activation of the host's immune response, whether it be rejection or autoimmunity, within an allogeneic transplantation setting, the same result may not be necessarily affordable to xenografts. In particular, small-size molecules, or "shed" antigens, released from the enveloped islets, could seep through the microcapsule, even within a membrane's molecular weight cut-off ranging from 50 to 100 kD, and trigger the indirect pathway of the immune reaction.[8] Additionally, there would be no membrane capable of interdicting access to such mediators of the inflammatory reaction as nitric oxide, and free oxygen radicals, whose harmful effects on islet cells are well known.[9] It should be also emphasized that the majority of microencapsulated islet grafts, regardless of the recipients' species, have been performed intraperitoneally, owing to either ease of this grafting procedure, or large final encapsulated islet transplant volume which would only fit the peritoneal cavity. However, an alternative transplantation site for microencapsulated islets would possibly prevent local delivery of "shed" antigens, or other dangerous molecules outflowing the capsular barrier, which, especially in some regions, could very well activate the cascade of immune events fatally leading to islet graft destruction. In this regard, we have employed, in the past, a specially designed, co-axial vascular chamber, directly anastomosed to blood vessels, embodying the microencapsulated islets. In this way, the encapsulated islets' secretory products, and eventually "shed" antigens, were directly diverted into the blood stream, thereby facilitating the transplant's metabolic effects, while attenuating the impact of antigens' signaling on the host's immune system. This set-up was proven to succeed, in our system, in terms of documented transplant function, and induced insulin-independency, in both canines and preliminarily diabetic patients undertaking no immunosuppressive therapy, although transplant functional life-span lasted for only a few months of follow-up.[10] We suspect that large size of the microcapsules employed in those vascular grafts (conventional-size microcapsules—CSM = 600–800 μm) prevented us from grafting a sufficient viable and functional islet cell mass.

Another common feature of early studies with microencapsulated islets was use of CSM,[11] which were certainly associated with clear advantages, with special regard to remarkable barrier properties associated with their thick gel core. However, the final microencapsulated islet transplant volume, in high mammalians, amounted an average 80 ml per dog and 120 ml per patient, if a sufficient, functional islet cell mass were to be grafted. Also, the peritoneal cavity is a known, highly reactive site which promptly responds to contact with foreign bodies, regardless of immunity. In light of this restraint, development of smaller-size microcapsules has become a prominent requirement for conducting islet transplantation trials in large-size mammals, in an attempt to prevent an initial inflammatory reaction which could then impair microencapsulated islet transplant survival and function. This sequence of events was observed in our microencapsulated canine islet autograft system, where, in absence of immune reactivity the huge mass of microencapsules elicited an intense inflammatory cell response that coincided with intracapsular islet cell death, after 3 months of transplant.[12]

## MINIMAL VOLUME MICROCAPSULES: PRINCIPLES, PROPERTIES, AND BACKGROUND STUDIES

Because of size-related problems associated with CSM, we addressed our efforts to developing new microcapsule prototypes, which would couple the already-tested CMS's physical/chemical and biocompatibility properties, to volume-sparing, small-size individual microspheres (MVC). If successful, this approach could either attenuate the burden of large, final encapsulated islet transplant mass on the peritoneal cavity, or permit access to alternative transplant sites which had been, so far, interdicted to the "huge" CSM. These MVC should be associated with improved insulin secretory kinetics of the enveloped islet cells, due to shorter distance between islets and the extra-capsular environment. On the other hand, by reducing the size of the microcapsules, some of the capsular physical-chemical features could be altered, beginning from thickness and porosity/permeability of the outer membrane, which directly regulate the capsule's immunobarrier competence. Also, changes in stoichiometric molar ratios of the microcapsule-forming polymers, which are required to fabricate smaller gel beads, or conformal coatings, could adversely affect the membrane's *ad hoc* tight MWCO. Finally, it should be ascertained that methods for pre-

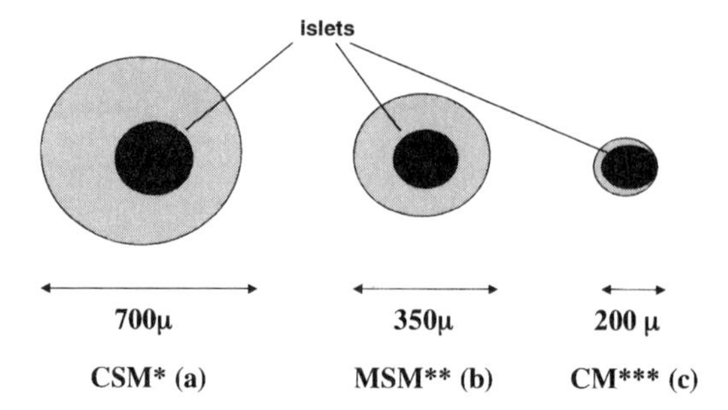


**FIGURE 1.** Types of microcapsules for islet transplant immunoisolation.

paring MVC do not possibly impair, in anyway, the enveloped islet cells' viability and functional competence. Over the past 4–5 years, we have generated, in our laboratory, two prototypes of MVC (FIG. 1):

(1) Coherent microcapsules (CM) are thin, skin-like, hydrogel films which tightly envelop each individual islet, with little idle, dead space being left between islet and the artificial coating membrane; the size of the CM equals or slightly exceeds that of the islets.

(2) Medium-size microcapsules (MSM) measure an equatorial diameter (average 350 μm) which is half the size of CSM; this type of capsule has been developed subsequent to initial results achieved, in our laboratory, by CM in higher mammal transplant trials.

### *Fabrication of Coherent Microcapsules and Medium-Size Microcapsules*

For both prototypes of MVCs we continued to employ the same polymer blend, comprised of high purity grade, low viscosity, endotoxin-free Na alginate (NAG) complexed with poly-L-ornithine (PLO) in a sandwich-like fashion, with NAG constituting both the inner core and the outer layer, and PLO forming the middle layer of the microcapsules. However, we had to surmount a few technical problems, when fabricating CM with the NAG/PLO complex, since the preparative process for making coherent microcapsules is completely different from that for medium-size and conventional-size microcapsules.

#### *Coherent Microcapsules*

As elsewhere reported,[13] these conformal coatings were prepared by a two-phase aqueous emulsification procedure, employing NAG, ficoll, and poly-ethylene glycol. The islet suspension was co-incubated with the emulsified reagents, on a rotating plate, so as to permit engulfment of each individual islet within the emulsion microdroplets. These were subsequently gelled in calcium chloride, and the resulting gel microbeads were overlayered with PLO and NAG which completed fabrication of CM. Empty CM, which resulted from the microemulsification process, were easily discarded. The PLO concentration was carefully titered in order to avoid any membrane's collapse. At the end of the process, CM enveloped each individual islet within a coherent, skin-like hydrogel cast, which occasionally was so thin to be invisible under inverted phase microscopy examination.

*Medium-Size Microcapsules*

This microcapsule's prototype was fabricated subsequently to CM, in order to assess whether retention of some idle space, within the microspheres, could result in a stronger immunobarrier, in comparison with CM, while occupying a final transplant volume which would still be acceptable, and certainly incomparably lower than CSM. Briefly, by adjusting physical and chemical parameters of the classical spray-gelling encapsulation method previously employed to fabricate CSM,[12] with special regard to air flow rate, reagents' temperature, and velocity of the islet suspension's extrusion through the microdroplet generator, we were able to obtain microspheres, measuring an average 350–400 µm in equatorial diameter, that entrapped each individual islet.

### *Quality Control of Islet-containing Coherent and Medium-Size Microcapsules*

Both procedures resulted in formation of intact, transparent and mechanically robust micromembranes, as assessed by light, electron (scanning + transmission) and laser confocal microscopy examination. We found no islets protruding through the membrane, an issue which could impair immunoisolation provided by microcapsules. Moreover, all islets contained in both CM and MSM fully retained their viability, as assessed by examination of either histological or fresh tissue samples, the latter after incubation with ethidium bromide and fluorescein diacetate, under fluorescence microscopy. The encapsulation procedure never adversely affected *in vitro* glucose-stimulated insulin release from the enveloped islets, thus fully proving

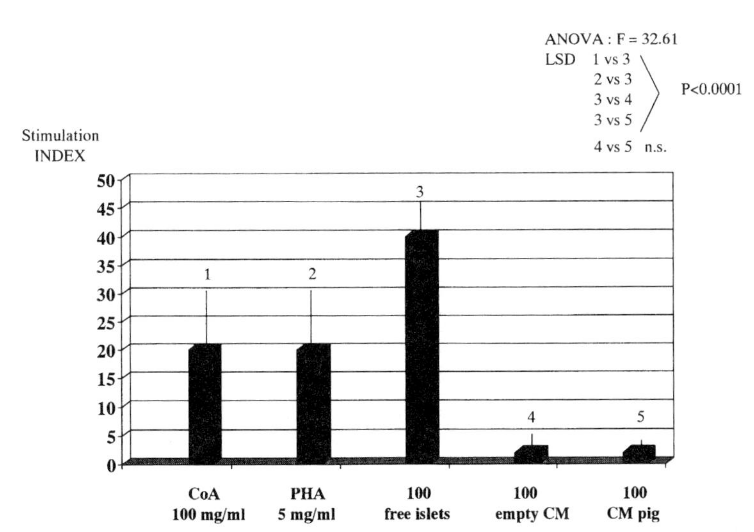


**FIGURE 2.** *In vitro* mixed xenogeneic human lymphocyte/free or coherent microcapsule (CM)–enveloped porcine islets. Lymphocyte controls were incubated with concanavalin-A (Con-A) and phytoemoagglutinin (PHA).

harmlessness of this procedure for islet transplant purposes. *In vitro* immunobarrier competence of both CM and MSM was demonstrated by assessing proliferation rate of mononuclear cells in mixed either allo- (W/F rat) or xenogeneic (pig) islet/splenocyte (LW rat) or lymphocyte (human) co-cultures (FIG. 2), respectively. The microcapsules were shown to fully prevent incorporation of $3H^3$-thymidine into the mononuclear cells, co-cultured with either allo- or xenogeneic islets. Additionally, the capsular membrane was proven to be impenetrable to Ig, when microencapsulated islet cells were exposed to ICA + human sera: a FITC-conjugated second antibody revealed that no Ig crossed the capsular barrier and bound to the encapsulated islets. On the contrary, unencapsulated islets were targeted by the FITC-conjugated second antibody/ICA complex, and as expected, resulted in a classic immunofluorescence pattern, under fluorescence microscopy examination.[14]

### In Vivo *Rodent Studies*

We had previously documented that 30-day transplant of empty both CM and MSM, in the sub-capsular renal space or in the peritoneal cavity, respectively, was associated with retrieval of intact microspheres, which were not overgrown with inflammatory cells, thereby reflecting the biometarials' elevated biocompatibility. *In vivo* the immunobarrier competence of CM had also been demonstrated by implanting xenogeneic non-discordant rat islets beneath the kidney capsule of normal mice: the islets fully retained their viability throughout 30 days of transplant, in the absence of any peri-capsular inflammatory cell overgrowth. Finally, hyperglycemia had been fully corrected in either LW rats or CD-1 mice, with STZ-induced diabetes, receiving allogeneic, or, respectively, non-discordant xenogeneic W/F rat islets within CM, intraperitoneally, throughout 140 days of transplant.

### In Vivo *Studies in Higher Mammals*

We have shown preliminary results, in normal adult pigs, that 30-day graft of empty CM into multiple sites, including parenchymatous organs, such as liver, spleen, sub-capsular renal space or the omentum, once interdicted to CSM because of size restrictions, was associated with complete absence of any inflammatory cell reaction, thus proving biocompatibility of these micromembranes even in a high mammalian system, and in sites which were alternative to the peritoneal cavity.[15] Initial 30-day transplant of allogeneic porcine islet–containing CM, in the same multiple sites used for empty microcapsules, was associated with both retrieval of fully viable islet cells and a lack of membrane inflammatory cell overgrowth,[16] at level of both, liver (FIG. 3) and omentum (FIG. 4).

## MINIMAL VOLUME MICROCAPSULES: TRIALS IN HIGHER MAMMALS

Information collected by background rodent and initial pig studies, encouraged us to proceed ahead with transplant of MVC, in particular by addressing the issue of whether these micromembranes could be suitable for correction of hyperglycemia in diabetic large-size mammals. Initially, we planned to evaluate whether CM would

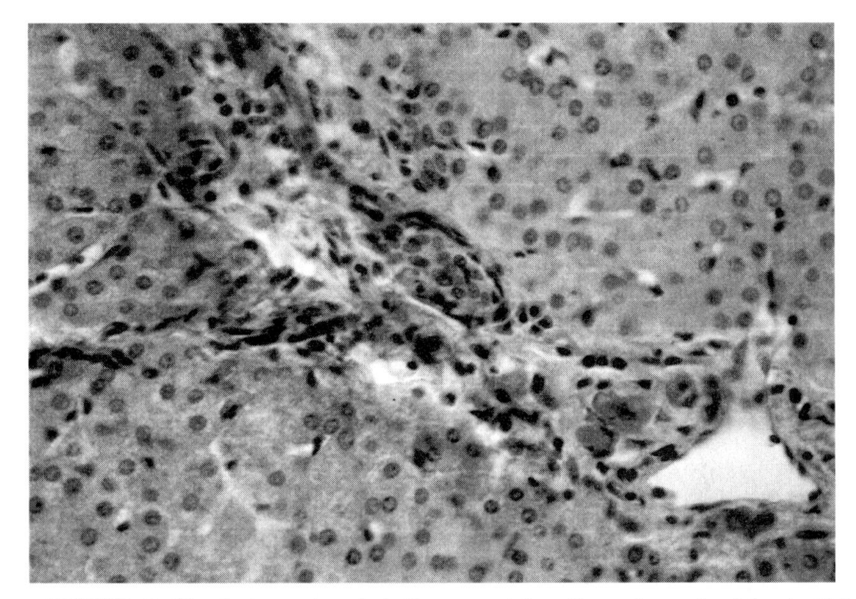

**FIGURE 3.** Histologic section of pig liver containing allogeneic porcine islets in CM at 30 days of transplant (H&E, 25×).

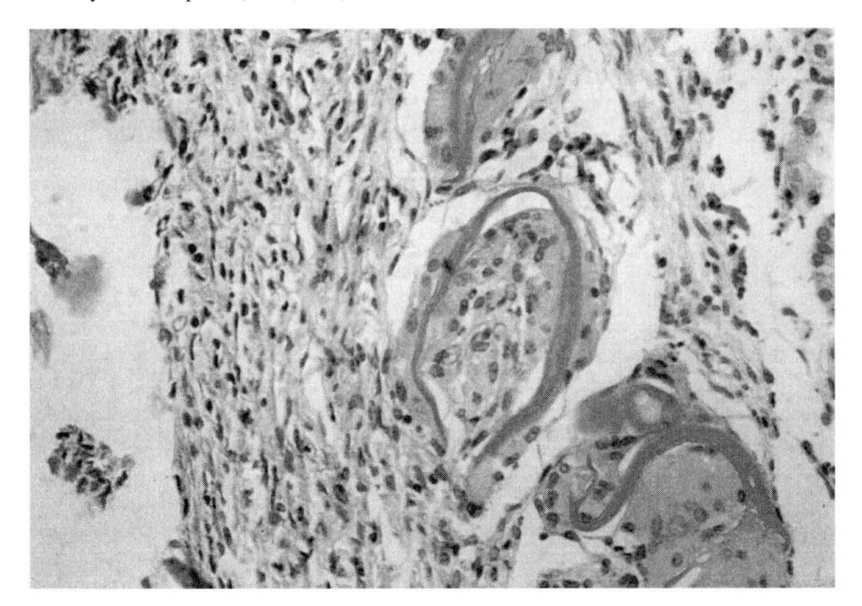

**FIGURE 4.** Histologic section of pig omentum containing allogeneic porcine islets in CM at 30 days of transplant (H&E, 25×).

prevent immune destruction of islet xenografts, after success had been achieved with allografts.

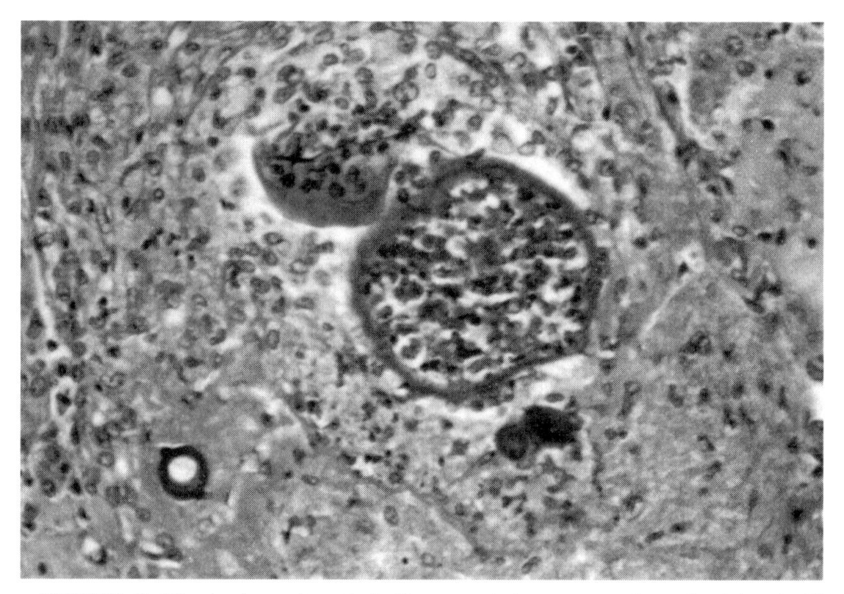

**FIGURE 5.** Histologic section of pig liver containing xenogeneic canine islets in CM at 15 days of transplant (H&E, 25×).

### *Survival of Xenogeneic Canine Islet-containing Coherent Microcapsules Transplanted into Multiple Sites of Adult Pigs*

Sub-therapeutic doses of highly purified canine islets (15,000/recipient) were grafted, upon envelopment into CM, according to the above reported method, in 10 normal adult pigs, into the following sites (3 ml/site):

(1) liver (via vena porta embolization);

(2) artificial omental pouch.

In this trial, we did not employ the spleen or the sub-capsular renal space as transplant sites, since in the previous pig studies, we had found it difficult to retrieve the CM grafted in these regions. Grafts were explanted at 15 and 30 days after transplant, because we wished to monitor any development of islet xenograft-directed immune response. Retrieved tissue samples were fixed in 10% buffered formaldehyde, sequentially dehydrated in ethanol, and finally embedded in paraffin. Histologic sections were then stained with hematoxilin and eosin (H&E). Liver and omentum sections showed that, at 15 days of transplant, the islets were very viable within CM that were not overgrown with fibrotic tissue (FIG. 5). However, at 30 days of transplant, a thick layer of dense inflammatory cell tissue which encased CM that once contained viable canine islets (FIG. 6) was observed. These findings occurred in both the liver and the omentum, although histologic features were different in the two sites: in the former, an excess of mononuclear cells infiltrating the grafts was noticed, whereas in the latter, fibroblasts and foreign body tissue prevailed on other cell populations, and islet viability was, at least, very poor (FIG. 7). The possible explanations for islet-containing CM xenograft failure are being scrutinized at this time. We may pose a preliminary hypothesis that:

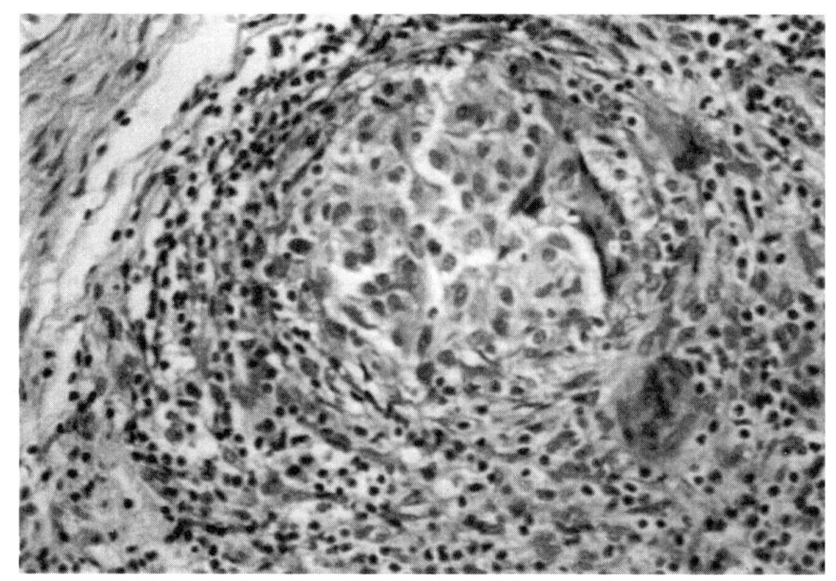

**FIGURE 6.** Histologic section of pig liver containing xenogeneic canine islets in CM at 30 days of transplant (H&E, 25×).

(1) The liver may constitute an angry environment for microcapsules embodying xenogeneic islet cells, since it comprises several cell populations which are deeply involved in immunodefense mechanisms. Moreover, the liver is a solid organ, and CM could have very well undergone some rupture problems, within the microcapillary network, under blood pressure gradients. Such a hypothesis seems to be corroborated by the fact that the nature of the histologic reaction in the omentum was significantly different, and it did not seem to include immune cells within the infiltrating tissue.

(2) The thin membrane of CM may not suffice to provide these capsules with appropriate immunobarrier competence in a particularly difficult transplant setting such as xenotransplantation.

If these speculations are proven to be true, we will address to strenghten the CM's immunobarrier properties, by either thickening the outer coat or incorporating additional molecules within the gel film.

### *Canine Islet-containing Medium-Size Microcapsule Allografts in Spontaneously Insulin-dependent Diabetic Dogs*

While an investigation is underway to assess and possibly surmount problems encountered with islet containing CM xenografts in adult pigs, we decided to restart studies with a NA/PLO gel-spraying microcapsule prototype (MSM). As mentioned in the preceeding section, these microcapsules are similar to the old-fashioned CSM, in terms of basic fabricative procedure, with the major difference being that MSM measure half the CSM's equatorial diameter (average 350 vs. 700 μm). Therefore the

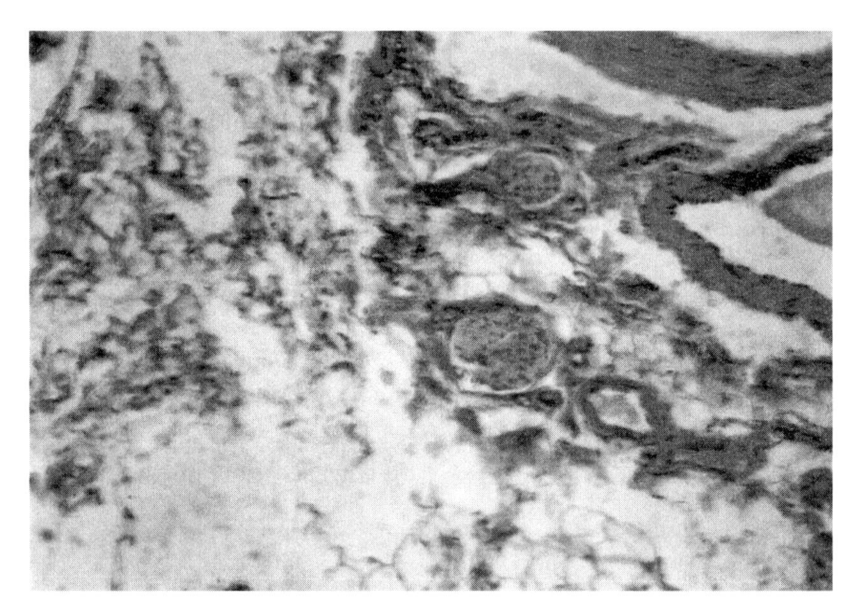

**FIGURE 7.** Histologic section of the pig omentum containing xenogeneic canine islet in CM at 30 days of transplant (H&E, 25×).

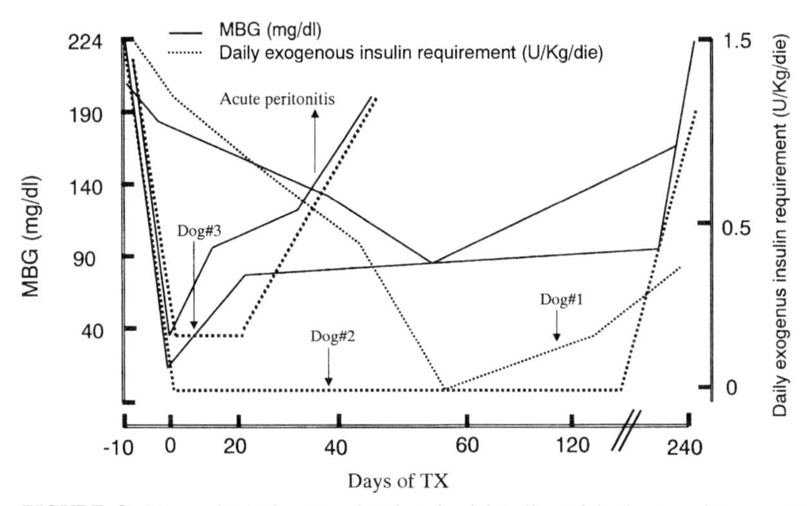


**FIGURE 8.** Intraperitoneal encapsulated canine islet allograft in three nonimmunosuppressed dogs with spontaneous diabetes mellitus.

final transplant volume of islet-containing MSM would be bearable also for a stringent transplant site as the peritoneal cavity. We estimated that transplant mass, within these capsules, would not exceed 10 ml/dog and 30 ml per patient, as compared with the incomparably higher CSM aliquots/recipient.

We began with canine islet-containing MSM allograft in 3 dogs that were spontaneously diabetic for at least two years. All these animals were on a daily insulin schedule, ranging from 1 to 1.5 U/Kg., and showed evidence of ongoing complications of diabetes such as cataracts in both eyes. Under local anesthesia, the 3 animals received intraperitoneal injection of approximately 80,000 canine islets enveloped in MSM, with their blood glucose (BG), as well as other metabolic parameters, being monitored throughout several weeks of post-transplant follow-up. All recipients showed evidence of transplant function in terms of both, decline in BG levels and exogenous insulin requirements (FIG. 8), with some differences that can be summarized as follows:

*Dog 1*

This dog showed a slow, but progressive decrease in insulin requirements and BG levels throughout the first 4 weeks post-transplant, then the animal suspended exogenous insulin, while normoglycemic. Insulin supplementation resumed after 10 days and continued on, although at lower daily doses, throughout 200 days of follow-up. The animal gained weight and his HbA1c levels decreased after the transplant.

*Dog 2*

This was the most successful case. Immediately after transplant the animal went into hypoglycemia (BG = 40 mg/dl) which required emergency treatment with e.v. 50% glucose solution infusion. Exogenous insulin was immediately suspended and never restarted for 4 months post transplant, during which the animal was cured from diabetes, and remained in excellent health. At 140 days after transplant, BG started drifting up and exogenous insulin supplementation resumed.

*Dog 3*

In spite of an initial response to the islet allograft, in terms of transplant-induced hypoglycemia (40 mg/dl) in the first few hours of transplant, and subsequent achievement of normoglycemia, for a few days, this animal started showing signs of abdominal discomfort, with intense vomiting, acute dehydration, and recurrent hyperglycemia. Upon abdominal CT scan, the animal was diagnosed with acute peritonitis and underwent surgery. A packet of dense connective tissue, with the appearance of a foreign body granuloma (FIG. 9), was found adjacent to the stomach and excised away. The animal fully recovered after the operation, but his BG levels remained high and he went back to his original daily exogenous insulin schedule. Retrospectively, the surgeon in charge of the graft procedure had experienced problems during the intraperitoneal microcapsule delivery which might have then caused the peritonitis.

The lessons we have learned from the above reported dog trial are multiple. First of all, the peritoneal cavity could still be retained as a potential transplant site, provided that the final encapsulated islet mass does not equal the huge volume reached in the past by CSM. In this regard, MSM could fulfill the task of providing the microcapsules with the right size, while complying with strict immunobarrier competence's requirements. In the best conditions, which comprise sufficient mass of viable islet cells, no errors in microcapsule fabrication, and correct surgical graft procedure, intraperitoneal islet allograft in MSM, may result in full reversal of dia-

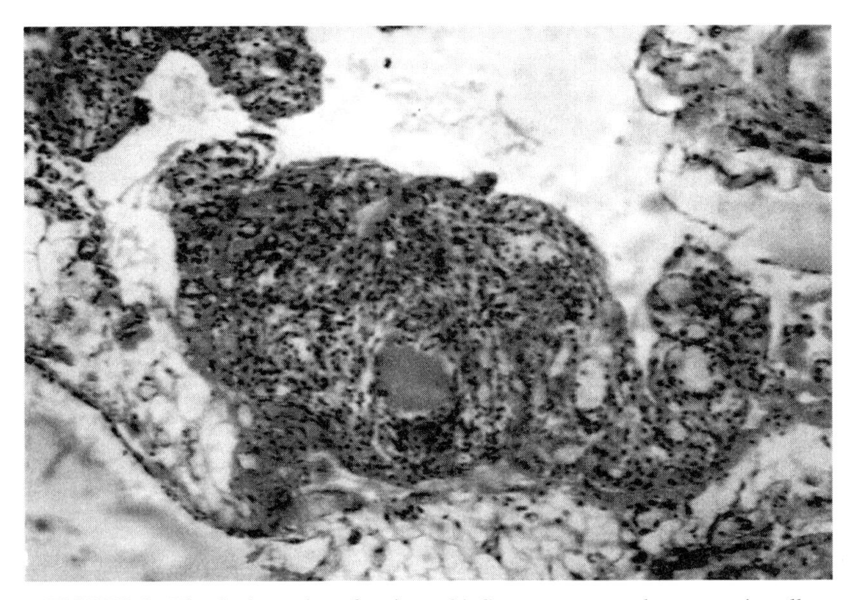

**FIGURE 9.** Histologic section of peritoneal inflammatory granuloma encasing allogeneic canine islet-containing MSM (H&E, 5×).

betes in higher mammals. These data could possibly apply also to humans. However, we will rapidly learn if MSM will also function, in a xenogeneic (i.e., porcine) islet cell transplant setting, in spontaneously diabetic dogs. This major challenge will unfold whether only size adjustments of the original CSM, so as to obtain MSM, will be compatible with success of islet xenografts, in higher mammals, with no other kind of immune intervention. After expanding our allografted dog population, we plan to initiate SPF porcine islet xenografts in dogs with spontaneous diabetes. SPF status is a *sine qua non* condition to embark on porcine islet xenograft trials in canines, in order to explore transplant conditions which could potentially be extended, in the future, to humans.

## CONCLUSION

Our long-standing work with islet transplant immunoisolation within microcapsules, as a frontier strategy to circumvent the host's immune response, had taught us that in order to initiate human clinical trials we needed to create new prototypes of microcapsules.[17] The new capsules had to be significantly smaller than the traditional CSM so as to provoke as minimal traumatization, and site-related inflammatory reaction as possible, upon transplant, while retaining strict immunobarrier competence and biocompatibility which had been largely associated with the initial CSM types. Downscaling the microcapsules'size would also help address other issues, such as exploration of multiple, potential transplant sites, and eventual replacement of an encapsulated islet graft whose function was exhausted. Along this research line we have generated CM, a NAG/PLO polymer complex, which was fabricated using a *de novo* method. As a result, we developed a microcapsule prototype which permitted us to embody each individual islet within a tiny hydrogel cast which was almost invisible and contained no dead space. This prototype was associated with immunobarrier competence *in vitro* and *in vivo*, in either rodents or adult pigs. CM were able to reverse hyperglycemia in STZ-diabetic rodents and protected porcine islet allografts from rejection upon transplant into adult pigs, for periods up to 30 days, when the studies were terminated. However, CM were not shown to provide long-term immunoprotection to canine islet xenografts into pigs. Assessment of the causes for this initial failure, which requires further sudy, is in progress.

Meanwhile, we wished to launch a new version of CSM, the MSM, which did not share with the former the extra size, a negative hallmark of those microcapsules. MSM allowed us to re-explore the peritoneal cavity which had been abandoned, in our laboratory, for a transplantation site owing to CSM-associated volume problems. The idea was proven to be correct, since we obtained, using intraperitoneally grafted allogeneic islet containing MSM, the first full, long-term remission of hyperglycemia in a dog with spontaneous, insulin-dependent diabetes. Whether MSM will be also suitable for islet xenografts will require further study.

In light of the experimental data so far collected, it may be possible that the optimal microcapsule size stands in between the large conventional 600–800 μm and the last generation, conformal 200 μm microcapsules. A moderate idle dead space between capsule's wall and islet surface, could help counteracting the effects of dangerous molecules, such as cytokines or nitric oxide which may result in islet cell transplant destruction. Moreover, a mid-size microcapsule could be easily implanted into the peritoneal cavity, with a good chance to prevent an inflammatory response, provided that both islets and membrane's constituent polymers would comply with state-of-the-art requirements. Nonethless, CM are extremely attractive, because their size virtually coincident with that of islets, would make it possible to graft these capsules virtually everywhere, also minimizing the risks of surgical grafting procedures. Potential transplant sites, which may be better than the peritoneal cavity, in terms of metabolic and nutrient supply advantages, could be then accessible. However, we showed that if potentially suitable for allografts, CM may not perform as well with xenografts, although further study is required to clearly prove this assumption. Moreover, CM are very suitable for membrane's chemical alterations, which suggests the possibility of easily modifying the capsule's composition. Possibly, addition of appropriate molecules to the basic polymer blend could help CM to counterbalance the increased vulnerability to noxious agents which derives from their thinner structure as compared to MSM and CSM.

Ongoing studies with MVC prototypes, and further progress in their formulation, will hopefully indicate us which is the ideal capsular barrier to fully immunoprotect islet allo- and xenografts for the cure of IDDM.

## ACKNOWLEDGMENT

This work was supported by a grant from the Juvenile Diabetes Foundation International (No. 196011).

## REFERENCES


1. FAN, M.Y., Z.P. LUM, X.W. FU & A.M. SUN. 1990. Reversal of diabetes in BB rats by transplantation of encapsulated pancreatic islets. Diabetes **39:** 519–522.
2. LUM, Z.P., I.T. TAI, M. KRESTOW, J. NORTON, I. VACEK & A.M. SUN. 1991. Prolonged reversal of diabetic state in NOD mice by xenografts of microencapsulated rat islets. Diabetes **40:** 1511–1516.
3. COLE, D.R., M. WATERFALL & L. MCINTYRE. 1991. Microencapsulated islet grafts in BB/E rqats : a possible role for cytokines in graft failure. Diabetologia **35:** 231–237.
4. CALAFIORE, R., KOH, F. CIVANTOS, F.L. SHIENVOLD, S.D. NEEDELL & R. ALEJANDRO. 1986. Xenotransplantation of microencapsulated canine islets in diabetic mice. Trans. Assoc. Am. Phys. **99:** 28–33.
5. SUN, Y., X. MA, D. ZHOU, I. VACEK & A.M. SUN. 1996. Normalization of diabetes in spontaneously diabetic cynomologus monkeys by xenografts of microencapsulated porcine islets without immunosuppression. J. Clin. Invest. **98:** 1417–1422.
6. SOON-SHIONG, P., R. HEINTZ, N. MERIDETH, Q.X. YAO, Z. YAO, T. ZHENG, M. MURPHY, M.K. MOLONEY, M. SCHMEHL. M. HARRIS, R. MENDE, R. MENDEZ & P. SANFORD. 1994. Insulin-independence in a type I diabetic patient after encapsulated islet transplantation. Lancet **343:** 950–951.
7. TYDEN, G., F.P. REINHOLT, G. SUNDKVIST & J. BOLINDER. 1996. Recurrence of autoimmune diabetes mellitus in recipients of cadaveric pancreatic grafts. N. Engl. J. Med. **335**: 888–889.
8. GILL, R.G. & L. WOLF. 1995. Immunobiology of cellular transplantation. Cell Transplant. **4**(4)**:** 361–370.
9. COLTON, C. K. 1995. Implantable biohybrid artificial organs. Cell Transplant. **4**(4)**:** 415–436.
10. CALAFIORE, R. 1992. Transplantation of microencapsulated pancreatic human islets for the therapy of diabetes mellitus : a preliminary report. Am. Soc. Artif.l Internal Organs J. **38:** 34–37.
11. LIM, F., & A.M. SUN. 1980. Microencapsulated islets as bioartificial endocrine pancreas. Science **210:** 908–910.
12. CALAFIORE, R. & G. BASTA. 1995. Microencapsulation of pancreatic islets: theoretical principles, technologies and practice. *In* Methods in Cell Transplantation. C. Ricordi, Ed.: 587–609. Landes. New York.
13. CALAFIORE, R., G. BASTA, L. OSTICIOLI, G. LUCA, C. TORTOIOLI & P. BRUNETTI. 1995. Coherent microcapsules for pancreatic islet transplantation: a new potential approach for bioartificial pancreas. Transplant. Proc. **28**(2)**:** 822–823.
14. CALAFIORE, R., G. BASTA, P. SARCHIELLI, G. LUCA, C. TORTOIOLI & P. BRUNETTI. 1996. A rapid qualitative method to assess in vitro immunobarrier competence of pancreatic islets containing alginate/polyaminoacidic microcapsules. Acta Diabetol. **33:** 150–153.
15. CALAFIORE, R., G. BASTA, C. BOSELLI, A. BUFALARI, G.M. GIUSTOZZI, G. LUCA, C. TORTOIOLI & P. BRUNETTI. 1997. Effects of alginate/polyaminoacidic coherent microcapsules (CM) transplantation in adult pigs. Transplant. Proc. **29:** 2126–2127.
16. CALAFIORE, R., G. BASTA, G. LUCA, C. BOSELLI, A. BUFALARI, G.M. GIUSTOZZI, R. GIALLETTI, F. MORICONI & P. BRUNETTI. 1998. Transplantation of allogeneic/xenogeneic pancreatic islet containing coherent microcapsules in adult pigs. Transplant. Proc. **30:** 482–483.
17. CALAFIORE, R. 1997. Perspectives in pancreatic and islet cell transplantation for the therapy of IDDM. Diabetes Care **45**: 889–896.

# Evaluation of Graft-Host Response for Various Tissue Sources and Animal Models

COLLIN J. WEBER,[a] SUSAN SAFLEY, MARY HAGLER, AND JUDITH KAPP

*Emory University School of Medicine, Departments of Surgery and Ophthalmology, Atlanta, Georgia 30322, USA*

**ABSTRACT: The efficacy of pancreatic islet transplants in correcting hyperglycemia and slowing the progression of complications in diabetics has been confirmed by many experimental and clinical studies. Unfortunately, the availability of human islets is extremely limited and, therefore, treatment of large numbers of human diabetic patients will almost certainly require either the use of islets harvested from animals (xenografts) or the use of insulin-secreting genetically modified cells of either human or animal origin. There is currently no effective regimen which will allow long-term survival of xenogeneic islets from widely unrelated donor-recipient combinations, such as pig-to-rodent, pig-to-dog, or pig-to-primate. There is considerable interest in the development of immunoisolation techniques for protection of donor islets. However, most materials used in immunoisolation devices are relatively bio-incompatible. Poly-L-lysine-alginate microcapsules are biocompatible and provide an optimal geometry for transmembrane diffusion of insulin and nutrients. Microcapsules allow long-term survival of xenogeneic islets in diabetic rodents or dogs with induced diabetes. However, mice and rats with spontaneous diabetes destroy encapsulated islet grafts within 2 to 3 weeks. Biopsies reveal large numbers of macrophages, immunoglobulins and limited numbers of helper and cytotoxic T-cells in the peri-microcapsule environment of the peritoneal cavity. Cytokines have been identified in peritoneal fluid from mice with islet grafts and may play a role in encapsulated islet destruction. Targeted immunomodulation by treatment of recipients with either anti-helper T-cell antibodies, or fusion proteins which block costimulatory interactions between antigen presenting cells and host T-cells have demonstrated synergy in significant prolongation of encapsulated islet xenograft survival in NOD mice with spontaneous diabetes. Technical improvements in microcapsule design also have contributed to prolonged graft survival. "Double-wall" microencapsulation provides a more durable microcapsule and islet pretreatment prior to encapsulation reduces the frequency of defective capsules with islets entrapped in the membrane. Long-term durability of encapsulated islet grafts remains a concern and further improvements in microcapsule design are a prerequisite to clinical trials.**

[a]Author for correspondence: Emory University School of Medicine, Department of Surgery, 1639 Pierce Dr., Room 5105, Woodruff Memorial Building, Atlanta, GA 30322; 404-727-0084 (voice); 404-727-3660 (fax); cweber@surgery.eushc.org (e-mail).

## BACKGROUND

### *The Rationale for Microencapsulated Islet Xenografts*

Clinical research in the last decade has generated considerable new data on the effects of therapies for insulin-dependent diabetes mellitus (IDDM). The Diabetes Control and Complications Trial (DCCT) found that intensive insulin therapy delayed the onset and slowed progression of retinopathy, nephropathy, and neuropathy in patients with IDDM.[1] Unfortunately, even with careful monitoring, DCCT patients had increased episodes of hypoglycemia.[1] Results of the DCCT support the rationale for pancreas and islet transplantation. Since the inception of islet transplant experiments, it has been postulated that such grafts could supply insulin homeostatically and that 'near-normal' modulation of carbohydrate metabolism might prevent the secondary complications of IDDM.[2] Clinical pancreas allografts have had improved outcomes in recent years, and near normal restoration of glucose homeostasis follows most pancreatic allo- and autografts.[3] However, since the first-year mortality of a human pancreatic allograft recipient remains relatively high (5–10%) and immunosuppression is required, limited numbers of pancreatic transplants are being done worldwide.[2,4]

Islet transplantation is an attractive therapy for patients with IDDM, since problems related to the exocrine pancreas may be avoided. However, allografts of donor human islets have not been successful long term,[3] and availability and yield of human islets are quite limited. Therapeutic islet transplants for large numbers of patients almost certainly will require donor islets harvested from animals (xenografts) or the use of insulin-secreting, genetically modified, immortalized cells. [2–8]

The possibility of use of an unlimited supply of genetically engineered human cells to provide glucose-stimulated insulin release is exciting. Substantial progress has been made over the last several years in regulation of proliferation and differentiation of β-cell lines. However, since engineering glucose-stimulated insulin release has proven extremely difficult,[7,8] these techniques are unlikely to become a clinical reality in the near future. Therefore, the use of islets harvested from animals (xenograft donors) has received considerable attention recently.

The optimal source of xenogeneic islets for clinical use remains controversial. Islets have been isolated from subhuman primates and xenografted into immunosuppressed, diabetic rodents, with short-term reversal of diabetes.[2] However, there are ethical issues surrounding use of primates. Other promising donor islet sources are porcine, bovine and rabbit islets, all of which function remarkably well (i.e., maintaining normoglycemia), in diabetic rodents until transplant rejection occurs.[9–11] Long-term human, bovine and porcine islet xenograft survival has been documented in nude mice and rats, suggesting that sufficient islet-specific growth factors are present in xenogeneic recipients.[12–17]

Adult porcine islets are difficult to isolate and to maintain *in vitro*; nevertheless, they are extremely promising for eventual clinical application since their glucose-responsiveness is similar to that of humans.[9,10] Isolation of bovine islets is technically easier (than porcine islets), and calf islets are glucose-responsive;[10] however, adult bovine islets are relatively insensitive to glucose.[10] Rabbit pancreas is an attractive source of islets since rabbit insulin differs from human insulin at only one amino acid and rabbit islets are glucose responsive.[11] The relatively small size of the rabbit pancreas is a disadvantage, when considering islet xenotransplantation to humans, but it is nonetheless currently feasible to consider isolation of relatively large numbers of donor islets for human diabetic recipients from either calves, pigs or rabbits.

Recently, pigs have been studied intensively as islet donors, including development of a technique for preparation of neonatal porcine islet cell clusters.[18] In addition, porcine islets within microcapsules have been reported to correct diabetes in cynomolgus monkeys.[19] Elaborate studies are in progress to engineer a "perfect pig", lacking certain porcine and α-1-gal antigens, and having adequate levels of complement-inhibiting factors.[20] Thus, porcine donors are perhaps most likely to provide islets for an inaugural human xeno-islet trial.

However, there is significant current concern regarding the potential for transmission of infectious agents from porcine organ donors to human xenograft recipients, and to the population at large. The risks of transmission of most pathogens can be minimized by "pathogen-free" animal colonies. However, pigs have an endogenous retrovirus (PERV) within their germ line. PERV has about 60% homology with the gibbon ape leukemia virus, and PERV has been shown to be released from porcine cells *in vitro*, and to infect human cell lines.[21–23] This is an extremely serious potential concern for the transplant community. Fortunately, careful studies of possible PERV transmission to human recipients of fetal porcine islets have been negative.[23] Further investigations of risks of porcine-to-human xenotransplants are ongoing, prompted by the severe shortage of human organs; and continued studies of islet xenotransplants are essential because of the large numbers of insulin-dependent diabetic patients who may benefit from islet grafts.

### *Advantages of Immunoisolation in Islet Xenotransplantation*

The most significant obstacle to islet xenotransplantation in human IDDM is the lack of an effective immunosuppressive regimen to prevent cross-species graft rejection. Recently, it has been reported that human islets will survive long-term in streptozotocin (STZ)-diabetic mice treated either with an anti-CD4 antibody,[15] or with CTLA4Ig, a high affinity fusion protein which blocks CD28-B7 interactions,[12] or by exposure of donor islets to purified high affinity anti-HLA $F(ab)_2$.[24] Unfortunately, with the exception of these studies, indefinite survival of islet xenografts has rarely been achieved, except with the aid of porous, mechanical barriers. Both intra-and extravascular devices are under development. However, potential clinical complications, such as bleeding, coagulation, technical problems, and bioincompatibility contraindicate their current use in diabetic patients.[25] For example, acrylic-copolymer hollow fibers placed subcutaneously maintained viability of small numbers of allogeneic human islets for two weeks (50 islets per 1.5 cm fiber–65,000 MW permeability).[26] However, to implant 500,000 islets would require >150 meters of these hollow fibers, which is not clinically feasible.[25]

One of the most promising islet envelopment methods is the polyamino-acid-alginate microcapsule. A large number of recent studies have shown that intraperitoneal xenografts of encapsulated rat, dog, or pig islets into STZ-diabetic mice or rats promptly normalized blood glucose for 10–100+ days.[16,17,27–31] Reversal of hyperglycemia by microencapsulated canine islet allografts, porcine islet xenografts, and one human islet allograft has been reported.[19,32,33] The mechanisms by which microcapsules protect islet xenografts from host destruction are not fully understood.

However, it has been suggested that prevention of cell-cell contact with host immunocytes may be a factor.[34] The marked prolongation of widely unrelated encapsulated islet xenografts in rodents with induced diabetes has prompted studies in animals with spontaneous diabetes.

### *The Spontaneously Diabetic NOD Mouse as a Model of Human IDDM*

Nonobese diabetic (NOD) mice develop diabetes spontaneously, beginning at approximately three weeks of age. NOD mice are an appropriate model for studying the feasibility of islet xenotransplants because their disease resembles human IDDM in several ways. Macrophage, dendritic cell and lymphocytic infiltration of islets precedes overt hyperglycemia.[35–38] NOD diabetes is T-lymphocyte–dependent[35–37] and it is associated with (MHC) Class II genes.[39,40] Cytotoxic T cells and antibodies specific for β cells or for insulin have been identified, characterized, and cloned from NOD mice.[36,37] Loss of tolerance to islet antigens in NOD mice correlates with appearance of Th1 immune responses to glutamic acid decarboxylase, a factor which has been reported to be a primary auto-antigen in human IDDM. [41,42] The disease can be induced in non-diabetic, syngeneic mice by transfer of both $CD8^+$ and $CD4^+$ T cells or T-cell clones from NOD mice,[36,43] and inhibition of NOD macrophages or $CD4^+$ T lymphocytes or treatment with anti-Class II monoclonal antibodies prevents or delays diabetes onset in NOD mice.[44,45] It has been suggested that helper T-cells function to activate $CD8^+$ cells, which damage β cells by direct cytotoxic attack. However, some recent studies have suggested that β-cell killing may be indirect, from a nonspecific inflammatory response which initially involves $CD4^+$ macrophages, which release cytokines and oxygen free-radicals (particularly nitric oxide), known β-cell toxins. Because of similarities to IDDM, NOD mice are the best model in which to study islet xenografts.

### *Islet Xenografts into NOD Mice*

Unlike mice with STZ-induced diabetes, NOD mice rapidly reject unencapsulated islet xenografts, allografts and isografts.[16,27,29] Immunosuppressive regimens have little effect on this reaction.[46] Several laboratories have reported that intraperitoneal microencapsulated islets (allo-and xenogeneic) function significantly longer than non-encapsulated controls, but eventually are destroyed also by recipients with spontaneous (autoimmune) diabetes (NOD mice or BB rats).[16,17,29,27] Rejection is accompanied by an intense cellular reaction, composed primarily of macrophages and lymphocytes, which entraps islet-containing microcapsules and is coincident with recurrence of hyperglycemia within 21 days, in both NOD and BB recipients.[17,29,47–51] The mechanism of encapsulated islet rejection by animals with spontaneous diabetes remains incompletely understood, but the fact that it rarely occurs in mice with induced (STZ) diabetes suggests that anti-islet autoimmunity may be involved in islet graft destruction.

### *Mechanisms of NOD Destruction of Encapsulated Islet Xenografts: Macrophages, T Cells, and Cytokines*

It has been suggested by several investigators that microcapsules, like other bioartificial membrane devices, promote survival of xenogeneic and allogeneic islets by: a) preventing or minimizing release of donor antigen(s), thereby reducing host sensitization, and/or b) preventing or reducing host effector mechanisms (i.e., T-cell contact, anti-graft antibody binding, cytokine release).[25,34,50,52]

Most studies of rejection of islets in microcapsules and other membrane devices have focused on effector mechanisms. For example, Halle[34] and Darquy and Reach[52] reported that microcapsules protected donor islets from host immunoglobulins, specifically human anti-islet antibodies and complement effects, *in vitro*. Although complement components are too large ($\gg$150,000 MW) to enter conventional poly-L-lysine microcapsules, it is possible that antibodies might combine with shed donor antigens, forming complexes which bind to the FcR of macrophages *in vivo* (in the peritoneal cavity), which could initiate cytokine release and thereby cause encapsulated islet destruction.[53] Complement could facilitate binding of these antigen-antibody complexes to macrophages via the C3b receptor or by the release of chemotactic peptides that could increase the number of macrophages within the peritoneal cavity.

Involvement of NOD T-lymphocytes in rejection of islets was proposed by Iwata *et al.*, who found significant prolongation of encapsulated hamster-to-NOD mouse encapsulated islet xenografts when NOD recipients were treated with deoxyspergualin (DSG), a T-cell immunosuppressant.[54] These data are consistent with prior findings of several laboratories, that treatment of NOD mice with monoclonal antibodies directed against $CD4^+$ helper T cells prolonged function of both encapsulated and nonencapsulated rat-to-NOD mice islet xenografts[20,25,29] and these findings are similar to observations of Auchincloss and Sachs,[20] Pierson,[55] and Gill[56] that $CD4^+$ T cells play a dominant role in xenoreactivity.

Several investigators have reported a predominance of macrophages/monocytes in the peri-microcapsular infiltrates of encapsulated islet allografts and xenografts in NOD mice and BB rats.[27,29,49,50,51] Cytokines known to be products of macrophages, including IL-1 and TNF $\alpha$,[57–64] may be involved in destruction of encapsulated islets. Both IL-1 $\alpha$ and TNF $\alpha$ have been reported to reduce insulin secretion and cause damage to islet cells *in vitro*.[57,59,61,64] Cytokine-mediated injury might occur directly or indirectly, by activation of an intraperitoneal inflammatory response. For example, IL-1 induces nitric oxide synthase (NOS),[58,59] with resultant generation of nitric oxide (NO), which causes injury to mitochondria and to DNA in $\beta$ cells.[58,59] Furthermore, this pathway of islet damage is worsened by TNF.[63,64] Theoretically, macrophages from either the peritoneal cavity or within donor islets themselves could be involved in cytokine-mediated damage.

Studies of cytokine messenger RNA profiles in pig-to-mouse islet xenografts have found selective increases in "Th2" cytokines (IL-4, IL-5, IL-10) and no change from normal in IL-2.[65] These results are different from those of O'Connell *et al.*,[66] who reported IL-2 messenger RNA in biopsies of rejecting nonencapsulated islet allografts, and also are distinct from the known NOD "Th1" anti-islet immune response.[41,42,67] The "Th2" response is characteristic of evoked antibody responses to foreign antigens, and thus humoral reactions to encapsulated xenografts may be important in graft destruction.

### *Costimulatory Molecules, APCs and Islet Xenograft Destruction by NOD Mice*

Involvement of APCs in immune responses to islet xenografts is suggested by recent studies of Lenschow *et al.*,[12] who found that blockade of the costimulatory molecule, B7, with the soluble fusion protein, CTLA4Ig, prolonged human-to-mouse islet xenografts in STZ-diabetic mice. Several studies, *in vitro* and *in vivo*, have shown that foreign molecules, which interact with the T-cell receptor (peptide/MHC, specific antibodies, mitogens), fail on their own to stimulate naïve T cells to proliferate[68] and may induce antigen-specific anergy.[69] An additional (costimulatory) signal is required, and it is delivered by APCs. In mice, one such costimulatory pathway involves the interaction of the T-cell surface antigen, CD28, with either one of two ligands, B7-1 and B7-2, on the APCs.[68–70] Once this full interaction of T cells and APCs occurs, however, subsequent re-exposure of T cells to peptide/MHC, mitogen, etc. may result in proliferation in the absence of costimulation.[71] CTLA-4 is a cell-surface protein that is closely related to CD28; however, unlike CD28, CTLA-4 is expressed only on activated T cells. It has been suggested that CTLA4 may modulate functions of CD28.[69–71]

CTLA4Ig is a recombinant soluble fusion protein, combining the extracellular binding domain of the CTLA4 molecule with the constant region of the IgG-1 gene.[70] Administration of CTLA4Ig to mice has been shown to induce antigen-specific unresponsiveness (in a murine lupus model) and long-term acceptance of murine cardiac allografts.[71–73] Recent studies have further illuminated helper T-cell-APC interactions, with recognition of the importance of binding of the APC-CD40 antigen to its ligand, GP39, on helper T cells.[75] A monoclonal hamster anti-murine GP39 antibody (MRI) blocks helper T-cell interactions with APCs, macrophages, effector T cells and B lymphocytes.[75] Thus, these relatively nontoxic agents (CTLA4Ig and MRI) may prove to be quite useful in modifying host immune responses to xenogeneic islet grafts.

### *The Immunogenicity of Encapsulated Islets and Mechanisms of Graft Destruction*

Empty microcapsules have been reported to elicit no cellular responses.[17,27,29,31,32,47] On the other hand, other investigators have found reactions to empty capsules.[51,76–78] Impurities in reagents such as contamination with endotoxin or high concentrations of mannuronate may contribute to bioincompatibility.[78] It is also apparent that some formulations of poly-L-lysine microcapsules are biocompatible and some are not. Until standardized reagents are available, immunologic studies of microencapsulated islets should include empty microcapsule controls which document their biocompatibility.

Recently, de Vos *et al.*[79] reported incomplete encapsulation or actual protrusion of islets through microcapsule membranes in some microcapsules and suggested that this biomechanical imperfection may be a factor in microcapsule destruction. Similar observations have been made by Chang,[80] who found incorporation of islets and hepatocytes within the walls of poly-L-lysine alginate microcapsules. Several other investigators have published photomicrographs of encapsulated islets showing obvious entrapment of islets in capsule walls, but did not comment on this problem.[19,34,81,82] Incomplete encapsulation would be anticipated to result in premature capsule fracture and exposure of donor islets to host cells; but there are no reports analyzing this as a source of donor antigen exposure and sensitization of the recipient.

Relatively few studies have focused on the role of donor islet antigen(s) released from microcapsules in initiating host immune responses. Ricker *et al.*[27] reported similar, intense cellular reactions by NOD mice to rat insulinoma, hepatoma, and pheochromocytoma cell lines in microcapsules and concluded that the NOD immune reaction was not islet-specific. Horcher *et al.*[83] reported 15-week survival of 6/7 encapsulated Lewis rat islet isografts, compared to failure of 8/10 encapsulated Wistar-to-Lewis islet allografts within 56 days. Isograft biopsies showed viable islets, intact capsules, and no pericapsular immune reaction, while biopsies of failed allografts revealed pericapsular cellular responses and nonviable islets.[83] This is the only report in the literature with encapsulated islet isograft controls. Although the Lewis rat model is not one with autoimmune diabetes, the results are significant, and suggest that donor antigen(s) are the stimulus for subsequent host responses.

### *Recent Studies from Our Laboratory: Microencapsulated Islet Grafts in NOD Mice*

For the last several years, our laboratory has been focused on studies of the efficacy and function of poly-L-lysine-alginate microencapsulated islet iso-, allo-, and xenografts in spontaneously diabetic NOD mice, as a model for eventual encapsulated islet xenotransplantation in man. We have investigated the function of human, porcine, rabbit, rat, mouse, and NOD islets in this model. Techniques of islet isolation have been reported previously.[16,17,28,29,47,48,84–87] In addition, purified adult canine and neonatal pig islets have been provided by Drs. R. Rajotte and G. Korbutt (Edmonton).

## EXPERIMENTAL

### *Preparation of Microcapsules*

We have developed a formulation of poly-L-lysine-alginate microencapsulation which involves forming a "double-wall" outer membrane.[17,29,84] This "double wall" microcapsule has increased durability. Our technique of microencapsulation utilizes alginate (β-D-mannpyroanospyluronic acid and α-L-fulopyranosyluornic acid) (Kelco low viscosity, low bacterial count, Delco Div. Merck, San Diego, CA) in aqueous phase, under conditions which are physiological, with regard to pH and temperature (24°C).[17]

Briefly, isolated islets are suspended 1:10 (v/v) in 2.0% sodium alginate in 0.9% saline. Droplets containing islets in alginate are produced by extrusion (1.7 ml/min) through a 22 gauge airjet needle (airflow 5 L min). Droplets fall 2 cm into a 20 ml beaker containing 10 ml of 1.1% $CaC1_2$ in 0.9% saline, pH 7.1. Gelled droplets are decanted and transferred to a 50 ml centrifuge tube, filled completely with 1.1% $CaC1_2$ for each 2–4 ml of microcapsules; then the tube is rotated gently, end-over-end, one revolution each 10 seconds for 10 minutes. Microcapsules are allowed to settle; supernatant is aspirated; and then microcapsules are washed in 0.5% $Cl_2$ followed by 0.28% $CaC1_2$ (in 0.9% saline, pH 7.1). After a final wash in 0.9% saline, poly-L-lysine (Sigma, St. Louis, MO), (MW 18,000) 0.5 mg/ml in saline is added (to fill the tube); and the tube is rotated for six minutes. Microcapsules are allowed to settle, and then are washed in 0.1% CHES in saline, pH 8.2, followed by another wash in 0.9% saline. Next, 0.2% sodium alginate is added, and the microcapsules are rotated again for 4 minutes. Thereafter, alginate is aspirated and discarded, microcapsules and washed in 0.9% saline. A final wash in 55 mM sodium citrate is used to solubilize any alginate not reacted with poly-L-lysine. This technique produces "single-wall" microcapsules, which are similar to those reported from several other laboratories.[27,34,49–52]

We found that "single-wall" capsules are fragile. In order to make microcapsules more resilient, we added several additional steps to the protocol prior to final the sodium citrate step. In essence, reincubation of capsules with both poly-L-lysine and dilute alginate are done, to prepare "double-wall" microcapsules.[84] Specifically, additional poly-L-lysine (0.5 mg/ml in saline) is added. Microcapsules are rotated for an additional six minutes, then washed again in 0.1% CHES (in 0.9% saline, pH 8.2) and then in saline, after which they are reincubated on the rotator, in dilute 0.2% sodium alginate for 4 min. Microcapsules then are washed in 0.9% saline, followed by addition of 55 mM sodium citrate in saline, pH 7.4, in which the microcapsules are rotated for an additional six minutes. Finally, microcapsules are washed three times in 0.9% saline, and then transferred to conventional tissue culture medium. This technique results in "double-wall" microcapsules. "Single-wall" microcapsules are translucent, measuring approximately 700 microns, while "double-wall" microcapsules are slightly smaller (~500 microns) and somewhat opaque.

## RESULTS

### *Characterization of Microcapsules*

We have characterized our current microcapsule perm-selectivity, and have found that "double-wall" microcapsules prepared with 2.0% alginate do not allow IgG (MW = 145,000) to traverse the membrane, whereas hemoglobin (MW = 68,000) is freely released from these microcapsules.[84]

We have found that "double-wall" poly-L-lysine microcapsules are well-tolerated within the peritoneal cavity in mice, rats and monkeys, for periods of 3–6 months.[17,29,85] A limited host cellular reaction is evident around spontaneously fractured microcapsules. However, intact empty microcapsules may be recovered by biopsy (lavage) and are uniformly free of host peritoneal cellular reaction.

### *"Double-Wall" 2.0% Alginate Microcapsules Allow Prolonged Islet Xenograft Survival*

Comparative studies of encapsulated rat and rabbit islet survival in NODs have shown that "double-wall" microcapsules prepared with 2.0% alginate were superior to microcapsules prepared with either "single-wall" technique or with a lower (1.85%) alginate concentration (see TABLE 1). The most substantial difference we have detected, which may explain improved results, is that "double-wall" microcapsules prepared with 2.0% alginate exclude immunoglobulin. As shown in TABLE 1, rat-to-NOD mice encapsulated islets survival increased from 19 ± 13 days to 86 ± 24 days when alginate was increased from 1.85% to 2.0%.

**TABLE 1.** Islet iso-, allo- and xenografts in diabetic NOD mice

| Group Islet Donor Recipient | Site | Capsule Type | Mouse Rx | Graft Survival (Days) (BG < 250. mg/dl) (N) | X ± SEM | Reaction (0–4+) |
|---|---|---|---|---|---|---|
| Le RAT→NOD | I.P. | SW, 1.85 | (–) | 10 | 13 ± 1* | + |
| Le RAT→NOD | I.P. | DW, 1.85 | (–) | 9 | 19 ± 3*‡‡ | 4+ |
| Le RAT→NOD | S | (–) | (–) | 5 | 5 ± 0.5 | 4+ |
| Le RAT→B10. | I.P. | DW, 1.85 | (–) | 5 | 132 ± 17‡ | 0 |
| Le RAT→B10. | S | (–) | (–) | 5 | 10 ± 0.6‡ | 4+ |
| Le RAT→NOD | I.P. | DW, 2.0 | (–) | 8 | 79 ± 15## | 1+# |
| Le RAT→NOD | I.P. | PT, DW, 2.0 | (–) | 7 | 126 ± 47## | 1+# |
| RABBIT→NOD | I.P. | DW, 2.0 | (–) | 7 | 20 ± 2 | 4+# |
| RABBIT→NOD | I.P. | PT, DW, 2.0 | (–) | 4 | 31 ± 6@ | 4+# |
| RABBIT→NOD | I.P. | DW, 2.0 | 10–2.16 | 5 | 15 ± 1 | 4+# |
| RABBIT→NOD | I.P. | DW, 2.0 | 53–6.7 | 4 | 22 ± 6 | 3+# |
| RABBIT→NOD | I.P. | DW, 2.0 | CyA | 4 | 22 ± 3** | 4+# |
| RABBIT→NOD | I.P. | DW, 2.0 | 14–4-4 | 4 | 55 ± 29** | 3+# |
| DOG→NOD | I.P. | DW, 2.0 | (–) | 3 | 14 ± 4 | 3+# |
| BALB/C→NOD | I.P. | DW, 2.0 | (–) | 4 | 73 ± 31 | 0–1+# |
| BALB/C→NOD | I.P. | (–) | (–) | 2 | 5, 5 | 4+ |
| NOD→NOD | I.P. | DW, 2.0 | (–) | 3 | 44 ± 7 | 0–1+# |
| NOD→NOD | S | (–) | (–) | 3 | 7 ± 1 | 4+ |

NOTATION: I.P. = intraperitoneal encapsulated islets; S = intrasplenic (islets not encapsulated); * = $p < .001$ vs. intrasplenic control; ‡ = $p < .001$ vs. NODs; SW, 1.85 = "single-wall," 1.85% alginate; DW, 1.85 = "double-wall," 1.85% alginate; DW, 2.0 = "double-wall," 2.0% alginate; ## = $p < .002$ vs. DW, 1.85%; Cyclosporine = 30. mg/kg, s.c., day −1, then daily 14.4.4 = 100. mcg, i.p., day −5, +2, then weekly; PT, DW, 2.0 = Islet pretreatment, "double-wall," 2% alginate; 53.6.7 = 100. mcg, i.p., day −5, +2, then weekly; ‡‡ = $p < .01$ vs. SW, 1.85%; ** = $p$ = not significant vs. DW, 2.0%; @ = $p < .02$ vs. DW, 2.0%; # = excludes IgG.

### *Technical Difficulties in Islet Encapsulation*

We have observed that a small percentage (2–5%) of microcapsules are obviously defective, being misshapen, oblong, or fractured, immediately after their preparation. In addition, we have found that islets or islet cells are either attached to or embedded in the microcapsule membrane (see FIG. 1). We have postulated that these microcapsule defects may allow islet exposure and host sensitization to the graft, as well as reducing the durability of the microcapsule membrane. To address this technical issue, recently, we have made another modification in capsule methodology, namely, "pretreating" (PT) islets in dilute alginate, prior to "double-wall" encapsulation.[85] We developed this pretreatment technique in order to minimize defective

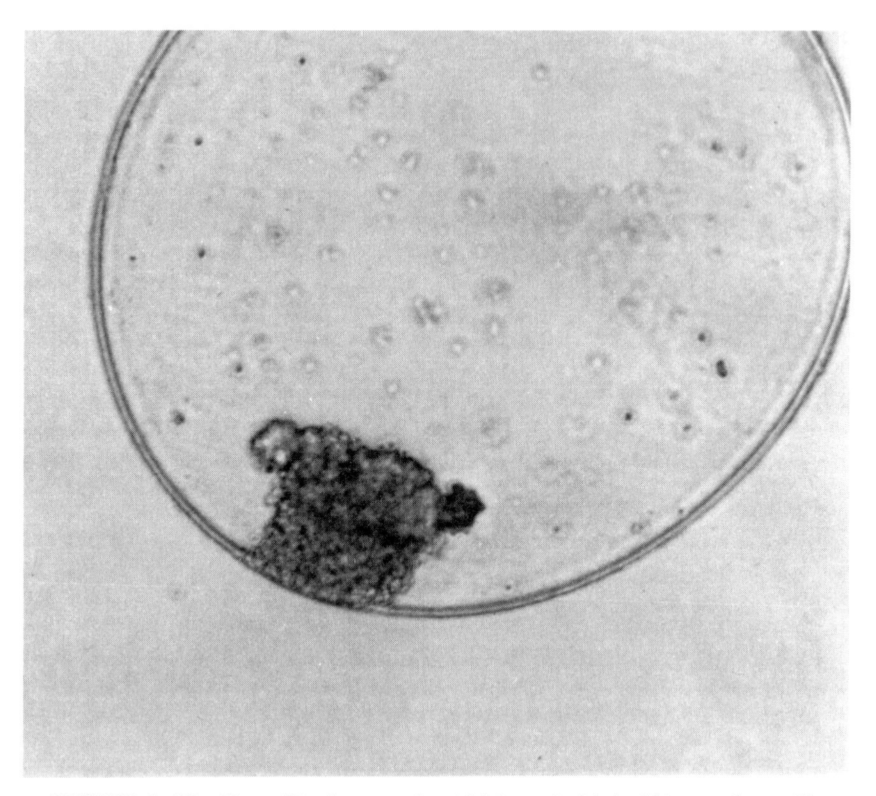

**FIGURE 1.** "Double-wall" microcapsule with islet embedded within membrane. Phase contrast, ×250.

microcapsules, with islets embedded within the microcapsule membrane, a difficulty reported by deVos[79] and Chang.[80] Briefly, the pretreatment technique is as follows. Cells are washed in Hank's balanced salt solution (HBSS), allowed to settle and excess HBSS is removed, leaving a pellet of cells and approximately 0.2 cc of HBSS. Thereafter, 1.5 mL of 2% alginate and 13.5 mL normal saline (NS) are added to produce a final concentration of 0.2% alginate. Cells in this liquid are then rotated for 10 minutes to mix. Thereafter, they are centrifuged to pellet the islets, at 2000 rpm for 3 minutes. Supernatant is removed and cells washed 3× in normal saline and spun to pellet as above 3×. Thereafter, the cell pellet is resuspended in 0.2 cc NS and then 15 ml of 1.1% calcium chloride is added and incubated for 10 minutes rotating. Thereafter, they are washed 2× in normal saline.

This procedure constitutes a precoating of cells with alginate and calcium chloride, which results in a thin layer of cross-linked alginate surrounding each islet. Thereafter, these precoated cells are processed to form conventional double-wall microcapsules. We have found that this technique is more effective than the re-encapsulation method of Chang,[80] the large final outer capsules of which are fragile and unstable. This maneuver has reduced the incidence of defective capsules having islets incorporated within capsule membranes from approximately 30% to 3–5% as assessed by phase and confocal microscopy and by FITC-labeled, islet-specific lectin staining.[85] With this refinement in microcapsule preparation, we have observed significantly prolonged survival of rabbit-to-NOD islet xenografts (from 19 ± 3 days for DW, 2.0% capsules to 31 ± 6 days for PT, DW, 2.0% capsules) ($p < .02$) (see TABLE 1).

### *Characterization of NOD Immune Responses to Encapsulated Islet Xenografts*

Functioning and rejected encapsulated xenografts from the peritoneal graft sites of spontaneously diabetic NOD mice were biopsied, on days 4-to-50 post transplantation. Controls included normal mouse peritoneal fluid and peritoneal fluid from NOD mice bearing empty microcapsules. Total peritoneal (pericapsular and free) cells were unchanged from controls by either empty capsules or capsules with functioning (recipient normoglycemic) islets.[17,29,47] However, cell number increased dramatically at rejection. Flow cytometric analyses revealed that 20–50% of non-adherent peritoneal cells were $B220^+$ (B cells), and that the majority of free peritoneal cells and cells adherent to microcapsules were $Mac1^+$.[17,47] The percentages of $CD4^+$ and $CD8^+$ peritoneal cells were low (4–9%). By FACS analysis the phenotype of peritoneal Mac1 cells shifted from predominantly $Gran1^-$ to Gran $1^+$ during rejection of xenogeneic islets in microcapsules (vs. empty capsules)[47] (see FIG. 2). These findings were confirmed by immunocytochemistry.[17] In addition, immunocytochemistry documented IgG and IgM around microcapsules, and IL-1 α and TNF α both around and within microcapsules.[47] Empty microcapsules biopsied from NOD recipients after 6 months *in vivo* were negative for both IgG and IgM reactivity.[86]

### *Analyses of Cytokine Messenger RNA (mRNA) in Encapsulated Islet Xenograft Biopsies from NOD Mice*

mRNA was extracted from recipient NOD peritoneal cells and expression of mRNA for IL-2, IL-4, and IL-10 was studied by RT-PCR, as previously described.[87] Integrity of RNA samples was assessed by inspection of northern transfer and hybridization with the probe for the 3′ untranslated region of β actin.[87] IL-4 was detected in the majority of xenografts undergoing rejection. IL-10 expression was variable. IL-2 was detected during autoimmune destruction of NOD isografts, but only rarely in rejecting xenografts.

### *Dependence of NOD Islet Graft Destruction on Helper T Cells*

Since a number of recent studies have suggested that interference with host helper T cells will prolong islet allo- and xenograft survival, we tested the effects of anti-CD4 antibody (GK 1.5) therapy on survival of encapsulated rat and canine islet xenografts in NOD mice.[29] Antibody treatment alone (without donor islet encapsulation) resulted in only modest prolongation of graft survival. However, treatment with GK 1.5 plus donor islet encapsulation resulted in markedly prolonged xenograft survival in NOD mice. Unfortunately, after cessation of chronic treatment with antibody, grafts were subsequently rejected, suggesting absence of tolerance.

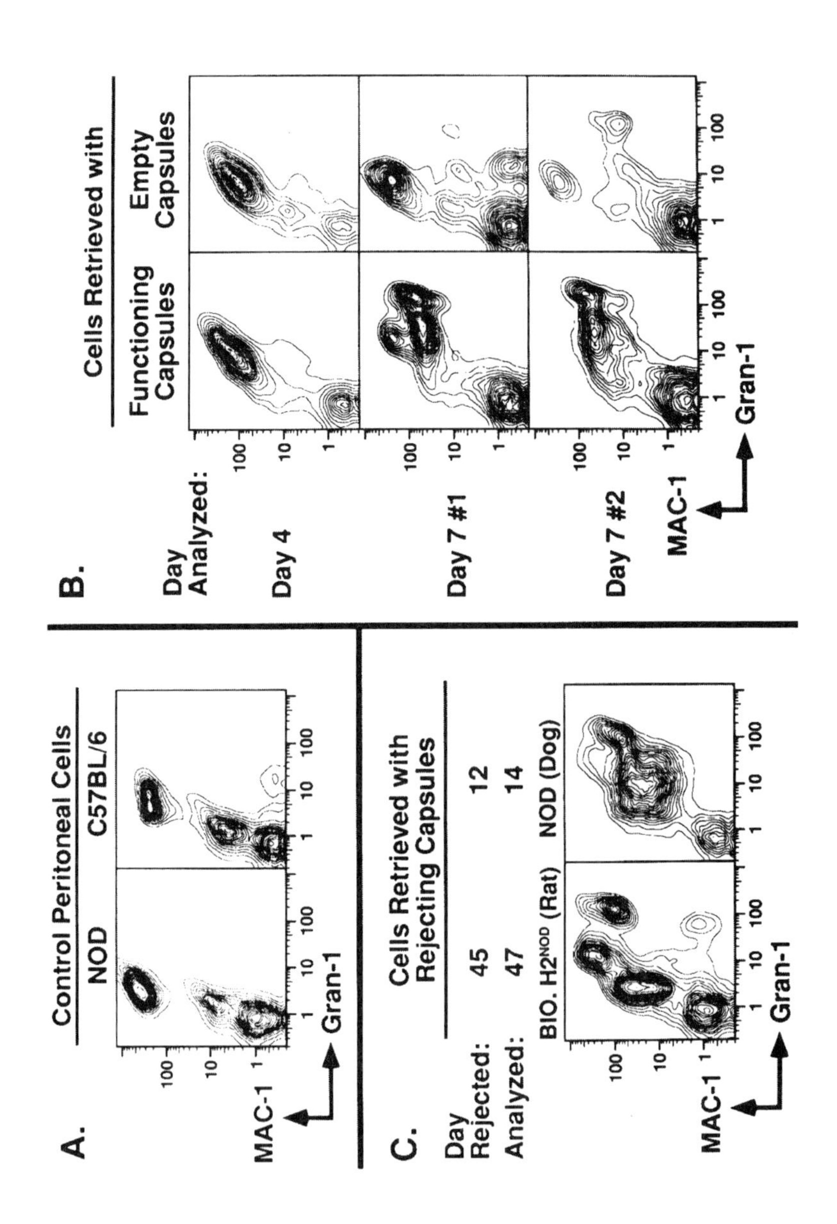

A.
Control Peritoneal Cells
NOD
C57BL/6
MAC-1
Gran-1
B.
Cells Retrieved with
Functioning Capsules
Empty Capsules
Day Analyzed:
Day 4
Day 7 #1
Day 7 #2
MAC-1
Gran-1
C.
Cells Retrieved with Rejecting Capsules
Day Rejected: 45 12
Analyzed: 47 14
BIO. H2NOD (Rat)
NOD (Dog)
MAC-1
Gran-1

Nonetheless, these studies did suggest that the NOD reaction to xenogeneic islets was helper T-cell–dependent.

### *$CD8^+$ T-Cell Depletion Does Not Protect Encapsulated Islet Xenografts in NOD Mice*

We have found that treatment of NOD recipients of encapsulated rabbit islets with either monoclonal antibody 53.6.7 (anti-CD8) (100 μg i.p. day −5 and then twice weekly) or cyclosporine, 30 mg/kg, s.c., daily had no effect on graft survival (TABLE 1). $CD8^+$ T-cell depletion was confirmed by flow cytometry of NOD spleen and peritoneal cells. Biopsies of failed grafts revealed intense host cellular responses and non-viable islets within intact microcapsules. These data are consistent with prior observations, that $CD4^+$ (but not $CD8^+$) T cells play a dominant role in non-encapsulated islet xenograft rejection.[56]

### *Comparisons of Encapsulated Islet Iso-, Allo-, and Xenograft Survival in NOD Mice*

We have found that microencapsulation allowed islet xenograft survival in NOD mice of 20 ± 2 days (N = 7) for rabbit islets and 14 ± 4 (N = 3 ) for dog islets (TABLE 2), with similar peri-microcapsule NOD cell accumulations at rejection. NODs also rejected encapsulated, allogeneic Balb/c islets in 73 ± 31 days (N = 4), Lewis rat islet, in 79 ± 2 days (N = 8) and encapsulated isologous NOD islets in 44 ± 7 days (N = 4) (TABLE 1). However, biopsies of these allo- and isologous grafts, at rejection, have shown few host macrophages adherent to microcapsules, while free peritoneal cells (thus far not characterized) were present. Thus, encapsulated islet xenograft rejection is distinct from iso- or allograft rejection in this model.

### *The NOD-MHC Is Necessary for Rejection of Encapsulated Islet Xenografts*

Both NOD and (STZ-diabetic) B10.H-$2^{g7}$ mice (which express the NOD-MHC-linked disease allele) rejected encapsulated rat islets, while NOD.H-$2^b$ mice, (which express all of the non-MHC-linked diabetes susceptibility genes), accepted encapsulated rat islets for <100 days. (similar to B10 controls)[48] (see FIG. 3). This suggests that the NOD-MHC may contribute to destructive responses against encapsulated islets which are distinct from diabetes susceptibility, since neither B10.H-$2^{g7}$ nor NOD.H-$2^b$ mice develop diabetes spontaneously.[48]

---

**FIGURE 2.** Flow cytometric analyses of cells obtained from NOD and control mice. **(A)** Mac-1 vs Gran-1 comparing control NOD and C57BL/6 mice with no microcapsules. **(B)** Analyses of Mac-1 vs. Gran-1 for cells retrieved from NOD mice bearing microcapsules containing Lewis rat islets on days 4 and 7 following transplantation compared with capsules retrieved from NOD mice bearing empty microcapsules for a similar period of time. Note increasing Gran-1 positivity following transplantation of capsules containing islets compared to empty microcapsules. **(C)** Examples of Mac-1 and Gran-1 positivity from a B10.H-$2^{NOD(g7)}$ mouse bearing microcapsules containing Lewis rat islets (*left*) and an NOD mouse bearing canine islets in microcapsules (*right*).

**TABLE 2.** Survival of microencapsulated (MC) adult rabbit and neonatal pig islets in NOD mice: effects of NOD treatment with CTLA4Ig

| Donor | Technique | Rx | Graft Survival (Days)(BG < 250 mg/dl) | | |
|---|---|---|---|---|---|
| | | | (N) | X ± S.E. | Days |
| Rabbit | MC/IP | None | 7 | 20 ± 2 | 12,16,18,18,20,28,28 |
| Rabbit | MC/IP | CTLA4-Ig[a] | 8 | 108 ± 24* | 37,43,47,58,148,151,173, 205 |
| Rabbit | MC/IP | CTLA4-Ig[b] | 4 | 70 ± 8* | 48,66,81,83 |
| Rabbit | Splenic | CTLA4-Ig[a] | 3 | 6 ± 1* | 5,6,6 |
| Rabbit | Splenic | None | 2 | — | 5,6 |
| Neonatal Pig | MC/IP | None | 8 | 27 ± 36 | 9,10,12,12,14,18,23,118[s] |
| Neonatal Pig | MC/IP | CTLA4-Ig[c] | 10 | 115 ± 19* | 61,74[s],80[s],101[s],108, 137[s],161[s], 266[s] |
| Neonatal Pig | MC/IP | CTLA4-Ig[c,d] | 10 | 103 ± 28 | 12,32,55,63,75,78,83,103, 239,287 |
| Neonatal Pig | Splenic | CTLA4-Ig[c] | 3 | 5 ± 1 | 4,5,5 |
| Neonatal Pig | Splenic | Non-encapsulated | 3 | 6 ± 1 | 5,6,7 |

NOTATION: IP = intraperitoneal; CTLA4Ig, 200 mcg I.P., QOD; * = $p$ >.04 vs. MC alone.
[a]×92 days; [b]×14 days; [c]×21 days; [s]sacrifice for biopsy; [d]"mutant" CTLA41g, which does not fix complement.

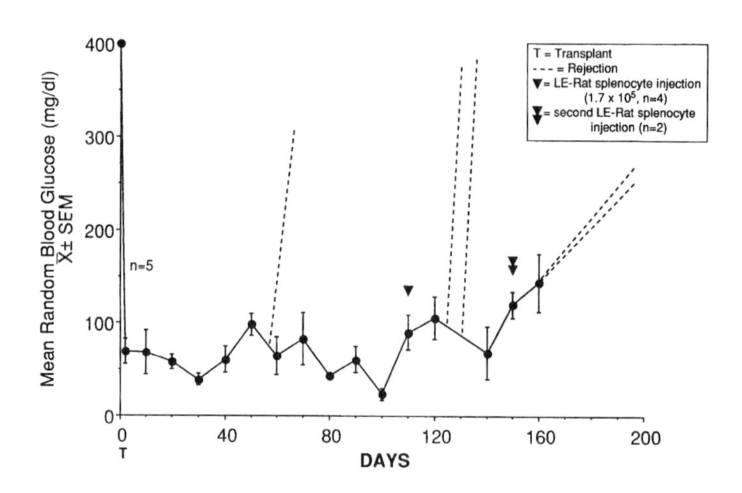


**FIGURE 3.** i.p. xenografts: Encapsulated LE-rat islets into unmodified STZ-diabetic NOD.H-$2^b$ mouse recipients. Administration of $1.7 \times 10^5$ donor LE-rat splenocytes (i.v.) resulted in graft rejection in 2/4 animals, and in 2/2 animals following a second challenge.

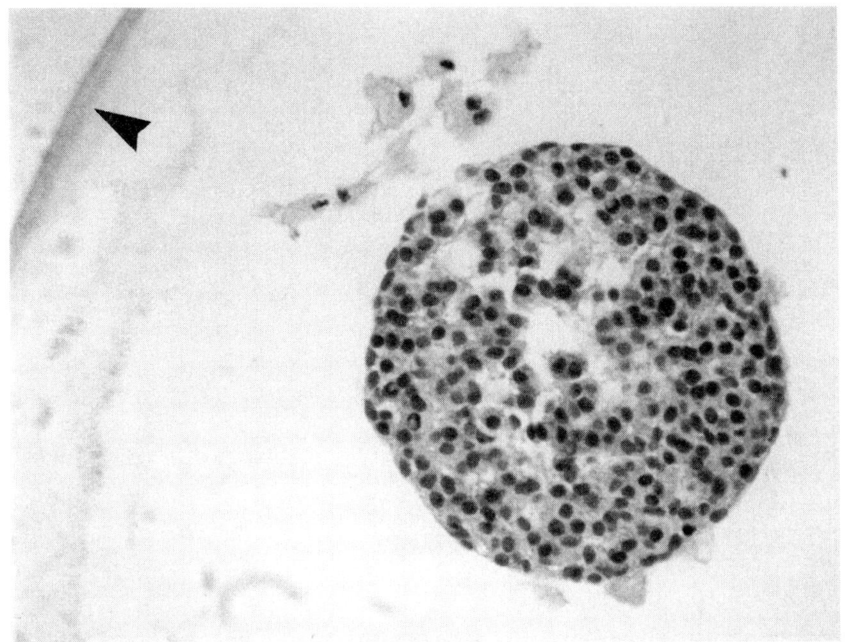

FIGURE 4A.

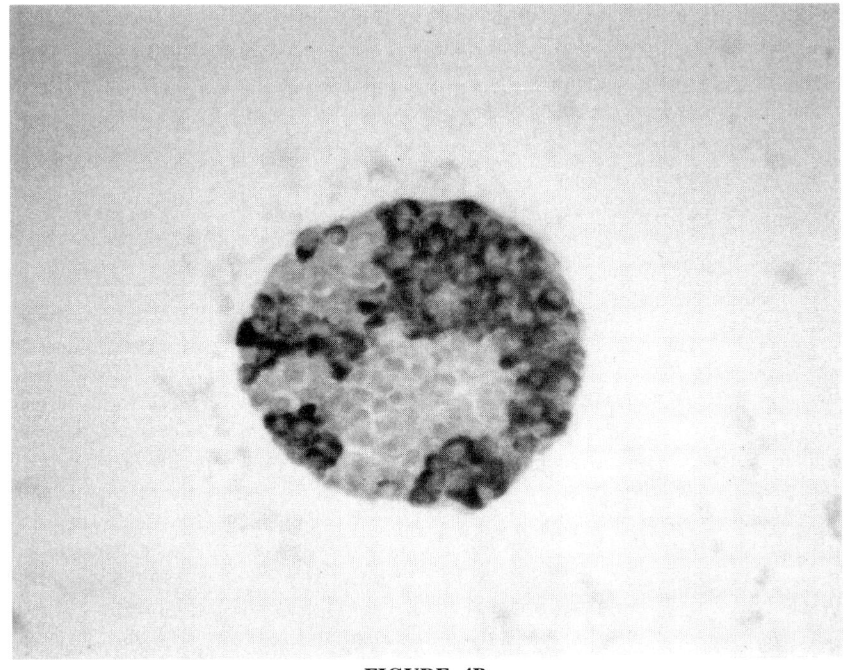

FIGURE 4B.
(Legend on p. 248.)

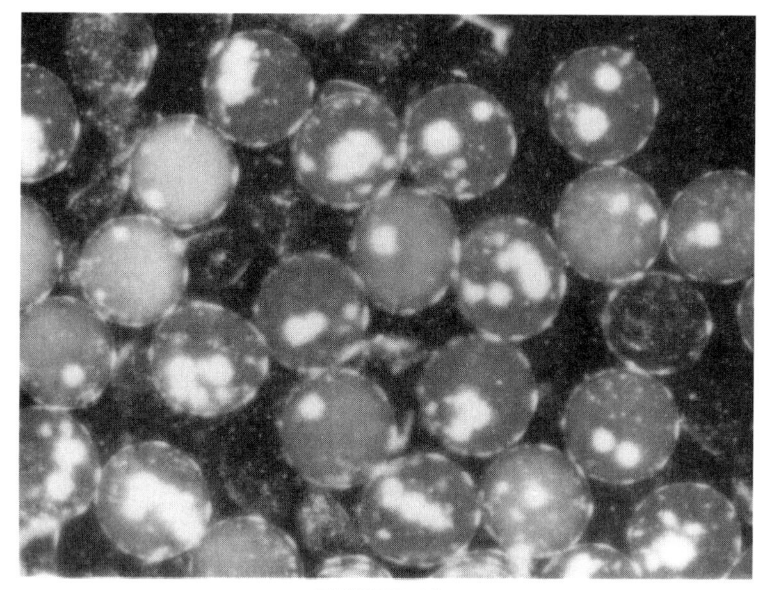

FIGURE 4C.

**FIGURE 4.** **(A)** Microencapsulated neonatal pig islet long-term functioning graft, biopsied on day 104 after xenotransplantation i.p. to spontaneously diabetic NOD mouse. CTLA4Ig, 200 μg i.p. Q.O.D., days 0–21. *Arrow* points to inside of intact microcapsule wall. No pericapsular NOD cellular response. H.& E. ×400. **(B)** Same biopsy as **A**. Anti-insulin immunohistochemistry demonstrates mosaic of β cells ×400. **(C)** Same biopsy as **A**, dark field microscopy, ×60, showing intact microcapsules and minimal pericapsular host reaction. Note islets within microcapsule.

### *Costimulatory Blockade Prolongs Encapsulated Islet Xenografts in Diabetic NOD Mice*

We have found that a combination of microencapsulation of donor adult rabbit or neonatal pig islets plus treatment of recipient nonobese diabetic (NOD) mice with murine CTLA4Ig results in prompt and long-term reversal of spontaneous diabetes, allowing islets to survive and function in these recipient mice for 60–200 days[88,89] (see TABLE 2 and FIG. 4). These data demonstrate synergy between CTLA4Ig treatment and islet encapsulation, since neither encapsulation nor CTLA4Ig alone were effective. To analyze the mechanism of action of CTLA4Ig in this model, we have substituted a recently developed mutant CTLA4Ig which does not bind complement (P. Linsley, personal communication). As shown in TABLE 2, both native CTLA4Ig and mutant CTLA4Ig were effective and synergized with islet microencapsulation in this model. This suggests that an "indirect" pathway of antigen presentation is dominant in NOD responses to encapsulated islet xenografts. Unlike findings with human islet→STZ-diabetic mice,[12] CTLA4Ig alone did not increase nonencapsulated intrasplenic or renal subcapsule rabbit or rat islet survival in NOD mice (TABLE 1), suggesting that encapsulation and CTLA4Ig both were required to prolong graft survival. We believe that this approach holds great promise for treatment of patients with diabetes, since human CTLA4Ig is available, since pig islets are plentiful, and since our microcapsules are durable and biocompatible.

## SUMMARY

Significant questions remain regarding the optimal preparation of xenogeneic beta cells. Processes for preparation, manipulation, expansion, and monitoring of donor porcine islet preparations are still in a developmental phase. The potential risks of transfer of infectious agents such as retroviruses from porcine donors is an issue which is a focus for intensive investigation currently. It is conceivable that islet cell lines from other sources, including human donors, might become practical and plentiful. Nonetheless, an effective and durable technique for islet or islet cell encapsulation may be clinically essential for any of the above donor islet sources.

Further refinements in the technology of islet cell encapsulation may be envisioned in the near future. These improvements may involve new reagents or new technologies or both. To date, the alginate-polyamino-acid microcapsule methodology has been the most widely studied and most effective technique for protection of donor islets placed in a xenogeneic host. The technique has allowed proof of the principle that cross species β-cell grafts can function to normalize hyperglycemia even when not revascularized. This technique provides hope for the future of clinical pancreatic islet xenotransplantation.

Immunoisolation affords the only currently effective method for protection of widely unrelated islet xenografts in a diabetic host. Although various immunoisolation designs are under development, microencapsulation offers an optimal geometry for transmembrane insulin delivery and nutrient uptake by donor islets. Poly-L-lysine alginate microcapsules were the first such devices developed and remain appealing because of their biocompatibility and because long-term islet graft survival has been achieved by many laboratories studying this technique.

Unfortunately, animals with spontaneous diabetes are able to circumvent the immunoisolation membrane and destroy donor islets within 2–3 weeks in most studies. Our laboratory has documented the presence of large numbers of macrophages, immunoglobulins, and cytokines in the peritoneal fluid adjacent to rejected encapsulated islet xenografts. In addition, we have found that this immunologic reaction to donor antigens released from encapsulated islets may be prevented by blockade of costimulatory interactions between host antigen-presenting cells and T cells. Thus, it would appear that prevention of host sensitization by graft tissue is essential for long-term survival of encapsulated islet xenografts. In addition, we have found that reductions in microcapsule membrane perm-selectivity enhance graft survival and pre-treatment of donor islets in dilute alginate reduces the number of defective microcapsules by preventing incorporation of islets themselves within the membrane being formed at the surface of the microcapsule. Further improvements in microcapsule design may be anticipated. It is particularly important to document long-term durability of microencapsulated islets *in vivo* prior to clinical trials with this technique.

## ACKNOWLEDGMENT

The authors acknowledge the expert assistance of Mrs. Gloria Colley in the preparation of this manuscript.

## REFERENCES

1. THE DIABETES CONTROL AND COMPLICATIONS TRIALS RESEARCH GROUP. 1993. The effect of intensive treatment of diabetes on the development and progression of long-term complications in insulin-dependent diabetes mellitus. New Engl. J. Med. **329:** 977–986.
2. LACY, P. 1993. Status of islet cell transplantation. Diabetes Rev. **1:** 76–92.
3. BARKER, C. & A. NAJI. 1992. Perspectives on islet transplantation for diabetes—cures or curiosities? New Engl. J. Med. **327:** 1861–1868.
4. WARNOCK, G. & R. RAJOTTE. 1992. Human pancreatic islet transplantation. Transplant. Rev. **6:** 195–208.
5. LIPES, M., R. COOPER, R. SKELLY, C. RHODES, E. BOSCHETTI, G. WEIR & A. DAVALLI. 1996. Insulin-secreting non-islet cells are resistant to autoimmune destruction. Proc. Natl. Acad. Sci. USA **93:** 8595–8600.
6. GROS, L., MONTOLIU, E. RIU, F. LEBRIGAND & F. BOSCH. 1997. Regulated production of mature insulin by non-β-cells. Human Gene Ther. **8:** 2249–2259.
7. MITANCHEZ, D., B. DOIRON, R. CHEN & A. KAHA. 1997. Glucose-stimulated genes and prospects of gene therapy for type I diabetes. Endocrine Rev. **18:** 520–540.
8. DOCHERTY, K. 1997. Gene therapy for diabetes mellitus. Clin. Sci. **92:** 321–330.
9. RICORDI, C., E. FINKE & P.A. LACY. 1986. Method for the mass isolation of islets from the adult pig pancreas. Diabetes **35:** 649–653.
10. GIANNARELLI, R., P. MARCHETTI, G. VILLANI, A. DE CARLO, S. COSIMI, M. ANDREOZZI, L. CRUSHELLI, P. MASIECO, A. COPPELLI & P. NAVALESI. 1994. Preparation of pure, viable porcine and bovine islets by a simple method. Transplant. Proc. **26:** 630–631.
11. JOS, V., J. CONNOLLY, D. DEARDON, R. PEARSON, N. PARROTT & R. JOHNSON. 1994. A simple method for islet isolation from the rabbit pancreas. Transplantation **58:** 390–392.
12. LENSCHOW, D., Y. ZENG, J. THISTLETHWAITE, A. MONTAG, W. BRADY, M. GIBON, P. LINSLEY & J. BLUESTONE. 1992. Long-term survival of xenogeneic pancreatic islet grafts induced by CTLA41g. Science **257:** 789–795.
13. WEBER, C., R. HARDY, S. RIVER, D. BAILEY-BRAXTON, R. MICHLER, W. THOMAS, J. CHABOT, F. PI-SUNYER, M. WOOD & K. REEMTSMA. 1986. Diabetic mouse bioassay for functional and immunologic human and primate islet xenograft survival. Transplant. Proc. **18**: 823–828.
14. AKITA, L., M. OGAWA & T. MANDEL. 1994. Effect of FK506 and anti-CD4 therapy on fetal pig pancreas xenografts and host lymphoid cells in NOD/Lt, CBA, and BALB/c mice. Cell Transplant. **3:** 61–73.
15. RICORDI, C., P. LACY, K. STERBENZ & M. DAVIE. 1987. Low-temperature culture of human islets plus in vivo treatment of L3T4 antibody produces a marked prolongation of islet human-to-mouse xenograft survival. Proc. Natl. Acad. Sci. USA **84**: 8080–8084.
16. WEBER, C., M. COSTANZO, S. ZABINSKI, S. KREKUN, T. KOSCHITZKY, V. D'AGATI, L., WICKER, R. RAJOTTE & K. REEMTSMA. 1992. Zenografts of microencapsulated rat, canine, porcine, and human islets into streptozotocin (SZN)—and spontaneously diabetic NOD mice. *In* Pancreatic Islet Transplantation. C. Ricordi, Ed.: 177–190. R.G. Landes. Austin, TX.
17. WEBER, C. & K. REEMTSMA. 1994. Microencapsulation in small animals-II: Xenografts. *In* Pancreatic Islet Transplantation Series: Vol. III: Immunoisolation of Pancreatic Islets. R. Lanza & W. Chick, Eds.: 59–79. R. Landes. Austin, TX.

18. KORBUTT, G., J. ELLIOTT, Z. AO, D. SMITH, G. WARNOCK & R. RAJOTTE. 1996. Large scale isolation, growth, and function of porcine neonatal islet cells. J. Clin. Invest. **97:** 2119–2129.
19. SUN, Y., X. MA, D. ZHOU, I. VACEK & A. SUN. 1996. Normalization of diabetes in spontaneously diabetic cynomologus monkeys by xenografts of microencapsulated porcine islets without immnosuppression. J. Clin. Invest. **98:** 1417–1422.
20. AUCHINCLOSS, H., JR. & D. SACHS. 1998. Xenogeneic transplantation. Annu. Rev. Immunol. **16:** 433–470.
21. PATIENCE, C., T. TAKEUCHI & R. WEIS. 1997. Infection of human cells by an endogenous retrovirus of pigs. Nature-Med. **13:** 282–286.
22. FISHMAN, J. 1994. Miniature swine as organ donors for man: strategies for prevention of xenotransplant-associated infections. Xenotransplantation **1:** 47–57.
23. HENEINA, W., A. TIBELL, W. STITZER, P. SANDSTROM, G. VAZQUEZ ROSALES, A. MATTHEWS, O. KORSGREN, T. CHAPMAN, C. FOLKS & C. GROTH. 1998. No evidence of infection with porcine endogenous retrovirus in recipients of porcine islet-cell xenografts. Nature **352:** 695–699.
24. FAUSTMAN, D. & C. COE. 1991. Prevention of xenograft rejection by marking donor HLA class I antigens. Science **252:** 1700–1702.
25. COLTON, C. & E. AVGOUSTINIATOS. 1991. Bioengineering in development of the hybrid artificial pancreas. J. Biochem. Eng. **113:** 152–170.
26. SCHARP, D., C. SWANSON, B. OLACK, P. LATTA, O. HEGRE, E. DOHERTY, F. GENTILE, K. FLAVIN, M. ANSARA & P. LACY. 1994. Protection of encapsulated human islets implanted without immunosuppression in patients with Type I or Type II diabetes and in nondiabetic control subjects. Diabetes **43:** 1167–1170.
27. RICKER, A., S. STOCKBERGER, P. HALBAN, G. EISENBARTH & S. BONNER-WEIR. 1986. Hyperimmune response to microencapsulated xenogeneic tissue in non obese diabetic mice. *In* The Immunology of Diabetes Mellitus. M. Jaworski, Ed.: 193–200. Elsevier. Amsterdam.
28. WEBER, C., S. ZABINSKI, J. NORTON, T. KOSCHITZKY, V. D'AGATI & K. REEMTSMA. 1989. The future role of microencapsulation in xenotransplantation. *In* Xenograft 25. M. Hardy, Ed.: 297–308. Elsevier. Amsterdam.
29. WEBER, C., S. ZABINSKI, T. KOSCHITZKY, R. RAJOTTE, L. WICKER, V. D'AGATI, L. PETERSON, J. NORTON & K. REEMTSMA. 1990. The role of $CD4^+$ helper T cells in destruction of microencapsulated islet xenografts in NOD mice. Transplantation **49:** 396–404.
30. SIEBERS, U., T. ZEKORN, A. HORCHER, G. KLOCK, R. HOUBEN, H. FRANK, R.G. BRETZEL, U. ZIMMERMANN & K. FEDERLIN. 1994. Microencapsulated transplantation of allogeneic islets into specifically presensitized recipients. Transplant. Proc. **26:** 787–788.
31. LANZA, R., W. KUHTREIBER, D. ECKER, J. STARUK & W. CHICK. 1995. Xenotransplantation of porcine and bovine islets without immunosuppression using uncoated alginate microspheres. Transplantation **59:** 1377–1384.
32. SOON-SHIONG, P., E. FELDMAN, R. NELSON, J. KOMTEBEDDE, O. SMIDSROD, G. SKUAK-BRAEK, T. ESPEVIK, R. HEINTZ & M. LEE. 1992. Successful reversal of spontaneous diabetes in dogs by intraperitoneal microencapsulated islets. Transplantation **54:** 769–774.
33. SOON-SHIONG, P., R.E. HEINTZ, N. MERIDETH, Q.X. YAO, Z. YAO, T. ZHENG, M. MURPHY, M.K. MOLONEY, M. SCHMEHL, M. HARRIS, R. MENDEZ & P.A. SANDFORD. 1994. Insulin independence in a type 1 diabetic patient after encapsulated islet transplantation. Lancet **343:** 950–951.
34. HALLE, J., S. BOURASSA, F. LEBLOND, S. CHEVALIER, M. BEAUDRY, A. CHAPDELAINE, S. COUSINEAU, J. SAINTONGE & J. YALE. 1993. Protection of islets of Langerhans from antibodies by microencapsulation with alginate-poly-l-lysine membranes. Transplantation **44:** 350–354.
35. JARPE, A., M. HICKMAN & J. ANDERSON. 1990. Flow cytometric enumeration of mononuclear cell populations infiltrating the islets of Langerhans in prediabetic NOD mice: development of model of autoimmune insulitis for Type I diabetes. Regional Immunol. **3:** 305–317.

36. MILLER, B., M. APPEL, J. O'NEIL & L. WICKER. 1988. Both the Lyt-$2^+$ and L3T$4^+$ T cell subsets are required for the transfer of diabetes in nonobese diabetic mice. J. Immunol. **140:** 52–58.
37. HASKINS, K., M. PORTAS & B. BRADLEY. 1988. T-lymphocyte clone specific for pancreatic islet antigen. Diabetes **37:** 1444–1448.
38. JANSEN, A., F. HOMO-DELARCHE, H. HOOIJKAAS, P. LEENEN, M. DARDENNE & H. DREXHAGE. 1994. Immunohistochemical characterization of monocytes-macrophages and dendritic cells involved in the initiation of the insulitis and B-cell destruction in NOD mice. Diabetes **43:** 667–674.
39. GELBER, C., L. PABROSKY, S. SINGER, D. MCATEER, R. TISCH, C. JOLICOEUR, R. BUELOW, H. MCDEVITT & G. FATHMAN. 1994. Isolation of nonobese diabetic mouse T-cells that recognize novel autoantigens involved in the early events of diabetes. Diabetes **43:** 33–39.
40. PODOLIN, R., A. PRESSEY, N. DELARAATO, P. FISCHER, L. PETERSON & L. WICKER. 1993. I-E+ nonobese diabetic mice develop insulitis and diabetes. J. Exp. Med. **178:** 803.
41. KAUFMAN, D., M. CLARE-SALZLER & J. TIAN. 1993. Spontaneous loss of T-cell tolerance to glutamic acid decarboxylase in murine insulin-dependent diabetes. Nature **365:** 69–72.
42. TISCH, R., X. YANG, S. SINGER, R. LIBLAU, L. FUGGER & H. MCDEVITT. 1993. Immune response to glutamic acid decarboxylase correlates with insulitis in nonobese diabetic mice. Nature **366:** 72–75.
43. DYLAN, D., R. GILL, N. SCHLOOT & D. WEGMANN. 1995. Epitope specificity, cytokine production profile and diabetogenic activity of insulin-specific T cell clones isolated from NOD mice. Eur. J. Immunol. **25:** 1062.
44. WANG, Y., L. HAO, R. GILL & K. LAFFERTY. 1987. Autoimmune diabetes in NOD mouse is L3T4 T-lymphocyte dependent. Diabetes **36:** 535–538.
45. BOITARD, D., A. BENDELAC, M. RICHARD, C. CARNAUD & J. BACH. 1988. Prevention of diabetes in nonobese diabetic mice by anti-I-A monoclonal antibodies: transfer of protection by splenic T cells. Proc. Natl. Acad. Sci. USA **85:** 9719–9723.
46. LAFFERTY, K. 1988. Circumventing rejection of islet grafts: an overview. *In* Transplantation of the Endocrine Pancreas in Diabetes Mellitus. R.Van Shilfgaarde & M. Hardy, Eds.: 279–291. Elsevier. Amsterdam.
47. WEBER, C., J. PRICE, M. COSTANZO, A. BECKER & A. STALL. 1994. NOD mouse peritoneal cellular response to poly-l-lysine-alginate microencapsulated rat islets. Transplant. Proc. **26:** 1116–1119.
48. WEBER, C., A. TANNA, M. COSTANZO, J. PRICE, L. PETERSON & L. WICKER. 1994. Effects of host genetic background on survival or rat→mouse islet xenografts. Transplant. Proc. **26:** 1186–1188.
49. WIJSMAN, J., P. ATKINSON & R. MAZHERI. 1992. Histological and immunopathological analysis of recovered encapsulated allogeneic islets from transplanted diabetic BB/W rats. Transplantation **54:** 588–592.
50. COLE, D., M. WATERFALL, M. MCINTYRE & J. BAIRD. 1992. Microencapsulated islet grafts in the B/E rat: a possible role for cytokines in graft failure. Diabetologia **35:** 231–237.
51. MAZAHERI, R., P. ATKINSON, C. STILLER, J. DUPRE, J. VOSE & G. O'SHEA. 1991. Transplantation of encapsulated allogeneic islets into diabetic BB/W rats: effects of immunosuppression. Transplantation **51:** 750–754.
52. DARQUY, S. & G. REACH. 1985. Immunoisolation of pancreatic B cells by microencapsulation. Diabetologia **28:** 776–780.
53. BALDWIN, W., S. PRUITT, R. BRAUER, M. DAHA & F. SANFILIPPO. 1995. Complement in organ transplantation. Transplantation **59:** 797–808.
54. IWATA, H., T. TAKAGI & H. AMEMIYA. 1992. Marked prolongation of islet xenograft survival (hamster-to-mouse) by microencapsulation and administration of 15-deoxyspergualin. Transplant. Proc. **24:** 1517–1518.
55. PIERSON, R., H. WINN, P. RUSSELL & H. AUCHINCLOSS. 1989. CD-4 positive lymphocytes play a dominant role in murine xenogeneic responses. Transplant. Proc. **21:** 519–521.

56. GILL, R., L. WOLF, D. DANIEL & M. COULOMBE. 1994. $CD4^+$ T cells are both necessary and sufficient for islet xenograft rejection. Transplant. Proc. **26:** 1203–1204.
57. RABINOVITCH, A., W. SUMOSKI, R. RAJOTTE & G. WARNICK. 1990. Cytotoxic effects of cytokines on human pancreatic islet cells in monolayer culture. J. Clin. Endocrinol. Metab. **71:** 152–156.
58. BERMANN, L., K. KRONCKE, D. SUSCHE, H. KOLB & V. KOLB-BACHOFEN. 1990. Cytokines on human pancreatic islet cells in monolayer culture. J. Clin. Endocrinol. Metab. **71:** 152–156.
59. ANDERSEN, H., K. JORGENSEN, J. EGEBERG, T. MANDRUP-POULSEN & J. NERUP. 1994. Nicotinamide preents Interleukin-I effects on cumulated insulin release and nitric oxide production in rat islets of Langerhans. Diabetes **43:** 770–777.
60. CIRULLI, V., P. HALBAN & D. ROUILLER. 1993. Tumor necrosis factor-a modifies adhesion properties of rat islet B cells. J. Clin. Invest. **92:** 1868–1876.
61. CAMPBELL, I., A. ISCARO & L. HARRISON. 1988. Interferon gamma and tumor necrosis factor alpha: cytotoxicity to murine islets of Langerhans. J. Immunol. **141:** 1325–1329.
62. RABINOVITCH, A. 1994. Immunoregulatory and cytokine imbalances in the pathogenesis of IDDM. Diabetes **43:** 613–621.
63. ABLAMUNITS, V., F. BARANOVA, T. MANDRUP-POULSEN & J. NERUP. 1994. In vitro inhibition of I insulin release by blood mononuclear cells from insulin-dependent diabetic and healthy subjects: synergistic action of IL-1 and TNF. Cell Transplant. **3:** 55–60.
64. MANDRUP-POULSEN, T., K. BENDTZEN, C. DINARELLO & J. NERUP. 1987. Human tumor necrosis factor potentiates interleukin-1 mediated rate of pancreatic B-cell cytotoxicity. J. Immunol. **39:** 4077–4082.
65. MORRIS C., M. FUNG, S. SIMEONOVIC, D. WILSON & A. HAPEL. 1994. Cytokine expression in CDA/H mice following xenotransplantation of fetal pig proislets. Transplant. Proc. **26:** 1304–1305.
66. O'CONNELL, P., A. PACHEOCO-SILVA, P. NICKERSON, R. MUGGIA, M. BASTOS, V. KELLEY & STROM. 1993. Unmodified pancreatic islet allograft rejection results in preferential expression of certain T cell activation transcripts. J. Immunol. **150:** 1093- 1104.
67. AGUILAR-DIOSDADA, M., D. PARKINSON, J. CORBETT, G. KWON, C. MARSHALL, R. GINGERICH, J. SANTIAGO & M. MCDANIEL. 1994. Potential autoantigens in IDDM: expression of carboxypeptidase-H and insulin but not glutamate decarboxylase on the B-cell surface. Diabetes **43:** 418–425.
68. JENKINS, M. 1994. The ups and downs of T cell costimulation. Immunity **1:** 443–446.
69. HARDING, F., J. MCARTHUR, J. GROSS, D. RAULET & J. ALLISON. 1992. CD28-mediated signaling co- stimulates murine T cells and prevents induction of anergy in T-cell clones. Nature **356:** 607–609.
70. HATHCOCK, K., G. LASZIO, H. DICKLER, J. BRADSHAW, P. LINSLEY & R. HODES. 1993. Identification of an alternative CTLA-4 ligand costimulatory for T cell activation. Science **262:** 905–907.
71. GUERDER, S., J. MEYERHOFF & R. FLAVELL. 1994. The role of the T cell costimulatory B7-1 in autoimmunity and the induction and maintenance of tolerance of peripheral antigen. Immunity **1:** 155–166.
72. BOLLING, S., L. TURKA, R. WEI, P. LINSLEY, C. THOMPSON & H. LIN. 1994. Inhibition of B7-induced CD28 T-cell activation with CTLA4Ig prevents cardiac allograft rejection: evidence for costimulation. Transplantation **57:** 413–415.
73. PEARSON, T., D. ALEXANDER, K. WINN, P. LINSLEY, R. LOWRY & C. LARSEN. 1994. Transplantation of tolerance induced by CTLA4-Ig. Transplantation **57:** 1701–1706.
74. LENSCHOW, D., S. HO, H. SATTAR, L. RHEE, G. GRAY, N. NABAVI, K. HEROLD & J. BLUESTONE. 1995. Differential effects of anti-B7-1 and anti-B7-2 monoclonal antibody treatment on the development of diabetes in the nonobese diabetic mouse. J. Exp. Med. **181:** 1145–1155.

75. DURIE, F., R. FAVA, T. FOY, A. ARUFFO, J. LEDBETTER & R. NOELLE. 1993. Prevention of collagen-induced arthritis with an antibody to gp39, the ligand for CD40. Science **261:** 1328–1330.
76. GIN, H., C. CADIC, C. BAQUEY & B. DUPUY. 1992. Peritoneal exudates from microencapsulated rat islets of Langerhans xenografted mice presenting characteristics of potentially cytotoxic non-specific inflammation. J. Microencapsulation **9:** 489–494.
77. CLAYTON, H., N. LONDON, P. COLLOBY, P. BELL & R. JAMES. 1991. The effect of capsule composition on the biocompatibility of alginate-poly-l-lysine capsules. J. Microencapsulation **8:** 221–233.
78. SOON-SHIONG, P., M. OTERLIE, G. SKJAK-BRAEK, O. SMIDSROD, R. HEINTZ, R.P. LANZA & T. ESPEVIK. 1991. An immunologic basis for the fibrotic reaction to implanted microcapsules. Transplant. Proc. **23:** 758–759.
79. DE VOS, P., G. WOLTERS & R. VANSCHILFGAARDE. 1994. Possible relationship between fibrotic overgrowth of alginate-polylysine-alginate microencapsulated pancreatic islets and the microcapsule integrity. Transplant. Proc. **26:** 782–783.
80. CHANG, T. 1992. Artificial cells in immobilization biotechnology. Artif. Cells & Immob. Biotechnol. **20:** 1121–1143.
81. LUM, Z., I. TAI, M. KRESTOW, J. NORTON, I. VACEK & A. SUN. 1991. Prolonged reversal of diabetic state in NOD mice by xenografts of microencapsulated rat islets. Diabetes **40:** 1511–1516.
82. CHICHEPORTICHE, D. & G. REACH. 1988. In vitro kinetics of insulin release by microencapsulated rat islets: effect of the size of the microcapsules. Diabetologia **31:** 54–57.
83. HORCHER, A., T. ZEKORN, U. SIEBERS, G. KLOCK, H. FRANK, R. HOUBEN, R.G. BRETZEL, U. ZIMMEERMAN & K. FEDERLIN. 1994. Transplantation of microencapsulated islets in rate: evidence for induction of fibrotic overgrowth by islet alloantigens released from microcapsules. Transplant. Proc. **26:** 784–786.
84. WEBER, C., M. COSTANZO, S. KREKUN & V. D'AGATI. 1993. Causes of destruction of microencapsulated islet grafts: characteristics of a 'double-wall' poly-l-lysine–alginate microcapsule. Diabetes Nutr. Metab. **1:** 167–171.
85. WEBER, C.J., J.A. KAPP, M.K. HAGLER, S. SAFLEY, J.T. CHRYSSOCHOOS & E.L. CHAIKOF. 1999. *In* Encapsulation and Immobilization Techniques. R.Lanza, W. Chick & W. Kutreiber, Eds. Springer-Verlag. New York. In press.
86. WEBER, C., V. D'AGATI, L. WARD, M. COSTANZO, R. RAJOTTE & K. REEMTSMA. 1993. Humoral reaction to microencapsulated rat, canine, porcine islet xenografts in spontaneously diabetic NOD mice. Transplant. Proc. **25:** 462–463.
87. WEBER, C., M. HAGLER, B. KONIECZNY, J. CHRYSSOCHOOS, R. RAJOTTE, F. LAKKIS & R. LOWRY. 1995. Encapsulated islet iso-, allo-, and xeno-grafts in diabetic NOD mice. Transplant. Proc. **27:** 3308–3311.
88. WEBER, C., M. HAGLER, J. CHRYSSOCHOOS, C. LARSEN, T. PEARSON, P. JENSEN, J. KAPP & P. LINSLEY. 1996. CTLA4-Ig prolongs survival of microencapsulated rabbit islet xenografts in spontaneously diabetic NOD mice. Transplant. Proc. **28:** 821–823.
89. WEBER, C., M. HAGLER, J. CHRYSSOCHOOS, G. KORBUTT, R. RAJOTTE, P. LINSLEY & J. KAPP. 1997. CTLA4-Ig prolongs survival of microencapsulated neonatal porcine islet xenografts diabetic NOD mice. Cell Transplant. **6:** 505–508.

# Antigen Presentation Pathways for Immunity to Islet Transplants

## Relevance to Immunoisolation

RONALD G. GILL[a]

*Barbara Davis Center for Childhood Diabetes, University of Colorado Health Sciences Center, 4200 East 9th Avenue, Box B-140, Denver, Colorado 80262, USA*

**ABSTRACT: Tremendous advances have been made over the past several years in the development of diverse biocompatible materials and structural designs for the implantation of immunoisolated cells and tissues. This area of bioengineering has clear application to insulin-dependent diabetes for which the implantation of micro- or macroencapsulated pancreatic islets or surrogate β cells has great potential therapeutic benefit. This discussion concentrates on three antigen-specific immunologic processes that impede the application of islet transplantation as a therapy for insulin-dependent diabetes: (1) Allograft immunity, (2) Xenograft immunity, and (3) Autoimmune pathogenesis of Type I diabetes. Special emphasis is placed on the potential impact of these immune pathways on immunoisolated tissues.**

### THE TWO-SIGNAL HYPOTHESIS OF T-CELL ACTIVATION: "DIRECT" AND "INDIRECT" PRESENTATION OF GRAFT ANTIGENS

T lymphocytes generally recognize antigens as peptide fragments presented in association with major histocompatibility complex (MHC) molecules. CD8 T cells recognize antigens presented in association with class I MHC molecules, while CD4 T cells generally recognize antigens presented by class II MHC molecules. However, a key tenet regarding immune responses is that *two* signals are required for T-lymphocyte activation.[1] Signal one is supplied by engagement of the antigen-specific T-cell receptor (TCR) while the second signal, or costimulator, is provided by non-antigen–specific inductive signals from the antigen-presenting cell(s) (APC). In recent years it has become apparent that costimulation is a complex process involving the contribution of a number of inter-related cell surface receptor-ligand interactions. Major participants in this process are the B7.1/B7.2 molecules (CD80/CD86) expressed by APC that bind the CD28 co-receptor molecule on T cells. However, interactions between CD40 on APC with CD40L (CD154) on T cells also contribute important costimulatory signals,[2] possibly for the enhanced expression of B7 molecules on APC. The relevance of these molecules to the induction of islet rejection is

[a]303-315-6390 (voice); 303-315-4124 (fax); ron.g.gill@uchsc.edu (e-mail).

illustrated by studies in which blocking B7/CD28[3,4] or CD40/CD40L[5] interactions *in vivo* can result in indefinite islet allograft or xenograft survival.

Of special relevance to this discussion is that there are two primary forms of graft antigen presentation that can fulfill this two-signal requirement for T-cell activation:

(1) "Direct"(or donor MHC-restricted) antigen presentation in which T cells engage native MHC molecules directly on the surface of donor-derived APC, and

(2) "Indirect" (or host MHC-restricted) antigen presentation in which donor-derived antigens are captured by recipient APC, degraded and re-presented in association with recipient MHC molecules.

Importantly, exogenous antigens are generally processed and presented by class II MHC molecules and so invoke a predominantly CD4 T-cell response. The distinction between these two antigen-presentation pathways is of great importance with regard to immunoisolated tissues. T cells of direct specificity for MHC antigens on the surface of donor cells require a cognate interaction with the graft, while T cells specific for donor-derived peptides presented by MHC on the surface of host APC do not. Thus, while tissue isolation strategies that prevent cell-cell contact between donor cells and host immune cells are expected to block the direct pathway as defined above, the indirect pathway is expected to be more problematic. That is, while the direct pathway may be excluded by immunoisolation, there is still the potential for peptide antigens to traverse the isolating membrane and be presented by host-type APC. The extent and consequence of this type of response to immunoisolated tissues may be considerable, depending on the type of isolation technology and the nature of tissue grafted.

## ALLOGRAFT IMMUNITY

The two-signal hypothesis of T-cell activation had a major impact on current concepts of allograft immunity. Since costimulation was presumed to be a property of hematopoietic APC, Lafferty and colleagues proposed that the majority of tissue immunogenicity was due to "passenger-leukocytes" resident within the transplant.[6] Experimental verification of this concept came from studies showing that tissue pretreatment could deplete donor-type APC and facilitate the acceptance of islet allografts in non-immunesuppressed mice.[7,8] Recent studies clearly show that the acceptance of pretreated islet allografts is due to a reduction of donor-derived costimulatory activity and not to a reduction of MHC expression by the graft.[9]

Such studies suggest that the predominant pathway of islet allograft rejection is through direct antigen presentation by donor-type APC. Further evidence for the role of direct antigen presentation is shown by the fact that CD8 T cells specific for donor class I MHC antigens are important for islet allograft rejection. Either depleting the recipient of CD8 T cells[10] or grafting class I MHC-deficient islets[11] leads to prolonged allograft acceptance. Thus, while it is clear that islet allograft rejection requires the participation of class II MHC-restricted CD4 T cells,[12,13] allograft rejection appears to be greatly dependent on CD8 T cells that directly engage donor cells. Perhaps equally important is the implication that indirect presentation of donor antigens is not a major pathway for acute islet allograft rejection. Thus, allogeneic tissues would be expected to have considerable benefit from strategies that exclude cell-cell contact with the graft.

## XENOGRAFT IMMUNITY

The T-cell response to xenografts differs greatly from the response to allografts. Islet xenograft rejection appears to be less dependent on donor APC than allograft rejection; depletion of passenger leukocytes has little benefit for the graft.[10] Also, while CD8 T cells play a central role for islet allograft rejection, CD8 T cells are not required for acute xenograft rejection.[14,15] Rather, CD4 T cells appear to be the predominant T-cell subset involved in xenograft rejection; CD4 T cells can trigger acute xenograft rejection independently of either CD8 T cells or antibody-producing B cells.[14,15] Furthermore, we have recently found that this CD4-mediated rejection of xenografts requires recipient class II MHC expression (Yang *et al.*, in preparation), indicating that the xenograft response is mediated predominantly by the 'indirect' pathway of antigen presentation. It is noteworthy that 'indirect' CD4 T cells are also the predominant helper cells for B cells, and so this pathway is also expected to drive a graft-specific antibody response.

The distinction between the T-cell–dependent responses to islet allografts and xenografts may also apply for responses to immunoisolated tissues. For example, Loudovaris *et al.* have found that macro-encapsulation permits allograft acceptance but not xenograft acceptance *in vivo.*[16] These investigators also found that CD4 T cells were both necessary and sufficient to trigger rejection of the immunoisolated xenografts. Previous studies also showed that CD4 T are required for the response to microencapsulated xenografts.[17] Taken together, such studies suggest that a major concern regarding immunoisolated xenografts is the potential for graft-derived antigens to sensitize the host via a CD4-dependent 'indirect' response. Although such CD4 T cells cannot directly engage grafted cells, an interaction with host APC by this pathway may trigger a significant inflammatory response *in vivo*. Though it is assumed that tissue damage by this process is mediated by soluble mediators such as cytokines and oxygen free radicals that can traverse the isolation membrane, the exact mechanism of immune injury to immunoisolated tissues remains unclear. In fact, the consequence of the indirect pathway on immunoisolated xenografts may be variable. Some studies have demonstrated dramatic prolongation of even discordant encapsulated xenografts,[18–20] although the degree of host immune sensitization in most cases is unclear. Thus, some forms of immunoisolation may also provide protection from the indirect pathway of antigen presentation.

## AUTOIMMUNE DISEASE PATHOGENESIS

An important problem for islet transplantation in Type I diabetes is the recurrence of the underlying autoimmune pathogenesis that triggers the disease. It is clear that disease pathogenesis can recur and destroy transplanted islets in both man[21] and in animal models of autoimmune diabetes.[22,23] Although the nature of disease pathogenesis remains controversial, there is evidence to suggest that T-cell–dependent autoimmune islet injury behaves much like the xenograft response described above. That is, islet damage can be triggered by autoreactive CD4 T cells specific for islet-associated antigens processed and presented by APC, analogous to the 'indirect' response to transplant antigens.

Both CD4 and CD8 T cells are required for disease onset in autoimmune-prone non-obese diabetic (NOD) mice.[24,25] However, the recurrence of disease in islet transplants in spontaneously diabetic NOD mice appears to be CD4 T-cell–dependent and CD8 T-cell–independent.[26] Several CD4 cell clones derived from NOD mice have been generated that recognize islet-antigens and, importantly, have been shown to be pathogenic *in vivo.*[27–30] In some cases, islet-specific CD4 T cells are sufficient to trigger overt islet destruction *in vivo.*[29–31] Pathogenic CD8 T cells have also been isolated from NOD mice,[26,32] indicating that this pathway can also contribute to islet damage. While immunoisolated islet cells would expected to be protected from CD8 T cells specific for class I MHC expressed by the transplanted β cells, pathogenic CD4 T cells specific for β-cell antigens presented by autologous APC could still mount an inflammatory response. For example, the insulin molecule itself has been shown to be an important target antigen for NOD CD4 T cells,[30,33] and so may be targeted by the autoimmune host regardless of the immunoisolation technology. The ability of different immunoisolation strategies to protect islet transplants from autoimmune recognition will need to be empirically determined.

## CONCLUSIONS

Perhaps the most significant conclusion from this discussion is that encapsulation technologies may best be described as 'cell-isolation' rather than 'immuno-isolation'. That is, while preventing cell-cell contact between host leukocytes and donor tissues is a common feature of isolation strategies, it is unlikely that all immune sensitization can be prevented, especially considering that some potential target antigens may be required to traverse the isolating membrane (e.g., insulin). Allografts, which appear to be rejected predominantly by direct antigen presentation and cognate interaction between responding T cells and target cells, would be expected to benefit most by immunoisolation strategies. Protection of xenografts by immunoisolation, however, would appear to be challenging since this response may involve a more significant component of indirect antigen presentation and inflammatory tissue damage. This pathway may also be a major component of autoimmune-mediated tissue injury. Thus, consistent long-term islet survival in autoimmune recipients achieved through immunoisolation alone, especially for xenografts, may prove to be difficult. However, some combinatorial approaches using immunoisolation with adjunct immune manipulation may prove beneficial as has been demonstrated for encapsulated islets in spontaneously diabetic NOD mice plus CTLA4-Ig treatment[34] or co-encapsulation of islets with immune-modulating Sertoli cells.[35]

## REFERENCES

1. LAFFERTY, K.L. & A.J. CUNNINGHAM. 1975. A new analysis of allogeneic interactions. Aust. J. Exp. Biol. Med. Sci. **53:** 27–42.

2. GREWAL, I.S. *et al.* 1996. Requirement for CD40 ligand in costimulation induction, T cell activation, and experimental allergic encephalomyelitis. Science **273:** 1864–1867.
3. LENSCHOW, D.J. *et al.* 1992. Long-term survival of xenogeneic pancreatic islet grafts induced by CTLA4Ig. Science **257:** 789–792.
4. TRAN, H. *et al.* 1997. Distinct mechanisms for the induction and maintenance of allograft tolerance with CTLA4-Fc treatment. J. Immunol. **159:** 2232–2239
5. PARKER, D. *et al.* 1995. Survival of mouse pancreatic islet allografts in recipients treated with allogeneic small lymphocytes and antibody to CD40 ligand. Proc. Natl. Acad. Sci. USA **92:** 9560–9564.
6. LAFFERTY, K.J., S.J. PROWSE & C.J. SIMEONOVIC. 1983. Immunobiology of tissue transplantation: a return to the passenger leukocyte concept. Annu. Rev. Immunol. **1:** 143–173.
7. BOWEN, K., L. ANDRUS & K. LAFFERTY. 1980. Successful allotransplantation of mouse pancreatic islets to nonimmunosuppressed recipients. Diabetes. **29** (Suppl. 1): 98–104.
8. FAUSTMAN, D. *et al.* 1981. Prolongation of murine islet allograft survival by pretreatment of islets with antibody directed to Ia determinants. Proc. Natl. Acad. Sci. USA **78:** 5156–5159.
9. COULOMBE, M. *et al.* 1996. Tissue immunogenicity. the role of MHC antigen and the lymphocyte costimulator B7-1. J. Immunol. **157:** 4790–4795.
10. WOLF, L.A., M. COULOMBE & R.G. GILL. 1995. Donor antigen-presenting cell-independent rejection of islet xenografts. Transplantation **60:** 1164–1170.
11. MARKMANN, J.F. *et al.* 1992. Indefinite survival of MHC class I-deficient murine pancreatic islet allografts. Transplantation **54:** 1085–1089.
12. SHIZURU, J.A. *et al.* 1987. Islet allograft survival after a single course of treatment of recipient with antibody to L3T4. Science **237:** 278–280.
13. HAO, L. *et al.* 1987. Role of the $L3T4^+$ T cell in allograft rejection. J. Immunol. **139:** 4022–4026.
14. PIERSON III, R.N. *et al.* 1989. Xenogeneic skin graft rejection is especially dependent on $CD4^+$ T cells. J. Exp. Med. **170:** 991–996.
15. GILL, R. *et al.* 1994. CD4 T cells are both necessary and sufficient for islet xenograft rejection. Transplant. Proc. **26:** 1203.
16. LOUDOVARIS, T., T.E. MANDEL & B. CHARLTON. 1996. $CD4^+$ T cell mediated destruction of xenografts within cell-impermeable membranes in the absence of $CD8^+$ T cells and B cells. Transplantation **61:** 1678–1684.
17. WEBER, C.J. *et al.* 1990. The role of $CD4^+$ helper T cells in the destruction of microencapsulated islet xenografts in NOD mice. Transplantation **49:** 396–404.
18. LANZA, R.P. *et al.* 1993. Biohybrid artificial pancreas. Long-term function of discordant islet xenografts in streptozotocin diabetic rats. Transplantation **56:** 1067–1072.
19. SUN, Y. *et al.* 1996. Normalization of diabetes in spontaneously diabetic cynomologus monkeys by xenografts of microencapsulated porcine islets without immunosuppression. J. Clin. Invest. **98:** 1417–1422.
20. YANG, H. *et al.* 1997. Long-term function of fish islet xenografts in mice by alginate encapsulation. Transplantation **64:** 28–32 .
21. SUTHERLAND, D.E.R. *et al.* 1984. Twin-to-twin pancreas transplantation: reversal and reenactment of the pathogenesis of type I diabetes. Transplant Assoc. Am. Physicians **97:** 80–87.
22. TERADA, M., K. LENNARTZ & Y. MULLEN. 1987. Allogeneic and syngeneic pancreas transplantation in non-obese diabetic mice. Transplant. Proc. **19:** 960–961.
23. NAJI, A. *et al.* 1981. Prevention of diabetes in rats by bone marrow transplantation. Ann. Surg. **194:** 328–338.
24. BENDELAC, A. *et al.* 1987. Syngeneic transfer of autoimmune diabetes from diabetic NOD mice to healthy neonates. Requirement for both $L3T4^+$ and $Lyt\text{-}2^+$ T cells. J. Exp. Med. **166:** 823–832.
25. MILLER, B.J. *et al* . 1988. Both the $Lyt\text{-}2^+$ and $L3T4^+$ T-cell subsets are required for the transfer of diabetes in nonobese diabetic mice. J. Immunol. **140:** 52–58.

26. WANG, Y. *et al.* 1991. The role of CD4+ and CD8+ T cells in the destruction of islet grafts by spontaneously diabetic mice. Proc. Natl. Acad. Sci. USA **88:** 527–531.
27. HASKINS, K. *et al.* 1988. T-lymphocyte clone specific for pancreatic islet antigen. Diabetes. **37:** 1444–1448.
28. HASKINS, K. & M. MCDUFFIE. 1990. Acceleration of diabetes in young NOD mice with a CD4+ islet-specific T cell clone. Science **249:** 1433–1436.
29. WEGMANN, D.R. *et al* . 1993. Establishment of islet-specific T-cell lines and clones from islet isografts placed in spontaneously diabetic NOD mice. J. Autoimmun. **6:** 517–527.
30. DANIEL, D. *et al.* 1995. Eptiope specificity, cytokine production profile and diabetogenic activity of insulin-specific T cell clones isolated from NOD mice. Eur. J. Immunol. **25:** 1056–1062.
31. KURRER, M. *et al.* 1997. Beta cell apoptosis in T cell-mediated autoimmune diabetes. Proc. Natl. Acad. Sci. USA **94:** 213–218.
32. SANTAMARIA, P. *et al.* 1995. Beta-cell-cytotoxic CD8+ T cells from nonobese diabetic mice use highly homologous T cell receptor α-chain CDR3 sequences J. Immunol. **154:** 2494–2503.
33. WEGMANN, D.R., M. NORBURY-GLASER & D. DANIEL. 1994. Insulin-specific T cells are a predominant component of islet infiltrates in pre-diabetic NOD mice. Eur. J. Immunol. **24:** 1853–1857 .
34. WEBER, C. *et al.* 1997. CTLA4-Ig prolongs survival of microencapsulated neonatal porcine islet xenografts in diabetic NOD mice. Cell Transplant. **6:** 505–508.
35. KORBUTT, G. *et al.* 1998. Coencapsulation of allogeneic islets with allogeneic Sertoli cells prolongs graft survival without systemic immunosuppression. Transplant. Proc. **30:** 419.

# Factors in Xenograft Rejection

SIMON C. ROBSON,[a] JAN SCHULTE AM ESCH II, AND FRITZ H. BACH

*Beth Israel Deaconess Medical Center, Harvard Medical School, Boston, Massachusetts 02215, USA*

**ABSTRACT: Important mechanisms underlying immediate xenograft loss by hyperacute rejection (HAR), in the pig-to-primate combination, have been recently delineated. There are now several proposed therapies that deal with the problem of complement activation and xenoreactive natural antibody (XNA) binding to the vasculature that have been shown to prevent HAR. However, vascularized xenografts are still lost, typically within days, by delayed xenograft rejection (DXR), alternatively known as acute vascular rejection (AVR). This process is characterized by endothelial cell (EC) perturbation, localization of XNA within the graft vasculature, host NK cell and monocyte activation with platelet sequestration and vascular thrombosis. Alternative immunosuppressive strategies, additive anti-complement therapies with the control of any resulting EC activation processes and induction of protective responses have been proposed to ameliorate this pathological process.**

**In addition, several potentially important molecular incompatibilities between activated human coagulation factors and the natural anticoagulants expressed on porcine EC have been noted. Such incompatibilities may be analogous to cross-species alterations in the function of complement regulatory proteins important in HAR. Disordered thromboregulation is potentially relevant to the progression of inflammatory events in DXR and the disseminated intravascular coagulation seen in primate recipients of porcine renal xenografts. We have recently demonstrated the inability of porcine tissue factor pathway inhibitor (TFPI) to adequately neutralize human factor Xa (FXa), the aberrant activation of both human prothrombin and FXa by porcine EC and the failure of the porcine natural anticoagulant, thrombomodulin to bind human thrombin and hence activate human protein C. The enhanced potential of porcine von Willebrand factor to associate with human platelet GPIb has been demonstrated to be dependent upon the isolated A1 domain of von Willebrand factor. In addition, the loss of TFPI and vascular ATPDase/CD39 activity following EC activation responses would potentiate any procoagulant changes within the xenograft. These developments could exacerbate vascular damage from whatever cause and enhance the activation of platelets and coagulation pathways within xenografts resulting in graft infarction and loss.**

**Analysis of these and the other putative factors underlying DXR should lead to the development and testing of genetic approaches that, in conjunction with selected pharmacological means, may further prolong xenograft survival to a clinically relevant extent.**

[a]Corresponding author: Beth Israel Deaconess Medical Center and Harvard Medical School, Research North Building, Room 370, 99 Brookline Avenue, Boston, MA 02215; 617-632-0831 (voice); 617-632-0880 (fax); Srobson@bidmc.harvard.edu (e-mail).

## INTRODUCTION

The proposed use of a unlimited supply of animal organs in clinical practice, viz. xenotransplantation, could provide a bridge to a successful allograft in a critically ill patient, or more optimistically, may even substitute for an allograft and provide long-term survival.[1–3] Unfortunately, the clinical application of xenotransplantation, to date, has resulted in global failure. Still, recent developments in the field of xenotransplantation biology have greatly expanded our understanding of the mechanisms by which xenografts are rejected and have given new hopes that this treatment may become a clinical reality.[1,3–6] Recently however, these advances have been coupled with sobering public health questions regarding the importance of potential zoonoses in xenograft recipients[7,8] that fall outside the scope of this article but have been addressed elsewhere.[9,10]

Xenoreactive natural antibodies (XNA) directed at α-galactosyl residues of xenogeneic glycoproteins[11] and associated complement (C) activation by the classical pathway,[12] appear to be the major immediate mediators of hyperacute rejection (HAR) and graft endothelial cell injury in the discordant swine-to-primate combination.[13–15] Discordant porcine organs can function for several days in primates following the inhibition of C and/or removal of XNA.[3,16–19] However, a xenograft rejection process still ensues.[20] Novel molecular biological techniques have allowed the production of donor animals (pigs/mice) with human transgenes directed toward amelioration of the C activation[21] and more recently XNA interaction.[22,23] Xenograft rejection events appear to be universally associated with the deposition of xenoreactive antibodies, local generation of procoagulants, vascular thrombosis and ultimate graft loss in a process termed delayed xenograft rejection (DXR)[20,24] or acute vascular rejection.[25,26] Recently described studies by White and colleagues have been rather more optimistic with respect to graft survival outcomes.[17,27–30] However, in general terms, AVR/DXR with development of vascular thrombosis must be considered major barriers to xenograft acceptance at this time.[20,25,26]

AVR/DXR is composed of many separate elements that result in various manifestations of xenograft rejection.[3,4,20] Vascular EC activation processes with the accompanying prothrombotic and inflammatory changes are important manifestations of experimental xenograft rejection.[20,31] This response may be associated with NK-cell and monocyte (Mo) mediated endothelial cell (EC) activation[32,33] and xenoreactive antibody interactions.[26] The role of the T cell in mediating AVR/DXR is controversial.[34–36]

## MECHANISMS OF DISCORDANT XENOGRAFT REJECTION

### *Hyperacute Rejection*

Following transplantation of a vascularized discordant xenograft (pig-to-primate), pre-formed XNA are bound to EC, resulting in C activation, vascular damage, intravascular thrombosis and finally ischemic necrosis. Depending on the species combination, hyperacute rejection (HAR) is either initiated by the rapid deposition of XNA from recipients within the graft and the subsequent activation of the classical pathway of C activation (e.g., pig-to-primate),[37] or is mediated by direct activation of host C through the graft endothelium (e.g., guinea pig-to-rat combination).[38] In addition to the activation of C, neutrophil adherence, and vasoconstriction all may contribute to the pathogenesis of HAR in various models of xenograft rejection.[24,39,40] One of the major complications that accompanies HAR relates to thrombosis of the graft microvasculature with platelet sequestration.[24] This development may be associated with ongoing inflammatory responses linked to C activation[41–44] or to other inflammatory mediators in certain vascular beds, such as that of the lung.[45]

The activation of C on xenogeneic surfaces is largely unregulated by vascular complement regulatory proteins because of certain functional incompatibilities between the pig and certain primate species, including man.[46,47] Effective regulation of C activation in xenografts may be obtained using human regulatory proteins viz. CD55 (Decay Accelerating Factor or DAF), CD59 and CD46 or pharmaceutical approaches with anti-complement strategies.[28,48,49] These approaches may all successfully abrogate HAR.[50,51]

In addition, techniques to down-regulate the expression of the major porcine xenoantigen for binding XNA, α-(1,3) gal, have been developed in transgenic pigs that express H-transferase or other glycosyltransferases.[22,23,52,53] The EC from these animals may effectively downregulate C activation though inhibition of XNA binding, but the ability to inhibit direct natural killer or NK cell interactions remains unclear.[54]

### *Acute Vascular Rejection or Delayed Xenograft Rejection*

When primate recipients are pre-treated to avert HAR by either effective blockade of C activation and/or by removing or inhibiting XNA, then porcine xenografts survive for several days. Such organs are still rejected by a process designated as acute vascular rejection or delayed xenograft rejection (AVR/DXR) that has been observed in several models of discordant xenotransplantation,[39] such as clinically relevant pig-to-baboon heart and kidney xenotransplantation.[3,16,20] Morphologically, AVR/DXR is characterized by a progressive infiltration with mononuclear cells (MNC), occurring over 2–4 days post-transplant and a process of intravascular thrombosis. These events are paralleled by a progressive activation of EC, including the upregulation of inflammatory cytokines and evolution of a procoagulant environment.[24]

The activation of EC is associated with induction of adhesion molecules, as well as stimulation of a procoagulant state through upregulation of tissue factor on Mo and graft EC, and downregulation of anticoagulant molecules, including thrombomodulin, tissue factor pathway inhibitor and antithrombin.[55–58] Downregulation of thrombomodulin expression, resulting in a markedly reduced capacity of EC to bind thrombin and activate protein C, may further enhance Mo cytokine production. Activated protein C appears to have a key role in inhibition of Mo activation.[59] Fibrin generation, local hypoxia, the deleterious effects of TNF, IL-1α plus other cytokines generated in response to activated C components and activated coagulation factors may cause substantial graft injury. The effects of MNC binding to EC, mediated through XNA binding, may synergize to result in the profound vascular injury observed with AVR/DXR.[24,58]

Mo and NK cells that are found at the site of rejection in recipients treated with the C activator and depleting agent, cobra venom factor, might recognize and bind to xenogeneic EC directly and cause cellular activation. Potential receptors have been described for both of these major cell types: Mo express carbohydrate binding factors or lectins and NK cells have receptors with specific lectin-binding domains.[32,33] NK cells have been shown to have the potential to cause damage to endothelium.[32,35,60–63] T cells do not appear to alter the principal features leading to DXR in small animal models; in addition, kinetics of host Mo and NK cell infiltration are not significantly influenced either by the absence or presence of T cells.[64]

Currently, it is uncertain what further features would emerge if AVR/DXR could be abrogated or suitably controlled. It has been suggested that the equivalent of the T-cell–mediated rejection of an allograft would occur in a discordant graft. Evidence from concordant xenografting of organs in man implies that processes of xenoreactive cellular responses would be more aggressive than that of the comparable alloreactive combinations.[34,37,65–67] Thus, to develop an optimal therapeutic regimen that will permit long-term function of a xenograft may require not only inhibition of XNA and C but also specific interference of processes related to EC perturbation in addition to Mo, NK, and lymphocyte infiltration and activation.

## ENDOTHELIAL CELL ACTIVATION

EC activation may be a critical factor in orchestrating the immune response while balancing hemostasis.[68] This process may be responsible for key elements underlying the rejection of discordant xenografts. Relationships of EC activation to regulation of platelet aggregation may further exacerbate the development of vascular thrombosis. Quiescent vascular EC inhibit platelet aggregation, at least in part because they express an ecto-enzyme that hydrolyzes ADP, a powerful extracellular agonist for platelet aggregation, and ATP, a potential EC agonist.[69] The presumed function of vascular ATP-diphosphohydrolase (ATPDase/CD39) is to prevent the accumulation of certain purinergic mediators and therefore modulate platelet aggregation and other inflammatory phenomena. Activated EC lose ATPDase activity as a consequence of oxidative stress as seen with xenograft rejection and thus become permissive for platelet aggregation.[70]

EC activation could be triggered by the binding of low levels of XNA or of elicited xenoreactive antibodies.[71–73] Elicited xenoreactive antibodies may interact with β1 and β3 integrins on EC and mediate tyrosine kinase phosphorylation. This event may represent an early event in a novel signaling pathway of EC activation that includes activation of MAPK and nuclear translocation with transactivation of the transcription factor NF-κB that is relevant for the transformation to a procoagulant EC phenotype.[73] Alternatively, minimal complement activation to assembly of the terminal complexes and expression of IL-1α may lead to EC perturbation and upregulation of procoagulants such as tissue factor[41,42] with thrombin generation.[74] Human NK cells and Mo both of which are present in an apparently activated state in rejecting xenografts, each have the potential through TNFα to activate porcine EC in co-cultures *in vitro.*[32,33,63,75]

The transcription factor NF-κB appears to play a pivotal role in EC activation and many of the genes associated with EC activation have one or more NF-κB binding sites within their promoters.[76] Thrombin, which is present in many situations, activates EC in a NF-κB–dependent manner; thrombin and TNF act synergistically in this regard.[74] Reactive oxygen species are generated in many situations and would activate NF-κB thereby leading to type II EC activation.[77] The NF-κB pathway also contributes to the induction of anti-apoptotic genes following exposure to TNF. Treatment of EC overexpressing IκBa results in apoptosis severely limiting this strategy to inhibit xenograft rejection.[31] A novel approach pursued by Anrather *et al.* is based on a mutated form of NF-κB[78] and is not complicated by apoptosis. Strategies for directly modulating EC activation and inducing protective type responses have been reviewed recently and will not be addressed in any further detail here.[31]

## INVOLVEMENT OF LEUKOCYTES IN DISCORDANT XENOGRAFT REJECTION

### *Polymorphonuclear Leukocytes*

Polymorphonuclear leukocytes (PML) appear to represent the major leukocyte type in HAR.[79–81] PML may infiltrate xenografts more rapidly than NK cells and T-cells because they adhere to P-selectin,[82–85] unlike NK cells, which utilize ICAM-1, VCAM-1 and possibly E-selectin.[61,86,87] Human neutrophils have been shown to directly recognize xenogeneic endothelium.[81] The implication that neutrophils participate in xenograft rejection is further strengthened by immunohistological studies that show significant infiltrates of leukocytes consisting predominantly of neutrophils, macrophages, and T cells, with occasional B cells and NK cells in the setting of porcine hyperacute rejection.[79,88]

### *Monocytes*

Mo are considered to be important effector cells during early xenograft rejection.[33,58,89] These cells may exacerbate the procoagulant potential of the graft vasculature by the heightened expression of tissue factor, thus promoting thrombotic occlusion of the vessels.[90,91] In addition, Mo may activate xenogeneic EC by direct cellular contact potentially by membrane bound TNF; xenogeneic Mo-EC contacts result in upregulation of E-selectin, IL-8 and monocyte chemotactic protein-1 while increasing plasminogen activator inhibitor type-1 expression within the co-cultures.[33] These cytokines and chemokines would result in further transendothelial migration of Mo and/or their activation causing inflammation, thrombosis and organ infarction.[24]

### *Natural Killer Cells*

Human anti-pig cellular responses may lead to xenograft rejection and natural killer (NK) cells appear to contribute to the human anti-porcine xenogeneic cytotoxicity.[79,87] Allogeneic as well as autologous normal cells are not susceptible to NK cell-mediated cytotoxicity because they express certain MHC class I molecules that give a negative signal to NK cells through specific inhibitory receptors.[92] It has been suggested that xenogeneic target cells may be susceptible to NK cell-mediated lysis because their MHC class I molecules are not recognized by these receptors. *Ex vivo* cardiac perfusion experiments suggest that the combination of NK cells and XNA are the major cause of organ injury.[61,79] These and other findings in xenogeneic islet transplantation, implicate NK cells in cell-mediated xenograft rejection.[64] However, no definitive proof currently exists that NK cells are obligatory for the evolution of this process in vascularized discordant xenografts.

### *T and B Lymphocytes*

Most of the available data suggest that the direct cytotoxic response of human lymphocytes to porcine cells appears to be largely heterogeneous.[34,37,65–67,93–95] Lysis of xenogeneic targets can be significantly inhibited by anti-CD3 or anti-CD8 antibody and partially inhibited by anti-CD2 antibody; anti-CD2 or anti-CD4 antibodies had little effect in allogeneic control experiments. Human anti-pig cell-mediated cytotoxic response appear comparable to allogeneic reactions, and has been shown to be restricted by swine leukocyte antigens (SLA) class I and class II.[34,67,93,94.] B cells have been detected in rejecting porcine xenografts.[88] However, little is known of the nature of elicited B-cell responses to xenoantigen viz. α-Gal. T-cell–independent B cells may be central in this event but this remains controversial.

## PUTATIVE MOLECULAR INCOMPATIBILITY OF CYTOKINES

There are several cytokines that are documented not to function across wide species' barriers. Whereas TNF and IL-1α have been shown to be fully functional across species, others may not have this lack of specificity. Two other human cytokines that are of potential importance in xenografting of porcine organs and are produced by the infiltrating mononuclear cells in AVR/DXR are IFNγ and IL-1β. These two human cytokines do not stimulate porcine EC.[32,89] However, while such incompatibilities may have benefits in xenotransplantation, they could still contribute to activation of the host immune system.

## DERANGEMENTS IN HEMOSTASIS AND DYSREGULATION OF BLOOD COAGULATION IN XENOTRANSPLANTATION

There are several precedents for the development of coagulation abnormalities and thrombocytopenia in association with solid organ xenograft rejection performed under certain experimental situations.[96,97] In many of the more recent reports detailing pig-to-primate xenotransplantation, graft survival has been determined in days and coagulation parameters have not been examined in detail.[18,98–100] Recently, we have determined that activation of coagulation factors by the xenograft vasculature, modulated in this instance by low levels of C activation via the classical pathway, has the potential to generate serious systemic hemostatic abnormalities with localized xenograft vascular injury progressing to a form of disseminated intravascular coagulation (DIC) (Transplantation, in press). Platelet sequestration within the xenograft may be pathogenetically linked to the expression of porcine vWF that interacts with human platelet receptors with high affinity and causes activation responses.[101–103]

There are additional and more recent clinical data for the association between disorders in hemostasis and exposure to xenogeneic vasculature. Hemoperfusion of porcine renal explants by human volunteers has resulted in significant thrombocytopenia with rapid onset of vascular injury;[104] similar events have been described with *ex vivo* porcine liver hemoperfusions.[105] The development of DIC and the observation of the Shwartzman phenomenon in antibody-mediated rejection of homografts[106,107] support the hypothesis that antibody-mediated vascular injury may be implicated in the perturbation of coagulation seen with xenograft injury[26] (Transplantation, in press). Saadi *et al.* have established that humoral injury to the vasculature, with the development of a procoagulant phenotype, is related to C activation; after the assembly of membrane attack complex, the production of tissue factor and initiation of coagulation in a blood vessel depend on the production of IL-1 and on its availability to stimulate vascular EC.[41] However, our recent observations with specific α-galactosyl epitope-mediated stimulation of suggest that xenoreactive antibodies may directly induce activation responses in the total absence of complement.[71–73]

### *Putative Molecular Incompatibility of Natural Anticoagulants*

Quiescent EC express effective anticoagulant and platelet antiaggregatory mechanisms that maintain circulatory homeostasis and vascular integrity under physiological conditions.[108] In addition to their modulation during cell activation,[70,109] it is possible that these factors may not be completely effective across species barriers because of molecular incompatibilities between activated coagulation components and their inhibitors.[110,111] This scenario could be considered analogous to the highly specific porcine endothelial complement inhibitors that are inoperative against activated human complement components.[12,112] Several of these antiproteases and natural anticoagulants are also expressed by Mo. [91,113]

Certain relevant porcine natural anticoagulants have been characterized. Data derived from the use of factor VII- or factor XII-deficient human plasmas or neutralizing anti-factor VII/VIIa antibodies in the context of porcine TF derived from EC preparations has demonstrated that the TF interaction with factor VII(a) is predominant in generating the procoagulant process *in vitro.*[24] The expression and very prominent presence of tissue factor and fibrin in histological sections of hearts rejected at 3–5 days is in keeping with the observations that the TF-mediated pathway of coagulation is implicated in the thrombosis observed in xenorejection processes.[58] We have recently shown that porcine tissue factor pathway inhibitor (TFPI) does not neutralize human factor Xa (FXa)[58,91] and there is aberrant activation of both human prothrombin and factor X by porcine EC *in vitro*[114] and *ex vivo.*[43] In addition, the porcine natural anticoagulant, thrombomodulin does not adequately bind human thrombin and hence fails to activate human protein C.[114,115] These incompatibilities contribute to substantial generation of human thrombin from prothrombin by porcine EC[114,116] that is also observed following *ex vivo* perfusion of pig hearts by human blood.[43]

Abnormal levels of thrombin generation could arise because of the inhibitory effects of the protein C system on TF-induced thrombin generation;[117,118] specifically the synergistic effects of thrombomodulin and TFPI.[119] Thrombin both initiates clotting and is an important mediator of EC activation[74] or xenogeneic platelet aggregation.[44] Further evidence for the importance of coagulation mediators in vascular inflammation can be inferred by the beneficial effects of their inhibition that have been noted in models of discordant xenograft rejection to be comparable to complement inhibition.[120,121]

In addition, the loss of TFPI[58] and vascular ATPDase/CD39 activity following EC activation responses *in vivo*[70,122] would potentiate any procoagulant changes within the graft.[20] Such developments could exacerbate vascular damage from whatever cause and potentiate the activation of platelets and coagulation pathways within xenografts resulting in graft infarction.[31]

### *Platelet Activation and Thromboregulation*

The relationship between xenograft rejection and platelet reactivity is highly complex.[123] Initiation of platelet activation and aggregation, may lead to recruitment of the several systems that appear to be involved in the rejection process. For instance, platelet binding to the activated complement component C1q could result in the activation of the platelet fibrinogen receptor (GPIIbIIIa) with consequent expression of P-selectin, and development of procoagulant activity on the platelets.[124] Additionally, expression of the platelet adhesion molecule P-selectin might promote platelet-leukocyte interactions resulting in expression of coagulation stimulated by monocyte TF.[125]

Endothelial-platelet interactions and development of platelet aggregates appear to be prominent factors in xenograft rejection.[44,123] The enhanced potential of porcine von Willebrand factor (vWF) to associate with human platelet GPIb through the porcine vWF A1 domain suggests that this will represent an important barrier to xenograft acceptance as this receptor triggers platelet activation *ab initio*.[126] Hence, exposure and expression of vWF in the xenogeneic sub-endothelium following EC retraction or injury could result in massive activation of circulating platelets with formation of aggregates even prior to activation of coagulation,[20] in a manner similar to that seen in TTP.

In addition, vascular damage, activation of platelets and coagulation with thrombosis within the xenograft vasculature could be exacerbated by the associated loss of vascular ATPDase/CD39, a putative thromboregulatory factor.[69,70] Inhibition of platelet aggregation by treatment of xenograft recipients with antagonists to the platelet fibrinogen receptor, GPIIbIIIa,[80,127] by the use of P-selectin or PAF antagonists,[84,128,129] or by administration of a soluble ATPDase[130] has been generally shown to prolong graft survival in several discordant xenotransplantation models.

### *Fibrinolytic Abnormalities*

Early reports have suggested abnormalities in the regulation of human plasminogen activators by porcine plasminogen activator inhibitor type I (PAI-1; associated with vascular EC);[131] these may compromise fibrinolytic pathways and further promote vascular occlusion in xenografts. However, recent expression and cloning of

PAI-1 has demonstrated that there are no obvious functional differences between the recombinant human and porcine PAI-1 (Declerck 1997).

## THERAPEUTIC OPTIONS AND ENDEAVORS

As discussed above, xenografts are rejected even where the evidence suggests that C is blocked; we would expect alternative patterns of rejection if both C and XNA actions are both abrogated. The precise definition of mechanisms that contribute to processes of xenograft rejection, including EC and platelet activation, thrombosis, and MNC mediated inflammation is essential for the development of therapeutic strategies to overcome such problems or to prevent these complications.

Immunosuppressive agents are associated with significant morbidity and mortality by increasing the risk of infection and the development of cancers. Despite life-threatening doses of cyclophosphamide in combination with cyclosporine, rejection of transgenic porcine organs in primates has not been halted. The possibility exists that other therapeutic agents such as FK506 and deoxyspergualin may be of more utility in xenograft rejection and that mixed xenogeneic chimerism with induction of tolerance may become a reality.[6] Application of such further therapeutic strategies, potentially including an approach to abrogating EC activation by involving both genetic manipulation and conventional therapeutic agents directed at specific targets in the overall rejection apparatus, should contribute to achieving long-term survival of a xenograft. It must remain a theoretical concern that accelerated chronic rejection may manifest in xenografted organs.

## CONCLUSIONS

There are several proposed therapies for dealing with the problem of C activation, XNA and elicited xenoreactive antibodies in addition to the genetic engineering approach. Adequate immunosuppression, other interventions such as plasmapheresis, anti-complement therapies and the control of any resulting EC activation process following binding of xenoreactive antibodies will be of crucial import.

The concept of AVR/DXR, involving a greater understanding of the mechanisms of inflammation and thrombosis, and appreciation of molecular incompatibilities, has led to novel ideas that may translate into approaches to therapy. As these forms of xenograft rejection are overcome, it is assumed that effective therapy for subsequent, graft-specific cellular responses will be necessary. However, whether all of this will lead to clinical trials of xenografting of immediately vascularized discordant organs must await the appropriate experimentation.

## REFERENCES

1. Taniguchi, S. & D. Cooper. 1997. Clinical xenotransplantation—past, present and future [Review]. Ann. Royal Coll. Surg. **79:** 13–19.
2. Platt, J.L. & F.H. Bach. 1991. Discordant xenografting: challenges and controversies. [Review]. Clin. Opin. Immunol. **3:** 735–739.

3. PLATT, J. L. 1996. Xenotransplantation—recent progress and current perspectives [Review]. Clin. Opin. Immunol. **8:** 721-728.
4. PARKER, W., S. SAADI, S.S. LIN, Z.E. HOLZKNECHT, M. BUSTOS & J.L. PLATT. 1996. Transplantation of discordant xenografts—a challenge revisited [Review]. Immunol. Today **17:** 373–378.
5. DORLING, A. & R.I. LECHLER. 1994. Prospects for xenografting [Review]. Clin. Opin. Immunol. **6**: 765–769.
6. AUCHINCLOSS, H. & D.H. SACHS. 1998. Xenogeneic Transplantation [Review]. Ann. Rev. Immunol. **16:** 433–470.
7. AKIYOSHI, D.E., M. DENARO, H.H. ZHU, J. L. GREENSTEIN, P. BANERJEE & J.A. FISHMAN. 1998. Identification of a full-length cDNA for an endogenous retrovirus of miniature swine. J. Virol. **72:** 4503–4507.
8. PATIENCE, C., Y. TAKEUCHI & R.A. WEISS. 1997. Infection of human cells by an endogenous retrovirus of pigs. Nature Med. **3:** 282–286.
9. BACH, F.H., J.A. FISHMAN, N. DANIELS, J. PROIMOS, B. ANDERSON, C. B. CARPENTER, L. FORROW, S.C. ROBSON & H.V. FINEBERG. 1998. Uncertainty in xenotransplantation: individual benefit versus collective risk. Nature Med. **4:** 141–144.
10. SACHS, D.H., R.B. COLVIN, A.B. COSIMI, P.S. RUSSELL, M. SYKES, C.G.A. MCGREGOR & J.L. PLATT. 1998. Xenotransplantation—caution, but no moratorium. Nature Med. **4:** 372.
11. GALILI, U. 1993. Interaction of the natural anti-gal antibody with alpha-galactosyl epitopes—A major obstacle for xenotransplantation in humans. Immunol. Today **14:** 480–482.
12. DALMASSO, A.P., G.M. VERCELLOTTI, R.J. FISCHEL, R.M. BOLMAN, F.H. BACH & J.L. PLATT. 1992. Mechanism of complement activation in the hyperacute rejection of porcine organs transplanted into primate recipients. Am. J. Pathol. **140:** 1157–1166.
13. COOPER, D., Y. YE, M. NIEKRASZ, *et al.* 1993. Specific intravenous carbohydrate therapy — a new concept in inhibiting antibody-mediated rejection experience with abo-incompatible cardiac allografting in the baboon. Transplantation **56:** 769–777.
14. COOPER, D.K.C., E. KOREN & R. ORIOL. 1994. Alpha-galactosyl oligosaccharides and discordant xenografting. Xenotransplantation **2:** 13–18.
15. PLATT, J.L., G.M. VERCELLOTTI, A.P. DALMASSO, A.J. MATAS, R.M. BOLMAN, J.S. NAJARIAN & F.H. BACH. 1990. Transplantation of discordant xenografts: a review of progress [Review]. Immunol. Today. **11:** 450–456.
16. MCCURRY, K.R., L.E. DIAMOND, D.L. KOOYMAN, G.W. BYRNE, M.J. MARTIN, J.S. LOGAN & J.L. PLATT. 1996. Human complement regulatory proteins expressed in transgenic swine protect swine xenografts from humoral injury. Transplant. Proc. **28:** 2.
17. WHITE, D.J.G. 1996. hDAF transgenic pig organs: are they concordant for human transplantation. Xenotransplantation **4:** 50–54.
18. DAVIS, E.A., S.K. PRUITT, P.S. GREENE, S. IBRAHIM, T.T. LAM, J.L. LEVIN, W.M. BALDWIN & F. SANFILIPO. 1996. Inhibition of complement, evoked antibody, and cellular response prevents rejection of pig-to-primate cardiac xenografts. Transplantation **62:** 1018–1023.
19. PRUITT, S.K., R.R. BOLLINGER, B.H. COLLINS, H.C. MARSH, J.L. LEVIN, A.R. RUDOLPH, W.M. BALDWIN & F. SANFILIPPO. 1996. Continuous complement (C) inhibition using soluble C receptor type 1 (SCR1)—effect on hyperacute rejection (HAR) of pig-to-primate cardiac xenografts. Transplant. Proc. **28:** 321.
20. BACH, F.H., H. WINKLER, C. FERRAN, W.W. HANCOCK & S.C. ROBSON. 1996. Delayed Xenograft Rejection [Review]. Immunol. Today **17:** 379–384.
21. ROSENGARD, A.M., N.R. CARY, G.A. LANGFORD, A.W. TUCKER, J. WALLWORK & D.J. WHITE. 1995. Tissue expression of human complement inhibitor, decay-accelerating factor, in transgenic pigs. A potential approach for preventing xenograft rejection. Transplantation **59:** 1325–1333.

22. SANDRIN, M.S., W.L. FODOR & E. MOUHTOURIS, *et al.* 1995. Enzymatic remodelling of the carbohydrate surface of a xenogenic cell substantially reduces human antibody binding and complement-mediated cytolysis. Nature Med. **1:** 1261–1267.
23. SANDRIN, M.S., W.L. FODOR, S. COHNEY, E. MOUHTOURIS, N. OSMAN, S.A. ROLLINS, S. P. SQUINTO & I. MCKENZIE. 1996. Reduction of the major porcine xenoantigen gal-alpha(1,3)gal by expression of alpha(1,2)fucosyltransferase. Xenotransplantation **3:** 134–140.
24. BACH, F.H., S.C. ROBSON, C. FERRAN, *et al.* 1994. Endothelial cell activation and thromboregulation during xenograft rejection [Review]. Immunol. Rev. **141:** 5–30.
25. PLATT, J.L. 1998. New directions for organ transplantation [Review]. Nature **392:** 11–17.
26. LIN, S.S., B.C. WEIDNER, G.W. BYRNE, *et al.* 1998. The role of antibodies in acute vascular rejection of pig-to-baboon cardiac transplants. J. Clin. Invest. **101:** 1745–1756.
27. SCHMOECKEL, M., G. NOLLERT, M. SHAHMOHAMMADI, J. MULLERHOCKER, V.K. YOUNG, W. KASPERKONIG, D.J.G. WHITE, C. HAMMER & B. REICHART. 1997. Transgenic human decay accelerating factor makes normal pigs function as a concordant species. J. Heart Lung Transplant. **16:** 758–764.
28. TUCKER, A.W., C.A. CARRINGTON, A.C. RICHARDS, S.C. ROBSON & D.F.G. WHITE. 1997. Endothelial cells from human decay acceleration factor transgenic pigs are protected against complement mediated tissue factor expression in vitro. Transplant. Proc. **29:** 888.
29. WHITE, D.J.G., M. SCHMOECKEL, E. COZZI, G. CHAVEZ & G. LANGFORD. 1997. Genetic engineering of pigs for xenogeneic heart transplantation [French]. Biodrugs **8:** 33–36.
30. COZZI, E., A.W. TUCKER, G.A. LANGFORD, *et al.* 1997. Characterization of pigs transgenic for human decay-accelerating factor. Transplantation **64:** 1383–1392.
31. BACH, F.H., C. FERRAN, M. SOARES, C.J. WRIGHTON, J. ANRATHER, H. WINKLER, S. C. ROBSON & W.W. HANCOCK. 1997. Modification of vascular responses in xenotransplantation - inflammation and apoptosis. Nature Med. **3:** 944–948.
32. GOODMAN, D.J., M. VON ALBERTINI, A. WILLSON, M.T. MILLAN & F.H. BACH. 1996. Direct activation of porcine endothelial cells by human natural killer cells. Transplantation **61:** 763–771.
33. MILLAN, M.T., C. GECZY, K.M. STUHLMEIER, D.J. GOODMAN, C. FERRAN & F.H. BACH. 1997. Human monocytes activate porcine endothelial cells, resulting in increased E-selectin, interleukin-8, monocyte chemotactic protein-1, and plasminogen activator inhibitor-type-1 expression. Transplantation **63:** 421–429.
34. YAMADA, K., J.D. SEEBACH, H. DERSIMONIAN & D.H. SACHS. 1996. Human anti-pig t-cell mediated cytotoxicity. Xenotransplantation **3:** 179–187.
35. SEEBACH, J.D., K. YAMADA, I.M. MCMORROW, D.H. SACHS & H. DERSIMONIAN. 1996. Xenogeneic human anti-pig cytotoxicity mediated by activated natural killer cells. Xenotransplantation **3:** 188–197.
36. CANDINAS, D., N. KOYAMADA, T. MIYATAKE, B.A. LESNIKOSKI, S.T. GREY, S.C. ROBSON, F.H. BACH & W.W. HANCOCK. 1995. Delayed xenograft rejection in complement depleted T cell deficient (nude) rat recipients of guinea pig xenografts. Abstract: Proceedings of 3rd International Xenotransplantation Congress, 1995.
37. AUCHINCLOSS, H. 1990. Xenografting: a review. Transplantation **48:** 14–20.
38. BALDWIN, W.M.I., S.K. PRUITT, R.B. BRAUER, M.R. DAHA & F. SANFILIPPO. 1995. Complement in organ transplantation. Transplantation **59:** 797–808.
39. HANCOCK, W.W., M.L. BLAKELY, W. VAN DER WERF & F.H. BACH. 1993. Rejection of guinea pig cardiac xenografts post-cobra venom factor therapy is associated with infiltration by mononuclear cells secreting interferon-gamma and diffuse endothelial activation. Transplant. Proc. **25:** 2932.
40. BACH, F.H., S.C. ROBSON, H. WINKLER, C. FERRAN, K.M. STUHLMEIER, C.J. WRIGHTON & W.W. HANCOCK. 1995. Barriers to xenotransplantation. Nature Med. **1:** 869–873.

41. SAADI, S., R.A. HOLZKNECHT, C.P. PATTE, D.M. STERN & J.L. PLATT. 1995. Complement-mediated regulation of tissue factor activity in endothelium. J. Exp. Med. **182:** 1807–1814.
42. SAADI, S. & J.L. PLATT. 1995. Transient perturbation of endothelial integrity induced by natural antibodies and complement. J. Exp. Med. **181:** 21–31.
43. ROBSON, S.C., V.K. YOUNG, N.S. COOK, *et al.* 1996. Thrombin inhibition in an ex vivo model of hyperacute xenograft rejection. Transplantation **61:** 862–868.
44. ROBSON, S.C., J.B. SIEGEL, B.A. LESNIKOSKI, C. KOPP, D. CANDINAS, U. RYAN & F.H. BACH. 1996. Aggregation of human platelets induced by porcine endothelial cells is dependent upon both activation of complement and thrombin generation. Xenotransplantation **3:** 24–34.
45. NORIN, A.J., R.J. BREWER, N. LAWSON, G.A. GRIJALVA, M. VAYNBLATT, W. BURTON, S.P. SQUINTO, S.L. KAMHOLZ & W.L. FODOR. 1996. Enhanced survival of porcine endothelial cells and lung xenografts expressing human cd59. Transplant. Proc. **28:** 797–798.
46. DALMASSO, A.P., G.M. VERCELLOTTI, J.L. PLATT & F.H. BACH. 1991. Inhibition of complement-mediated endothelial cell cytotoxicity by decay-accelerating factor. Potential for prevention of xenograft hyperacute rejection. Transplantation **52:** 530–533.
47. DALMASSO, A.P., J.L. PLATT & F.H. BACH. 1991. Reaction of complement with endothelial cells in a model of xenotransplantation. Clin. Exp. Immunol. **1:** 31–35.
48. WHITE, D. 1992. Transplantation of organs between species. Int. Arch. Allergy Immunol. **98:** 1–5.
49. WHITE, D., J. WALLWORK. 1993. Xenografting—probability, possibility, or pipe dream? Lancet **342:** 879–880.
50. BALDWIN, W.M., S.K. PRUITT, R.B. BRAUER, M.R. DAHA & F. SANFILIPPO. 1995. Complement in organ transplantation—contributions to inflammation, injury, and rejection [Review]. Transplantation **59:** 797–808.
51. PRUITT, S.K., A.D. KIRK, R.R. BOLLINGER, *et al.* 1994. The effect of soluble complement receptor type 1 on hyperacute rejection of porcine xenografts. Transplantation **57:** 363–370.
52. SANDRIN, M.S., H.A. VAUGHAN, P.L. DABKOWSKI & I. MCKENZIE. 1993. Studies on human naturally occurring antibodies to pig xenografts. Transplant. Proc. **25:** 2917–2918.
53. VAUGHAN, H.A., I. MCKENZIE & M.S. SANDRIN. 1995. Biochemical studies of pig xenoantigens detected by naturally occurring human antibodies and the galactose-alpha(1-3)galactose reactive lectin. Transplantation **59:** 102–109.
54. WATIER, H., J.M. GUILLAUMIN, F. PILLER, M. LACORD, G. THIBAULT, Y. LEBRANCHU, M. MONSIGNY & P. BARDOS. 1996. Removal of terminal alpha-galactosyl residues from xenogeneic porcine endothelial cells—decrease in complement-mediated cytotoxicity but persistence of igg1-mediated antibody-dependent cell-mediated cytotoxicity. Transplantation **62:** 105–113.
55. CONWAY, E.M. & R.D. ROSENBERG. 1988. Tumour necrosis factor suppresses transcription of the thrombomodulin gene in endothelial cells. Molec. Cell. Biol. **8:** 5588–5592.
56. ESMON, C.T. 1993. Cell mediated events that control blood coagulation and vascular injury [Review]. Ann. Rev. Cell Biol. **9:** 1–26.
57. CONWAY, E.M., R. BACH, R.D. ROSENBERG & W.H. KONIGSBERG. 1989. Tumor necrosis factor enhances expression of tissue factor mRNA in endothelial cells. Thromb. Res. **53:** 231–241.
58. KOPP, C.W., J.B. SIEGEL, W.W. HANCOCK, J. ANRATHER, H. WINKLER, C.L. GECZY, E. KACZMAREK, F.H. BACH & S.C. ROBSON. 1997. Effect of porcine endothelial tissue factor pathway inhibitor on human coagulation factors. Transplantation **63:** 749–758.
59. GREY, S., A. TSUCHIDA, C.L. ORTHNER, H.H. SALEM & W.W. HANCOCK. 1994. Selective inhibitory effects of the anticoagulant activated protein C on the responses of human mononuclear phagocytes to LPS, IFN-$\gamma$ or phorbol ester. J. Immunol. **153:** 3664–3672.

60. INVERARDI, L., M. SAMAJA, F. MARELLI, J.R. BENDER & R. PARDI. 1992. Cellular early immune recognition of xenogeneic vascular endothelium. Transplant. Proc. **24:** 459–461.
61. INVERARDI, L., M. SAMAJA, R. MOTTERLINI, F. MANGILI, J.R. BENDER & R. PARDI. 1992. Early recognition of a discordant xenogeneic organ by human circulating lymphocytes. J. Immunol. **149:** 1416–1423.
62. INVERARDI, L., B. CLISSI, A.L. STOLZER, J.R. BENDER, M.S. SANDRIN & R. PARDI. 1997. Human natural killer lymphocytes directly recognize evolutionarily conserved oligosaccharide ligands expressed by xenogeneic tissues. Transplantation **63:** 1318–1330.
63. MALYGUINE, A.M., S. SAADI, J.L. PLATT & J.R. DAWSON. 1996. Human natural killer cells induce morphologic changes in porcine endothelial, cell monolayers. Transplantation **61:** 161–164.
64. LIN, Y., M. VANDEPUTTE & M. WAER. 1997. Natural killer cell- and macrophage-mediated rejection of concordant xenografts in the absence of T and B cell responses. J. Immunol. **158:** 5658–5667.
65. AUCHINCLOSS, H. 1988. Xenogeneic transplantation [Review]. Transplantation **46:** 1–20.
66. MOSES, R.D., H.J. WINN & H.J. AUCHINCLOSS. 1992. Evidence that multiple defects in cell-surface molecule interactions across species differences are responsible for diminished xenogeneic T cell responses. Transplantation **53:** 203–209.
67. BREVIG, T. & T. KRISTENSEN. 1997. Direct cytotoxic response of human lymphocytes to porcine PHA-lymphoblasts and lymphocytes. APMIS **105:** 290–298.
68. VON ALBERTINI, M.A., D.M. STROKA, C. BROSTJAN, K.M. STUHLMEIER, F.H. BACH & S.C. ROBSON. 1997. Adenosine nucleotides induce E-selectin expression in porcine endothelial cells. Transplant. Proc. **29:** 1–2. (BBRC. In press).
69. KACZMAREK, E., K. KOZIAK, J. SEVIGNY, J.B. SIEGEL, J. ANRATHER, A.R. BEAUDOIN, F.H. BACH & S.C. ROBSON. 1996. Identification and characterization of CD39 vascular ATP diphosphohydrolase. J. Biol. Chem. **271:** 33116–33122.
70. ROBSON, S.C., E. KACZMAREK, J.B. SIEGEL, D. CANDINAS, K. KOZIAK, M. MILLAN, W.W. HANCOCK & F.H. BACH. 1997. Loss of ATP diphosphohydrolase activity with endothelial cell activation. J. Exp. Med. **185:** 153–163.
71. PALMETSHOFER, A., U. GALILI, A.P. DALMASSO, S.C. ROBSON & F.H. BACH. 1998. Alpha-galactosyl epitope-mediated activation of porcine aortic endothelial cells—type II activation. Transplantation **65:** 971–978.
72. PALMETSHOFER, A., U. GALILI, A.P. DALMASSO, S.C. ROBSON & F.H. BACH. 1998. Alpha-galactosyl epitope-mediated activation of porcine aortic endothelial cells—type I activation. Transplantation **65:** 844–853.
73. PALMETSHOFER, A., S.C. ROBSON & F.H. BACH. 1998. Tyrosine phosphorylation following lectin mediated endothelial cell stimulation. Xenotransplantation **5:** 61–66.
74. ANRATHER, D., M.T. MILLAN, A. PALMETSHOFER, S.C. ROBSON, C. GECZY, A.J. RITCHIE, F.H. BACH & B.M. EWENSTEIN. 1997. Thrombin activates nuclear factor-kappa-b and potentiates endothelial cell activation by TNF. J. Immunol. **159:** 5620–5628.
75. STROKA, D.M., J.T. COOPER, C. BROSTJAN, M.T. MILLAN, D.J. GOODMAN, C.J. WRIGHTON, F.H. BACH & C. FERRAN. 1997. Expression of a negative dominant mutant of human p55 tumor necrosis factor-receptor inhibits TNF and monocyte-induced activation in porcine aortic endothelial cells. Transplant. Proc. **29:** 12.
76. BAEUERLE, P.A. & D. BALTIMORE. 1988. Activation of DNA-binding activity in an apparently cytoplasmic precursor of the NF-kappaB transcription factor. Cell **53:** 211–217.
77. FERRAN, C., M.T. MILLAN, V. CSIZMADIA, J.T. COOPER, C. BROSTJAN, F.H. BACH & H. WINKLER. 1995. Inhibition of NF-κB by pyrrolidine dithiocarbamate blocks endothelial cell activation. BBRC **214:** 212–223.
78. ANRATHER, J., V. CSIZMADIA, C. BROSTJAN, M.P. SOARES, F.H. BACH & H. WINKLER. 1997. Inhibition of bovine endothelial cell activation in vitro by regulated expression of a transdominant inhibitor of NF-kappa-B. J. Clin. Invest. **99:** 763–772.

79. KIRK, A.D., J.S. HEINLE, J.R. MAULT & F. SANFILIPPO. 1993. Ex-vivo characterization of human anti-porcine hyperacute cardiac rejection. Transplantation **56:** 785–793.
80. ROBSON, S.C., V.K. YOUNG, N.S. COOK, G. KOTTIRSCH, J.B. SIEGEL, B.A. LESNIKOSKI, D. CANDINAS, D. WHITE & F.H. BACH. 1996. Inhibition of platelet GPIIbIIIa in an ex vivo model of hyperacute xenograft rejection does not prolong cardiac survival time. Xenotransplantation **3:** 43–52.
81. ALMOHANNA, F., K. COLLISON, R. PARHAR, *et al.* 1997. Activation of naive xenogeneic but not allogeneic endothelial cells by human naive neutrophils—a potential occult barrier to xenotransplantation. Am. J. Pathol. **151:** 111–120.
82. MULLIGAN, M.S., M.J. POLLEY, R.J. BAYER, M.F. NUNN, J.C. PAULSON & P.A. WARD. 1992. Neutrophil-dependent acute lung injury—requirement for P-selectin (GMP-140). J. Clin. Invest. **90:** 1600–1607.
83. SUGAMA, Y., C. TIRUPPATHI, K. JANAKIDEVI, T.T. ANDERSEN, J.W. FENTON & A.B. MALIK. 1992. Thrombin-induced expression of endothelial P-selectin and intercellular adhesion molecule-1—a mechanism for stabilizing neutrophil adhesion. J. Cell. Biol. **119:** 935–944.
84. COUGHLAN, A.F., M.C. BERNDT, L.C. DUNLOP & W.W. HANCOCK. 1993. In vivo studies of P-selectin and platelet activating factor during endotoxemia, accelerated allograft rejection, and discordant xenograft rejection. Transplant. Proc. **25:** 2930–2931.
85. PATEL, K.D., G.A. ZIMMERMAN, S.M. PRESCOTT, R.P. MCEVER & T.M. MCINTYRE. 1991. Oxygen radicals induce human endothelial cells to express GMP-140 and bind neutrophils. J. Cell. Biol. **112:** 749–759.
86. XING, Z., M. JORDANA, H. KIRPALANI, K.E. DRISCOLL, T.J. SCHALL & J. GAULDIE. 1994. Human NK cells expressing alpha 4 beta 1/beta 7 adhere to VCAM-1 without preactivation. Scand. J. Immunol. **39:** 131–136.
87. SEEBACH, J.D., G.L. WANECK. 1997. Natural killer cells in xenotransplantation [Review]. Xenotransplantation **4:** 201–211.
88. IBRAHIM, S., A.D. KIRK & F. SANFILIPPO. 1996. Phenotype of infiltrating cells in an ex vivo model of human antiporcine hyperacute cardiac xenograft rejection. Transplant. Proc. **28:** 2.
89. BACH, F.H., S.C. ROBSON, C. FERRAN, *et al.* 1995. Xenotransplantation: endothelial cell activation and beyond. [Review]. Transplant. Proc. **27:** 77–79.
90. NEMERSON, Y. 1992. The tissue factor pathway of blood coagulation. Semin. Hematol. **29:** 170–188.
91. KOPP, C.W., S.C. ROBSON, J.B. SIEGEL, J. ANRATHER, H. WINKLER, S. GREY, E. KACZMAREK, F.H. BACH & C.L. GECZY. 1998. Regulation of monocyte tissue factor activity by allogeneic and xenogeneic endothelial cells. Thromb. Haemost. **79:** 529–538.
92. SEEBACH, J.D., C. COMRACK, S. GERMANA, C. LEGUERN, D.H. SACHS & H. DERSIMONIAN. 1997. HLA-Cw3 expression on porcine endothelial cells protects against xenogeneic cytotoxicity mediated by a subset of human NK cells. J. Immunol. **159:** 3655–3661.
93. GONIAS, S.L. 1994. Demonstration of direct xenorecognition of porcine cells by human cytotoxic T lymphocytes. Immunology **81:** 268–272.
94. SPRINGER, T.A. 1994. Indirect presentation of MHC antigens in transplantation. Immunol. Today **15:** 32–38.
95. SULTAN, P., A.G. MURRAY, J.M. MCNIFF, M.I. LORBER, P.W. ASKENASE, A. BOTHWELL & J.S. POBER. 1997. Pig but not human interferon-gamma initiates human cell-mediated rejection of pig tissue in vivo. Proc. Natl. Acad. Sci. USA **94:** 8767–8772.
96. ROSENBERG, J.C., R.J. BROERSMA, G. BULLEMER, E.F. MAMMEN, R. LENAGHAN & B.F. ROSENBERG. 1969. Relationship of platelets, blood coagulation, and fibrinolysis to hyperacute rejection of renal xenografts. Transplantation **8:** 152–161.
97. BROERSMA, R.J., G.D. BULLEMER, J.C. ROSENBERG, R. LENAGHAN, B.F. ROSENBERG & E.F. MAMMEN. 1969. Coagulation changes in hyperacute rejection of renal xenografts. Thromb. Diath. Haem.–Supplementum **36:** 333–340.

98. DAVIS, E.A., F. JAKOBS, S.K. PRUITT, *et al.* 1997. Overcoming rejection in pig-to-primate cardiac xenotransplantation. Transplant. Proc. **29:** 938–939.
99. MCCURRY, K.R., D.L. KOOYMAN, C.G. ALVARADO, A.H. COTTERELL, M.J. MARTIN, J. S. LOGAN & J.L. PLATT. 1995. Human complement regulatory proteins protect swine-to-primate cardiac xenografts from humoral injury. Nature Med. **1:** 423–427.
100. BYRNE, G., K.R. MCCURRY, M.J. MARTIN, S.M. MCCLELLAN, J.L. PLATT & J.S. LOGAN. 1997. Transgenic pigs expressing human CD59 and decay-accelerating factor produce an intrinsic barrier to complement-mediated damage. Transplantation **63:** 149–155.
101. SCHULTE, J., J.B. SIEGEL, F.H. BACH & S.C. ROBSON. 1996. The A1 domain of von Willebrand factor expressed on cell membranes directly activates platelets. Blood **88** (Suppl.): 1290.
102. PARETI, F.I., M. MAZZUCATO, E. BOTTINI & P.M. MANNUCCI. 1992. Interaction of porcine von Willebrand factor with the platelet glycoproteins Ib and IIb/IIIa complex. Brit. J. Haematol. **82:** 81–86.
103. MAZZUCATO, M., L. DEMARCO, P. PRADELLA, A. MASOTTI & F.I. PARETI. 1996. Porcine von willebrand factor binding to human platelet GPIb induces transmembrane calcium influx. Thromb. Haemost. **75:** 655–660.
104. BREIMER, M.E., S. BJORCK, C.T. SVALANDER, A. BENGTSSON, L. RYDBERG, K. LIEKARLSEN, P.O. ATTMAN, M. AURELL & B.E. SAMUELSSON. 1996. Extracorporeal (ex vivo) connection of pig kidneys to humans. 1. Clinical data and studies of platelet destruction. Xenotransplantation **3:** 328–339.
105. COLLINS, B.H., R.S. CHARI, J.C. MAGEE, R.C. HARLAND, B.J. LINDMAN, J.S. LOGAN, R.R. BOLLINGER, W.C. MEYERS & J.L. PLATT. 1995. Immunopathology of porcine livers perfused with blood of humans with fulminant hepatic failure. Transplant. Proc. **27:** 280–281.
106. STARZL, T.E., H.J. BOEHMIG, H. AMEMIYA, C.B. WILSON, F.J. DIXON, G.R. GILES, K.M. SIMPSON & C. G. HALGRIMSON. 1970. Clotting changes, including disseminated intravascular coagulation, during rapid renal-homograft rejection. New Engl. J. Med. **283:** 383–390.
107. STARZL, T.E., R.A. LERNER, F.J. DIXON, C.G. GROTH, L. BRETTSCHNEIDER & P.I. TERASAKI. 1968. Shwartzman reaction after human renal homotransplantation. New Engl. J. Med. **278:** 642–648.
108. ROBSON, S.C., D. CANDINAS, W.W. HANCOCK, C. WRIGHTON, H. WINKLER, F.H. BACH. 1995. Role of endothelial cells in transplantation [Review]. Int. Arch. Allerg. Immunol. **106:** 305–322.
109. PLATT, J.L., G.M. VERCELLOTI, B.J. LINDMAN, T.R. OEGEMA, F.H. BACH, A.P. DALMASSO. 1990. Release of heparan sulfate from endothelial cells. J. Exp. Med. **171:** 1363–1368.
110. ROBSON, S.C. & C. KOPP. 1996. Disordered thromboregulation in discordant xenograft rejection. Life Sci. **6:** 34–38.
111. LAWSON, J.H. & J.L. PLATT. 1996. Molecular barriers to xenotransplantation. Transplantation **62:** 303–310.
112. DALMASSO, A.P. 1992. The complement system in xenotransplantation. Immunopharmacology **24:** 149–160.
113. GREY, S.T. & W.W. HANCOCK. 1996. A physiologic anti-inflammatory pathway based on thrombomodulin expression and generation of activated protein C by human mononuclear phagocytes. J. Immunol. **156:** 2256–2263.
114. SIEGEL, J.B., S.T. GREY, B. A. LESNIKOSKI, C.W. KOPP, M. SOARES, J. ESCH, F.H. BACH & S.C. ROBSON. 1997. Xenogeneic endothelial cells activate human prothrombin. Transplantation. **64:** 888–896.
115. LAWSON, J.H., L.J. DANIELS & J.L. PLATT. 1997. The evaluation of thrombomodulin activity in porcine to human xenotransplantation. Transplant. Proc. **29:** 884–885.
116. JURD, K.M., R.V. GIBBS & B.J. HUNT. 1996. Activation of human prothrombin by porcine aortic endothelial cells—a potential barrier to pig to human xenotransplantation. Blood Coag. Fibrinol. **7:** 336–343.
117. VANTVEER, C., N.J. GOLDEN, M. KALAFATIS & K.G. MANN. 1997. Inhibitory mechanism of the protein C pathway on tissue factor-induced thrombin generation—syn-

ergistic effect in combination with tissue factor pathway inhibitor. J. Biol. Chem. **272:** 7983–7994.

118. VANTVEER, C. & K.G. MANN. 1997. Regulation of tissue factor initiated thrombin generation by the stoichiometric inhibitors tissue factor pathway inhibitor, antithrombin-iii, and heparin cofactor-ii. J. Biol. Chem. **272:** 4367–4377.
119. VAN, 'T, VEER, C., T.M. HACKENG, C. DELAHAYE, J.J. SIXMA & B.N. BOUMA. 1994. Activated factor X and thrombin formation triggered by tissue factor on endothelial cell matrix in a flow model: effect of the tissue factor pathway inhibitor. Blood **84:** 1132–1142.
120. LESNIKOSKI, B.A., D. CANDINAS, I. OTSU, R. METTERNICH, F.H. BACH & S.C. ROBSON. 1997. Thrombin inhibition in discordant xenograft rejection. Xenotransplantation **4:** 140–146.
121. JAKOBS, F.M., E.A. DAVIS, T. WHITE, F. SANFILIPPO & W.M. BALDWIN. 1998. Prolonged discordant xenograft survival by inhibition of the intrinsic coagulation pathway in complement c6-deficient recipients. J. Heart Lung Transplant. **17:** 306–311.
122. CANDINAS, D., N. KOYAMADA, T. MIYATAKE, J. SIEGEL, W.W. HANCOCK, F.H. BACH & S.C. ROBSON. 1996. Loss of rat glomerular ATP diphosphohydrolase activity during reperfusion injury is associated with oxidative stress reactions. Thromb. Haemost. **76:** 807–812.
123. ROBSON, S.C. 1994. Platelets in xenograft rejection. Xenotransplantation **2:** 38–46.
124. PEERSCHKE, E.I.B., K.B.M. REID & B. GHEBREHIWET. 1993. Platelet activation by C1q results in the induction of αII/βIII integrins and the expression of P-selectin and procoagulant activity. J. Exp. Med. **178:** 579–587.
125. AMIRKHOSRAVI, A., M. ALEXANDER, K. MAY, D.A. FRANCIS, G. WARNES, J. BIGERSTAFF & J.L. FRANCIS. 1996. The importance of platelets in the expression of monocyte tissue factor antigen measured by a new whole blood flow cytometric assay. Thromb. Haemost. **75:** 87–95.
126. SCHULTE AM ESCH, J., J.B. SIEGEL, M. CRUZ, J. ANRATHER & S.C. ROBSON. 1997. The A1 domain of von Willebrand factor expressed on cell membranes directly activates platelets. Blood **90:** 4425–4437.
127. CANDINAS, D., B.A. LESNIKOSKI, W.W. HANCOCK, I. OTSU, N. KOYAMADA, A.P. DALMASSO, S.C. ROBSON & F.H. BACH. 1996. Inhibition of platelet integrinGPIIbIIIa prolongs survival of discordant cardiac xenografts. Transplantation **62:** 1–5.
128. MAKOWKA, L., F.A. CHAPMAN, D.V. CRAMER, S.G. QIAN, H. SUN & T.E. STARZL. 1990. Platelet-activating factor and hyperacute rejection. The effect of a platelet-activating factor antagonist, SRI 63-441, on rejection of xenografts and allografts in sensitized hosts. Transplantation **50:** 359–365.
129. OHAIR, D.P., A.M. ROZA, R. KOMOROWSKI, G. MOORE, R.P. MCMANUS, C.P. JOHNSON, M.B. ADAMS & G.M. PIEPER. 1993. Tulopafant, a PAF receptor antagonist, increases capillary patency and prolongs survival in discordant cardiac xenotransplants. J. Lipid Med. **7:** 79–84.
130. KOYAMADA, N., T. MIYATAKE, D. CANDINAS, P. HECHENLEITNER, J. SIEGEL, W.W. HANCOCK, F.H. BACH & S.C. ROBSON. 1996. Apyrase administration prolongs discordant xenograft survival. Transplantation **62:** 1739–1743.
131. FAY, W.P., J.G. MURPHY & W.G. OWEN. 1996. High concentrations of active plasminogen activator inhibitor-1 in porcine coronary artery thrombi. Arterioscl. Thromb. Vasc. Biol. **16:** 1277–1284.

# Encapsulated, Genetically Engineered Cells, Secreting Glucagon-like Peptide-1 for the Treatment of Non-insulin–dependent Diabetes Mellitus

RÉMY BURCELIN,[a] ERIC ROLLAND,[b] WANDA DOLCI,[a] STÉPHANE GERMAIN,[b] VÉRONIQUE CARREL,[b] AND BERNARD THORENS[a,c]

[a]*Institute of Pharmacology and Toxicology, University of Lausanne, 27, rue du Bugnon, CH-1005 Lausanne, Switzerland*

[b]*Modex Therapeutics, 27, rue du Bugnon, CH-1005 Lausanne, Switzerland*

**ABSTRACT: Non-insulin-dependent, or type II, diabetes mellitus is characterized by a progressive impairment of glucose-induced insulin secretion by pancreatic β cells and by a relative decreased sensitivity of target tissues to the action of this hormone. About one third of type II diabetic patients are treated with oral hypoglycemic agents to stimulate insulin secretion. These drugs however risk inducing hypoglycemia and, over time, lose their efficacy. An alternative treatment is the use of glucagon-like peptide-1 (GLP-1), a gut peptidic hormone with a strong insulinotropic activity. Its activity depends of the presence of normal blood glucose concentrations and therefore does not risk inducing hypoglycemia. GLP-1 can correct hyperglycemia in diabetic patients, even in those no longer responding to hypoglycemic agents. Because it is a peptide, GLP-1 must be administered by injection; this may prevent its wide therapeutic use. Here we propose to use cell lines genetically engineered to secrete a mutant form of GLP-1 which has a longer half-life *in vivo* but which is as potent as the wild-type peptide. The genetically engineered cells are then encapsulated in semi-permeable hollow fibers for implantation in diabetic hosts for constant, long-term, *in situ* delivery of the peptide. This approach may be a novel therapy for type II diabetes.**

## INTRODUCTION

Loss of glucose-induced insulin secretion by pancreatic β cells is a characteristic of non-insulin-dependent diabetes mellitus (NIDDM).[1] In the treatment of NIDDM, when diet and exercise are no longer able to correct the diabetic syndrome, postprandial insulin secretion is stimulated by administration of insulin secretagogues such as sulfonylureas.[2] These substances stimulate insulin secretion by directly inhibiting the activity of the $K^+_{ATP}$ channel thereby depolarizing the β-cell plasma membrane and stimulating insulin secretion. The initial efficacy of sulfonylureas however vanishes after a few years of treatment. This is thought to be due, in part, to β-cell ex-

[b]+41 21 692 54 50 (voice); +41 21 692 54 55 (fax).

[c]Author for correspondence: +41 21 692 53 90 (voice); +41 21 692 53 55 (fax); Bernard.thorens@ipharm.unil.ch (e-mail).

haustion resulting from the action of sulfonylureas solely on the stimulation of insulin secretion without a concomitant positive effect on insulin biosynthesis. New clinically useful insulin secretagogues are therefore required. The insulinotropic hormone glucagon-like peptide-1-(7–37) (GLP-1) is the most potent stimulator of glucose-induced insulin secretion so far characterized.[3–5] It is produced in the intestinal L cells as a proteolytic processing product of the preproglucagon molecule[6] and is secreted in the blood following nutrient ingestion, in particular glucose and fatty acids. GLP-1 binds to a specific β-cell plasma membrane receptor of the G protein-coupled receptor family which is linked to the activation of adenylyl cyclase.[7–9] GLP-1 insulinotropic activity is measurable with peptide concentrations as low as 1–10 pmole/l and is detected only in the presence of normal or elevated glycemic levels.[10–12] Beside its effect on insulin secretion, GLP-1 also stimulates the transcription of the insulin gene and the translation of the insulin mRNA.[13,14] Importantly, the insulinotropic effect of this peptide is preserved in patients with NIDDM, even those with secondary failure to sulfonylureas.[15–18] This, combined with the glucose-dependence of its action and its positive effects on insulin biosynthesis, makes GLP-1 an attracive potential new agent for the treatment of type II diabetes. A significant drawbacks in the therapeutic use of this peptide, however, is its short half-life *in vivo,* about 5 minutes.[19] This is due, in part, to a rapid inactivation by the circulating endopeptidase dipeptidylpeptidase IV (DPPIV),[20–22] which hydrolyzes peptides or protein after the second amino terminal residue, provided that the sequence is X-Pro/Ala. DPPIV action on GLP-1 produces GLP-1-(9–27), which is a relatively weak antagonist of the GLP-1 receptor.[23] Another problem in the use of GLP-1 is its peptidic nature which requires it to be administered by injections. In an effort to develop GLP-1 as a therapeutically useful molecule, this peptide was administrated either as subcutaneous injections[24–26] or as bucal tablets.[27] Although a good correction of the glycemic excursion could be obtained, the therapeutic efficacy of the peptide was also short-lived.

In the present paper we will describe first our effort at improving the stability of the peptide by making it resistant to degradation by the enzyme dipeptidylpeptidase IV. Second we will describe an approach that may be taken for the continuous *in situ* synthesis and delivery of GLP-1 based on the transplantation of encapsulated, genetically engineered cells secreting GLP-1.

## THE PREPROGLUCAGON MOLECULE

The preproglucagon molecule is synthesized both in pancreatic α cells and in the jejunum and colon L cells.[28] Preproglucagon is a 180 amino acid long prohormone and its sequence contains, in addition to glucagon, two sequences of related structure: glucagon-like peptide-1 and glucagon-like peptide-2[29,30] (FIG. 1). There is a cell-specific proteolytic maturation of preproglucagon.[4,6] In α cells, the principal secreted active peptide is glucagon (FIG. 1). The other peptides such as "glicentin-related polypeptide" (GRPP) and "major proglucagon fragment" (MPF), which contains the GLP-1 and GLP-2 sequences, do not have any known physiological function. In intestinal L cells, preproglucagon is cleaved by specific proteases so as to generate glicentin, oxyntomodulin and GLP-1 but not glucagon (FIG. 1). Stimula-

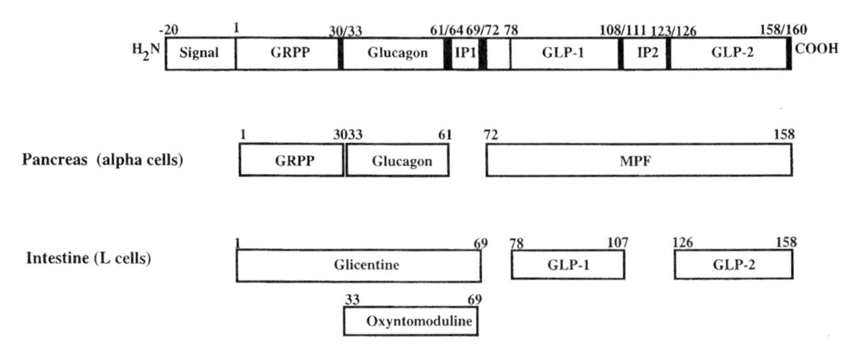


**FIGURE 1.** The preproglucagon molecule and its major proteolytic fragments. In pancreatic α cells, GRPP (glicentin-related polypeptide), glucagon and MPF (major proglucagon fragment) are the main products generated by cleavage of the proglucagon molecule at the sites indicated by the heavy vertical bars and which represent dibasic amino acid residues. In intestinal L cells, glicentin, GLP-1, GLP-2 and oxyntomodulin are the main products. In contrast to the other cleavage sites, the active form of GLP-1 (amino acid 78 to 107) is generated by proteolytic cleavage at the single arginine residue at position 78.

tory actions of oxyntomodulin on hydrochloric acid secretion by gastric parietal cells[31] and on insulin secretion[32] have been reported. These actions, which are observed at relatively high peptide concentrations, may be due to binding of oxyntomodulin to the GLP-1 receptor.[33]

GLP-1 (amino acid 72–108) of the preproglucagon molecule (FIG. 1) can be further proteolytically processed into GLP-1-(78–108) or GLP-1-(78–107)amide which are the only biologically active forms of the peptide. The amidated form represents about two thirds of the truncated GLP-1 present in porcine or human intestinal mucosa.[34,35] In the rest of this work, we will refer to the active forms of truncated GLP-1, which are also called GLP-1-(7–37) and GLP-1-(7–36)amide, as GLP-1.

The stimulatory action of GLP-1 on glucose-induced insulin secretion was first demonstrated in the perfused rat pancreas system.[10,11] In these experiments, GLP-1(7–37) or GLP-1(7–36)amide were shown to have identical effects on the β-cell secretory response. The stimulation of insulin secretion was detected at concentrations of peptide as low as 1 to 10 pM.[12] The stimulatory effect of these peptides was shown to be glucose-dependent. No insulin secretion could be elicited by GLP-1 with 2.8 mM glucose in the perfusate. However, with 6.6 mM glucose in the perfusate, a strong potentiation of insulin secretion was induced by GLP-1.

## GLP-1 AS A NOVEL THERAPEUTIC SUBSTANCE FOR NIDDM

Non-insulin-dependent, or type II diabetes mellitus, is characterized by a decreased responsiveness of β cells to elevations in blood glucose concentrations.[36–38] Interestingly, injections of GLP-1 at pharmacological levels (plasma concentrations of 50–100 pM) can produce a marked stimulation of insulin secretion in diabetic patients[15–17] and correct postprandial hyperglycemia. Even more striking, intravenous infusion of GLP-1 in fasted type II diabetic patients who were markedly hyperglycemic, completely corrected the blood glucose levels. This was provoked by a strong insulin secretory response which, however, waned as the glycemia returned to normal values.[18] In addition to its role on insulin secretion GLP-1 also stimulates insulin biogenesis. Thus, this may be a valuable new therapeutic tools in the control of hyperglycemia in NIDDM.

## IMPROVED STABILITY AND *IN VIVO* POTENCY OF A GLP-1 MUTANT

GLP-1 potential as a new agent for the treatment of type II diabetes is limited by its short half-life *in vivo*, about 5 minutes.[19] This is due, in part, to a rapid inactivation by the circulating endopeptidase dipeptidylpeptidase IV (DPPIV,[20–22] which hydrolyzes peptides or protein after the second amino terminal residue, provided that the sequence is X-Pro/Ala. DPPIV action on GLP-1 produces GLP-1-(9–27) which is a relatively weak antagonist of the GLP-1 receptor.[23]

We have demonstrated[42] that it was possible to substitute the second amino terminal amino acid by glycine, alanine, serine or threonine while preserving the capability of the peptide to stimulate cAMP production by a cell line transformed to express the cloned GLP-1 receptor (clone 5 cells). However, not all peptides were equipotent. We demonstrated that the glycine-substituted peptide, referred to as GLP-1-Gly8, was the best peptide. Binding of GLP-1-Gly8 to the GLP-1 receptor was evaluated in displacement experiments. Clone 5 cells were incubated in the presence of tracer amounts of radioiodinated GLP-1 and increasing concentrations of wild-type or mutant GLP-1 peptides. We showed that the $IC_{50}$s for displacement of bound radioiodinated GLP-1 by GLP-1 or GLP-1-Gly8 were not statistically different ($0.41 \pm 0.14$ nM vs. $1.39 \pm 0.61$ nM, respectively). The dose-dependent induction of cAMP accumulation in clone 5 cells by both peptides displayed also the same $EC_{50}$ ($0.25 \pm 0.05$ nM and $0.33 \pm 0.09$ nM for the wild-type and mutant peptide, respectively).

The resistance of GLP-1-Gly8 to degradation by dipeptidylpeptidase IV (DPPIV) was first evaluated by incubating the peptide in the presence of the purified enzyme and analyzing of the reaction products by HPLC. The intact peptides (GLP-1 and GLP-1-Gly8) eluted with a retention time of 7.5 minutes, whereas the cleaved products (GLP-1-(9–37)) had a retention time of 10.5 min. In conditions where 10% of GLP-1 was converted into GLP-1-(9–39), less than 0.1% GLP-1-Gly8 was recovered as cleaved peptide, indicating a marked resistance of the peptide to degradation by DPPIV. The stability of GLP-1-Gly8 was further analyzed by incubation of the peptide in the presence of fetal bovine serum (FBS), which naturally contains DPPIV activity.[39,40] Importantly, this assay was designed to measure the bioactivity of the remaining peptide by assessing the ability of the incubation medium to activate cAMP production by clone 5 cells. The half-life of GLP-1 was about 35 hours when incubated in the presence of FBS and this half-life was extended to 65 hours when diprotin A, a specific DPPIV inhibitor,[41] was added at the beginning of the experiment. In contrast, in the same conditions, GLP-1-Gly8 remained stable for more than 72 hours, even in the absence of diprotin A. Similar observations were made when the peptides were incubated in the presence of baby hamster kidney (BHK) cells cultured in the same medium.

## IMPROVED *IN SITU* POTENCY OF GLP-1-GLY8

To evaluate the potency of the mutant peptide, we used mice fed a high fat diet. C57Bl/6J mice were fed a normal chow (NC) or a high fat, carbohydrate-free, (HF) diet. Body weights become significantly higher in the HF group after 8 weeks of diet (30.2 ± 0.6 g vs. 28.1 ± 0.3 g, respectively) and remained about 30% higher than that of controls up to 26 weeks (38.5 ± 0.8 g vs. 30.3 ± 0.3 g, respectively). Fed blood glucose levels were lower in the HF than in the NC group since no carbohydrates were present in the HF diet. Fasting induced a rapid decrease in blood glucose concentrations in NC mice, whereas in the HF group glycemia remained at the same level (5.7 ± 0.2 mM and 7.2 ± 0.1 mM after 6 hours fast in NC and HF mice, respectively). Insulin levels in the fed state were lower in the HF as compared to the NC mice. Glucagon levels in the fed state were higher in HF than in NC mice, but not different after fasting. These data therefore indicate the presence of a diabetic phenotype induced by high fat. Furthermore, intraperitoneal glucose tolerance tests (IPGTT) showed a markedly impaired tolerance in the high-fat-fed mice.

The potency of GLP-1-Gly8 as compared with that of the wild-type peptide was evaluated by injecting the peptide and measuring the effect on the glucose tolerance as measured by an IPGTT. We showed that injection of 1 nanomole of GLP-1-Gly8 corrected completely the glucose intolerance of high-fat-fed mice even when injected up to 4 hours before the IPGTT. In contrast, when 1 nanomole of GLP-1 was injected 30 minutes before the tolerance test, its effect had already vanished. In another set of experiments, we injected decreasing amounts of the mutant peptide 2 hours before the IPGTT. We showed that as little as 0.1 nanomole of the peptide gave a significant improvement of the glucose intolerance. These data therefore demonstrate that GLP-1-Gly8 was at least 40-fold more potent that GLP-1 in its ability to correct glucose intolerance.

This last result is of great importance in planning a cell-based delivery system for the *in situ* release of GLP-1 for the treatment of NIDDM. From the published work cited above, it can be calculated that about 200 μg of GLP-1 a day would be needed for an adult diabetic patient. If this amount could indeed by reduced by 40-fold because of the highest potency of GLP-1-Gly8, this would impact on thc number of genetically engineered cells required for therapeutic efficacy.

## ENGINEERING OF GLP-1-GLY8–SECRETING CELLS

### *The Cell Line*

We choose the C2C12 murine (C3H) myoblast cells line as the cells to be engineered. These cells have several advantages. They grow fast in tissue culture and can be easily genetically engineered by classical techniques. Furthermore, when serum-deprived, they can fuse and thus enter a growth-arrest phase.

### *The Expression Vector*

GLP-1 is derived from the preproglucagon molecule. It therefore not possible to directly utilize the preproglucagon gene or cDNA for genetically engineering cells capable of secreting GLP-1 as several other peptides could be released. In particular, it is necessary to avoid simultaneous secretion of GLP-1 and glucagon since these peptides have partially antagonistic effects: GLP-1 is secreted to stimulate insulin secretion and induce glucose storage whereas glucagon induces glucose production in particular from liver, and therefore raises blood glucose levels.

We therefore designed an expression vector consisting of the GLP-1-Gly8 coding sequence placed downstream of a signal peptide and a 30-amino-acid-long prosequence. The signal peptide is required for targeting of the newly synthesized polypeptide into the secretory pathway. It is removed at the time of translocation into the endoplasmic reticulum by the signal peptidase. The prosequence has been added to improve the stability of the newly synthesized polypeptide. It however needs to be removed so that the bioactive peptide can be secreted by the cells. In order to ensure a proper cleavage of the prosequence, a furin cleavage site has been engineered between the GLP-1-Gly8 and prosequence. Furin is a proteolytic enzyme whose role is to process proteins when they passage through the secretory pathway. Its site of action is mostly in the trans-Golgi network. C2C12 express little furin activity. We therefore had to simultaneously engineer these cells so that the expression of furin was increased.

C2C12 cells were therefore first transfected with the furin construct. Selected clones were then further transfected with the GLP-1-Gly8 expression construct. Several hundred clones were analyzed for the secretion of GLP-1 using a biological assay based on the stimulation of cAMP production by the clone 5 cells, as previously mentioned. The expression level obtained based on this criteria was up to 0.5 $\mu$g/$10^6$ cells/day.

## ENCAPSULATION OF GLP-1-GLY8–SECRETING CELLS AND CLONE SELECTION

### *Metabolic Selection*

In a first set of selection for clones surviving encapsulation and transplantation, we evaluated the ability of several clones secreting high levels of GLP-1-Gly8 to survive at high cell density *in vitro*. The surviving clones were then directly selected after encapsulation in polyethylene sulfone semi-permeable hollow fibers and subcutaneous transplantation in syngeneic mice. Following a three week implantation period, the capsules were retrieved and viability of the cells assessed by histological examination. Whereas some clones did not survive, some survived extremely well and maintained secretion of GLP-1-Gly8. These clones were then evaluated for their survival in different strains of mice (allogeneic transplantation) using the same encapsulation devices. The same clones showed very good survival in, for instance, C57Bl/6 mice.

### *Transplantation in High-Fat-Fed Diabetic Mice*

Capsules containing GLP-1-Gly8 secreting cells were prepared. A fairly reproducible loading of the capsules was obtained with ~220 ng GLP-1-Gly8 being released per day per capsule. Mice were implanted with two capsules and kept for several weeks. Initial experiments demonstrated that glucose intolerance could be improved in mice receiving engineered cells, but not in those receiving nonengineered cells.

## CONCLUSIONS

Our work has demonstrated that GLP-1 potency could be greatly increased by substituting the second amino acid by glycine. This increases the resistance of the peptide to the degradation by dipeptidylpeptidase IV without affecting its affinity for the GLP-1 receptor nor its efficacy in stimulating cAMP formation by target cells expressing this receptor. The extent of improvement could be evaluated to be approximately 40-fold. This has important consequences for the development of a cell-based delivery system. Indeed, it can be calculated that about 5–10 μg of the modified peptide could be sufficient for the daily treatment of a diabetic patient. We are expecting that genetically engineered cells, similar to the one we already have or with some improvements that we are now developing, may secrete about 1–2 μg of peptide a day. This will therefore require the use of devices capable of containing 3–10 million cells. This may be achievable with presently available technology.

An important other outcome of the present study is the observation that, in addition to the immune problems faced when performing cellular transplantation, even in encapsulated form, there are a number of variables which may permit the cells to survive. Clearly apparent from our clonal selection experiments, not all cell clones, even though they are derived from the same cell population, can survive transplantation after encapsulation in hollow fibers. We believe that this indicates the existence of a "metabolic fitness" of these particular clones, which is distinct from immunological tolerance problems. Indeed, our selection was first based on transplantation in syngeneic mice where immune problems should be minimal, if present at all. The clones selected in these conditions were then shown to be able to survive as well in allogeneic conditions. We also obtained good survival in the peritoneal cavity of rats, using capsules with smaller cut-off properties (64 kD instead of 280 kD).

Initial experiments at using the selected GLP-1-Gly8-secreting cells to correct glucose intolerance in high fat fed mice demonstrated improvement of the diabetic phenotype. We believe that future experiments will confirm our initial data and that in situ delivery of this peptide by encapsulated, genetically engineered cells may become a novel therapeutic approach for the treatment of NIDDM.

## REFERENCES

1. DEFRONZO, R.A. 1988. The triumvirate: β-cell, muscle, liver. A collusion responsible for NIDDM. Diabetes **37:** 667–687.
2. KAHN, C.R. & Y. SHECHTER. 1990. Insulin, oral hypoglycemic agents, and the pharmacology of the endocrine pancreas. *In* The Pharmacological Basis of Therapeutics. A. G. Gilman, T. W. Rall, A. S. Nies & P. Taylor, Eds. : 1463–1494. Pergamon Press. New York, Oxford.
3. SHIMIZU, I., M. HIROTA, C. OHBOSHI & K. SHIMA. 1987. Identification and localization of glucagon-like peptide-1 and its receptor in rat brain. Endocrinol. **121:** 1076–1082.
4. ØRSKOV, C. 1992. glucagon-like peptide-1, a new hormone of the entero-insular axis. Diabetologia **35:** 701–711.

5. THORENS, B. & G. WAEBER. 1993. Glucagon-like peptide-1 and the control of insulin secretion in the normal state and in NIDDM. Diabetes **42:** 1219–1225.
6. MOJSOV, S., G. HEINRICH, I.B. WILSON, M. RAVAZZOLA, L. ORCI & J. F. HABENER. 1986. Preproglucagon gene expression in pancreas and intestine diversifies at the level of post-translational processing. J. Biol. Chem. **261:** 11880–11889.
7. GÖKE, R. & J.M. CONLON. 1988. Receptors for glucagon-like peptide-1(7-36)amide on rat insulinoma-derived cells. J. Endocrinol. **116:** 357–362.
8. THORENS, B. 1992. Expression cloning of the pancreatic beta cell receptor for the gluco-incretin hormone glucagon-like peptide I. Proc. Natl. Acad. Sci. USA **89:** 8641–8645.
9. WIDMANN, C., E. BÜRKI, W. DOLCI & B. THORENS. 1994. Signal transduction by the cloned glucagon-like peptide-1 receptor. Comparison with signalling by the endogenous receptors of β cell lines. Mol. Pharmacol. **45:** 1029–1035.
10. HOLST, J.J., C. ØRSKOV, O. VAGN NIELSEN & T.W. SCHWARTZ. 1987. Truncated glucagon-like peptide 1, an insulin-releasing hormone from the distal gut. FEBS Lett. **211:** 169–174.
11. MOJSOV, S., G.C. WEIR & J.F. HABENER. 1987. Insulinotropin: glucagon-like peptide 1(7-37) co-encoded in the glucagon gene is a potent stimulator of insulin release in the perfused rat pancreas. J. Clin. Invest. **79:** 616–619.
12. WEIR, G.C., S. MOJSOV, G.K. HENDRICK & J.F. HABENER. 1989. Glucagon-like peptide 1 (7-37) actions on endocrine pancreas. Diabetes **38:** 338–342.
13. DRUCKER, D.J., J. PHILIPPE, S. MOJSOV, W.L. CHICK & J.F. HABENER. 1987. Glucagon-like peptide I stimulates insulin gene expression and increases cyclic AMP levels in rat islet cell line. Proc. Natl. Acad. Sci. USA **84:** 3434–3438.
14. FEHMANN, H.-C. & J.F. HABENER. 1992. Insulinotropic hormone glucagon-like peptide-I(7-37) stimulation of proinsulin gene expression and proinsulin biosynthesis in insulinoma bTC-1 cells. Endocrinology **130:** 159–166.
15. NATHAN, D.M., E. SCHREIBER, H. FOGEL, S. MOJSOV & J.F. HABENER. 1992. Insulinotropic action of glucagonlike peptide-1-(7-37) in diabetic and nondiabetic subjects. Diabetes Care 15:270–276.
16. GUTNIAK, M., C. ØRSKOV, J.J. HOLST, B. AHRÉN & S. EFENDIC. 1992. Antidiabetogenic effect of glucagon-like peptide-1 (7-36)amide in normal subjects and patients with diabetes mellitus. N. Engl. J. Med. **326:** 1316–1322.
17. NAUCK, M.A., M.M. HEIMESAAT, C. ØRSKOV, J.J. HOLST, R. EBERT & W. CREUTZFELD. 1993. Preserved incretin activity of glucagon-like peptide 1 (7-36) amide but not of synthetic human gastric inhibitory polypeptide in patients with type-2 diabetes mellitus. J. Clin. Invest. **91:** 301–307.
18. NAUCK, M.A., N. KLEINE, C. ØRSKOV, J.J. HOLST, B. WILLMS & W. CREUTZFELD. 1993. Normalization of fasting hyperglycaemia by exogenous glucagon-like peptide 1 (7-36 amide) in type 2 (non-insulin-dependent) diabetic patients. Diabetologia **36:** 741–744.
19. ØRSKOV, C., A. WETTERGREN & J.J. HOLST. 1993. Biological effects and metabolic rates of glucagon-like peptide-1 7-36 amide and glucagonlike peptide-1 7-37 in healthy subjects are indistinguishable. Diabetes **42:** 658–661.
20. PAULY, R.P., F. ROSCHE, M. WERMANN, C.H.S. MCINTOSH, R. A. PEDERSON & H.-U. DEMUTH. 1996. Investigation of glucose-dependent insulinotropic polypeptide-(1-42) and glucagon-like peptide-1(7-36) degradation in vitro by dipeptidyl peptidase IV using matrix-assisted laser desorption/ionization-time of flight mass spectrometry. A novel kinetic approach. J. Biol. Chem. **271:** 23222–23229.
21. DEACON, C.F., M.A. NAUCK, M. TOFT-NIELSEN, L. PRIDAL, B. WILLMS & J.J. HOLST. 1995. Both subcutaneously and intravenously administered glucagon-like peptide 1 are rapidly degraded from the NH2-terminus in type II diabetic patients and in healthy subjects. Diabetes **44:** 1126–1131.
22. MENTLEIN, R., B. GALLWITZ & W.E. SCHMIDT. 1993. Dipeptidyl peptidase IV hydrolyses gastric inhibitory polypeptide, glucagon-like peptide-1-(7-36)amide, peptide histidine methionine and is responsible for their degradation in human serum. Eur. J. Biochem. **214:** 829–835.

23. KNUDSEN, L.B. & L. PRIDAL. 1996. Glucagon-like peptide-1-(9-39) amide is a major metabolite of glucagon-like peptide-1-(7-36)amide after in vivo administration to dogs, and it acts as an antagonist of the pancreatic receptor. Eur. J. Pharmacol. **318:** 429–435.
24. GUTNIAK, M.K., B. LINDE, J.J. HOLST & S. EFENDIC. 1994. Subcutaneous injection of the incretin hormone glucagon-like peptide 1 abolishes postprandial glycemia in NIDDM. Diabetes Care **9:** 1039–1044.
25. JUNTTI-BERGGREN, L., J. PIGON, F. KARPE, A. HAMSTEN, M. GUTNIAK, L. VIGNATI & S. EFENDIC. 1996. The antidiabetogenic effect of GLP-1 is maintained during a 7-day treatment period and improves diabetic dyslipoproteinemia in NIDDM patients. Diabetes Care **19:** 1200–1206.
26. TODD, J.F., J.P.H. WILDING, C.M.B. EDWARDS, F.A. KHAN, M.A. GHATEI & S.R. BLOOM. 1997. Glucagon-like peptide-1 (GLP-1): a trial of treatment in non-insulin-dependent diabetes mellitus. Eur. J. Clin. Invest. **27:** 533–536.
27. GUTNIAK, M.K., H. LARSSON, S.J. HEIBER, O.T. JUNESKANS, J.J. HOLST & B. AHREN. 1996. Potential therapeutic levels of glucagon-like peptide-1 achieved in human by a buccal tablet. Diabetes Care **19:** 843–848.
28. EISSELE, R., R. GÖKE, H.-P. HARTHUS, H. VERMEER, R. ARNOLD & B. GÖKE. 1992. Glucagon-like peptide-1 cells in the gastrointestinal tract of pancreas of rat, pig and man. Eur. J. Clin. Invest. **22:** 283–291.
29. BELL, G.I., R.F. SANTERRE & G.T. MULLENBACH. 1983. Hamster preproglucagon contains the sequence of glucagon and two related peptides. Nature **302:** 716–718.
30. BELL, G.I., R. SANCHEZ-PESCADOR, P.J. LAYBOURN & R.C. NAJARIAN. 1983. Exon duplication and divergence in the human preproglucagon gene. Nature **304:** 368–371.
31. JAROUSSE, C., H. NIEL, M.-P. AUDOUSSET-PUECH, J. MARTINEZ & D. BATAILLE. 1986. Oxyntomodulin and its C-terminal octapeptide inhibit liquid meal-stimulated acid secretion. Peptides **7:** 253–256.
32. JAROUSSE, C., D. BATAILLE & B. JEANRENAUD. 1984. A pure enteroglucagon, oxyntomodulin (glucagon 37), stimulates insulin release in perfused rat pancreas. Endocrinol. **115:** 102–105.
33. GROS, L., B. THORENS, D. BATAILLE & A. KERVRAN. 1993. Glucagon-like peptide-1-(7-36)amide, oxyntomodulin, and glucagon interact with a common receptor in a somatostatin-secreting cell line. Endocrinol. **133:** 631–638.
34. ØRSKOV, C., M. BERSANI, A.H. JOHNSEN, P. HQJRUP & J.J. HOLST. 1989. Complete sequences of glucagon-like peptide-1 from human and pig small intestine. J. Biol. Chem. **264:** 12826–12829.
35. MOJSOV, S., M.G. KOPZYNSKI & J.F. HABENER. 1990. Both amidated and nonamidated forms of glucagon-like peptide-1 are synthesized in the rat intestine and the pancreas. J. Biol. Chem. **265:** 8001–8008.
36. CERASI, E., R. LUFT & S. EFENDIC. 1971. Decreased sensitivity of the pancreatic b cells to glucose in prediabetic and diabetic subjects. Diabetes **21:** 224–234.
37. ROBERTSON, R.P. & D. PORTE JR. 1973. The glucose receptor: a defective mechanism in diabetes mellitus distinct from the beta adrenergic receptor. J. Clin. Invest. **52:** 870–876.
38. ARONOFF, S.L., P.H. BENNETT, N.B. RUSHFORTH, M. MILLER & R.H. UNGER. 1976. Normal glucagon response to arginine infusion in "prediabetic" Pima Indians. J. Clin. End. Metab. **43:** 279–286.
39. GORNE, R.C., J. HIENS, H. HILSE & P. OEHME. 1983. Dipeptidyl peptidase activities in various organs of the Wistar rat. Pharmazie **38:** 112.
40. GOSSRAU, R. 1979. Histochemical and biochemical distribution of dipeptidyl peptidasc IV. Histochcmistry **60:** 231.
41. HANSKI, C., T. HUHLE & W. REUTTER. 1985. Involvement of plasma membrane dipeptidyl peptidase IV in fibronectin-mediated adhesion of cells on collagen. J. Biol. Chem. **266:** 1169–1176.
42. BURCELIN, R., W. DOLCI & B. THORENS. 1999. Long-lasting antidiabetic effect of a dipeptidyl peptidase IV-resistant analogue of GLP-1. Metabolism **48:** 252–258.

# Genetically Engineered Pancreatic β-Cell Lines for Cell Therapy of Diabetes

SHIMON EFRAT[a]

*Department of Molecular Pharmacology, Albert Einstein College of Medicine, 1300 Morris Park Avenue, Bronx, New York 10461, USA and*
*Department of Human Genetics and Molecular Medicine, Sackler School of Medicine, Tel Aviv University, Ramat Aviv, 69978 Tel Aviv, Israel*

**ABSTRACT: The optimal treatment of insulin-dependent diabetes mellitus (IDDM), which is caused by the autoimmune destruction of pancreatic islet β cells, would require the regulated delivery of insulin by transplantation of functional β cells. β-cell transplantation has so far been restricted by the scarcity of human islet donors. This shortage would be alleviated by the development of differentiated β-cell lines, which could provide an abundant and well-characterized source of β cells for transplantation. Using conditional transformation approaches, our laboratory has generated continuous β-cell lines from transgenic mice. These cells produce insulin amounts comparable to those of normal islets and release insulin in response to physiological stimuli. Cell replication in these β cells can be tightly controlled both in culture and *in vivo*, allowing regulation of cell number and cell differentiation. Another challenge to cell therapy of IDDM is the protection of transplanted cells from immunological rejection and recurring autoimmunity. By employing adenovirus genes which downregulate antigen presentation and increase cell resistance to cytokines, β-cell transplantation across allogeneic barriers was achieved without immunosuppression. In principle, similar β-cell lines can be derived from isolated human islets using viral vectors to deliver conditionally regulated transforming and immunomodulatory genes into β cells. The combination of these approaches with immunoisolation devices holds the promise of a widely available cell therapy for treatment of IDDM in the near future.**

## INTRODUCTION

The delivery of bioactive proteins by transplantation of primary cells, or engineered cell lines which secrete them, represents a promising therapeutic approach to a number of human diseases characterized by the deficiency of a secreted factor. The development in recent years of cell encapsulation techniques has turned this approach into a realistic possibility. Cell transplantation is likely to gradually replace protein delivery by injections, which is often inefficient, costly, and plagued by side effects and, most importantly, escapes the fine-tuned control mechanisms provided by the natural secretion system.

Insulin-dependent diabetes mellitus (IDDM) is a good example of a disease that can benefit from cell therapy. IDDM is an autoimmune disorder caused by a combi-

[a]Address correspondence to Dr. Efrat in Israel: 972-3-640-7701 (voice); 972-3-640-9900 (fax); sefrat@post.tau.ac.il (e-mail).

nation of mostly unknown genetic and environmental factors. The disease results from a lymphocyte-mediated destruction of the insulin-producing β cells in the pancreatic islets of Langerhans, which leads to insulin deficiency. Current research efforts center on developing early detection methods, identifying the antigenic target for the autoimmune response, and understanding the mechanisms by which the β cells are destroyed. These efforts may open the way for antigen-specific tolerization, as well as genetic engineering of the β cells to resist the autoimmune attack and disable the immune effector cells. A better understanding of genes and factors involved in islet development may allow induction of islet regeneration, coupled with ways to prevent recurring autoimmunity against the newly-formed islets. However, these research avenues are likely to require much additional work before they can lead to novel therapeutic approaches.

IDDM has been treated in the past 75 years by insulin injections. Although this therapy is life-saving, the exact insulin dosage is difficult to determine, leading to episodes of hyperglycemia or hypoglycemia. As a result of hyperglycemia, many IDDM patients develop in the long term severe complications. Insulin delivery to IDDM patients would be immensely improved if it could be continuously adjusted to the changing physiological needs, such as through transplantation of glucose-sensitive β cells.

Cell therapy of IDDM has faced several obstacles, including:

(1) The availability of a reliable and abundant cell source.

The cell mass required to maintain islet function of an entire pancreas is in the order of $10^8$–$10^9$ cells. The scarcity of human islet donors has severely limited allograft islet transplantation. Furthermore, the use of xenogeneic islets faces enormous immunological and physiological problems, and has raised safety concerns regarding zoonosis. The reproducible isolation and preservation of functional islets on a large scale remains difficult, costly and laborious.

(2) The need for regulated insulin secretion.

A number of groups have attempted to develop insulin gene therapy for diabetes by introducing into non-β cells, such as pituitary cells or hepatocytes, the capacity to produce proinsulin and process it to mature insulin.[1–3] The major advantage of autologous insulin-producing non-β cells is in avoiding the immunological problems associated with transplant rejection and with autoimmunity to β cells. However, the greatest difficulty in this approach has been to reconstruct in non-β cells the highly regulated insulin secretion of normal β cells, without which this approach would not offer a significant advantage over insulin injections. The islet β cells are uniquely equipped not only with the ability to produce insulin, but also with sensing and coupling mechanisms to regulate its release in response to changes in the blood concentration of a variety of molecules, most notably glucose.[4] Thus, the optimal treatment of IDDM is likely to be the replacement of the damaged β cells with intact β cells.

(3) Protection of the transplanted cells from immune rejection by the host.

In addition to graft rejection, the IDDM host is primed to destroy β cells, therefore recurring autoimmunity is a major concern. The experimental approaches developed in recent years to prevent transplant rejection, such as encapsulation, induction of donor-specific tolerance,[5,6] and various genetic manipulations of the donor cells to resist immune attacks,[7,8] may not be sufficient in an autoimmune environment.

(4) IDDM usually develops in young children, therefore any alternative therapy would need to offer a life-long solution.

The limitations on β-cell transplantation due to cell supply would be eliminated by the development of universal donor β-cell lines. Such cell lines would provide an abundant and reproducible source of β-cell material for transplantation. The cells could be selected in culture for optimal function and could be further modified by gene transfer to improve their properties and survival. They could be extensively screened for pathogens to assure transplant safety.

## REGULATION OF β-CELL GROWTH AND FUNCTION

A number of growth factors are known to be mitogenic to β cells, however they do not allow massive cell expansion in culture. The development of β-cell lines has depended on oncogenic transformation to induce replication of the quiescent, differentiated β cells. We have engineered, in recent years, a number of highly differentiated β-cell lines derived by expression of the SV40 T antigen (Tag) oncoprotein under control of the insulin promoter in transgenic mice,[9–12] termed β-tumor cells (βTC).

There is a dual challenge in employing transformed β cells in cell therapy:

(1) Maintaining a high level of differentiation with respect to insulin biosynthesis and regulated secretion over a prolonged period of propagation in culture and following transplantation.

βTC cells produce high amounts of insulin and respond to all the physiological stimuli of insulin secretion. However, they tend to dedifferentiate during proliferation in culture. One particular deviation from the normal phenotype, which appears usually during the first 20 passages in culture, is the induction of the low-$K_m$ glucose-phosphorylating enzyme hexokinase,[11,12] which leads to an insulin secretory response to subphysiological glucose levels. Glucose phosphorylation is considered the main mechanism for glucose sensing in β cells, which couples the amounts of secreted insulin to the extracellular glucose levels. Normal β cells express mainly the high-$K_m$ glucokinase isotype, which triggers insulin secretion only when extracellular glucose concentration exceeds a physiological threshold. The mechanism responsible for the increase in hexokinase mRNA and activity is not known; however it is thought that the upregulation results from the increased metabolic requirements of the dividing cells, as hexokinase may be more efficient than glucokinase in providing energy from glucose metabolism to the proliferating β cells. The increase in hexokinase activity represents a serious obstacle in the development of β-cell lines for cell therapy of diabetes, since transplantation of such cells may result in hypoglycemia.

(2) Regulation of cell replication.

Safety and functional considerations mandate a tight control of cell number. Transplantation of cells which proliferate in an unregulated manner can cause hypoglycemia and raise safety concerns, even when implanted within an encapsulation device.

To address both of these issues we have designed a strategy of reversible transformation, by placing the Tag oncogene under a conditional gene expression system. This system allows regulated cell expansion or growth arrest, as needed. The hope was not only to be able to prevent unregulated cell proliferation, but also to enhance the function of the growth-arrested β cells, given that most β cells in adult islets do not replicate under normal conditions.

This approach depends on 3 key elements:

(1) A tight regulatory system for gene expression.

We utilized the bacterial tetracycline (Tc) operon regulatory system, developed by Gossen and Bujard,[13] to control the expression of Tag.[14] The tetracycline repressor (tetR) recognizes a short palindromic operator sequence (tet-op) and binds to it. This interaction is inhibited by binding of the Tc ligand to the repressor. By fusing the tetR with the activating domain of the herpes simplex virus VP16 protein, Gossen and Bujard have turned the repressor into a potent Tc-controlled transactivator (tTA), which turns on genes flanked by the specific tet-op sites.[13] We generated transgenic mice with the tTA gene under control of the insulin gene regulatory region (RIP-tTA) (14). In a separate lineage of transgenic mice, the Tag gene was introduced under control of a minimal promoter combined with tet-op sequences (tet-Tag). This promoter by itself is not sufficient for expression of the gene, and neither of the two types of transgenic mice developed a phenotype. The two lines of mice were crossed to generate double-transgenic mice. In these mice the tTA protein activated transcription of the Tag gene specifically in β cells. This resulted in the development of β-cell tumors, which were cultured to derive a stable cell line, denoted βTC-tet. In the presence of Tc, Tag expression is completely blocked.[14]

(2) A complete dependence of β-cell proliferation on Tag expression.

During the cell transformation process other oncogenes can be activated in the cells, which could free them from dependence on Tag. However, this does not seem to be the case in the βTC-tet cells. The cells undergo complete growth arrest, both in culture and *in vivo*, in the absence of Tag (and in the presence of Tc).

(3) Reversibility of regulation.

Cells can be repeatedly induced to replicate and undergo growth arrest. This allows more flexibility in regulating cell numbers *in vivo*.

After demonstrating that cell replication can be tightly controlled, it was of interest to determine whether growth arrest affected cell function. Proliferating βTC-tet cells manifest correct responsiveness to glucose in the physiological concentration range,[15] and growth arrest does not change this response considerably. The most apparent effect of prolonged growth arrest (longer than 2–3 weeks) is a severalfold increase in insulin content. This change occurs without significant changes in proinsulin biosynthesis and may involve a more efficient processing of proinsulin to mature insulin. Another effect of growth arrest relates to the changes in glucose phosphorylation patterns described above. Following more than 60 passages *in vitro*, βTC-tet cells develop a high hexokinase activity, resulting in an insulin secretory response to subphysiological glucose levels. However, following 2–4 weeks of growth arrest, which presumably decreases the metabolic requirements of the cells, the hexokinase activity was downregulated severalfold.[15] This finding confirms the correlation between cell proliferation and high hexokinase activity in the βTC lines, and demonstrates that growth arrest allows restoration of the normal pattern of glucose phosphorylation, which is key to correct glucose sensing and accurate insulin secretion.

To evaluate their capacity to maintain glucose homeostasis *in vivo*, βTC-tet cells were implanted into streptozotocin-treated diabetic syngeneic recipients.[14] The cell implantation led to correction of hyperglycemia, demonstrating the ability of βTC-tet cells to function as normal β cells *in vivo*. As observed in the past with other βTC lines, the implanted cells continued to proliferate in mice not treated with Tc, which resulted in hypoglycemia and premature death. In contrast, in mice implanted with slow-release Tc pellets, blood glucose levels were stabilized in the normal range. The normal blood glucose levels were maintained for as long as the mice were followed, 4 months after Tc implantation. These results indicate that the cells undergo growth arrest as a result of Tc-induced inhibition of Tag expression, but remain viable and capable of normal glucose sensing and insulin production and secretion. The treatment was reversible: when the Tc pellets were removed from the mice at the end of the 4-month period of treatment, cell proliferation resumed, resulting in the development of hypoglycemia and tumors within an additional one month. This finding indicates that the βTC-tet cells maintain a proliferative capacity during a prolonged period of growth arrest, which allows renewed cell replication once Tag expression is restored.

To determine whether the transplanted cells were capable of responding to changes in plasma glucose by adjusting their insulin secretion, we subjected the diabetic mice implanted with βTC-tet cells to hyperglycemic clamp studies.[15] In this assay, awake, unrestrained mice are infused through an indwelling catheter, pre-implanted into the jugular vein, with a glucose solution which raises their steady-state plasma glucose levels to 16–17 mmol/L. Insulin secretion is monitored over a 2-h period in plasma samples obtained from the tail vein. βTC-tet cells responded to the hyperglycemia by increasing their insulin release up to 13-fold. Glucose-induced insulin secretion was similar in proliferating and both short-term (8–10 days) and long-term (5–8 weeks) growth-arrested cells. These findings demonstrate that the growth arrested cells maintain an ability for correct glucose sensing and insulin secretion *in vivo*.

The main disadvantage of the approach described above is the need for a constant presence of Tc for maintaining growth arrest for long periods *in vivo*. Using a mutant tetracycline repressor developed by Bujard, which requires Tc for DNA binding,[16] will permit to induce cell growth in culture in the presence of Tc, and cause growth arrest by removing Tc upon transplantation *in vivo*. This approach is currently being tested in our transgenic system.

## MODULATION OF β-CELL IMMUNOGENICITY

Cell encapsulation may not be efficient enough in protecting the transplanted cells from small immune effector molecules, such as cytokines, which can penetrate the device through its pores. β cells are particularly sensitive to cytokine effects, which include inhibition of cell function and induction of apoptosis. We have explored genetic approaches for protecting encapsulated cells from the effect of cytokines.

A number of viruses have evolved intricate mechanisms to avoid immune destruction of infected cells. One example is human adenoviruses. The adenovirus (Ad) early region 3 (E3) genes code for at least 4 proteins that inhibit the host immune responses mediated by cytotoxic T lymphocytes and tumor necrosis factor α (TNF). One of these is a 19kD glycoprotein (gp19), which has been shown to bind to the heavy chain of selected class I MHC haplotypes and prevent its transport out of the endoplasmic reticulum.[17] Because of the decreased expression of class I MHC on the plasma membrane, the recognition of Ad-infected cells by cytotoxic T cells is inhibited. In addition to gp19, three other Ad2 E3 region polypeptides have immunoregulatory activity. A protein of 14.7 kD, or the combination of the 10.4 kD and 14.5 kD proteins, can inhibit TNF-induced cytolysis of Ad-infected cells.[17,18] All of the E3 polypeptides are produced from transcripts generated from a common viral promoter by alternative splicing.

To evaluate the potential use of these immunoregulatory viral functions in facilitating allogeneic cell transplantation, we expressed the Ad E3 genes in pancreatic β cells in transgenic mice under control of the insulin gene regulatory region (RIP-E3), and transplanted transgenic islets under the renal capsule of allogeneic recipients.[19] The islets survived for over 3 months, which was the last time point examined. In contrast, non-transgenic allogeneic islets were all rejected within 2–4 weeks. Transplantation efficiency varied among different strains, which is consistent with the varying ability of gp19 to bind different class I MHC heavy chain haplotypes.[20,21] These findings indicate that the Ad E3 genes may be useful in engineering β-cell lines to reduce their immunogenicity and extend their survival in allotransplantation.

## CONCLUSIONS

Our work has demonstrated that transformed β-cell lines can maintain their differentiated functions of insulin biosynthesis and regulated secretion. By employing tight control of cell proliferation, it became possible to use these cells in restoring and maintaining euglycemia in diabetic animals. Furthermore, we have shown that cells engineered with viral genes that reduce their immunogenicity can be successfully transplanted across allogeneic barriers without immunosuppression or immunoisolation. These genetic manipulations can be applied to cultured human islets, using viral vectors for delivery of conditionally regulated transforming and immunomodulatory genes into β cells, to derive a universal donor human β-cell line. Although differentiated human β cells have been difficult to transform and propagate *in vitro*,[22] it is conceivable that such difficulties can eventually be overcome. Immunoisolation devices containing engineered human β cells are likely in the future to replace insulin injections as an accurate, convenient, and safe way to maintain euglycemia in IDDM patients in the long term.

## ACKNOWLEDGMENTS

This work has been supported by the Juvenile Diabetes Foundation International, by a Career Scientist Award from the Irma T. Hirschl Foundation, and by an NIDDK James A. Shannon Director's Award.

## REFERENCES


1. VALERA, A., C. FILLAT, C. COSTA, *et al.* 1994. Regulated expression of human insulin in the liver of transgenic mice corrects diabetic alterations. FASEB J. **8:** 440–447.
2. KOLODKA, T.M., M. FINEGOLD, L. MOSS, *et al.* 1995 Gene therapy for diabetes mellitus in rats by hepatic expression of insulin. Proc. Natl. Acad. Sci. USA **92:** 3293–3297.
3. LIPES, M.A., E.M. COOPER, R. SKELLY, *et al.* 1996. Insulin-secreting non-islet cells are resistant to autoimmune destruction. Proc. Natl. Acad. Sci. USA **93:** 8595–8600.
4. HOLZ, G.G. & J.F. HABENER. 1992. Signal transduction crosstalk in the endocrine system: pancreatic β cells and the glucose competence concept. Trends Biochem. Sci. **17:** 388–393.
5. POSSELT, A.M., C.F. BARKER, J.E. TOMASZEWSKI, *et al.* 1990. Induction of donor-specific unresponsiveness by intrathymic islet transplantation. Science **249:** 1293–1295.
6. POSSELT, A.M., J.S. ODORICO, C.F. BARKER, *et al.* 1992. Promotion of pancreatic islet allograft survival by intrathymic transplantation of bone marrow. Diabetes **41:** 771–775.
7. LAU, H.T., M. YU, A. FONTANA, *et al.* 1996. Prevention of islet allograft rejection with engineered myoblasts expressing FasL in mice. Science **273:** 109–112.
8. PEARSON, T.C., D.Z. ALEXANDER, R. HENDRIX, *et al.* 1996. CTLA4-Ig plus bone marrow induces long-term allograft survival and donor-specific unresponsiveness in the murine model. Evidence for hematopoietic chimerism. Transplantation **61:** 997–1004.
9. EFRAT, S., S. LINDE, H. KOFOD, *et al.* 1988. Beta-cell lines derived from transgenic mice expressing a hybrid insulin gene-oncogene. Proc. Natl. Acad. Sci. USA **85:** 9037–9041.
10. D'AMBRA, R., M. SURANA, S. EFRAT, *et al.* 1990. Regulation of insulin secretion from β-cell lines derived from transgenic mice insulinomas resembles that of normal β-cells. Endocrinology **126:** 2815–2822.
11. EFRAT, S., M. LEISER, M. SURANA, *et al.* 1993. Murine insulinoma cell line with normal glucose-regulated insulin secretion. Diabetes **42:** 901–907.
12. KNAACK, D., D.M. FIORE, M. SURANA, *et al.* 1994. Clonal insulinoma cell line which stably maintains correct glucose responsiveness. Diabetes **43:** 1413–1417.
13. GOSSEN, M. & H. BUJARD. 1992. Tight control of gene expression in mammalian cells by tetracycline-responsive promoters. Proc. Natl. Acad. Sci. USA **89:** 5547–5551.
14. EFRAT, S., D. FUSCO-DEMANE, H. LEMBERG, *et al.* 1995. Conditional transformation of a pancreatic β-cell line derived from transgenic mice expressing a tetracycline-regulated oncogene. Proc. Natl. Acad. Sci. USA **92:** 3576–3580.
15. FLEISCHER, N., C. CHEN, M. SURANA, *et al.* 1998. Functional analysis of a conditionally-transformed pancreatic β-cell line. Diabetes **47:** 1419–1425.
16. GOSSEN, M., S. FREUNDLIEB, G. BENDER, *et al.* 1995. Transcriptional activation by tetracyclines in mammalian cells. Science **268:** 1766–1769.
17. WOLD, W.S.M. & L.R. GOODING. 1991. Region E3 of adenovirus: a cassette of genes involved in host immunosurveillance and virus-cell interactions. Virology **184:** 1–8.

18. WOLD, W.S.M. 1993. Adenovirus genes that modulate the sensitivity of virus-infected cells to lysis by TNF. J. Cell. Biochem. **53:** 329–335.
19. EFRAT, S., G. FEJER, M. BROWNLEE, *et al.* 1995. Prolonged survival of murine pancreatic islet allografts mediated by adenovirus early region 3 immunoregulatory transgenes. Proc. Natl. Acad. Sci. USA **92:** 6947–6951.
20. COX, J.H., J.W. YEWDELL, L.C. EISENLOHR, *et al.* 1990. Antigen presentation requires transport of MHC class I molecules from the endoplasmic reticulum. Science **247:** 715–718.
21. BEIER, D.C., J.H. COX, D.R. VINING, *et al.* 1994. Association of human class I MHC alleles with the adenovirus E3/19K protein. J. Immunol. **152:** 3862–3872.
22. WANG, S., G. BEATTIE, M. MALLY, *et al.* 1997. Isolation and characterization of a cell line from the epithelial cells of the human fetal pancreas. Cell Transplant **6:** 59–67.

# Re-engineering the Functions of a Terminally Differentiated Epithelial Cell *in Vivo*

BRUCE J. BAUM,[a,d] SONGLIN WANG,[a] EDNA CUKIERMAN,[b]
CHRISTINE DELPORTE,[a] HIDEAKI KAGAMI,[a] YITZHAK MARMARY,[a]
PHILIP C. FOX,[a] DAVID J. MOONEY,[c] AND KENNETH M. YAMADA[b]

[a]*Gene Therapy and Therapeutics Branch and* [b]*Craniofacial Developmental Biology and Regeneration Branch, National Institute of Dental and Craniofacial Research, National Institutes of Health, Bethesda, Maryland 20892, USA*

[c]*Department of Chemical Engineering, University of Michigan, Ann Arbor, Michigan 48109–2136, USA*

**ABSTRACT: Because of their easy access, and important role in oral homeostasis, mammalian salivary glands provide a unique site for addressing key issues and problems in tissue engineering. This manuscript reviews studies by us in three major directions involving re-engineering functions of salivary epithelial cells. Using adenoviral-mediated gene transfer *in vivo*, we show approaches to i) repair damaged, hypofunctional glands and ii) redesign secretory functions to include endocrine as well as exocrine pathways. The third series of studies show our general approach to develop an artificial salivary gland for clinical situations in which all glandular tissue has been lost.**

## INTRODUCTION

An age-old clinical axiom states that the mouth is the gateway to the body. Indeed, many systemic diseases present with clinical signs easily recognizable in the open mouth.[1] Analogously, the mouth provides several advantages for the applied scientist or clinician interested in tissue engineering, but none is more important than ease of access.

For many years, we have been studying mechanisms by which salivary glands produce their secretions.[2,3] Salivary glands have provided a valuable experimental model for generations of scientists interested in neurofunctional controls, from Claude Bernard and Ivan Pavlov to the present day. They are highly responsive epithelial tissues whose function can be readily and non-invasively measured.[4,5]

In humans there are three major pairs of salivary glands (parotid, submandibular, and sublingual). These glands consist almost entirely of well-differentiated epithelial cells that exist as a monolayer bordering on an extensively arborized lumen.[6] Each of these major glands has a direct exit into the mouth through a single main excretory duct. Thus, from an open mouth the cannulation of the duct orifice, a procedure which in humans requires no anesthesia, affords direct access to the luminal membrane of virtually every epithelial cell in this secretory tissue. It is our belief that

[d]Author for correspondence: GTTB, NIDCR, NIH, 10 Center Drive, MSC 1190, Building 10, Room 1N113, Bethesda, MD 20892; 301-496-1363 (voice); 301-402-1228 (fax); bruce_j_baum@nih.gov (e-mail).

this situation provides a valuable model for addressing several important issues in tissue engineering. In this manuscript we will review results from two distinct areas of our tissue-engineering studies: i) the *in vivo* repair of salivary glands considered to be irreversibly damaged owing to irradiation and ii) the *in vivo* redesign of salivary glands to function in an endocrine capacity. Additionally, we will describe very new efforts in a third direction, the replacement of destroyed glands with a "first generation" artificial salivary gland.

## GENERAL APPROACH

Our studies directed at *in vivo* re-engineering of salivary epithelial cells (i.e., for repair or redesign of function) have utilized replication-deficient recombinant adenoviruses to transfer genes into the target cells. After introduction of recombinant adenoviruses to the glands via intraductal delivery through the excretory duct orifice, these vectors readily infect both ductal and acinar cells in rodent glands, typically resulting in ~20–30% of the cells transduced.[7,8] While adenoviral vectors are extremely efficient at transferring genes to, and thus changing the phenotype of, a salivary cell *in vivo*, they are not without negative features. The two most significant drawbacks of recombinant adenoviral vectors are i) their inability to integrate their DNA into the host cell chromosome and ii) their induction of a potent immune response involving innate, cellular and humoral immunity.[9,10] As in other parenchymal tissues, the consequence of these drawbacks in salivary glands is the quite transient expression of the transgene.[11,12] Nonetheless, recombinant adenoviral vectors are extremely useful for proof of principle experiments.

Our studies directed at the replacement of destroyed gland tissue utilize more traditional tissue-engineering concepts.[13] Our goal is to create a functional new tissue using allogeneic graft cells grown and appropriately organized on a suitable biocompatible substratum.

## *IN VIVO* GLAND REPAIR

Each year in the U.S. ~30,000 individuals undergo therapeutic ionizing radiation to their salivary glands during radiation therapy for head and neck maligancies.[14] Acinar cells, the fluid-, salt- and protein-secretory cell type in the glands, are most sensitive to radiation and are readily destroyed.[15] Patients whose salivary glands are thus rendered hypofunctional suffer from rampant dental caries (decay), frequent mucosal infections (such as oral Candidiasis), dysphagia (swallowing difficulties), as well as considerable pain and discomfort. At present, there is no conventional effective therapy for this condition.

Several years ago, we began examining a strategy which sought to convert the irradiation-surviving absorptive ductal epithelial cells into a secretory, water-permeable phenotype. We hypothesized that remaining ductal epithelial cells would be capable of generating a $KHCO_3$-rich fluid, in the absence of acinar cells, if they are transduced with (and express) a gene encoding a facilitated water permeability pathway, a water channel.[16] We chose to test this hypothesis by constructing a recombi-

**TABLE 1.** Effect of AdhAQP1 on fluid secretion from irradiated rat submandibular glands[a]

| Treatment | Saliva Flow (μl/100g body weight in 15 min) ± SEM |
|---|---|
| Sham IR + Addl312 | 36.6 ± 6.8 (4) |
| IR + Addl312 | 12.2 ± 3.7 (6) |
| IR + AdhAQP1 | 30.6 ± 3.5 (9) |

[a]Data modified from presentation in Delporte *et al.*[16] IR = 21 Gy irradiation. Addl312 is a control virus encoding no transgene while AdhAQP1 encodes human AQP1. Numbers in parentheses = number of animals studied. Irradiation (or sham treatment) was performed and 4 months later the indicated virus was administered to the submandibular glands. Saliva was collected 3 days later.

nant, type 5 adenovirus encoding aquaporin-1 (AQP1).[16] AQP1 is the archetypal mammalian water channel and generally exists in a non-polarized distribution about the plasma membrane.[17] The pivotal experiment tested the ability of the recombinant virus, termed AdhAQP1, to enhance fluid secretion from rat submandibular glands which had been exposed 4 months earlier to 21 Gy X-irradiation (TABLE 1). Animals receiving a control virus showed ~65% reduction in salivary flow rates when compared to animals that had been sham-irradiated. However, animals receiving AdhAQP1 after irradiation secreted saliva at control levels.[16] Furthermore, the saliva secreted was significantly higher in [$K^+$] than control saliva, consistent with our hypothesized secretory mechanism.

These results provide considerable encouragement towards the possible utility of this approach for the effective clinical treatment of patients with radiation-induced salivary hypofunction. Further, the data are suggestive of the possible re-engineering of a cellular phenotype *in vivo* from a non-fluid secreting to a fluid secreting phenotype. Our recent work suggests that near maximal, osmotically obligated transepithelial water movement can be realized at low levels of cellular transduction, at least in an *in vitro* model system.[18] While this general approach, utilizing adenoviral-mediated gene transfer, is not yet ready for clinical use (especially because of the transient expression as described above), we believe it represents a significant achievement. Currently, we are examining the safety and efficacy of the strategy in a non-human primate model.

## *IN VIVO* GLAND REDESIGN

For much of this century, there have been reports suggesting that salivary glands were capable of secreting in an endocrine (directly to the bloodstream) as well as exocrine (saliva to the mouth) manner.[19,20] While this is not a widely accepted view, physiologically, if true it would offer many significant therapeutic opportunities using gene transfer.[21] We directly tested the ability of rat salivary glands to secrete a foreign transgene product, human α1-antitrypsin (hα1AT), a secretory protein made in the liver, into the bloodstream. We administered a recombinant adenovirus, AdMLPhα1AT, to adult rats and measured hα1AT levels in serum, saliva, and gland extracts.[22] We detected hα1AT in all compartments for 4–7 days. On day 4, peak lev-

**TABLE 2.** Levels of h$\alpha$1AT in serum from rat submandibular gland arterial and venous blood after administration of AdMLPh$\alpha$1AT[a]

| Sample | h$\alpha$1AT (ng/ml) |
|---|---|
| Carotid Artery | 19.4 ± 10.6 |
| Submandibular Vein | 67.9 ± 27.2 |

[a]Data modified from presentation in Kagami *et al.*[22] These represent results (mean ± SEM) obtained with 7 animals whose right carotid arteries and submandibular veins were sampled 24 hours after admistration of AdMLPh$\alpha$1AT ($5 \times 10^9$ pfu) to the right submandibular gland. The range of h$\alpha$1AT levels in sera from carotid arteries was 0–70.7 ng/ml, while for sera from submandibular veins the levels were 5.5–223.4 ng/ml. In each of the 7 animals, the venous level of h$\alpha$1AT was greater than the arterial level.

els achieved were ~5 ng/ml (serum), ~70 ng/ml (saliva), and ~10 ng/mg protein (gland extract). Furthermore, we were able to show that the concentration of h$\alpha$1AT in venous blood exiting the gland was consistently higher than that in arterial blood entering the gland (TABLE 2). These studies unequivocally demonstrated that h$\alpha$1AT could be secreted in an endocrine manner from rat salivary glands.[22]

The h$\alpha$1AT studies did not, however, demonstrate that the transgene product secreted from the glands was functional systemically. Recently, we showed that this was possible using a different recombinant virus, AdCMVhGH, encoding human growth hormone (hGH).[21] Effective therapeutic levels of GH are ~5 ng/ml in serum, comparable to what was achieved with h$\alpha$1AT. Importantly, hGH can bind to, and activate, rodent GH receptors. Forty-eight hours after intraductal administration of AdCMVhGH to rat submandibular glands, serum hGH levels were ~16 ng/ml versus background levels of ~1 ng/ml seen in control rats. We also observed a concomitant increase in serum insulin-like growth factor levels (~33%), serum triglycerides (~twofold), and the serum BUN/creatinine ratio (~35%) indicating the hGH secreted from the salivary glands was physiologically functional and systemically active.

These aggregate results strongly support the notion that salivary glands may provide a useful target site for the therapeutic delivery of transgene products for systemic use. This view also has been supported by the recent studies of Goldfine *et al.*[23] Following the retrograde instillation of plasmid DNA into salivary glands, they observed measurable levels of endocrine hormones in rat serum. Although not yet demonstrated clearly, there appears to be a constitutive secretory routing pathway to the bloodstream in glandular epithelial cells. However, our studies with h$\alpha$1AT show that a transgene product can be secreted simultaneously by both the exocrine (saliva) and endocrine (serum) pathways. Currently, we are attempting to determine if there are protein-based sorting signals which we can utilize to direct a transgene product preferentially into one or the other pathway.

## AN ARTIFICIAL SALIVARY GLAND?

There are many patients who effectively have lost all functional salivary epithelium, both acinar and ductal, and experience severe salivary hypofunction. These include many irradiated patients (above) as well as individuals with Primary Sjögren's

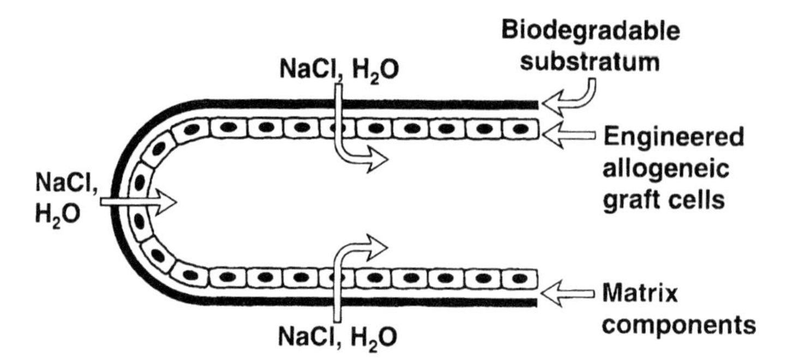


**FIGURE 1.** Schematic depiction of a first generation artificial salivary gland constructed as a blind-end tube. The design requirements for such a device include i) a porous, slowly biodegradable substratum; ii) matrix components (peptides or macromolecules) that promote formation of a polarized epithelial cell monolayer; iii) allogeneic epithelial cells genetically engineered to secrete water and salt unidirectionally; and iv) an overall form easily implantable in the buccal mucosal with an "exit" to the oral cavity. See text for additional detail.

syndrome, an autoimmune exocrinopathy. In the absence of any glandular epithelial tissue to manipulate by gene transfer, an alternative patient management strategy is needed. Although it is possible to transplant mammalian salivary glands,[24] this option would likely prove to be clinically inadequate because of an insufficient donor supply, the continuous need for immunosuppression, as well as the surgical difficulty. Using well-accepted tissue-engineering principles,[13] we are exploring the development of an orally implantable, artificial fluid-secreting device, a "first-generation" artificial salivary gland (FIG. 1).

The initial device which we have envisioned would consist of a blind-end tube made of a salt and water-permeable, somewhat porous, slowly biodegradable substrate. Previously, while investigating an approach to engineer intestinal tissue, Mooney *et al.* reported the construction of a tubular and biodegradable substrate which promoted vascularization following implantation.[25] This type of substrate could be engineered to contain suitable matrix components necessary to promote the polarization, growth and organizational behavior of allogeneic graft cells. The graft cells would be genetically engineered to be capable of unidirectional salt and water movement in response to autonomic neurotransmitter stimulation.[3]

Since native salivary epithelia exist essentially as a monolayer lining a lumen,[6] the substrate ideally should induce the polarized cells to form a monolayer affording complete coverage of its internal surface. Such a device also should be small enough to implant conveniently into the buccal mucosa with a maintained intra-oral exit.

Much of our initial effort has focused on the allogeneic graft cell. We have chosen to use a human submandibular gland cell line, termed HSG.[26] The phenotype of these cells is known to be highly responsive to different extracellular matrix components.[27–29] Further, they are useful targets for gene transfer methods[7] and can utilize established salivary gland cell-specific promoter elements.[30] Clearly, much additional work is needed before such an artificial fluid-secreting device can be realized, but we believe that it is conceptually feasible.

## SUMMARY

This manuscript has provided an overview of three directions for our tissue-engineering studies using salivary glands as a model tissue. While salivary glands are not often considered in tissue-engineering efforts, they present an inviting target because of their easy access and organizational structure. Additionally, salivary glands suffer significant clinical disease for which there is no effective conventional therapy available. We believe that the spectrum of studies reviewed herein demonstrate salivary glands are valuable models to address key issues and problems in tissue engineering.

## ACKNOWLEDGMENTS

We wish to thank our many excellent colleagues who have contributed to the concepts and efforts described herein.

## REFERENCES

1. BRICKER, S.L., R. P. LANGLAIS & C.S. MILLER, Eds. 1994 Oral Diagnosis, Oral Medicine and Treatment Planning. Lea & Febiger. Philadelphia, PA.
2. BAUM, B.J., I.S. AMBUDKAR, J. HELMAN, V.J. HORN, J.E. MELVIN, L.M. MERTZ & R. J. TURNER. 1990. Dispersed salivary gland acinar cell preparations for use in studies of neuroreceptor-coupled secretory events. Methods Enzymol. **192:** 26–37.
3. BAUM, B.J, 1993. Principles of saliva secretion. Ann. N.Y. Acad. Sci. **694:**17–23.
4. YOUNG, J.A. & E.W. VAN LENNEP. 1979. Secretion of salivary and salt glands. *In* Membrane Transport in Biology, Vol 4: 563–674. B. G. Giebisch, D.C. Tosteson & H.H. Ussing, Eds. Springer-Verlag. Berlin/New York.
5. MANDEL, I.D. 1989. The role of saliva in maintaining oral homeostasis. J. Am. Dent. Assoc. **119:** 298–304.
6. COOK, D.I., E.W. VAN LENNEP, M.L. ROBERTS & J.A. YOUNG. 1994. Secretion by the major salivary glands. *In* Physiology of the Gastrointestinal Tract. L.R. Johnson, Ed.: 1061–1117. Raven. New York.
7. MASTRANGELI, A., B.C. O'CONNELL, W. ALADIB, P.C. FOX, B.J. BAUM & R.G. CRYSTAL. 1994. Direct in vivo adenovirus-mediated gene transfer to salivary glands. Am. J. Physiol. **266:** G1146–G1155.
8. DELPORTE, C., R.S. REDMAN & B.J. BAUM. 1997. Relationship between the cellular distribution of the $\alpha_v\beta_{3/5}$ integrins and adenoviral infection in salivary glands. Lab. Invest. **77:** 167–173.
9. KOZARSKY, K.F. & J. M. WILSON. 1993. Gene therapy: adenovirus vectors. Curr. Opin. Genetics Develop. **3:** 499–503.
10. BRAMSON, J.L., F.L. GRAHAM & J. GAULDIE. 1995. The use of adenoviral vectors for gene therapy and gene transfer in vivo. Curr. Opin. Biotechnol. **6:** 590–595.
11. ADESANYA, M.R., R.S. REDMAN, B.J. BAUM & B.C. O'CONNELL. 1996. Immediate inflammatory responses to adenovirus-mediated gene transfer in rat salivary glands. Hum. Gene Ther. **7:** 1085–1093.
12. KAGAMI, H., J.C. ATKINSON, S.M. MICHALEK, B. HANDELMAN, S. YU, B.J. BAUM & B.C. O'CONNELL. 1998. Repetitive adenovirus administration to the parotid gland: role of immunological barriers and induction of oral tolerance. Hum. Gene Ther. **9:** 305–313.
13. MOONEY, D.J. & J.A. ROWLY. 1997. Tissue engineering: integrating cells and materials to create functional tissue replacements. *In* Controlled Drug Delivery. K. Park, Ed.: 333–346. ACS Books. Washington, DC.

14. SILVERMAN, S. JR. 1992. Precancerous lesions and oral cancer in the elderly. Clin. Geriatric Med. **8:** 529–541.
15. KASHIMA, H.K., W.R. KIRKHAM & J.R. ANDREWS. 1965. Postradiation sialadenitis. A study of the clinical features, histopathologic changes and serum enzyme variations following irradiation of human salivary glands. Am. J. Roentgenol. Radium Ther. Nucl. Med. **94:** 271–291.
16. DELPORTE, C., B.C. O'CONNELL, X. HE, H.E. LANCASTER, A.C. O'CONNELL, P. AGRE & B.J. BAUM. 1997. Increased fluid secretion after adenoviral-mediated transfer of the aquaporin-1 cDNA to irradiated rat salivary glands. Proc. Natl. Acad. Sci. USA **94:** 3268–3273.
17. PRESTON, G.M. & P. AGRE. 1991. Isolation of the cDNA for erythrocyte integral membrane protein of 28 kilodaltons: member of an ancient channel family. Proc. Natl. Acad. Sci. USA **88:** 11110–11114.
18. DELPORTE, C., A.T.M.S. HOQUE, J.A. KULAKUSKY, V.R. BRADDON, C.M. GOLDSMITH, R.B. WELLNER & B.J. BAUM, 1998. Relationship between adenovirus-mediated aquaporin-1 expression and fluid movement across epithelial cells. Biochem. Biophys. Res. Commun. **246:** 584–588.
19. LAWRENCE, A.M., S. TAN, S. HOJVAT & L. KIRSTEINS. 1977. Salivary gland hyperglycemic factor: an extrapancreatic source of glucagon-like material. Science **195:** 70–72.
20. TIECHE, J.M., J. LEONORA & R.R. STEINMAN. 1980. Isolation and partial characterization of a porcine parotid hormone that stimulates dentinal fluid transport. Endocrinology **106:** 1994–2004.
21. HE, X., C.M. GOLDSMITH, Y. MARMARY, R.B. WELLNER, A.F. PARLOW, L.K. NIEMAN & B.J. BAUM. 1998. Systemic action of human growth hormone following adenovirus-mediated gene transfer to rat submandibular glands. Gene Ther. **5:** 537–541.
22. KAGAMI, H., B.C. O'CONNELL & B.J. BAUM. 1996. Evidence for the systemic delivery of a transgene product from salivary glands. Hum. Gene Ther. **7:** 2177–2184.
23. GOLDFINE, I.D., M.S. GERMAN, H.-C. TSENG, J. WANG, J.L. BOLAFFI, J.-W. CHEN, D.C. OLSON & S.S. ROTHMAN. 1997. The endocrine secretion of human insulin and growth hormone by exocrine glands of the gastrointestinal tract. Nature Biotechnol. **15:** 1378–1382.
24. EID, A., D.W. NITZAN, E. SHILONI, A. NEUMAN & Y. MARMARY. 1997. Salivary gland transplantation: a canine model. Transplantation **64:** 679–683.
25. MOONEY, D.J., G. ORGAN, J.P. VACANTI & R. LANGER. 1994. Design and fabrication of cell delivery devices to engineer tubular tissues. Cell Transplant. **3:** 203–210.
26. SHIRASUNA, K., M. SATO & T. MIYAZAKI. 1981. A neoplastic epithelial duct cell line established from an irradiated human salivary gland. Cancer **48:** 745–752.
27. ROYCE, L.S., M.C. KIBBEY, P. MERTZ, H.K. KLEINMAN & B.J. BAUM. 1993. Human neoplastic submandibular intercalated duct cells express an acinar phenotype when cultured on a basement membrane matrix. Differentiation **52:** 247–255.
28. HOFFMAN, M.P., M.C. KIBBEY, J.J. LETTERIO & H.K. KLEINMAN. 1996. Role of laminin-1 and TGF-beta 3 in acinar differentiation of a human submandibular gland cell line (HSG). J. Cell Sci. **109:** 2013–2021.
29. LAFRENIE, R.M., S.M. BERNIER & K.M. YAMADA. 1997. Adhesion to fibronectin or collagen I gel induces rapid, extensive biosynthetic alternations in epithelial cells. J. Cell. Physiol. **175:** 163–173.
30. ZHENG, C., M.P. HOFFMAN, T. MCMILLAN, H.K. KLEINMAN & B.C. O'CONNELL. 1998. Growth factor regulation of the amylase promoter in differentiating salivary gland acinar cells. J. Cell. Physiol. **177:** 628–635.

# Reverse Engineering of Bioadhesion in Marine Mussels

J. HERBERT WAITE[a]

*Marine Biology/Biochemstry Program, University of Delaware, Newark, Delaware USA*

**ABSTRACT: Marine mussels (*Mytilus*) are experts at bonding to a variety of solid surfaces in a wet, saline and turbulent environment. Bonding is rapid, permanent, versatile and protein-based. In mussels, adhesive bonding takes the form of a byssus—a bundle of extracorporeal threads—each connected to living tissues of the animal at one end and secured by an adhesive plaque at the other. We have investigated the composition and formation of byssal plaques and threads with the hope of discovering technologically relevant innovations in chemistry and materials science. All proteins isolated from the byssus to date share the quality of containing the unusual amino acid, 3,4-dihydroxyphenylalanine. This residue appears to have a dual functionality with significant consequences for adsorption and cohesion. On the one hand, it forms a diverse array of weaker molecular interactions such as metal chelates, H-bonds, and π-cations: these appear to dominate in surface behavior (adsorption). On the other hand, 3,4-dihydroxyphenylalanine and its redox couple, dopaquinone, can mediate formation of covalent cross-links among byssal proteins (cohesion). One of the challenges in making functional biomimetic versions of byssal adhesion is to understand how these two reactivities are balanced.**

## INTRODUCTION

For organisms inhabiting wave-swept environments in the sea, a strong and environmentally resilient attachment offers adaptive advantages for survival. It may also offer valuable technological insights for improving bonding practices in the presence of water. A closer examination of intertidal rock surfaces reveals a variety of sessile organisms including barnacles, oysters, mussels, limpets, tube polychaetes, and macroalgae. What makes the adhesive strategies of these organisms interesting is that they are opportunistic and bond to almost any available hard wet surface. This includes, for example, mineral, paraffin, polyacrylate, Teflon, steel, glass, tooth, and bone.[1] Bonding strengths range from 0.1 to $10 \times 10^6$ $Nm^{-2}$ depending on the substratum among other factors.

The adhesive strategy of marine mussels *Mytilus edulis* is hardly representative of all the others, but it does provide a particularly good model system for studying opportunistic adhesion.[2] Mussels attach to wet surfaces by making a byssus, which is an extracorporeal bundle of tiny tendons that are attached distally to a foreign substratum and proximally by insertion of the stem root into the byssal retractor muscles

[a]Current address: Marine Science Institute, MCD Biology Department, University of California at Santa Barbara, Santa Barbara, CA 93106; 805-893-7998 ( fax); waite@lifesci.ucsb.edu (e-mail).

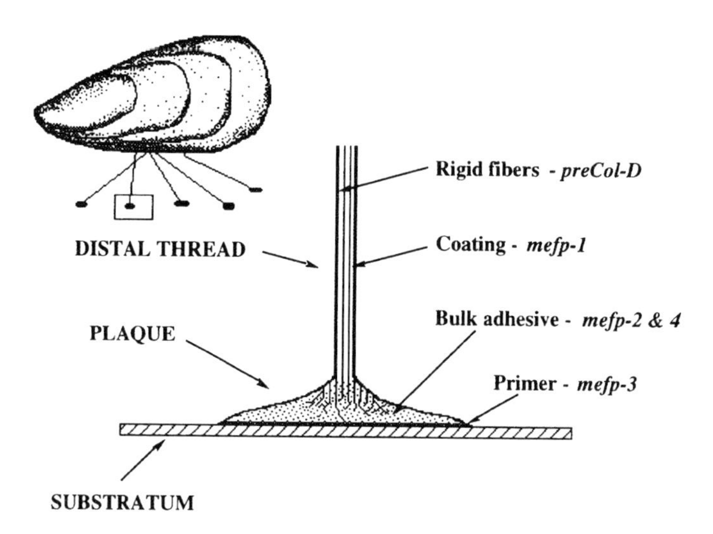


**FIGURE 1.** Cartoon of a marine mussel (inset, *upper left*) attached by way of a byssus, one plaque of which is enlarged to show morphological nomenclature (*left*) and proposed protein distribution (*right*).

(FIG. 1). There is much that is extraordinary about the properties and composition of byssal threads, but the focus of this report will be limited to the adhesive plaques.

Byssal adhesive plaques have diameters of 2–3 mm and, except where the plaque meets the thread, a thickness of 0.15 mm or less. Transmission electron microscopy of plaque sections reveals structures that resemble microcellular solids with closed cell diameters of 1–3 μm and trabecular walls of 50 nm thickness.[3] Presumably this structure is formed by a phase inversion of a dispersion of protein precursors in sea water; however, details of the process remain speculative. The plaque surface facing the sea water is coated with a protective lacquer or cuticle about 10 μm thick. The plaque substrate-interface in sectionned materials, in contrast, is composed of a continuous trabecular sheet that is indistinguishable from the microcellular interior of the plaque.

Chemical characterization of byssal plaques has been hampered by the almost complete insolubilization that accompanies maturation. Recent progress in retarding the "curing" or cross-linking of plaques has allowed greater recovery and identification of plaque precursor proteins.[4] These are usually extracted from plaques by trituration in 5% (v/v) acetic acid with 8 M urea. Four polymorphic protein families and one collagen have been detected following acid-urea polyacrylamide gel electrophoresis. These are summarized in TABLE 1. Note that all share the redox functional group, 3,4-dihydroxyphenyl-L-alanine (DOPA). The enzyme-catalyzed oxidation of DOPA to peptidyl dopaquinone undoubtedly leads to curing but the precise reaction pathways are not yet known.[5]

**TABLE 1.** A comparison of the redox-active proteins in the adhesive plaques and foot of *Mytilus edulis*

| Protein | Mass (kDa) | DOPA (mol%) | Repeat Unit (freq) | Cachet[a] |
|---|---|---|---|---|
| mefp-1 | 110 | 10–15 | AK**P**S**YPP**T**Y**K (80) | 4-Hydroxyproline<br>3,4-Dihydroxyproline |
| mefp-2 | 40 | 2–3 | EGF motif (11) | Cystine |
| mefp-3 | 6 | 20–25 | none | 4-Hydroxyarginine<br>Tryptophan |
| mefp-4 | 80 | 3–4 | ? | Histidine |
| preCol-D | 80 | <0.1 | Gly-X-Y | Silk-domains |

[a]Cachet denotes a quality that distinguishes each mefp from the others.

## PROTEINS OF THE PLAQUE

Most plaque proteins follow a simple nomenclature in which the first two letters denote the species of mussel (e.g., Me for *Mytilus edulis*) to which is added fp for foot protein. Mefp-2 is the most abundant plaque protein (up to 40% by weight). Its complete primary structure was first elucidated in *M. galloprovincialis* by Inoue *et al.*[6] using partial peptide sequence maps from *M. edulis*[7] and shown to consist of 11 tandem repeats of an epidermal growth factor (EGF) motif sandwiched between acidic and DOPA-enriched N- and C- termini, e.g.,

x x **N** x **C** x **P N P C K N** x **G** x **C** – – x x x **G** x x x **Y** x **C** x **C** x x **G Y** x **G** x x **C**

where bold letters represent conserved residues, x is any amino acid, and – denotes a gap. Since Cys (**C**) residues are completely conserved in this structure, EGF homology is likely to extend to disulfide pairing thus predicting that each repeat motif is, like EGF, internally stabilized by three pairs of disulfide bonds. These may, however, undergo some randomization following reduction and interfacial denaturation. Indeed, disulfide randomization is believed to contribute to foam stability in a variety of food proteins.[8] Polyphenols such as DOPA also enhance foam stabilization.[9]

Mefp-1 is the largest of the plaque precursors and not, in fact, limited to the plaques.[10] The latter finding was paradoxical because mefp-1 was shown to be strongly adhesive *in vitro*; moreover, its commercial utility as a cell and tissue culture adhesive (BioGlue, Sigma) contibuted to the popular notion that it was "the" plaque adhesive. The dominant feature of mefp-1 is a tandemly repeated decapeptide with up to 80 repeats:[10]

[AK**P**S**YPP**T**Y**K]$_{80}$

This repeat is highly basic and hydrophilic with a 20% occurrence of trans-4-hydroxyproline (**P**) and 10% *trans*-2,3-*cis*-3,4-dihydroxyproline (**P**).[11] DOPA (**Y**) occurs as often as twice per repeat and probably contributes to quinone cross-linking as well as the high affinity complexation of Fe (III), i.e., log stability constant >39 at pH 7.5 and 20°C.[12] Fifty to 75 ferric ions can be bound per molecule of mefp-1 *in vitro.*[13] An ironclad byssus may be an adaptation to improve durability and resistance to degradation. Other transition metals may be equally well-bound.

Mefp-3 is the smallest of the plaque proteins and has the highest DOPA (**Y**) content in mole %. Mefp-3 is also arginine-rich and many of these residues are modified to 4-hydroxy-L-arginine (**R**). At least 10 electrophoretic variants of mefp-3 can be detected in individual mussels; only one of these, variant F, has been completely sequenced:[4]

AD**YY**GPN**Y**GPP**RRY**GGGN**Y**N**RY**NG**Y**GGG**RRY**GG**Y**KGWNNGWN**R**G**RR**GK**Y**W

Other studies[14] including unpublished results in this lab predict eighteen additional variant sequences (mature protein mass range 5–7 kD) from the cDNA of a single mussel. All variants share a conserved N-terminus and an overall composition that is dominated by G, N, **Y**, and **R**.

Mefp-4 belongs to a family of proteins with a mass range of 70–80 kD. All have a common N-terminus and contain elevated levels of glycine, arginine and histidine. DOPA occurs at about 5 mol %. This molecule may contain tandemly repeated tyrosine-rich octapeptides.[4]

The fifth major plaque protein, preCol-D, is actually the predominant molecular species in the distal portion of each byssal thread. Because the tensile elements of the threads are "rooted" in the cellular solid of the plaque,[3] a considerable amount of collagen in the form of preCol-D occurs in plaques. PreCols have a unique block copolymer structure. They are trimeric in which the central domain forms a collagen triple helix representing more than 50% of the mass.[15] Arrayed on either side of this are the silk-like domains that contain polyalanine runs punctuated by GGX sequences that resemble spider dragline silk proteins. The DOPA residues are located exclusively at the N- and C-termini in the His-rich domains. The mechanism of fiber formation by preCols is not known for certain, but one model has been proposed based on available evidence.[16]

## CURING PLAQUE PROTEINS

The debate about the mechanism of DOPA-protein curing in the byssus is a longstanding one. Many researchers have favored quinone-tanning as the basis for curing,[5,17,18] but this suffers from a lack of direct evidence. There is no doubt that byssal attachment strength increases with maturation,[19] that peptidyl-DOPA residues of the mefps are enzymatically oxidized to peptidyl-quinones, and that the quinones are involved in cross-link formation *in vitro*. The latter is particularly well-illustrated by the data in FIGURE 2. Here, an mefp-1-derived decapeptide, AKPSY<u>**P**</u>**PY**K ($MH^+$ 1200.3), has been oxidized by catecholoxidase. Following a 1-hour incubation, the abundance of parent peptide is reduced giving rise instead to a family of multimers up to octamers (8X). Since molecular interactions weaker than covalent bonds are labile to the conditions of MALDI TOF, the multimer formation must be mediated by quinone-derived cross-links (scheme A).

R / OH / OH —Catechol oxidase→ R / O / O ——→ Cross-linking

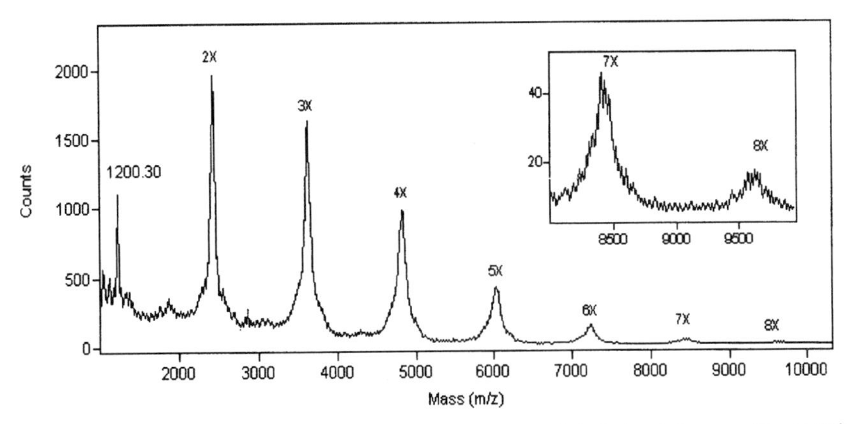


**FIGURE 2.** Enzymatic cross-linking of a tryptic mefp1-derived decapeptide ($MH^+$ =1200.3) as detected by MALDI-TOF mass spectrometry. *Enzyme*: Sigma catecholoxidase (weight ratio E:S = 1:20); *Buffer*: 0.1 M phosphate pH 7.5; *Temperature*: 20°C; *Time*: 60 min.

However, identification of quinone-derived cross-links and a connection between these and tensile strength in byssus await confirmation. Michael-type addition products between DOPA and lysine or histidine are well-characterized in other proteins,[21,22] as are polyphenolic coupling reactions.[5,22] Solid-state REDOR NMR analyses of $^{13}C$, $^{2}H$, and $^{15}N$-labeled byssal plaques detected few if any nucleophilic adducts or phenolic coupling products.[23,24] However, the byssal threads and plaques analyzed in these studies were taken from mussels maintained in stationary sea water which probably shielded the secreted byssal threads from the normal flow or turbulence required for curing. Recent NMR analyses of *flow-stressed* byssal threads are showing a different picture. The diphenoxy label in the $^{13}C$ spectrum at 145 ppm has $^{2}H$ diphenoxy label nearby; this may suggest dismutative coupling between DOPA and DOPA-quinone residues (unpublished data).

In a study designed to model curing *in vitro*, mefp-1 adsorbed to highly oriented pyrolytic graphite was treated with catecholoxidase. Resistance of the film to displacement was measured by atomic force microscopy in contact mode.[25] Results indicate that catechol oxidase treatment enhances the resistance to displacement of adsorbed films of mefp-1 from about 20 nN to over 600 nN—a 30-fold increase! Since catecholoxidase catalyzes the formation of quinones from DOPA, the displacement resistance of mefp-1 probably reflects quinone-derived intermolecular cross-links between adsorbed mefp-1 molecules. The formation of cross-links across the protein-substratum interface are improbable.

## PROBING THE PLAQUE INTERFACE

The characterization of the major plaque proteins begs the ultimate adhesive question: How do byssal plaques adhere? Any attempt to describe the adhesive mechanism requires knowledge about the structure and distribution of proteins with-

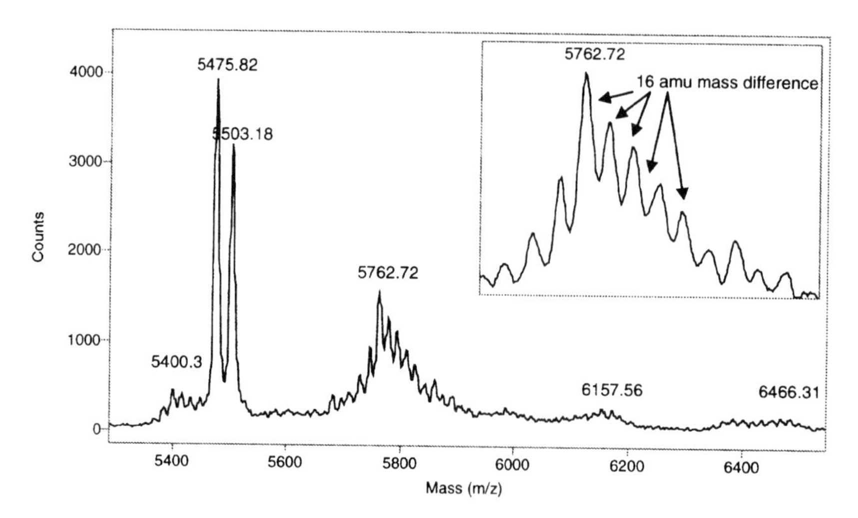


**FIGURE 3.** A MALDI TOF mass spectrogram of the underside (interface) of a freshly secreted byssal adhesive plaque removed from a stainless steel substratum. The plaque was prepared with sinapinic acid as matrix and irradiated at 330 nm at a laser power of 2355. The peak clusters at M/z = 6466, 6157, 5762, 5400 etc. represent mefp-3 variants and exhibit different degrees of post-translational hydroxylation, i.e., peaks in each cluster are separated from one another by 16 daltons (inset M/z cluster at 5762).

in the plaques. The maturation of the plaque precursors by hydroxylation, oxidation, cross-linking and metal complexation reactions tends to modify or conceal the epitopes of the precursors and thus renders the results of an immunohistochemical approach inconclusive. Using specific polyclonal antibodies, for example, mefp-1 was shown to be distributed in the byssal cuticle and at the plaque-substratum interface.[26] While this is possible, it seems improbable that one protein would serve two rather different functions, i.e., a coating and adhesive. Clearly other approaches are necessary to dissect such ambiguities.

We have recently observed that plaques can be delaminated from smooth surfaces so that their bonding faces can be directly subjected to laser desorption.[27] Preliminary results using matrix-assisted laser desorption ionization mass spectrometry with time-of-flight in the mass range 1 to 100 kD suggest that mefp-3 is the only major protein species to desorb near the plaque-substratum interface (FIG. 3). Perhaps mefp-3 functions as an adhesive primer. Since individual mussels express as many as 20 different variants and only a fraction of these seem to be deposited on any given surface (unbublished results), the following question is appropriate: Are variants specifically selected for certain surfaces? This question is undergoing further scrutiny in our laboratory.

Of the remaining proteins, mefp-1 has been localized to the lacquer-like cuticle covering the outer surface of the plaque and byssus generally.[3,28] Here it must serve to protect underlying structural components from wear and microbial attack. By undergoing cross-linking and chelating large amounts of ferric ions, it is transformed into a very tough and dense finish. We suspect, but have yet to prove, that mefp-2

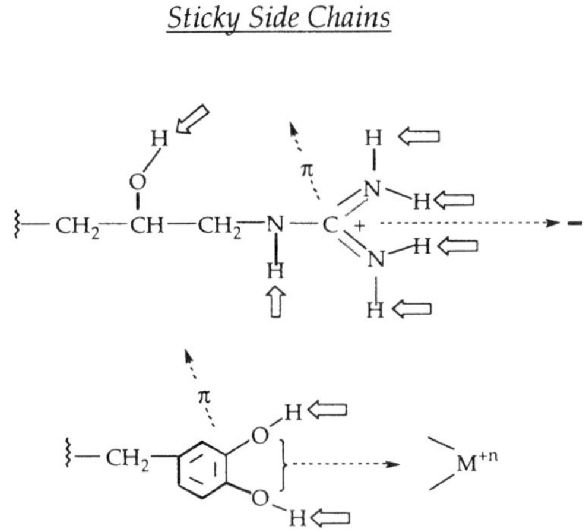

Sticky Side Chains

**FIGURE 4.** Summary of the potential interactions of two common functional groups in mefp-3. Hydroxyarginine (*top*) engages in 5 H-bonds, π-, and coulombic interactions, while DOPA can form H-bond, chelate, and π-interactions.

and -4 are located in the bulk adhesive of the plaque. Mefp distributions are tentatively summarized on the right-hand side of FIGURE 1.

## CHEMISTRY OF THE INTERFACE

Given the proteins involved, an adhesive interface rich in DOPA and basic residue side-chains seems inescapable. FIGURE 4 shows these key residues and the manifold interactions they are capable of participating in. DOPA engages in H-bonding, metal complexation, π-π and π-cation interactions. Hydroxyarginine (mefp-3) can form up to six H-bonds as well as π-π, π-cation and coulombic interactions. Such functionality is well-adapted for bonding to diverse polar surface types: organometallic complexes 13, 29 on metal and mineral surfaces; π-π and π-cation interactions on aromatic surfaces 30, and electrostatic interactions on surfaces with negative charges.

Unfortunately, none of these interactions suffice to explain the significant byssal adhesion on nonpolar surfaces. A recent test is noteworthy in this regard: An aqueous solution of mefp-3 was applied to a silicone release coating (Dow-Corning #3140) and dried. The strength of adsorption was measured by a standard peel test in the velocity range of 1–500 μm $sec^{-1}$. Peel force on the untreated release coating never exceeded 5 $Nm^{-1}$, whereas on release coating with preadsorbed mefp-3, it ranged from 100 to 300 $Nm^{-1}$.[31] XPS analysis of the surfaces suggested that mefp-3 was delaminated from the release coating; however, it contained significant amounts of Si. The latter is suggested to be derived from polydimethylsiloxane uprooted from the release coating. Thus, failure may actually be occurring within the silicone itself.

Intertidal marine invertebrates practice a variety of opportunistic adhesive strate gies that, if understood, may have profound philosophical and technological significance. Recent progress in the analysis of byssal adhesion in mussels suggests that at least four protein families are involved and that the mechanism of adhesion is chemically and structurally complex.

## ACKNOWLEDGMENTS

I thank the the National Institute of Dental Research (Biomaterials) and the U.S. Office of Naval Research for their support of this research.

## REFERENCES

1. WAITE, J.H. 1987. Nature's underwater adhesive specialist. Int. J. Adhesion & Adhesives **7:** 9–17.
2. WAITE, J.H. 1992. The formation of mussel byssus: anatomy of a natural manufacturing process. Results Probl. Cell Diff. **19:** 27
3. BENEDICT, C.V. & J.H. WAITE. 1986. Composition and ultrastructure of the byssus of *Mytilus edulis*. J. Morphol. **189:** 261–270.
4. PAPOV, V.V., T.V. DIAMOND, K. BIEMANN & J.H. WAITE. 1995. Hydroxyarginine-containing polyphenolic proteins in the adhesive plaques of the marine mussel *Mytilus edulis* J. Biol. Chem. **270:** 20183–20192.
5. WAITE, J.H. 1990. The phylogeny and chemical diversity of quinone tanned glues and varnishes. Comp. Biochem. Physiol. **97B:** 19–29.
6. INOUE, K., Y. TAKEUCHI, D. MIKI & S. ODO. 1995. Mussel adhesive plaque protein is a member of epidermal growth factor like gene family. J. Biol. Chem. **270:** 6698–6702.
7. RZEPECKI, L.M., K.M. MUELLER & J.H. WAITE. 1992. Chracterization of a cystine-rich polyphenolic protein family from the blue mussel *Mytilus edulis*. L. Biol. Bull. **183:** 123–133.
8. KITABATAKE, N. & E. DOI. 1987. Conformational change of hen egg ovalbumin during foam formation detected by 5,5′dithiobis(2-nitrobenzoic acid). J. Agric. Food Chem. **35:** 953–957.
9. SARKER, D.K., P.J. WILDE & D.C. CLARK. 1995. Control of surfactant induced destabilization of foams through polyphenol-mediated protein-protein interactions. J. Agric. Food Chem. **45:** 295–300.
10. LAURSEN, R. 1992. Reflections on the structure of mussel adhesive proteins. Results Probl. Cell Diff. **19:** 52–72.
11. TAYLOR, S.W., J.H. WAITE, M.M. ROSS, J. SHABANOWITZ & D.F. HUNT. 1994. *Trans* 2,3-*cis*-3,4-Dihydroxyproline in the tandemly repeated consensus decapeptides of an adhesive protein from *Mytilus edulis*. J. Am. Chem. Soc. **116:** 10803–10804.
12. TAYLOR, S.W., G.W. LUTHER & J.H. WAITE. 1994. Polarographic and spectrophotometric investigation of Fe (III) complexation to 3,4-dihydroxyphenylalanine-containing peptides and proteins from *Mytilus edulis*. Inorg. Chem. **33:** 5819–5824.
13. TAYLOR, S.W., D.B. CHASE, M.H. EMPTAGE, M.J. NELSON & J.H. WAITE. 1996. Ferric ion complexes of a DOPA-containing adhesive protein from *Mytilus edulis*. Inorg. Chem. **35:** 7572–7577.
14. INOUE, K., Y. TAKEUCHI, D. MIKI, S. ODO, S. HARAYAMA & J.H. WAITE. 1996. Cloning, sequencing, and sites of expression for the hydroxyarginine-containing plaque protein of the mussel *Mytilus galloprovincialis*. Eur. J. Biochem. **239:** 172-176.
15. QIN, X., K.J. COYNE & J.H. WAITE. 1997. Tough tendons: Mussel byssus has collagen with silk-like domains. J. Biol. Chem. **272:** 32623–32627.

16. QIN, X.X. & J.H. WAITE. 1998. A collagenous precursor that may mediate block copolymer gradients in mussel byssal threads. Proc. Nat. Acad. Sci. USA **95:** 10517–10522.
17. BROWN, C.H. 1950. Some structural proteins of *Mytilus edulis*. Quart. J. Microsc. Sci. **91:** 331-339.
18. PRYOR, M.G.M. 1962. Sclerotization. Comp. Biochem. **4:** 371–396.
19. DOLMER, P. & I. SVANE. 1994. Attachment and orientation of *Mytilus edulis* L. in flowing water. Ophelia **40:** 63–74.
20. WANG, S.X., M. MURE, K.F. MEDZIHRADSKY, A.L. BURLINGAME, D.E. BROWN, D.M. DOOLEY, A.J. SMITH, H.K. KAGAN & J.P. KLINMAN. 1996. A cross-linked cofactor in lysyl oxidase: Redox function for amino acid side chains. Science **273:** 1078–1084
21. XU, R., X. HUANG, T.L. HOPKINS & K.J. KRAMER. 1997. Catecholamine and histidyl protein cross-linked structures in sclerotized insect cuticle. Insect Biochem. Molec. Biol. **27:** 101–108.
22. ANDERSEN, S.O., J.P. JACOBSEN, G. BOJESEN & P. ROEPSTORFF. 1992. Phenoloxidase-catalysed coupling of catechols. Identification of novel coupling products. Biochim. Biophys. Acta **1118:** 134–138.
23. HOLL, S.M., D.C. HANSEN, J.H. WAITE & J. SCHAEFER. 1993. Solid state NMR analysis of cross-linking in a mussel protein glue. Arch. Biochem. Biophys. **302:** 255–258.
24. KLUG, C.A., L.A. BURZIO, J.H. WAITE & J. SCHAEFER. 1996. *In situ* analysis of peptidyl Dopa in mussel byssus using rotational-echo double-resonance NMR. Arch. Biochem. Biophys. **333:** 221–224.
25. HANSEN, D.C., S.G. CORCORAN & J.H. WAITE. 1998. Enzymatic tempering of a mussel adhesive protein film. Langmuir **14:** 743–746.
26. BENEDICT, C.V. & J.H. WAITE. 1986. Location and analysis of byssal structural proteins of *Mytilus edulis*. J. Morphol. **189:** 171-181.
27. ROSS, M.M., S.W. TAYLOR & J.H. WAITE. 1995. Mass spectrometry of marine biomolecules. Proceedings of the 43rd ASMS Conference on Mass Spectrometry & Allied Topics, p. 298.
28. MIKI, D., Y. TAKEUCHI, K. INOUE & S. ODO. 1996. Expression sites of two byssal protein genes of *Mytilus galloprovincialis*. Biol. Bull. **190:** 213–217.
29. HANSEN, D.C., S.C. DEXTER & J.H. WAITE. 1995. The inhibition of corrosion of S30403 stainless steel by a naturally occurring catecholic polymer. Corrosion Sci. **37:** 1423–1441.
30. BATEY, A.M., P.K.LEAVITT, C. A. SIEDLECKI, B.J. TYLER, P.A. SUCI, R.E. MARCHANT & G. GEESEY. 1997. Adsorption of adhesive proteins from the marine mussel, *Mytilus edulis,* on polymer films in the hydrated state using angle dependent X-ray photoelectron spectroscopy and atomic force microscopy. Langmuir **13:** 5702–5710.
31. WAITE, J.H. 1997. Marine bioadhesion: Unravelling the chemistry. J. Adhes. Soc. Japan **33:** 186–193.

# Overview of Extracorporeal Liver Support Systems and Clinical Results

BRIAN E. McLAUGHLIN, CHRISTINE M. TOSONE, LINDA M. CUSTER, AND CLAUDY MULLON[a]

*Circe Biomedical, Inc., Lexington, Massachusetts 02421, USA*

**ABSTRACT:Patients with acute liver failure (ALF) continue to have an almost 50% mortality rate despite improvements associated with the use of orthotopic liver transplantation (OLT). Numerous *ex vivo* methods have been developed in attempts to improve patient survival. These methods can be divided into three groups: detoxification (e.g., dialysis, charcoal adsorption, plasma exchange), which only provides excretory function; *ex vivo* liver perfusion (e.g., whole organ or tissue perfusion), which provides some metabolic function; and bioartificial or cell-based systems, which combine elements of the first two methods. Clinical trials have shown minimal efficacy of the various detoxification methods in terms of ALF patient survival, while the relative success of OLT has shown the importance of providing metabolic as well as excretory functions. Attempts to provide those additional functions with *ex vivo* tissue perfusion have been fraught with complications such as clotting and acute tissue rejection, leading to the conceptual development of cell-based bioreactor systems. A number of these bioartificial systems have been clinically evaluated, and the preliminary patient survival rates have encouraged further work in this area.**

## INTRODUCTION

Numerous therapies have been developed and evaluated for the treatment of acute liver failure (ALF), the most successful of which has been orthotopic liver transplantation (OLT). However, the mortality rate for ALF patients undergoing OLT continues to be high. In order to increase patient survival, various extracorporeal methods have been clinically investigated. These methods are intended to temporarily replace some of the functions of the failed liver and support patients to recovery or bridge them to transplantation. *Ex vivo* blood treatments can be divided into three categories: passive detoxification, *ex vivo* liver perfusion, and bioartificial or cell-based systems. The advent of the newest of these treatments, cell-based systems, was a progression from the former two, which in some cases have shown benefit but have limitations. Detoxification systems do not incorporate tissue and are thereby passive, providing only excretory liver function. The relative success of OLT has demonstrated the importance of not only detoxification but of synthetic and metabolic functions. Attempts have been made to provide these functions through *ex vivo* perfusion of whole livers and tissue sections, but these methods remain a challenge owing to immune reactions and blood clotting. This has led to the development of bioreactors

[a]Author for correspondence: Circe Biomedical, Inc., 99 Hayden Avenue, Lexington, MA 02421; 781-863-8720 (voice); 781-861-7936 (fax); mullon@circebio.com (e-mail).

incorporating hepatocytes, and early clinical results have encouraged further work in this area.

This review will discuss those therapies which have been clinically evaluated in each of the three categories above and look at the clinical effectiveness of each in terms of patient survival.

## BLOOD PURIFICATION METHODS

A variety of *ex vivo* detoxification methods have been tested clinically in attempts to remove waste products and toxins. Such methods include hemodialysis, hemoperfusion, hemofiltration, hemodiabsorption, plasmapheresis, high volume plasmapheresis, albumin dialysis, and strategies combining multiple methods (TABLE 1). None of these treatments has gained wide acceptance. Most techniques used with patients in hepatic coma permit the return to consciousness but do not save the lives of the patients. Consequently, morbidity and mortality remain high.[1]

### *Hemodialysis*

Conventional dialysis, with low-permeability membranes used to treat kidney failure, has failed to produce any significant improvements in the survival of patients with liver failure. High permeability poly(acrylonitrile) (PAN) dialysis membranes, which can clear intermediate molecular weight (500 to 5000 dalton) compounds, demonstrated promising results for hepatic support when used in a pig model. Based on this, Opolon and colleagues conducted a clinical study on 39 patients.[2] Recovery of consciousness was found in 17 patients, of whom nine survived (23%). Compared with a previous study of 117 patients without blood treatment, in which 26 patients survived (22%), no significant improvement in survival with hemodialysis was found. Two earlier clinical trials performed by Opolon[3] and by Silk[4] had similar outcomes.

### *Hemofiltration*

Continuous hemofiltration was applied to hepatic failure to avoid the high incidence of cerebral edema caused by rapid changes in plasma osmolality during the intermittent processes of hemodialysis and hemoperfusion.[5] Continuous hemofiltration has been used for body fluid control in cases of severe cardiac or pulmonary failure and has been proven to be capable of removing substances of molecular weight less than 10,000 dalton with PAN or poly(methyl methacrylate) (PMMA) membrane filters. In one clinical study, five patients with acute hepatic failure were treated by continuous hemofiltration with fluid replacement. Three of five treated patients (60%) survived, with two patients undergoing successful transplantation and one recovering hepatic function without transplantation.[6] Investigators have also combined hemofiltration with other therapies. Inaba *et al.*[7] reported the treatment of a patient with fulminant hepatic failure (FHF) using high-volume plasma exchange combined with hemofiltration. The patient was converted from hepatic encephalopathy grade IV to grade II, but later died. Okamoto *et al.*[8] reported on an additional case in which a patient who was admitted with grade II hepatic encephalopathy and

**TABLE 1.** Clinical results of various support methods for acute liver failure

| Method | Survival Rates | | Investigators | Year |
|---|---|---|---|---|
| | Treatment % (survive/tot) | Control % (survive/tot) | | |
| Hemodialysis | 21 (5/24) | — | Opolon | 1976 |
| | 31 (20/65) | 15 (8/53) | Silk | 1978 |
| | 23 (9/39) | 22 (26/117) | Opolon | 1981 |
| Hemofiltration | 60 (3/5) | — | Rakela | 1988 |
| —with plasmapheresis | 56 (38/68) | — | Yoshiba | 1996 |
| Plasmapheresis | 60 (6/10) | — | Inoue | 1981 |
| | 34 (15/45) | 14 (5/35) | Yamazaki | 1988 |
| | 27 (7/26) | 22 (4/18) | Soeda | 1991 |
| | 46 (5/11) | — | Kondrup | 1992 |
| | 60 (9/15) | — | Larsen | 1994 |
| Hemoperfusion | 24 (17/71) | 15 (8/53) | Silk | 1978 |
| | 65 (20/31)[a] | — | Gimson | 1982 |
| | 20 (9/45)[b] | — | Gimson | 1982 |
| | 51 (38/75)[a] | — | O'Grady | 1988 |
| | 37 (23/62)[b] | 39 (13/33) | O'Grady | 1988 |
| —Plasma perfusion | 19 (5/26) | — | McGuire | 1995 |
| Hemodiabsorption | 52 (8/15) | — | Ash | 1992 |
| —with plasma sorption | 20 (1/5) | 60 (3/5) | Hughes | 1994 |
| | 0 (0/1) | — | Ash | 1998 |
| Albumin dialysis | 67 (2/3)[c] | — | Seige | 1998 |
| | 71 (10/14)[c] | — | Stange | 1998 |
| Extracorporeal liver perfusion | 20 (2/10) | — | Abouna | 1973 |
| | 18 (2/11) | — | Tung | 1980 |
| | 57 (13/23) | — | Lie | 1990 |
| | 25 (1/4) | — | Chari | 1994 |
| —with hemodialysis | 27 (3/11) | — | Ozawa | 1982 |
| —with oxygenation | 50 (1/2) | — | Fox | 1993 |
| Cross circulation | 33 (1/3) | — | Burnell | 1967 |

[a]Grade III hepatic encephalopathy. [b]Grade IV hepatic encephalopathy. [c]Acute-on-chronic failure.

rapidly deteriorating neurological status was treated with a combination of plasmapheresis and continuous hemodiafiltration. The patient was successfully maintained for 54 days until liver transplantation was performed. Yoshiba *et al.*[9] reported the results of a larger study in which 68 patients with FHF were treated with the combination of hemodiafiltration and high-volume plasmapheresis. Thirty-eight of the patients (56%) survived and recovered fully without liver transplantation.

### *Plasmapheresis*

In plasmapheresis, plasma is separated from the cellular blood components and replaced with normal plasma constituents, allowing the removal of circulating toxins and waste products. Two different mechanisms are used, centrifugation and membrane filtration. Intermittent plasmapheresis has been used in patients with hepatic failure since the early 1970s. This approach has been found to reduce encephalopathy, though without any impact on overall survival.[10]

Continuous flow membrane plasmapheresis has been used with some success in humans. In a 10 patient study, 7 patients with FHF and 3 with cirrhosis were treated.[11] Three of the seven patients with FHF survived, and all three of the patients with cirrhosis regained consciousness and left the hospital. The authors suggested that recovery could be improved by starting the treatment before the onset of serious neurological symptoms. In another study of 80 patients with FHF, 45 were treated with plasma exchanges of five liters daily until they fully recovered or died.[12] The survival rate for the treated group was 34%, while that for the untreated group was 14%. However, the study was not randomized, and the patient population was not controlled with respect to the underlying etiology or disease severity.

The efficacy and limitations of plasma exchange compared to hemoperfusion were investigated in a study prompted by the low survival rate of patients with FHF treated with plasmapheresis. Mortality rates were analyzed for 44 patients with acute hepatic failure who were treated either primarily with plasmapheresis or primarily with hemoperfusion,[13] in which blood is passed through an absorption column to remove toxins. Plasma exchange using 3.2 liters of plasma was performed using membrane plasma separators. In the plasmapheresis group, the overall survival rate was 27% compared to 22% in the hemoperfusion group. The occurrence of biochemical indicators of liver failure was very similar between the treatment groups. The overall survival rate of standard plasma exchange remains low, and the usefulness of this approach is limited by the large amount of plasma needed.

### *High-Volume Plasmapheresis*

It has been theorized that the failure of plasmapheresis as a treatment for FHF may result, in part, from the assumption that all toxins responsible for hepatic encephalopathy are located in the plasma. Assuming a wider dispersion of the toxic substances resulting from liver failure, high-volume plasma exchange could hypothetically remove those toxins distributed throughout the body and not just in the plasma pool. Based on these assumptions, a clinical study was designed which used high-volume plasmapheresis to exchange a volume equal to the individual's extracellular water (20% of body weight).[14] Eleven patients were treated with three courses of plasmapheresis on consecutive days. Five of the 11 patients (46%) survived.

Larsen *et al.*[15] conducted an additional study of high-volume plasmapheresis in 15 patients with hepatic encephalopathy who were in grade III or IV coma. All patients were scheduled for transplantation and awaiting donor organs. A total of 33 plasmaphereses were performed from one to eight times in each patient with a mean volume of 9.9 L (range 5–16 L) per treatment. Overall, nine of fifteen patients (60%) survived including six of eleven patients (55%) in grade IV coma. All survivors underwent successful transplantation. Of the six patients who died, three died before a donor liver was available and three died following transplantation.

### *Hemoperfusion*

Hemoperfusion, in which toxins are removed from blood by sorption or ion exchange, has been used in the treatment of liver disease since the 1960s. Typically, blood is perfused through a column of charcoal particles which are coated with albumin or a hydrogel for hemocompatibility. Often ion exchange resins are used as well, to facilitate the removal of ionic compounds in addition to organic compounds.[16]

Patients with hepatic failure have been treated with charcoal hemoperfusion in numerous clinical studies.[4,17,18] In a series of 76 patients with hepatic failure caused primarily by acetaminophen overdose (46 patients) or viral hepatitis (23 patients), a 65% survival rate was found when patient treatment was initiated at grade III coma. The survival rate dropped to 20% when treatment was started after grade IV coma.[17] These results were compared to a previous study with a survival rate of 15% in a group of patients who received standard intensive care measures.[4]

Results from a clinical trial of 75 patients with grade III encephalopathy showed overall survival rates of 51% and 50% for patients who received 5 and 10 hours of hemoperfusion daily, respectively. Owing to the lack of a control group, it was unclear whether this hemoperfusion was of benefit, and the study did not demonstrate any benefit from longer treatments. In 62 patients with grade IV encephalopathy, the overall survival rates were 39% and 35%, respectively, for patients who received 5 and 10 hours of hemoperfusion daily.[19]

More recently, plasma perfusion, in which the plasma is first separated and then passed through an adsorbent device, has minimized the destruction of platelets and reduced bleeding complications associated with hemoperfusion. McGuire *et al.*[20] reported that this process was used in Japan to treat 26 patients with FHF with an overall survival rate of 19%.

### *Hemodiabsorption*

Hemodiabsorption is a hybrid process in which blood is passed through a hemodialyzer containing a suspension of sorbent material, such as charcoal or resin, in the extracapillary space. The process of adsorption of organic substances is similar to that in hemoperfusion, but a higher binding capacity is provided by the large surface area of fine particles in suspension and by continuous removal of toxin by dialysate flow; eliminating direct blood contact reduces clotting problems.[21]

The first hemodiabsorption device to be used in patient therapy was a HemoCleanse, Inc. (West Lafayette, Indiana, USA) sorbent suspension dialyzer. This device uses powdered charcoal and cation ion exchange resin in the dialyzer, and removes toxins from the sorbents by dialysate circulation. In a preliminary uncontrolled study, beneficial effects on neurological status were observed in 15 patients with liver failure. A randomized, controlled study was then performed using ten patients diagnosed with FHF and grade IV hepatic encephalopathy.[22] One of the five patients treated with hemodiabsorption (20%) survived, while three of five patients (60%) in the control group survived. More recently, hemodiabsorption has been combined with plasma perfusion, such that a second sorption component and a plasmapheresis membrane allow direct contact of the plasma and sorption materials, typically charcoal and silica. This system was fully evaluated in one patient, who did not survive.[23]

### *Albumin Dialysis*

Albumin is an abundant plasma protein, and many toxins bind to albumin and other proteins in the blood, making removal of those toxins across dialysis membranes difficult. Several centers are investigating albumin dialysis, in which a high-flux dialyzer is used in conjunction with albumin-containing dialysate. Patient blood is circulated through the device as in hemodialysis; protein-bound toxins are allowed to diffuse across the membrane and bind with albumin in the dialysate. In one study using single-pass dialysate flow, two of three patients (67%) with acute-on-chronic (AOC) liver failure were successfully bridged to transplant.[24] In another study using dialysate regeneration and recirculation, 10 of 14 AOC patients survived (71%).[25]

## *EX VIVO* PERFUSION

### *Extracorporeal Whole Liver Perfusion*

In extracorporeal liver perfusion, the patient's blood is perfused through a xenogeneic or allogeneic liver. Porcine livers were first used in clinical trials for the treatment of stage IV encephalopathy from FHF in the 1960s. Norman[26] reported 15 clinical porcine liver perfusions carried out on five patients, with one patient receiving five treatments over 18 days. Clinical and biochemical improvements were obtained with no antibody response demonstrated. In a study by Tung *et al.*,[27] 11 patients in hepatic coma were treated with 19 liver perfusions. None of the seven patients with preexisting liver conditions survived; two of the remaining four survived (18%).

Abouna[28] performed 33 clinical *ex vivo* liver perfusions in the treatment of 10 patients in stage IV hepatic coma using a variety of livers. The *ex vivo* livers came from 22 pigs, seven baboons, two human cadavers, one calf, and one Macaca monkey. Perfusions were maintained for 5 to 52 hours. Normal consciousness was restored in five of the patients, and two survived (20%). Serious complications were rare, and bleeding problems were not encountered. Immunologic complications occurred with the pig liver perfusions though, and histological observations showed acute humoral graft rejection with porcine but not with baboon livers. It was observed that while intermittent liver perfusions were capable of restoring consciousness on repeated occasions in the same patient, ultimate survival was dependent upon the degree of initial damage to the patient's own liver and on the development of extra-hepatic complications.

A clinical trial by Lie *et al.*[29] in which 23 patients with FHF were treated with 99 baboon liver perfusions showed long-term survival in 13 of these patients (57%). The improved results were thought to result from the longer perfusion times found to be possible with baboon livers, approximately one day for each treatment. A study by Chari *et al.*[30] treated four patients with liver failure by pig liver perfusion. All four showed improvement in biochemical and neurologic parameters, but three subsequently died.

In an attempt to better preserve the xenogeneic liver, extracorporeal perfusion was combined with hemodialysis.[31] A clinical trial using this technique for 11 patients in stage IV hepatic coma reported a mental status improvement rate of 45% and an overall survival rate of 27%. The duration of each cross-hemodialysis was at most eight hours. This study suggested that the extracorporeal liver could be better maintained by hemodialysis, which was reported to improve oxygenation. Extracorporeal liver perfusion was attempted with the addition of an oxygenator in the extracorporeal circuit. Two patients were treated for 48 hours and 72 hours, respectively.[32] The first patient was successfully transplanted; the second patient died.

### *Liver Tissue Hemoperfusion*

To simplify the technique of extracorporeal perfusion, attempts were made to use fresh or frozen liver slices or cubes rather than whole organs.[33,34] The liver pieces were enclosed within a stirred-tank reactor and were in direct contact with the recipient's blood. These systems were shown to be effective in lowering toxin concentrations and in producing synthetic factors *in vitro* and in animals for a few hours. Problems were encountered primarily in obtaining the tissue pieces and maintaining them with an adequate nutrient and oxygen supply: ischemic damage to the tissue hepatocytes was common.[35] Although this problem was partially overcome by perfusing the liver slices with oxygen-carrying fluorocarbons,[36] the use of liver pieces as artificial livers has remained elusive.

### *Cross-Circulation*

Cross-circulation is a dated technique in which a patient's circulation is connected to that of another human to allow the blood from one to be treated by the liver of the other. Human cross-circulation was reported to be successful in the treatment of one of three patients with acute liver failure,[37] though in each case the donor suffered from significant adverse reactions during the procedure.

## BIOARTIFICIAL LIVER SYSTEMS

### *Introduction*

The clinical results presented in TABLE 1 demonstrate that the benefits of detoxification systems for treating liver failure—those systems that mimic only excretory liver functions—are limited. In the few trials cited that had concurrent control groups, most did not show any benefit of the extracorporeal system over the standard-of-care. Extracorporeal liver perfusion is interesting, on the other hand, in that by using living liver tissue it may be possible to provide a broad array of liver functions, including not only excretory but synthetic and metabolic functions. However, many complications plague this method ranging from vessel leakage and blood clotting to adverse immune reactions. In many instances these complications are the result of the high degree of variability inherent in using whole organs, and also result from direct contact between the organ and patient blood. Given the established use of extracorporeal therapies such as hemodialysis, and the complications and potential benefits of whole liver perfusion, the merging of these two concepts to create a hybrid or bioartificial liver has appeal as a means of providing the best of both worlds.

In its most basic form, a bioartificial liver system combines viable liver tissue with a bioreactor in an extracorporeal circuit. Typically, isolated hepatocytes are used. These cells fall into any number of categories, including human and non-human, primary and immortal, and fresh and cultured, with each distinction having advantages and disadvantages. Human cells offer the advantage of eliciting minimal immune responses, but primary human cells are not readily available. Human cell lines provide an unlimited supply of cells, but generally there is a trade-off between differentiation and proliferation, such that cells which are capable of replicating are compromised in terms of cell-specific function. Non-human cells which have been used clinically include rabbit, rat, and pig hepatocytes. These cells are also readily available, though the actual animal source and procurement methods need to be tightly controlled to give a reproducible product. Since primary hepatocytes are used, increased liver-specific function is possible.

Cells can be used fresh or after culturing: Cells can be loaded into a bioreactor and used immediately to treat a patient, or first cultured in the reactor before treatment. Using fresh cells permits the cells to be cryopreserved following isolation and thawed at the time of patient treatment. This greatly simplifies the logistics of treatment, such as cell transportation and storage. Culturing cells in the reactor prior to treatment, on the other hand, can allow increased cell-to-cell interactions, producing a synergistic effect on function.

### *Bioreactor Design Issues*

The bioreactor in a bioartificial liver has several roles. Cells are contained in the reactor and maintained in an optimal environment, allowing the cells to function outside the body and to remain separate from the patient. Many reactors utilize membranes, which not only retain the cells but prevent direct hepatocyte–blood cell contact, isolating the cells to minimize immune responses. Reactors are designed to maximize mass transfer to the cells, so that not only toxins but oxygen and nutrients in the blood reach the cells, and metabolites and synthetic products are in turn added to the patient's circulation. In those reactors which have direct cell-blood contact, this means ensuring flow is uniform throughout the device and there is a large surface area of cells to contact. In membrane devices, the mass transfer is in large part determined by the pore size and porosity of the membrane for given flow rates and pressures. The trend with extracorporeal liver assist systems, both bioartificial and otherwise, has been towards pore sizes large enough to allow free passage of plasma proteins. This increases mass transfer by shifting the primary mode of transfer from diffusion to convection, and not only allows protein-bound toxins to contact the cells but also allows secreted macromolecules to circulate to the patient.

Many bioartificial liver systems incorporate a means of oxygenating the circulating blood or plasma in order to maintain cell function and viability. In some designs a means of oxygenation is included in the reactor; other systems use an ancillary oxygenation device in series in the extracorporeal circuit. Heat exchangers are generally placed in the circuit as well, to maintain the cells at physiological temperatures. Charcoal columns are also used in some systems, allowing certain organic compounds to be removed from the circuit prior to cell contact.

As alluded to above, some bioartificial liver systems treat whole blood directly, while in others the plasma is first separated from the blood cells and then circulated through the reactor. The latter can be accomplished by membrane separation or by centrifugation. The primary advantage to whole blood treatment is that the treatment process is simplified and the use of ancillary equipment reduced. By treating only plasma though, the need for anticoagulant use is reduced, and an additional level of isolation between the hepatocytes and the blood cells is provided.

### *Examples of Bioartificial Liver Reactors*

A broad array of reactor designs for bioartificial livers have been evaluated clinically or are presently in development. The prevalent designs are based on hollow fiber bioreactors, in which hollow fiber membranes packed in a cartridge provide a large surface area and minimal mass transfer distances between the inside and the outside of the fibers. Typically, blood or plasma circulates through the lumens of the fibers and cells are held in the extracapillary space. A hollow fiber device using primary porcine cells was evaluated in animal trials at the University of Pittsburgh,[39] and based on those results approval for clinical trials was recently granted. In a system developed at the University of Minnesota,[38] blood perfuses the outside of the fibers. Primary pig hepatocytes are cultured in a collagen gel in the fiber lumens; as the collagen polymerizes and the gel contracts a channel through the lumen is created, through which nutrient media is circulated. This three-compartment reactor has been evaluated in animals and a preliminary clinical trial is anticipated.

In addition to hollow fiber devices, systems in development incorporate a variety of other reactor designs. Clément[40] has described a fluidized bed reactor in which blood perfuses alginate-encapsulated porcine hepatocytes. Alginate polymer provides immunoisolation while keeping mass transfer resistances low. The system has shown benefit in an anhepatic pig model. Kawada *et al.*[41] placed porous glass bead microcarriers cultured with a human hepatoma cell line in a packed column reactor with radial flow. The device has been used *in vitro* with circulating media. While the device lacks an immune barrier for the cells, the use of a human cell line may minimize the need for that.

In stacked plate reactors, large surface area is obtained by alternately stacking flat membranes and spacers. In recent *in vitro* studies[42,43] cells were cultured on oxygenation membranes in monolayers or flat sheets to try to mimic liver structure. Perfusate through the spaces between membranes directly contacted the cells. Indicators of cell function, such as albumin secretion and urea formation, demonstrated liver-specific function. In another reactor design in which liver structure was mimicked, porcine hepatocytes were cultured in a rotary low-gravity system.[44] Cells in the rotating reactor, which was originally designed by NASA, formed aggregates and demonstrated liver metabolic activity *in vitro*.

### *Bioartificial Liver Clinical Results*

The first reported clinical use of a bioartificial liver took place in the mid-1980s when Matsumura *et al.*[45] treated a patient with hepatic failure due to carcinoma of the bile duct. Their device consisted of a Kiil plate dialyzer with a high-flux cellulose membrane seeded with $1 \times 10^{10}$ isolated rabbit hepatocytes. The patient recovered and was discharged (TABLE 2). During that same period Margulis *et al.*[46] conducted a controlled clinical trial of a simple bioartificial liver on patients with acute liver failure and hepatic encephalopathy. One group received standard intensive care, one was also treated with a hepatocyte perfusion device. A reservoir in se-

**TABLE 2.** Clinical trials of bioartificial liver support for acute liver failure

| Investigator | Year | Device configuration | Cell type | Survival rates: Treatment % (survive/tot) | Survival rates: Control % (survive/tot) |
|---|---|---|---|---|---|
| Matsumura | 1987 | Plate dialyzer, cell suspension | Rabbit hepatocytes | 100 (1/1) | — |
| Margulis | 1989 | AV shunt, cell suspension | Pig heptatocytes | 63 (37/59) | 41 (27/67) |
| Li<br>Li | 1993<br>1998 | Glass bead packed bed reactor | Pig hepatocytes | 67 (2/3) | — |
| Sussman<br>Ellis | 1994<br>1996 | Hollow fiber bioreactor | Cultured human hepatoma line | 45 (5/11)<br>78 (7/9)[a]<br>33 (1/3)[b] | —<br>75 (6/8)[a]<br>25 (1/4)[b] |
| Gerlach | 1997 | Multiple compartment hollow fiber bioreactor | Cultured pig hepatocytes | 100 (6/6) | — |
| Demetriou<br>Watanabe | 1995<br>1997 | Hollow fiber bioreactor | Pig hepatocytes | 89 (8/9)<br>94 (17/18)[c]<br>100 (3/3)[d] | —<br>—<br>— |

[a]Group not expected to need OLT. [b]Group expected to need OLT. [c]Fulminant hepatic failure group. [d]Primary non-function of transplant group.

ries with an arterio-venous shunt was seeded with charcoal and a suspension of $4 \times 10^7$ isolated porcine hepatocytes, which was retained in the device with nylon filters. Patient blood was perfused directly through the reservoir for an average of six hours, with devices being changed every hour. Thirty-seven of 59 patients in the test group survived (63%), while 27 of 67 patients in the control group survived (41%).

Researchers at Monsanto Company (St. Louis, Missouri, USA) developed and clinically evaluated a packed column reactor containing cultured porcine hepatocytes in three patients.[47–49] Devices were prepared by seeding the reactor with isolated hepatocytes and circulating them to cause cell aggregation and entrapment among the glass beads of the reactor. During treatment, patient blood was separated with a hollow fiber plasmapheresis device and plasma perfused through the reactor. Two of the three patients treated (67%) survived. At present, the technology for this bioartificial liver has been licensed by Monsanto to HemoCleanse, Inc. for use with their sorption systems. Sussman and Kelly[50] have developed a human hepatoblastoma cell line and a bioartificial liver using this line. The C3A cells, derived from a HepG2 line, were selected for biochemical activity such as albumin production and cytochrome P450 metabolism. Cells are seeded in two hemodialysis cartridges in series where they expand to fill the devices, each with approximately 200 g of cells. Prepared cartridges are transported to the point of patient treatment when needed; patient and devices are then connected to a whole blood extracorporeal circuit. This system was developed by Hepatix, Inc., now Vitagen, Inc. (La Jolla, CA, USA), and initially evaluated in an uncontrolled clinical trial.[50] Of eleven patients with FHF or primary non-function (PNF), four survived to receive transplants; a fifth recovered without needing OLT (45%). An expanded clinical trial with controls was then initiated.[51] Patients were placed in either of two sets: those expected to need OLT to survive, and those not. Each set was divided into test and control groups. In each case, no difference was seen between the survival rates in the test and the control groups. For those not expected to need OLT, 78% of nine patients survived with treatment, while 75% of eight patients survived with standard-of-care. For those expected to need OLT, one of three survived with treatment (33%) compared to one of four without (25%).

Gerlach[52] has developed and clinically evaluated a bioreactor with multiple hollow fiber compartments. Two sets of fibers are used to prepare and perfuse the device. When cells are first seeded into the extracapillary space, transmembrane pressure is used to hold cells against the membrane surface until they attach. Following this the device is cultured for days to weeks while cells form liver-like structures, and then removed from culture, transported, and connected to an extracorporeal circuit for patient treatment. Plasma flow through the device during treatment is directed into one set of fibers and out the second to force flow through the extracapillary space. A third set of fibers is for oxygenation. Hybrid Organ GmbH (Berlin, Germany), a company established to develop this liver system, reported all six patients in an initial clinical trial survived beyond 30 days post-treatment (100%).

Demetriou *et al.*[53] developed a hollow fiber bioreactor which used primary pig hepatocytes attached to microcarriers. Microcarriers and cells were seeded into the extracapillary space of the reactor and perfusion of plasma through the fibers was begun within a few hours. Nine patients with FHF or PNF received one or several six hour treatments. Eight of the nine survived (88%); seven were bridged to transplant and one recovered without OLT.

A research division of W.R. Grace and Company, presently Circe Biomedical, Inc. (Lexington, MA, USA), initiated development of a cell-based bioreactor in 1985.[54] This reactor used microporous poly(sulfone) hollow fibers (0.15 μm pore size) and isolated porcine hepatocytes. In 1993, Grace and Demetriou combined efforts and designs to create the HepatAssist® liver-assist system. In this system, patient plasma is fed into and out of a high flow recirculating loop. The loop consists of a pump, a charcoal adsorption column, a membrane oxygenator and heat exchanger, a reservoir, and the hollow fiber cartridge. The cartridge contains $5 \times 10^9$ viable porcine hepatocytes in a suspension with collagen-coated microcarriers, which provide surface area for cell attachment and promote spatial distribution of cells in the bioreactor.

Circe has recently completed a Phase I/II clinical trail of the HepatAssist® system.[53,55] Studies were conducted at Cedars-Sinai Medical Center of Los Angeles by Achilles Demetriou, at Paul Brousse Hospital of Paris by Henri Bismuth, and at UCLA Medical Center by Ronald Busuttil. The total clinical experience to date in treating PNF and FHF with stage III or IV hepatic encephalopathy has been 39 patients.[55,56] Thirty-five of those patients survived beyond 30 days post-treatment (90%), and six of those 35 recovered without needing OLT. Based on these results and on satisfactorily characterizing the safety of the system with regard to porcine endogenous retroviruses,[57] a Phase II/III, multicenter, randomized, controlled, parallel group clinical trial has been approved by the U.S. FDA and is underway. The study will seek to establish the efficacy of the system and will enroll approximately 150 patients.

### *Considerations*

Microporous fibers such as those used in the Circe system allow free exchange of proteins and macromolecules between the plasma and hepatocytes but prevent cell passage. This permits large or protein-bound toxins to pass to the cell side of the fibers and synthesized products like clotting factors to enter the plasma stream. This in turn allows the patient to realize the full benefit of the liver-specific functions of the cells. The membranes used by Sussman[50] and by Matsumura[45] were high flux dialysis membranes which reduced the passage of albumin and excluded higher molecular weight proteins. These membranes do, however, exclude antibodies, complements, and other immunological molecules, providing an immunoprotected environment for xenogeneic and allogeneic cells. Since artificial liver and whole liver perfusions have been well tolerated, though, and since treated patients have subsequently received transplants without complications,[58] the short-term use of microporous membranes with foreign cells appears safe. This is reinforced by findings by Ye[59] in which allograft transplants in primates following pig heart transplantation and pig blood transfusion functioned normally with no accelerated cellular rejection. This study and current observations from artificial liver use[58] suggest that bridging with xenografts does not prohibit subsequent organ allografting.

Apart from the HepatAssist® system, in all but the earliest clinically evaluated systems cells are cultured in the bioreactor prior to patient treatment. After cells are seeded in these systems, they must be maintained with circulating nutrient media for a given amount of time while the cells take on the proper configuration before a patient can be treated. To make such devices available on short notice, they must be prepared and continuously maintained at the clinical site. Devices can be maintained and shipped on demand by the manufacturer as well, at the expense of delaying patient treatment. By seeding the device at the time of treatment, however, cells can be cryopreserved for shipment and storage. This permits the liver-assist system to be prepared quickly with little notice and tremendously simplifies the logistics of supplying cells. Cryopreserved cells do not require nutrient or oxygen supplies during shipment or storage, and contamination risks during handling are minimized. In addition, storage shelf life is measured in years versus weeks. Because cryopreserved cells can be stored for long periods, they can be quarantined prior to release, permitting each lot to be fully characterized with respect to cell viability and function, microbiological and viral screens, and related quality control assays.

## CONCLUSIONS

The recent clinical successes with bioartificial liver treatments for patients with acute liver failure are very encouraging. The limited results suggest great promise for a treatment method for a disease with a high mortality rate. To date, however, the studies have not been randomized, most have not had control groups, and patient populations have not been stratified with regard to the underlying etiology or disease severity. Survival rates have been shown to vary with etiology[60,61] and with the point in disease progression at which treatment is initiated.[17,19] Given the current lack of understanding of the pathogenesis of hepatic encephalopathy and acute liver failure, clinical studies need to be undertaken which will take all these points into consideration. Not only is it hoped that the early positive results will be borne out on a larger scale with appropriate controls, but that the many facets of liver failure will be better understood so as to best care for patients affected by it.

## REFERENCES

1. Trey, C. 1972. The fulminant hepatic failure surveillance study. Brief review of the effects of presumed etiology and age of survival. Can. Med. Assoc. J. **106**(Suppl.): 525–527.
2. Opolon, P. 1981. Large pore hemodialysis in fulminant hepatic failure. *In* Artificial Liver Support. G. Brunner & F. W. Schmidt, Eds.: 126–131. Springer-Verlag
3. Opolon, P., J.R. Rapin, C. Huguet, A. Granger, M.L. Delorme, M. Boschat & A. Sausse. 1976. Hepatic failure coma (HFC) treated by polyacrylonitrile membrane (PAN) hemodialysis (HD). Trans. Am. Soc. Artif. Intern. Organs. **22:** 701–710.
4. Silk, D.B. & R. Williams. 1978. Experiences in the treatment of fulminant hepatic failure by conservative therapy, charcoal haemoperfusion, and polyacrylonitrile haemodialysis. Int. J. Artif. Organs **1:** 29–33.
5. Hughes, R.D. & R. Williams. 1993. Use of sorbent columns and haemofiltration in fulminant hepatic failure. Blood Purif. **11:** 163–169.
6. Rakela, J., S.B. Kurtz, J.T. McCarthy, R.A. Krom, W.P. Baldus, D.B. McGill, J. Perrault & D.S. Milliner. 1988. Postdilution hemofiltration in the management of acute hepatic failure: a pilot study. Mayo Clin. Proc. **63:** 113–118.
7. Inaba, S., T. Kishikawa, A. Zaitsu, H. Ishibashi, J. Kudo, R. Ogawa & M. Yoshiba. 1991. Continuous haemoperfusion for fulminant hepatic failure [letter]. Lancet. **338:** 1342–1343.
8. Okamoto, K., M. Kurose, Y. Ikuta, K. Ogata, T. Harada, K. Takeda & T. Sato. 1996. Prolonged artificial liver support in a child with fulminant hepatic failure. ASAIO J. **42:** 233–235.
9. Yoshiba, M., K. Inoue, K. Sekiyama & I. Koh. 1996. Favorable effect of new artificial liver support on survival of patients with fulminant hepatic failure. Artif. Organs **20:** 1169–1172.
10. Devictor, D., C. Tahiri, C. Lanchier, Y. Navelet, P. Durand & A. Rousset. 1995. Flumazenil in the treatment of hepatic encephalopathy in children with fulminant liver failure. Intensive Care Med. **21:** 253–256.
11. Inoue, N. 1981. Continuous flow membrane plasmapheresis utilizing cellulose acetate hollow fiber in hepatic failure. *In* Artificial Liver Support. G. Brunner & F. W. Scmidt, Eds.: 126–131. Springer-Verlag.
12. Yamazaki, Z., F. Kanai, Y. Idezuki & N. Inoue. 1987. Extracorporeal methods of liver failure treatment. Biomater Artif. Cells Artif. Organs **15:** 667–675.
13. Soeda, K., M. Odaka, Y. Tabata, S. Kobayashi, Y. Itoh & K. Isono. 1991. Efficacy and limitations of plasma exchange in patients with acute hepatic failure; comparing with hemoadsorption, and with impaired regeneration syndrome. Biomater. Artif. Cells Immobil. Biotechnol. **19:** 203–211.
14. Kondrup, J., T. Almdal, H. Vilstrup & N. Tygstrup. 1992. High volume plasma exchange in fulminant hepatic failure. Int. J. Artif. Organs. **15:** 669–676.
15. Larsen, F.S., B.A. Hansen, L.G. Jorgensen, N.H. Secher, P. Kirkegaard & N. Tygstrup. 1994. High-volume plasmapheresis and acute liver transplantation in fulminant hepatic failure. Transplant. Proc. **26:** 1788.
16. Seda, H.W., R.D. Hughes, C.D. Gove & R. Williams. 1984. Removal of inhibitors of brain $Na^+$, $K^+$-ATPase by hemoperfusion in fulminant hepatic failure. Artif. Organs **8:** 174–178.
17. Gimson, A.E., S. Braude, P.J. Mellon, J. Canalese & R. Williams. 1982. Earlier charcoal haemoperfusion in fulminant hepatic failure. Lancet **2:** 681-3.
18. Williams, R., R.Y. Calne, K. Rolles & R.J. Polson. 1985. Current results with orthotopic liver grafting in Cambridge/King's College Hospital series. Br. Med. J. (Clin. Res. Ed.) **290:** 49–52.

19. O'GRADY, J.G., A.E. GIMSON, C.J. O'BRIEN, A. PUCKNELL, R.D. HUGHES & R. WILLIAMS. 1988. Controlled trials of charcoal hemoperfusion and prognostic factors in fulminant hepatic failure. Gastroenterology **94:** 1186–1192.
20. MCGUIRE, B.M., T.D. SIELAFF, S.L. NYBERG, M.Y. HU, F.B. CERRA & J.R. BLOOMER. 1995. Review of support systems used in the management of fulminant hepatic failure. Dig. Dis. **13:** 379–388.
21. ASH, S. R. 1994. Hemodiabsorption in the treatment of acute hepatic failure. ASAIO J. **40:** 80–82.
22. HUGHES, R.D., A. PUCKNELL, D. ROUTLEY, P.G. LANGLEY, J.A. WENDON & R. WILLIAMS. 1994. Evaluation of the BioLogic-DT sorbent-suspension dialyser in patients with fulminant hepatic failure. Int. J. Artif. Organs **17:** 657–662.
23. ASH, S.R., D.E. BLAKE, D.J. CARR & K.D. HARKER. 1998. Push-pull sorbent based pheresis for treatment of acute hepatic failure. ASAIO J. **44:** 129–139.
24. SEIGE, M., U. SCHWEIGART, K.-F. KOPP, M. CLASSEN & B. KREYMANN. 1998. Long-term treatment of 3 patients with acute on chronic liver failure by albumin dialysis. ASAIO J. **44:** 90A.
25. STANGE, J., S. MITZNER, S. KLAMMT, P. PESZYNSKI, J. FREYTAG, S. ALDINGER, W. GERIKE, W. LAUCHART, T. RISLER, H. GÖHL & R. SCHMIDT. 1998. Hepatic recovery following extracorporeal detoxification in acute on chronic hepatic failure (AoCHF)—clinical experience. ASAIO J. **44:** 91A.
26. NORMAN, J.C., C.A. SARAVIS, M. BROWN & W. MCDERMOTT. 1966. Immunochemical observations in clinical heterologous (xenogeneic) liver perfusions. Surgery **60:** 179–190.
27. TUNG, L.C., R. HARING, J. WALDSCHMIDT & D. WEBER. 1980. [Experience in treating hepatic coma by extracorporal liver perfusion]. Zentralbl. Chir. **105:** 1195–1205.
28. ABOUNA, G.M., L.M. FISHER, K.A. PORTER & G. ANDRES. 1973. Experience in the treatment of hepatic failure by intermittent liver hemoperfusions. Surg. Gynecol. Obstet. **137:** 741–752.
29. LIE, T.S. 1990. Extracorporeal hemoperfusion over the baboon and human liver to treat fulminant hepatitis and its bridge role for liver transplantation. Jpn. J. Artif. Organs **19:** 1414–1422.
30. CHARI, R.S., B.H. COLLINS, J.C. MAGEE, J.M. DIMAIO, A.D. KIRK, R.C. HARLAND, R.L. MCCANN, J.L. PLATT & W.C. MEYERS. 1994. Brief report: treatment of hepatic failure with ex vivo pig-liver perfusion followed by liver transplantation. N. Engl. J. Med. **331:** 234–237.
31. OZAWA, K., Y. KAMIYAMA, K. KIMURA, M. UKIKUSA, Y. KONO, T. YAMATO, Y. SHIMAHARA, T. NAKATANI, M. ASANO, R. IRIE, S. KAWASHIMA, K. UCHIDA, M. OHTOSHI, H. AOYAMA, F. HIRAI, K. YASUDA & T. TOBE. 1982. Clinical experience of postoperative hepatic failure treatment with pig or baboon liver cross-hemodialysis with an interposed membrane. Artif. Organs **6:** 433–446.
32. FOX, I.J., A.N. LANGNAS, L.W. FRISTOE, M.S. SHAEFER, J.E. VOGEL, D.L. ANTONSON, J.P. DONOVAN, T.G. HEFFRON, R.S. MARKIN, M.F. SORRELL, *et al.* 1993. Successful application of extracorporeal liver perfusion: a technology whose time has come. Am. J. Gastroenterol. **88:** 1876–1881.
33. KIMURA, K., K.J. GUNDERMANN & T.S. LIE. 1980. Hemo Perfusion Over Small Liver Pieces For Liver Support. Artif. Organs **4:** 297–301.
34. KAWAMURA, A., J. MEGURO, K. KUKITA, M. YONEKAWA, F. KUMAGAI, J. UCHINO, Y. KURAOKA & T. TAMAKI. 1987. The development of a new hybrid hepatic support system using frozen liver pieces. Artif. Organs **11:** 311.
35. KOSHINO, I., F. CASTINO, K. YOSHIDA, C. CARSE, H. KAMBIC, K. SCHEUCHER, A.P. KRETZ, P.S. MALCHESKY & Y. NOSE. 1975. A biological extracorporeal metabolic device for hepatic support. Trans. Am. Soc. Artif. Intern. Organs **21:** 492–500.
36. KOSHINO, I., H. SAKAMOTO, Y. SHINADA, Y. TSUJI, T. KAWAMATA, M. MATSUSHITA, T. KON & Y. KASAI. 1979. Use of liver slices for an artificial liver. Trans. Am. Soc. Artif. Intern. Organs **25:** 493–496.
37. BURNELL, J.M., J.K. DAWBORN, R.B. EPSTEIN, R.A. GUTMAN, G.E. LEINBACH, E.D. THOMAS & W. VOLWILER. 1967. Acute hepatic coma treated by cross-circulation or exchange transfusion. N. Engl. J. Med. **276:** 935–943.

38. SIELAFF, T.D., S.L. NYBERG, M.D. ROLLINS, M.Y. HU, B. AMIOT, A. LEE, F.J. WU, W.S. HU & F.B. CERRA. 1997. Characterization of the three-compartment gel-entrapment porcine hepatocyte bioartificial liver. Cell Biol. Toxicol. **13:** 357–364.
39. MAZARIEGOS, G.V., R. LOPEZ, F. RIDDERVOLD, E. MOLMENTI, D. GERBER, A. HANNA, Y. ZHU, G.D. BLOCK, V.L. SCOTT, S. AGGARWAL, D.J. KRAMER, R.A. YIN, R.A. WAGNER, M.L. FULMER, B.P. AMIOT & J.F. PATZER II. 1998. Preclinical evaluation of a bioartificial liver assist device. ASAIO J. **44:** 92A.
40. CLÉMENT, B. 1997. Design of an extracorporeal bioartificial liver based on porcine hepatocytes entrapped within alginate gel. Presented at New Frontiers in the Treatment of Liver Disease, December 5–6, 1997, Padua, Italy.
41. KAWADA, M., S. NAGAMORI, H. AIZAKI, K. FUKAYA, M. NIIYA, T. MATSUURA, H. SUJINO, S. HASUMURA, H. YASHIDA, S. MIZUTANI & H. IKENAGA. 1998. Massive culture of human liver cancer cells in a newly developed radial flow bioreactor system: ultrafine structure of functionally enhanced hepatocarcinoma cell lines. *In Vitro* Cell Dev. Biol. Anim. **34:** 109–115.
42. BADER, A., L. DE BARTOLO & A. HAVERICH. 1997. Initial evaluation of the performance of a scaled up flat membrane bioreactor (FMB) with pig liver cells. Presented at New Frontiers in the Treatment of Liver Diseases, December 5–6, 1997, Padua, Italy.
43. SMITH, M.D., E. EKEVALL, I. AIRDRIE, M.H. GRANT, J.M. COURTNEY, R.B. COUSINS & J.D.S. GAYLOR. 1997. Development and characterization of a hybrid artificial liver bioreactor with integral membrane oxygen. Presented at New Frontiers in the Treatment of Liver Diseases, December 5–6, 1997, Padua, Italy.
44. DABOS, K.J., L.J. NELSON, J.N. PLEVRIS, M.M. DOLLINGER, C. HEWAGE, I.H. SADLER & P.C. HAYES. 1998. Microgravity environment in a rotary cell culture system (rccs) promotes cell aggregation and maintains differentiation and proliferation of primary porcine hepatocytes. J Hepatol. **28:** 62.
45. MATSUMURA, K.N., G.R. GUEVARA, H. HUSTON, W.L. HAMILTON, M. RIKIMARU, G. YAMASAKI & M.S. MATSUMURA. 1987. Hybrid bioartificial liver in hepatic failure: preliminary clinical report. Surgery. **101:** 99–103.
46. MARGULIS, M.S., E.A. ERUKHIMOV, L.A. ANDREIMAN & L.M. VIKSNA. 1989. Temporary organ substitution by hemoperfusion through suspension of active donor hepatocytes in a total complex of intensive therapy in patients with acute hepatic insufficiency. Resuscitation **18:** 85–94.
47. LI, A.P., G. BARKER, D. BECK, S. COLBURN, R. MONSELL & C. PELLEGRIN. 1993. Culturing of primary hepatocytes as entrapped aggregates in a packed bed bioreactor: a potential bioartificial liver. *In Vitro* Cell Dev. Biol. **29a:** 249–254.
48. CECCHIN, A. 1994. U.S. firms in high gear to build reliable artificial liver. Med. Tribune **35:** 10.
49. LI, A. P. 1998. Personal communication.
50. SUSSMAN, N.L., G.T. GISLASON, C.A. CONLIN & J.H. KELLY. 1994. The Hepatix extracorporeal liver assist device: initial clinical experience. Artif. Organs **18:** 390–396.
51. ELLIS, A.J., R.D. HUGHES, J.A. WENDON, J. DUNNE, P.G. LANGLEY, J.H. KELLY, G.T. GISLASON, N.L. SUSSMAN & R. WILLIAMS. 1996. Pilot-controlled trial of the extracorporeal liver assist device in acute liver failure. Hepatology **24:** 1446–1451.
52. GERLACH, J. C. 1997. Long-term liver cell cultures in bioreactors and possible application for liver support. Cell Biol. Toxicol. **13:** 349–355.
53. DEMETRIOU, A.A., J. ROZGA, L. PODESTA, E. LEPAGE, E. MORSIANI, A.D. MOSCIONI, A. HOFFMAN, M. MCGRATH, L. KONG, H. ROSEN, *et al.* 1995. Early clinical experience with a hybrid bioartificial liver. Scand. J. Gastroenterol. **208 (Suppl.):** 111–117.
54. JAUREGUI, H.O., C. MULLON, D. TRENKLER, S. NAIK, H. SANTANGINI, P. PRESS, T. E. MULLER & B.A. SOLOMON. 1995. In vivo evaluation of a hollow fiber liver assist device. Hepatology **21:** 460–469.
55. WATANABE, F.D., C. MULLON, W.R. HEWITT, N. ARKADOPOULOS, E. KAHAKU, S. EGUCHI, T. KHALILI, W. ARNAOUT, C.R. SHACKLETON, J. ROZGA, B. SOLOMON & A.A. DEMETRIOU. 1997. Clinical experience with a bioartificial liver in the treat-

ment of severe liver failure. A phase I clinical trial. Ann. Surg. **225:** 484–491; discussion 491–494.

56. MULLON, C. & Z. PITKIN. 1999. The HepatAssist® Bioartificial Liver Support System: clinical study and pig hepatocyte process. Exp. Opin. Invest. Drugs **8:** 229–235.
57. FOX, J. L. 1998. FDA seeks "comfort factors" before removing hold on porcine xenotransplantation trials. Nature Biotechnol. **16:** 224.
58. BAQUERIZO, A., A. MHOYAN, H. SHIRWAN, J. SWENSSON, R.W. BUSUTTIL, A.A. DEMETRIOU & D.V. CRAMER. 1997. Xenoantibody response of patients with severe acute liver failure exposed to porcine antigens following treatment with a bioartificial liver. Transplant. Proc. **29:** 964–965.
59. YE, Y., Y. LUO, T. KOBAYASHI, S. TANIGUCHI, S. LI, M. NIEKRASZ, S. KOSANKE, J. BAKER, L. MIELES, D. SMITH, *et al.* 1995. Secondary organ allografting after a primary "bridging" xenotransplant. Transplantation. **60:** 19–22.
60. RIORDAN, S.M. & R. WILLIAMS. 1997. Experience in design of controlled clinical trials in acute liver failure. *In* Bioartificial Liver Support Systems. The Critical Issues. G. Crepaldi, A. A. Demetriou & M. Muraca, Eds.: 104–115. CIDC Edizioni Internazionali. Rome.
61. WILLIAMS, R. 1996. Classification, etiology, and considerations of outcome in acute liver failure. Semin. Liver Dis. **16:** 343–348.

# Bioreactors for Hybrid Liver Support: Historical Aspects and Novel Designs

BENEDIKT BUSSE AND JÖRG C. GERLACH[a]

*Charité, Campus Virchow-Klinikum, Medizinische Fakultät der Humboldt Universität, Berlin, D-13353 Berlin, Germany*

**ABSTRACT: A novel bioreactor construction has been designed for the utilization of hepatocytes and sinusoidal endothelial cells. The reactor is based on capillaries for hepatocyte aggregate immobilization. Three separate capillary membrane systems, each permitting a different function are woven in order to create a three dimensional network. Cells are perfused via independent capillary membrane compartments. Decentralized oxygen supply and carbon dioxide removal with low gradients are possible. The use of identical parallel units to supply hepatocytes facilitates scale up.**

***In vitro* studies demonstrate long-term external metabolic function in primary isolated hepatocytes within bioreactors. These systems are capable of supporting essential liver functions. Animal experiments have verified the possibility of scaling-up the bioreactors for clinical treatment. However, since there is no reliable animal model for investigation of the treatment of acute liver failure, the promising results obtained from these studies have limited relevance. The small number of clinical studies performed so far is not sufficient to reach conclusions about improvements in the therapy of acute liver failure. Although important progress has been made in the development of these systems, various hepatocyte culture models and bioreactor constructions are being discussed in the literature, which indicates competition in this field of medical research.**

**An overview, which emphasizes the development of hepatocyte culture models for bioreactors, subsequent *in vitro* studies, animal studies, and clinical application, is also provided.**

## INTRODUCTION

Massive necrosis of hepatocytes in acute liver failure destroys synthesis, metabolism, and elimination pathways of the liver. In the recent development of the so-called "hybrid" or "bioartificial" liver support systems, liver cells are cultivated in bioreactors. The aim is the therapeutical use of the biological activity of liver cells in extracorporeal systems.[1] In this review, liver cell culture models for this purpose, bioreactor constructions based upon these models, animal experiments with hybrid liver support systems, and initial clinical applications are discussed.

[a]Author for correspondence: Charité, Campus Virchow-Klinikum, Medizinische Fakultät der Humboldt Universität Berlin, Chirurgische Klinik, Augustenburger Platz 1, D-13353 Berlin, Germany; +49-30-450-59002 (voice); +49-30-450-52900 (fax); joerg.gerlach@charite.de (e-mail).

## HEPATOCYTE CULTURE MODELS

Based upon advances in cell biology, several different culture models for maintenance of hepatocytes *in vitro* have been developed. These developments used basic cell culture methods and most of this expertise has now been transferred in the construction of bioreactors for large-scale investigations in extracorporeal hybrid liver support.

(1) Cells can be immobilized upon *artificial membranes*. Wolf *et al.* immobilized cells on synthetic polymer capillaries[2] and Jauregiou *et al.* used polystyrene Amicon XM-50 capillaries.[3]
(2) *Microcarriers* are artificial spherical bodies made from different materials, including dextran, polystyrene and glass,[4] to which cells can adhere. The carriers themselves can be cultured in suspension. The advantage of this technique,[5,6] compared to the standard monolayer culture in plastic flasks, is a larger surface for cell adhesion. Co-culturing of microcarriers with different cell types has also been investigated.[7]
(3) Another method of hepatocyte immobilization is the *encapsulation* of the cells within semipermeable membranes. With this technique, cells are protected from mechanical damage, and additionally, immunoisolation from xenogenic cells,[8,9] should be possible. Some groups use alginate-poly-lysine as a capsule material.[10,11] Results have also been reported with matrigel® as an additional adhesion substrate.[12] Other groups have used polyacrylate[13] or sodiumcelluloseacetate and polymethylammoniumchloride.[14]

Dunn *et al.*[15] developed a culture model which is described as a "collagen sandwich culture." Cells are spread on a monolayer and then covered with another collagen layer. The long-term maintenance of function[16] and integrity of the cytoskeleton[17] found by these workers has been attributed to more physiological cell-to-cell interactions in this model. Bader *et al.* have measured the metabolizing capacity of liver specific drugs in this type of cell culture.[18] Koebe *et al.* have made the sandwich culture easier to handle with the so called "immobilization gel" technique showing comparable results,[19] while at the same time offering greater stability of the cell culture in perfused systems with flow-induced shear stresses.[20]

The aggregate culture technique immobilizes cells without artificial materials.[21] Active self-aggregation of hepatocytes was used by Landry *et al.*[22] with neonatal hepatocytes and Tong *et al.*[23] with adult hepatocytes, respectively. Koide *et al.*[24] established a culture technique in which supplementary proteoglycans from reticular fibers of the rat liver are used. In this system, cells are maintained in spherical aggregates with a diameter of approximately 120 μm. This culture model has the advantage that a suspension of cells as free aggregates in the medium is possible, avoiding further artificial adhesion materials.[25] Glycosaminoglycans[26] in combination with insulin, epidermal growth factor[27] and other uncharacterized factors secreted by cells[28] were reported to influence cell morphology in these aggregates. Electron-microscopy of these multicellular spheroids reveals a well-differentiated cytoplasmic architecture and multiple bile-canaliculi-like structures. Also non-parenchymal cells and a newly synthesized extra cellular matrix were seen.[29] While albumin production decreases in normal monolayer culture after four days, this cell culture method maintains a steady albumin synthesis for 14 days.[30] Yuasa *et al.* have measured a reduced DNA-synthesis expression rate by increased synthesis of albumin in spheroid culture compared to the monolayer technique.[31] Spherical aggregates can be encapsulated or used in a bioreactor over several weeks.[32]

Other culture models have been developed, e.g., Miura *et al.* used calcium alginate for immobilization and measured protein synthesis[33] and detoxification,[34,35] and Yanagi *et al.*[36] retained hepatocytes in reticular sponge structures.

Implantable systems utilizing microcarriers, microcapsules or aggregates have also been developed. Transplantation into the peritoneum or the spleen has been performed. Henne-Bruns *et al.*[37] have described the technical problems of transplantation and could also demonstrate that, if a sufficient cell mass is to be provided, the location as well as the viability of transplanted cells becomes problematic.[38] Additionally, they stressed the problem of peritonitis and inflammation due to peritoneal irritations with subsequent intra-abdominal adhesions and the accompanying threat of mechanical ileus. The present contribution therefore is limited to devices which can be used as extracorporeal systems.

## BIOREACTOR CONSTRUCTION

Bioreactors enable the culture models described above to be operated in a large scale.[39,40] They enable the potential of hybrid type extracorporeal liver support systems to be developed.

The first capillary membrane liver cell bioreactor was constructed in 1972 by Knazek *et al.*,[41,42] with semipermeable capillary membranes for cell adhesion and metabolite exchange. Since then, three general categories of hepatocyte bioreactors have emerged:

(1) bioreactors for suspension culture without cell immobilization,
(2) bioreactors based on cell immobilization, and
(3) bioreactors with membranes which provide both mass transfer and cell immobilization functions.

The majority of developments of this principle have been used for non-anchorage–dependent cells, although some have been proposed for liver cells. Olumide *et al.* designed a two-chamber system which was divided by flat sheet cuprophan membranes.[43] An early clinical trial by Matsumura *et al.*[44] in 1987 was based upon a similar construction. One side of the reactor contained rabbit hepatocytes, and in the other side patients' blood was circulated. A large clinical study was performed by Margulis *et al.*[45,46] in which 20 ml capsules filled with pig hepatocytes in suspension were used.

The advantage of hepatocyte suspension bioreactors is their ability to incorporate a large number of cells in constructions which are simple to build and operate. However, since hepatocytes are anchorage-dependent cells, their viability and function are limited to a few hours after their isolation from the donor-organ.[47] This means that such systems are not very practicable for clinical treatment, since they would have to be changed several times each day.

To address this problem, some bioreactor constructions integrate certain materials for cell attachment. Biosolon® microcarriers were used to immobilize hepatocytes inside a blood-perfused column by Shnyra *et al.*[48] A similar approach aimed at producing a high adhesion surface area was taken by Uchino.[49] In a reactor, glass plates with a diameter of 20 × 10 cm were used to culture cells.[50,51] Yanagi *et al.* also used a flat sheet model with 40 rotating discs, where hepatocytes where immobilized in calcium alginate hydrogel.[52] The aggregate culture model produces self-immobilized cells. Takabatake *et al.* used this in an extracorporeal perfusion system[53] in which some 200 aggregates were perfused and oxygenated in a glass cylinder.

Capillary membrane devices are well established in other fields of medicine, e.g., in hemodialysis. Since hepatocytes can be immobilized upon membranes, such reactors can offer a large hepatocyte attachment surface. Membranes with different chemical and physical properties have been used.[54,55] Capillaries of these membranes each generate an intra- and extraluminal compartment with connection of the two compartments by pores of defined size. Hepatocytes are normally attached to the outer capillary wall,[56] or, as in the cases of Demetriou *et al.*[57] and Arnaout *et al.*,[58] in combination with microcarriers. Dixit *et al.* attach the cells to coated polysulfone capillaries, which are used for cell nutrition, and adjacent to neighboring cellulose acetate capillaries for blood circulation.[59] Intraluminal hepatocyte seeding is also possible, as demonstrated by Hu *et al.*[60] and Nyberg *et al.*[61–63]

Most of the culture models described above can be reproduced within hollow fiber bioreactors, and some techniques, such as microencapsulation[64] or the incorporation of special biological matrix layers,[65] find prospective application in membrane bioreactors. It remains to be seen whether it is essential for reactors to have an artificial surface for the immobilization of all inoculated hepatocytes. The aforementioned aggregate technique might possibly negate this requirement. In addition to cell immobilization, selective exchange of solutes between two compartments is possible with artificial membranes, so further technical functions can be provided inside a membrane reactor. A novel construction which utilizes capillary membrane technology for the immobilization of cells, which reorganize to aggregates, and incorporates different types of membranes to effect different functions, will be described in the following section.

## NOVEL REACTOR DEVELOPMENT

Available culture models produce a remarkable change in the local conditions of cells in comparison to their *in vivo* situation. If a culture model could ensure high cell densities[66] as well as a free three-dimensional cell rearrangement of the microenvironment of hepatocytes by hepatocyte self aggregation, the reconstruction of junctional complexes, relocalization of the cytotechnique in which the cells can reorganize themselves into three-dimensional structures, would be much easier.

Most culture models rely on diffusion for substrate exchange, while hepatocytes *in vivo* operate under perfusion conditions. The *in vivo* gradients of oxygen, carbon dioxide and metabolites are not usually given sufficient consideration. As a result, the metabolite transfer vectors in such models are often greatly distorted when com-

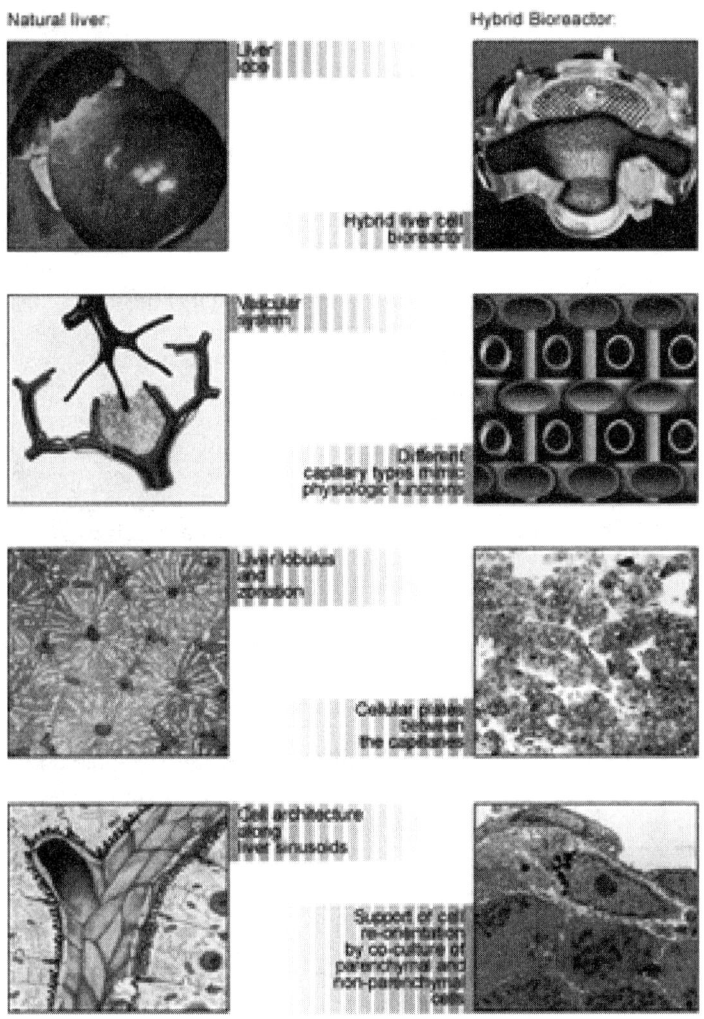


**FIGURE 1.** Schematization of the bioreactor.

pared to the *in vivo* situation. A culture technique which allows the cells to operate under more physiological conditions, e.g., flow conditions with low metabolite gradients, may result in a cell macro-environment more closely related to the physiological situation.

A culture model has been developed, which takes these requirements into consideration. Additional benefits, such as high culture densities,[67] decentralized metabolite exchange, and direct membrane contact oxygenation,[68] are also incorporated. In the novel bioreactor construction, hepatocyte immobilization is achieved via cell attachment supporting capillaries[69] and use of a cell compatible capillary potting material.[70] One specific feature of the model is that the woven capillaries enter and

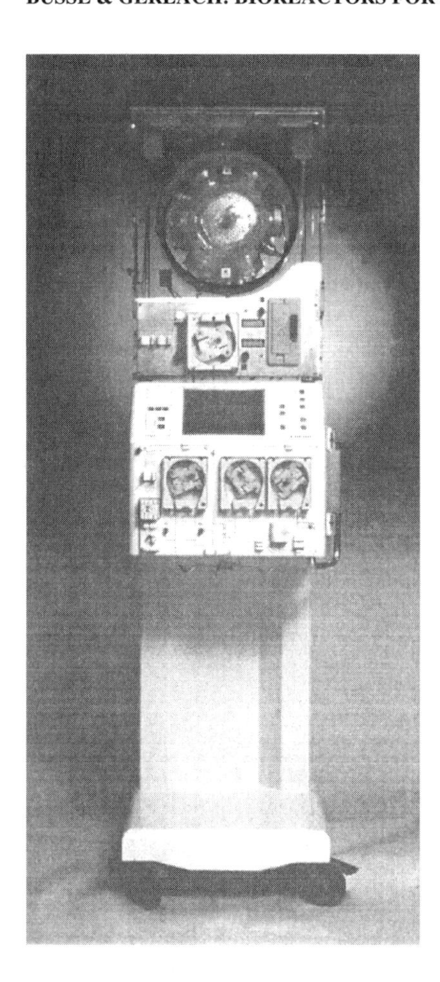

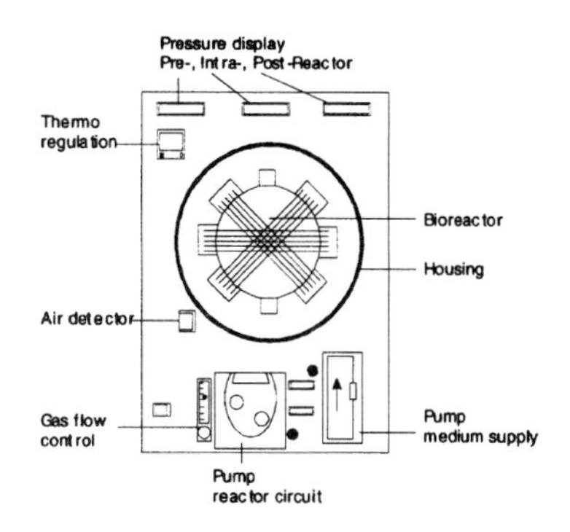


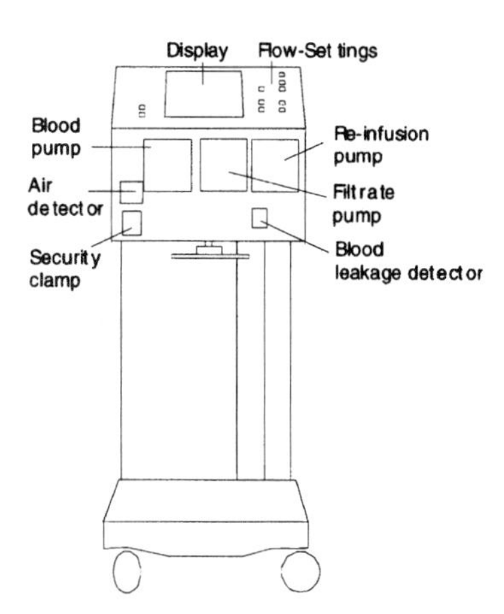


**FIGURE 2.** Prototype of the complete bioreactor.

leave the reactor in sorted, discrete bundles so that they can serve different functions. Independent plasma inflow, plasma outflow and oxygen supply/carbon dioxide removal are therefore possible. Each of many identical, parallel capillary units supplies only a few hepatocytes, resulting in perfusion with low gradients. The bioreactor is schematicized in FIGURE 1 with the photo of the prototype of the complete device given in FIGURE 2.

Results of *in vitro* investigations[71–74] demonstrate that primary hepatocyte cultures can be maintained over a period of several weeks *in vitro* and that they reorganize themselves to give tissue-like structures within the artificial system. The cells spontaneously form aggregates on, and between, the capillaries and reorganize into a three-dimensional array. Rebuilt cell junctions and the reconstitution of bile canaliculi-like

**TABLE 1.** Clinical applications of hybrid liver support systems

| Group | Patients | Classification | Survivors | Hepatic encephalopathy before application |
|---|---|---|---|---|
| Margulis | 59 (18–85 yr) | Acute: 35<br>acute-on-chronic: 6<br>secondary liver failure: 18 (cholestasis, leptospirosis, sepsis | 37 | III–IV (20/5 survivors)<br>I–II (39/32 survivors) |
| Matsumara | 1 (45 yr) | Bile duct carcinoma, end-stage | 3 weeks after application | I |
| Sussman | 23 (9–67 yr) | acute | 13 (5 LTx) | III–IV |
| Demetriou | 33 | acute: 19<br>primary graft failure (PGF): 3<br>acute-on-chronic: 11 | acute: 17 (16 LTx)<br>PGF: 3 (LTx)<br>acute-on-chronic: 3 (2 LTx) | III–IV |
| Neuhaus/ Gerlach | 8 | acute 5<br>subacute 2<br>hyperacute 1 | 8 (LTx) | III–IV |

structures were demonstrated in all reactors under investigation. Even after seven weeks of perfusion, the majority of the cells show an intact ultrastructure.[75]

## SIDE EFFECTS OF THERAPY WITH LIVER SUPPORT SYSTEMS

If blood or plasma is perfused through one compartment of a membrane reactor, this membrane can serve as an immunological barrier between the cultured cells on one side and the patient on the other.[76] In such an application, immunosuppression during and after a treatment with heterologous cells may be less important.[77] Incorporation of a plasmapheresis system in the extracorporeal circuit and the consequent perfusion of reactors with plasma only, avoids direct contact between the patients immunologically competent blood cells and the bioreactor.[78] This may further prevent activation of the patients' white blood cells.

During one set of experimental applications of hybrid liver support in pigs, side effects were not reported.[79] TNF-α liberation, as one marker of the activation of the cytokine system, was comparable with values obtained from therapy with other non-hybrid extracorporeal systems.[80]

The first clinical trial of a hybrid liver support system, was reported in 1987 by Matsumura *et al.*[81] In one patient, metabolic encephalopathy was treated temporarily with rabbit hepatocytes. In two controlled studies, Margulis *et al.*,[82,83] utilized a hybrid artificial liver support system based on porcine hepatocytes. More recently, Demetriou *et al.*[84–86] and Sussman *et al.*[87–89] have published case reports. Applications differed in terms of the technique of treatment (e.g., including charcoal perfusion and hypothermia) as well as in the overall duration and the mode (i.e., frequency of application) of the treatment. Recent studies by both groups have reported successful application of their systems in larger numbers of patients. Sussman *et al.*

**TABLE 2.** Technical features and application characteristics of hybrid liver support systems

| Group | Cell source and mass | Culture/ perfusion system | Membrane cutoff and surfaces | Blood flow/ plasma flow | Anti-coagulation | Time schedule for applications |
|---|---|---|---|---|---|---|
| Margulis | Freshly isolated porcine hepatocycles, $4 \times 10^7$ cells ≅ 0.68 g | PVC-cartridge (volume 20 mL), inner space-bordered by a nylone net, filled with charcoal granules | Direct blood contact | Arterio-venous blood perfusion of the cartridge: 80–100 mL/min | Heparin | Exchange of cartridges every hour, single application duration 6 h maximum of three applications in a single patient |
| Matsumara | Cryoconserved primary rabbit hepatocytes, $1 \times 10^{10}$ cells ≅ 100 g | Plate-dialyzer (Kiil-dialyzer) | Cellulose-membranes, MW 20,000, 1 $m^2$ | Arterio-venous blood flow through the blood compartment of the dialyzer | Heparin | Two intervals (4 and 6 h) |
| Sussman | Hep G2 C3A, proliferated within the device, cryoconserved, 2 × 200 g | Hollow-fiber-dialyzator | Celluloseacetate, MW 70,000, 2 $m^2$ | Veno-venous blood flow through the blood compartment of the dialyzer: 150–300 mL/min, microfiltration across the membranes 10 mL/min | Heparin | Continuous perfusion with a maximum of 9 days, single cartridges have been used between 3 and 58 h |
| Demetriou | Primary porcine hepatocytes, cryoconserved, $5 \times 10^9$ cells ≅ 50 g | Hollow-fiber-dialyzator, adhesion of cells on collagen coated microcarriers | Celluloseacetate, MW 60–80,000, 0.7 $m^2$ | Plasmaphereses by a centrifugal device, veno-venous blood flow: 100 mL/min, separation rate: 50 mL/min, plasma flow inside device circuit 400 mL/min | Citrat | Perfusion for 3–6 h per interva. A maximum of three intervals on following days |
| Neuhaus/ Gerlach | Primary porcine liver cells, mixed liver cell culture, stand-by cultivation up to two weeks, $2.5–5 \times 10^{10}$ cells ≅ 250–500 g | Aggregate parenchymal/non-parenchymal co-culture in a three dimension woven hollow fiber bioreactor with intergrated oxyengeator | Polyethersulfone, MW 200–400,000, 2 × 2.11 $m^2$ | Plasmaseparation by hollow-fiber technique, polyethersulfone membranes, cutoff 200 kD, surface 0.4 m2, blood flow 150–300 mL/min, filtration rate 30-60 mL/min, plasma flow inside reactor circuit 100 mL/min | Heparin | Continous perfusion of a single bioreactor up to 3 days |

used tumor-derived C3A-hepatoma cells,[90,91] whereas Demetriou *et al.*[92] used primary cultures of pig hepatocytes.

A phase I study started recently with our own development.[93] Eight patients were treated as a bridge to liver transplantation up to August 1998; all are already at home and well. In the clinical applications reported so far, as well as in our own experience, signs of acute immunological reactions were not observed. In particular, there were no hypersensitive reactions after repeated therapy in the same patient. TABLES 1 and 2 summarize the clinical trials to date along with the primary reactor characteristics and limitations.

## FUTURE PROSPECTS

In conclusion, the ideal bioreactor configuration, mode of use and the cell source and are still being debated. In addition to the further development of hybrid liver support devices, workers should also focus on the question which cell type would be appropriate and whether non-autologous cells in bioreactors cause side effects during clinical use.

In order to obtain sufficient "net" biological activity in bioreactors, rigorous analysis of the culture models is necessary. This is a prerequisite for the construction of scaled up systems.[94] Investigations of cell-perfusate mass transfer performance by diffusion and/or convective flow, the cell mass to reactor volume ratio, the distribution of medium and gas and their respective gradients, and the availability of oxygen for the cells have been investigated.[95,96] Hollow fiber reactors should provide a good ratio of perfusate flow,[97] adhesion surface/substrate-exchange surface,[98,99] oxygen supply[100,101] and bioreactor volume.

The standardization of the evaluation of pre-clinical and clinically used systems also appears to be an important pre-condition to answering questions of safety, efficacy, and biochemical activity.[102]

## REFERENCES

1. PAPPAS, S.C. 1988. Fulminant hepatic failure and the need for artificial liver support. Mayo Clin. Proc. **63:** 198–200.
2. WOLF, C.F.W. & B.E. MUNKELT. 1975. Bilirubin conjugation by an artificial liver composed of cultured cells and synthetic cappilaries. Trans. Am. Soc. Artif. Int. Organs **21:** 16–27.
3. JAUREGIOU, H.O., S. NAIK, B.A. SOLOMON, R.L. DUFFY, M. LIPSKY & P.M. GALETTI. 1983. Attachment of adult rat hepatocytes to modified Amicron XM-50 membranes. Trans. Am. Soc. Artif. Int. Organs **19:** 698–702.
4. CUNNINGHAM, J.M. & H.J. HODGSON. 1992. Microcarrier culture of hepatocytes in whole plasma for use in liver support bioreactors. Int. J. Artif. Organs **15**(3)**:** 162–167.
5. KASAI, S., M. SAWA, Y. NISHIDA, K. ONODERA, S. HIRAI, T. YAMAMOTO & M. MITO. 1992.. Cellulose microcarrier for high-density-culture of hepatocytes. Transplant. Proc. **24**(6)**:** 2933–2934.
6. SHYNRA, A., A. BOCHAROV, N. BOCHKOVA & V. SPIROV. 1990. Large-scale production and cultivation of hepatocytes on Biosolon microcarriers. Artif. Organs **14**(6)**:** 421–428.
7. VOSS, J.U. & H. SEIBERT. 1991. Microcarrier-attached rat hepatocytes as a xenobiotic-metabolizing system in cocultures. Cell Biol. Toxicol. **7**(4)**:** 387–399.

8. CHANG, T.M. 1992. Hybrid artificial cells: microencapsulation of living cells. ASAIO J. **38**(2)**:** 128–130.
9. SUGAMORI, M., A.H. BOAG, R.L. BROUGHTON & M.V. SEFTON. 1986. Microencapsulation of mammalian cells in polyacrylate membranes for metabolic prostheses. *In* Progress in Artificial Organs. Y. Nosè, C. Kjellstrand & P. Ivanovich, Eds. : 630–634. ISAO Press.
10. SUN, A.M., Z. CAI, Z. SHI, F. MA, G.M. O'SHEA & H. GHARAPETIAN. 1986. Micoencapsulated hepatocytes as a bioartificial liver. Trans. Am. Soc. Artif. Intern. Organs **32:** 39–41.
11. SUN, A.M., Z. CAI, Z. SHI, F. MA & G.M. O'SHEA. 1987. Microencapsulated hepatocytes: an in vitro and in vivo study. Biomater. Artif. Cells Artif. Organs **15:** 483–496.
12. DIXIT, V., M. ARTHUR, R. REINHARDT & G. GITNICK. 1992. Improved function of microencapsulated hepatocytes in a bioartificial liver support system. Artif. Organs **16:** 336–341.
13. SUGAMORI, M., A.H. BOAG, R.L. BROUGHTON & M.V. SEFTON. 1986. Microencapsulation of mammalian cells in polyacrylate membranes for metabolic protheses. *In* Progress in Artificial Organs, Y. Nosè. C. Kjellstrand & P. Ivanovich, Eds. : 630–634. ISAO Press.
14. STANGE, J., S. MITZNER, H. DAUTZENBERG, W. RAMLOW, M. KNIPPEL, M. STEINER, B. ERNST, R. SCHMIDT & H. KLINKMANN. 1993. Prolonged biochemical and morphological stability of encapsulated liver cells—a new method. Biomater. Artif. Cells Immobil. Biotechnol. **21**(3)**:** 343–352.
15. DUNN, J.C.Y., M.L. YARMUSH, H.G. KOEBE & R.G. TOMPKINS. 1989. Hepatocyte function and extracellular matrix geometry: long-term culture in a sandwich configuration. FASEB J. **3:** 174–177.
16. DUNN, J.C., R.G. TOMPKINS & M.L. YARMUSH. 1992. Hepatocytes in collagen sandwich: evidence for transcriptional and translational regulation. J. Cell Biol. **116**(4)**:** 1043–1053.
17. EZZEL, R.M., M. TONER, K. HENDRICKS, J.C. DUNN, R.G. TOMPKINS & M.L. YARMUSH. 1993. Effect of collagen gel configuration on the cytosceleton in cultured rat hepatocytes. Exp. Cell Res. **208**(2)**:** 442–452.
18. BADER, A., K. ZECH, O. CROME, U. CHRISTIANS, R. PICHLMAYR & K.F. SEWING. 1994. Use of organotypical cultures of primary hepatocytes to analyze drug biotransformation in man and animals. Xenobiotica **24:** 623–633.
19. KOEBE, H.G., S. PAHERNIK, P. EYER & F.W. SCHILBERG. 1994. Collagen gel immobilization: a usefull cell culture technique for long-term metabolic studies on human hepatocytes. Xenobiotica **24:** 95–107.
20. KOEBE, H.G., M. WICK, U. CRAMER, V. LANGE & F.W. SCHILDBERG. 1994. Collagen gel immobilization provides a suitable cell matrix for long term human hepatocyte cultures in hybrid reactors. Int. J. Artif. Organs **17**(2)**:** 95–106.
21. GERLACH, J., K. KLOEPPEL, C. MÜLLER, N. SCHNOY, M.D. SMITH & P. NEUHAUS. 1993. Hepatocyte aggregate culture technique in liver support systems. Int. J. Artif. Organs **16:** 785–788.
22. LANDRY, J., D. BERNIER & C. OUELLET. 1985. Speroidal aggregate culture of rat liver cells: histiotypic reorganization, biomatrix deposition, and maintainance of functional activities. J. Cell Biol. **101:** 914–923.
23. TONG, J.Z., O. BERNARD & F. ALVAREZ. 1990. Long term culture of rat liver cell spheroids in hormonally defined media. Exp. Cell Res. **189:** 87–92.
24. SHINJI, T., N. KOIDE & T. TSUJI. 1988. Glycosaminoglycans partially substitute for proteoglycans in spheroid formation of adult rat hepatocytes in primary culture. Cell Struct. Funct. **13**(2)**:** 179–188.
25. KOIDE, N., K. SAKAGUCCI & Y. KOIDE. 1990. Formation of multicellular spheroids composed of adult rat hepatocytes in dishes with positive charged surfaces and under other nonadherent environments. Exp. Cell Res. **186**(2)**:** 227–235.
26. SPRAY, D.C., M. FUJITA, J.C. SAEZ, H. CHOI, T. WATANABE, E. HERTZBERG, L.C. ROSENBERG & L.M. REID. 1987. Proteoglycans and glycosaminoglycans induce gap junction synthesis and function in primary liver culture. J. Cell Biol. **105:** 541–551.

27. KAWAGUCHI, M., N. KOIDE, K. SAKAGUCHI, T. SHINJI & T. TSUJI. 1992. Combination of epidermal growth factor and insulin is required for multicellular spheroid formation of rat hepatocytes in primary culture. Acta Med. Okayama **46**(3): 195–201.
28. SAKAGUCHI, K., N. KOIDE, K. ASANO, H. TAKABATAKE, H. MATSUSHIMA, T. TAKENAMI, R. ONO, S. SASAKI, M. MORI & Y. KOIDE. 1991. Promotion of spheroid assembly of adult rat hepatocytes by some factors present in the initial 6-hour conditioned medium of the primary culture. Pathobiology **59**(5): 351–356.
29. ASANO, K., N. KOIDE & T. TSUJI. 1989. Ultrastucture of multicellular spheroids formed in the primary culture of adult rat hepatocytes. J. Clin. Electron Microsc. **22**(2): 243–252.
30. KOIDE, N., T. SHINJI, T. TANABE, K. ASANO, M. KAWAGUCHI, K. SAKAGUCHI, Y. KOIDE, M. MORI & T. TSUJI. 1989. Continued high albumin production by multicellular spheroids of adult rat hepatocytes in the presence of liver derived proteoglycans. Biochem. Biophys. Res. Commun. **161**(1): 385–391.
31. YUASA, C., Y. TOMITA, M. SHONO, K. ISHIMURA & A. ICHIHARA. 1993. Importance of cell aggregation for expression of liver functions and regeneration demonstrated with primary cultured hepatocytes. J. Cell Physiol. **156**: 522–530.
32. TAKABATAKE, H., N. KOIDE & T. TSUJI. 1991. Encapsulated multicellular spheroids of rat hepatocytes produce albumin and urea in a spouted bed circulating culture system. Artif. Organs **15**(6): 474–480.
33. MIURA, Y., T. AKIMOTO, H. KANAZAWA & K. YAGI. 1986. Synthesis and secretion of protein by hepatocytes entrapped within calcium alginate. Artif. Organs **10**(6): 460–465.
34. MIURA, Y., T. AKIMOTO, N. YOSHIKAWA & K. YAGI. 1990. Characterization of immobilized hepatocytes as liver support. Biomater. Artif. Cells Artif. Organs **18**(4): 549–554.
35. THOMPKINS, R.G. & E.A. CARTER. 1988. Enzymatic function of alginate immobilized rat hepatocytes. Biotechnol. Bioeng. **31**: 11–18.
36. YANAGI, K., S. MIZUNO & N. OSHIMA. 1989. A high density culture of hepatocytes using a reticulated polyvinyl formal resin. Trans. Am. Soc. Artif. Intern. Organs **36**: 13–16.
37. HENNE-BRUNS, D., U. KRUGER, D. SUMPELMANN, W. LIERSE & B. KREMER. 1991. Intraperiotoneal hepatocyte transplantation: morphological results. Virchows Arch. A Pathol. Anat. Histopathol. **419**(1): 45–50.
38. HENNE-BRUNS, D. 1993. Problems and controversies with transplantation of isolated hepatocytes for artificial liver support. *In* Artificial Liver Support. G. Brunner & M. Mito, Eds. 2. Auflage: 313–323. Springer Verlag. Berlin, Heidelberg, New York.
39. VANHOLDER, R. & S. RINGOIR. 1991. Artificial organs: an overview. Artif. Organs **14**: 613–618.
40. VANHOLDER, R. & S. RINGOIR. 1991. Bioartificial pancreas and liver: a review. Artif. Organs **14**: 398–402.
41. KNAZEK, R.A., P.M. GULLINO, P.O. KOHLER & R.L. DEDRICK. 1972. Cell culture on artificial capillaries: an approach to tissue growth in vitro. Science **78**: 65–67.
42. KNAZEK, R.A., P.O. KOHLER & P.M. GULLINO. 1974. Hormone production by cells grown in vitro on artificial capillaries. Exp. Cell Res. **84**: 251–254.
43. OLUMIDE, F., A. ELIASHIV, N. KRALIOS, L. NORTON & B. EISEMAN. 1977. Hepatic support with hepatocyte suspension in a permeable membrane dialyzer. Surgery **82**: 599–606.
44. MATSUMURA, K.N., G.R. GUEVARA, H. HUSTON, W.L. HAMILTON, M. RIKIMARU, G. YAMASAKI & M.S. MATSUMURA. 1987. Hybrid bioartificial liver in hepatic failure: preliminary clinical report. Surgery **101**(1): 99–103.
45. MARGULIS, M.S., E.A. ERUKHIMOV, L.A. ANDREIMAN, K.A. KUZNETSOV, L.M. VIKSNA, A.I. KUZNETSOV & V.V. DEVYATOV. 1990. Hemoperfusion through suspension of cryopreserved hepatocytes in a treatment of patients with acute liver failure. Res. Surg. **2**: 99–102.
46. MARGULIS, M.S., E.A. ERUKHIMOV & L.A. ANDREIMAN. 1989. Temporary organ substitution by hemoperfusion through suspension of active donor hepatocytes in a

total complex of intensive therapy in patients witjh acute hepatic insufficiency. Resuscitation **18:** 85–94.

47. GERLACH, J., K. KLOEPPEL & H.H. SCHAUWECKER. 1989. Use of hepatocytes in adhesion and suspension cultures for liver support bioreactors. Int. J. Artif. Organs **12:** 788–792.
48. SHNYRA, A., A. BOCHAROV, N. BOCHKOVA & V. SPIROV. 1991. Bioartificial liver using hepatocytes on biosilon microcarriers: treatment of chemically induced acute hepatic failure in rats. Artif. Organs **15:** 189–197.
49. TUBURAYA, T., J. UCHINO & T. KOMAI. 1989. Can hepatocytes contribute to an advance of artificial liver? Artif. Organs **13**(4)**:** 381.
50. UCHINO, J., T. TSUBURAYA, F. KUMAGAI, T. HASE, T. HAMADA, T. KOMAI, A. FUNATSU, E. HASHIMURA, K. NAKAMURA & T. KON. 1988. A hybrid bioartificial liver composed of multiplated hepatocyte monolayers. ASAIO Trans. **34:** 972–977.
51. UCHINO, J., H. MATSUE, M. TAKAHASHI, Y. NAKAJIAMA, M. MATSUSHITA, T. HAMADA & E. HASHIMURA. 1991. A hybrid artificial liver. Function of cultured monolayer pig hepatocytes in plasma from hepatic failure patients. ASAIO Trans. **37:** 337–338.
52. YANAGI, K., K. OOKAWA, S. MIZUNO & N. OHSHIMA. 1989. Performance of a new hybrid artificial liver support system using hepatocytes entrapped within a hydrogel. ASAIO Trans. **35:** 570–572.
53. TAKABATAKE, H., N. KOIDE & T. TSUJI. 1991. Encapsulated multicellular spheroids of rat hepatocytes produce albumin and urea in a spouted bed circulating culture system. Artif. Organs **15**(6)**:** 474–480.
54. JAUREGUI, H.O., S. NAIK, J.L. DRISCOLL, B.A. SOLOMON & P.M. GALLETTI. 1983. Adult rat hepatocyte cultures as the cellular component of an artificial hybrid liver. *In* Biomaterials in Artificial Organs, Proceedings of a seminar on biomaterials held at the University of Strathclyde, Glasgow. J.P. Paul, J.D.S. Gaylor, J.M. Courtney & T. Gilchrist, Eds. : 130–140.
55. DEMETRIOU, A.A., W.S. ARNAOUT, G. BACKFISCH & A.D. MOSCIONI. 1993. Immobilized isolated liver cells on a biomatrix. *In* Artificial Liver Support. G. Brunner & M. Mito, Eds. 2. Auflage: 283–295. Springer Verlag. Berlin, Heidelberg, New York.
56. WOLF, C.F.W. & B.E. MUNKELT. 1976. Bilirubin conjugation by an artificial liver composed of cultured cells and synthetic capillaries. Trans. Am. Soc. Artif. Intern. Organs **21:** 16–27.
57. ROZGA, J., M.D. HOLZMANN, M.S. RO, D.W. GRIFFIN, D.F. NEUZIL, T. GIORGIO, A. MOSCIONI & A.A. DEMETRIOU. 1993. Development of a hybrid bioartificial liver. Ann. Surg. **217**(5)**:** 502–511.
58. ARNAOUT, W.S., A.D. MOSCIONI, R.L. BARBOUR & A.A. DEMETRIOU. 1990. Development of bioartificial liver: bilirubin conjugation in Gunn-rats. J. Surg. Res. **48:** 379–382.
59. DIXIT,V. 1994. Development of a bioartificial liver using isolated hepatocytes. Artif. Organs **18:** 371–384.
60. HU, W.S., S.L. NYBERG & R.A. SHATFORD. 1991. Cultivation of hepatocytes in a new entrapment reactor: a potential bioartificial liver. *In* Animal Cell Culture And Production of Biologicals. R. Sasaki & K. Ikura, Eds. : 75–80. Kluwer Academic Publishers. Dordecht, The Netherlands.
61. NYBERG, S.L., A. RUSSEL, R.A. SHATFORD, V. MADHUSUDAN, M.V. PESHWA, J.G. WHITE, F.B. CERRA & W.S. HU. 1993. Evaluation of a hepatocyte-entrapment hollow fiber bioreactor: a potential bioartificial liver. Biotechnol. Bioeng. **41:** 194–203.
62. SHATFORD, R.A., S.L. NYBERG, S.J. MEIER, J.G. WHITE, W.D. PAYNE, W.S. HU & F.B. CERRA. 1992. Hepatocyte function in a hollow fiber bioreactor: a potential bioartificial liver. J. Surg. Res. **53:** 549–557.
63. SCHOLZ, M. & W.S. HU. 1991. A two compartment cell entrapment bioreactor with three different holding times for cells, high and low molecular weight compounds. Cytotechnology **4:** 127–137.

64. MATTHEW, H.W., S.O. SALLEY, W.D. PETERSON, D.R. DESHMUKH, A. MUKHOPADHYAY & M.D. KLEIN. 1991. Microencapsulated hepatocytes. Prospects for extracorporeal liver support. ASAIO Trans. **37**(3): 328–330.
65. AKAIKE, T., S. TOBE, A. KOBAYASHI, M. GOTO & K. KOBAYASHI. 1993. Design of hepatocyte specific extracellular matrices for hybrid artificial liver. Gastroenterol. Jpn. **28** (Suppl. 4): 45–56.
66. CLAYTON, D.F., A.L. HARRELSON & J.E. DARNELL. 1985. Dependence of liver-specific transscription on tissue organisation. Mol. Cell Biol. **5:** 2623–2632.
67. GERLACH, J., M. SMITH & P. NEUHAUS. 1994. Hepatocyte culture between woven capillary systems—a microscopy study. Artif. Organs **18:** 226–230.
68. GERLACH, J., K. KLÖPPEL, P. STOLL, J. VIENKEN, C. MÜLLER & H.H. SCHAUWECKER. 1990. Gas supply across membranes in liver support bioreactors. Artif. Organs **14:** 328–333.
69. GERLACH, J., P. STOLL, N. SCHNOY & E.S.B. BÜCHERL. 1990. Membranes as substrate for hepatocyte adhesion in liver support bioreactors. Int. J. Artif. Organs **13:** 436–441.
70. GERLACH, J., H.H. SCHAUWECKER, E. HENNIG & E.S. BÜCHERL. 1989. Endothelial cell seeding on different polyurethanes. Artif. Organs **13:** 144–147.
71. GERLACH, J. & P. NEUHAUS. 1994. Culture model for primary hepatocytes. In Vitro Cell. Dev. Biol. **30A:** 640–642.
72. GERLACH, J., J. ENCKE, O. HOLE, C. MÜLLER, C.J. RYAN & P. NEUHAUS. 1994. Bioreactor for larger scale hepatocyte in-vitro perfusion. Transplantation **58:** 984–988.
73. GERLACH, J., J. ENCKE, O. HOLE, C. MÜLLER, J. COURTNEY & P. NEUHAUS. 1994. Hepatocyte culture between three dimensional arranged biomatrix-coated independent artificial capillary systems and sinusoidal endothelial cell co-culture compartments. Int. J. Artif. Organs **17:** 301–306.
74. GERLACH, J., M. FUCHS, M. SMITH, J. ENCKE, P. NEUHAUS & E. RIEDEL. 1996. Is a clinical application of hybrid liver support limited by an initial disorder in primary hepatocyte amino acid metabolism? Transplantation **62:** 224–228.
75. GERLACH, J., N. SCHNOY, J. ENCKE, C. MÜLLER, M. SMITH & P. NEUHAUS. 1995. Improoved hepatocyte in vitro maintainance in a culture model with woven multicompartment capillary systems: electron microscopic studies. Hepatology **22:** 546–552.
76. SULLIVAN, S.J., T. MAKI & K.M. BORLAND. 1991. Biohybrid artificial pancreas: long-term implantation studies in diabetic, pancreatectomized dogs. Science **252:** 718–721.
77. NYBERG, S.L., J.L. PLATT, K. SHIRABE, W.D. PAYNE, W.S. HU & F.B. CERRA. 1992. Immunoprotection of xenocytes in a hollow fiber bioartificial liver. ASAIO J. **38:** M463–M467.
78. GLEISNER, M., R. BORNEMANN, R. STEMEROWICZ, M. MEISLER, P. NEUHAUS & J. GERLACH. 1997. Immunisolation of hybrid liver support systems by semipermeable membranes. Int. J. Artif. Organs **20:** 644–649.
79. JANKE, J., J. GERLACH, D. KARDASSIS, C. BÖHMER & R. ROSSAINT. 1997. Effect of a hybrid liver support system on cardiopulmonary function in healty pigs. Int. J. Artif. Organs **20:** 570–576.
80. GERLACH, J., A. JÖRRES, O. TROST, O. HOLE, J. VIENKEN, J.M. COURTNEY, G.M. GAHL & P. NEUHAUS. 1993. Side effects of hybrid liver support therapy: TNF-α liberation in pigs, associated with extracorporeal bioreactors. Int. J. Artif. Organs **16:** 604–608.
81. MATSUMURA, K.N., G.R. GUEVARA, H. HUSTON, W.L. HAMILTON, M. RIKIMARU, G. YAMASAKI & M.S. MATSUMURA. 1987. Hybrid bioartificial liver in hepatic failure: preliminary clinical report. Surgery **101**(1): 99–103.
82. MARGULIS, M.S., E.A. ERUKHIMOV, L.A. ANDREIMAN, K.A. KUZNETSOV, L.M. VIKSNA, A.I. KUZNETSOV & V.V. DEVYATOV. 1990. Hemoperfusion through suspension of cryopreserved hepatocytes in a treatment of patients with acute liver failure. Res. Surg. **2:** 99–102.
83. MARGULIS, M.S., E.A. ERUKHIMOV & L.A. ANDREIMAN. 1989. Temporary organ substitution by hemoperfusion through suspension of active donor hepatocytes in a total

complex of intensive therapy in patients with acute hepatic insufficiency. Resuscitation **18:** 85–94.

84. ROZGA, J., M.D. HOLZMANN, M.S. RO, D.W. GRIFFIN, D.F. NEUZIL, T. GIORGIO, A. MOSCIONI & A.A. DEMETRIOU. 1993. Development of a hybrid bioartificial liver. Ann. Surg. **217**(5)**:** 502–511.
85. NEUZIL, D., J. ROZGA, A.D. MOSCIONI, M.S. RO, R. HAKIM, W.S. ARNAOUT & A.A. DEMETRIOU. 1993. Use of a novel bioartificial liver in a patient with acute liver insufficiency. Surgery **113**(3)**:** 340–343.
86. ROZGA, J., L. PODESTA, E. LE PAGE, A. HOFFMAN, E. MORSIANI, L. SHER, G.M. WOOLF, L. MAKOWKA & A.A. DEMETRIOU. 1993. Control of cerebral oedema by total hepatectomy and extracorporeal liver support in fulminant hepatic failure. Lancet **342:** 898–899.
87. SUSSMAN, N.L. & J.H. KELLY. 1993. Improved liver function following treatment with an extracorporeal liver assist device. Artif. Organs **17**(1)**:** 27–30.
88. SUSSMAN, N.L., M.J. FINEGOLD & J.H. KELLY. 1992. Recovery from syncytial giant-cell hepatitis (SCGH) following treatment with an extracorporal liver assist device (ELAD). Hepatology **16:** 51A.
89. WOOD, R.P., S.M. KATZ, C.F. OZAKI, H.P. MONSOUR, G.T. GISLASON, J.H. KELLY & N.L. SUSSMAN. 1993. Extracorporeal liver assist device (ELAD): a preliminary report. Transplant. Proc. **25**(4)**:** 53–54.
90. GISLASON, G.T., D.D. LOBDELL, J.H. KELLY & N.L. SUSSMAN. 1994. A treatment system for implementing an extracorporeal liver assist device. Artif. Organs **18**(5)**:** 385–389.
91. KELLY, J.H. & N.L. SUSSMAN. 1994. The hepatix extracorporeal liver assist device in the treatment of fulminant hepatic failure. ASAIO J. **1:** 83–85.
92. ROZGA, J., L. PODESTA, E. LEPAGE, E. MORSIANI, A.D. MOSCIONI, A. HOFFMAN, L. SHER, F. VILLAMIL, G. WOOLF, M. MCGRATH, L. KONG, H. ROSEN, T. LANMAN, J. VIERLING, L. MAKOWKA & A.A. DEMETRIOU. 1994. A bioatificial liver to treat severe acute liver failure. Ann. Surg. **219**(5)**:** 538–546.
93. GERLACH, J. Development of a hybrid liver support system—a review. 1996. Int. J. Artif. Organs **19:** 645–655.
94. LANGER, R. & J.P. VACANTI. 1993. Tissue engineering. Science **260:** 920–925.
95. MCLIMANS, W.F., L.E. BLUMENSON & K.V. TUNNAH. 1968. Kinetics of gas diffusion in mammalian cell culture systems. Biotechnol. Bioeng. **10:** 741–763.
96. GERLACH, J., K. KLÖPPEL, P. STOLL, J. VIENKEN, C. MÜLLER & H.H. SCHAUWECKER. 1990. Gas supply across membranes in liver support bioreactors. Artif. Organs **14**(5)**:** 328–333.
97. WOLF, C.F. & L.L. LAUFFER. 1986. Design and fabrication of a capillary cell culture chamber for study of convective flow. Int. J. Artif. Organs **9**(1)**:** 25–32.
98. DAVIS, M.E. & L.T. WATSON. 1985. Analysis of a diffusion-limited hollow fiber reactor for the measurement of effective substrate diffusivities. Biotechnol. Bioeng. **27:** 182–186.
99. SCHONBERG, J.A. & G. BELFORT. 1987. Enhancement nutrient transport in hollow fiber perfusion bioreactors: a theoreatical analysis. Biotechnol. Prog. **3:** 80–89.
100. PIRET, J.M. & C.L. COONEY. 1991. Model of oxygen transport limitations in hollow fiber bioreactors. Biotechnol. Bioeng. **37:** 80–92.
101. GIORGIO, T.D., A.D. MOSCIONI, J. ROZGA & A.A. DEMETRIOU. 1993. Mass transfer in a hollow fiber device used as a bioartificial liver. ASAIO J. **39:** 886–892.
102. HUGHES, R. & R. WILLIAMS. 1996. Assessment of bioartificial liver support in acute liver failure. *In* Acute Liver Failure. R. Williams & W.M. Lee, Eds. Cambridge.

# Novel Bioartificial Liver Support System: Preclinical Evaluation

JOHN F. PATZER II,[a–d,k] GEORGE V. MAZARIEGOS,[a,b] ROBERTO LOPEZ,[b,g] ERNESTO MOLMENTI,[b] DAVID GERBER,[b] FRIDTJOV RIDDERVOLD,[e,h] AJAI KHANNA,[b] WEN-YAO YIN,[b,i] YONG CHEN,[b] VICTOR L. SCOTT,[e] SHUSHMA AGGARWAL,[e] DAVID J KRAMER,[a,b,e] ROBERT A. WAGNER,[f] YUE ZHU,[a,b] MELISSA L. FULMER,[b] GEOFFREY D. BLOCK,[a] AND BRUCE P AMIOT[j]

[a]*Department of Surgery,* [b]*Thomas E Starzl Transplantation Institute,* [c]*Department of Chemical Engineering,* [d]*The McGowan Center for Artificial Organs,* [e]*Department of Anesthesiology, and* [f]*Central Animal Facility, University of Pittsburgh, Pittsburgh, Pennsylvania 15213-2582, USA*

[g]*Department of Surgery, Universidad de Monterrey, Monterrey, NL, Mexico*

[h]*Department of Anesthesiology, Rikshospitalet, University of Oslo, National University Hospital of Norway, N-0027 Oslo 1, Norway*

[i]*Tzu-Chi General Hospital, Hualien, Taiwan, ROC*

[j]*Excorp Medical, Inc., Suite 235, 7200 Hudson Boulevard, Oakdale, Minnesota 55128, USA*

**ABSTRACT: Preclinical safety and efficacy evaluation of a novel bioartificial liver support system (BLSS) was conducted using a D-galactosamine canine liver failure model. The BLSS houses a suspension of porcine hepatocytes in a hollow fiber cartridge with the hepatocytes on one side of the membrane and whole blood flowing on the other. Porcine hepatocytes harvested by a collagenase digestion technique were infused into the hollow fiber cartridge and incubated for 16 to 24 hours prior to use. Fifteen purpose-bred male hounds, 1–3 years old, 25–30 kg, were administered a lethal dose, 1.5 g/kg, of D-galactosamine. The animals were divided into three treatment groups: (1b) no BLSS treatment (n = 6); (2b) BLSS treatment starting at 24–26 h post D-galactosamine (n = 5); and (2c) BLSS treatment starting at 16–18 h post D-galactosamine (n = 4). While maintained under isoflurane anesthesia, canine supportive care was guided by electrolyte and invasive physiologic monitoring consisting of arterial pressure, central venous pressure, extradural intracranial pressure (ICP), pulmonary artery pressure, urinary catheter, and end-tidal $CO_2$. All animals were treated until death or death-equivalent (inability to sustain systolic blood pressure > 80 mmHg for 20 minutes despite massive fluid resuscitation and/or dopamine administration), or euthanized at 60 hours. All animals developed evidence of liver failure at 12–24 hours as evidenced by blood pressure lability, elevated ICP, marked hepatocellular enzyme elevation with microscopic massive hepatocyte necrosis and cerebral edema, elevated prothrombin time, and metabolic acidosis. Groups 2b and 2c marginally prolong survival compared with Group 1b (pairwise log rank censored survival time analysis, $p = 0.096$ and $p = 0.064$, respectively). Since survival times for Groups 2b and 2c are not sig-**

[k]Author for correspondence: Departments of Surgery and Chemical Engineering, 1249 Benedum Hall, University of Pittsburgh, Pittsburgh, PA 15261; 412-624-9819 (voice); 412-624-9639 (fax); patzer+@pitt.edu (e-mail).

**nificantly different ($p = 0.694$), the groups were combined for further statistical analysis. Survival times for the combined active treatment Groups 2b and 2c are significantly prolonged versus Group 1b ($p = 0.047$). These results suggest the novel BLSS reported here can have a significant impact on the course of liver failure in the D-galactosamine canine liver failure model. The BLSS is ready for Phase I safety evaluation in a clinical setting.**

## INTRODUCTION

The American Liver Foundation estimates that one in ten people has some form of liver disease.[1] Also, 43,967 people died in the United States from liver disease or its complications in 1996.[1] Patients with liver disease generally fall into two classifications: fulminant liver failure, defined as sudden onset (less than eight weeks) with no previous history of liver disease, and chronic liver disease. Both classifications have subclassifications that further define the etiology of the disease. Patients with either classification can progressively worsen until they require orthotopic liver transplantation (OLT), which is the only recognized effective treatment.[2] In 1996, the latest year for which statistics are available, 7,480 people were listed for liver transplantation while only 4,013 livers were available for transplant.[3] A medical need for a treatment modality that can "bridge" patients to transplant or slow or reverse the progression of acute liver disease clearly exists.

From an engineering viewpoint, the liver is a complex biochemical reactor that performs several functions: oxidative *detoxification*; intermediate *metabolism* and supply of nutrients; toxin and waste *excretion* through the bile; protein and macromolecule *synthesis*; and *modulation* of immune and hormonal systems. An implantable, long-term artificial liver would need to perform all of these functions. Treatment for liver failure, however, could focus on various aspects of liver function. Under the hypothesis that early removal of the putative (unknown) toxins associated with progressive liver failure would be sufficient for the liver to recover function on its own, treatment in the early stages of acute liver failure could supplement *detoxification* and *excretion* function by variants on extracorporeal hemodialysis directed toward removal of protein-bound toxins. Treatment modalities based on this hypothesis have been proposed and are in various stages of clinical evaluation.[4-6]

In many cases, a more fully functional bioartificial liver support system (BLSS) that provides active oxidative *detoxification*, intermediate *metabolism*, and additional *excretion* capabilities may be required to treat progressive liver failure. Several devices that rely on liver cells (hepatocytes) housed in an extracorporeal circuit to provide active biochemical processing to provide active metabolic support to patients with acute liver failure are in various stages of clinical,[7–15] preclinical,[16,17] and research[18–21] development. These devices use viable liver cells because they can provide necessary biochemical function without the requirement to identify the particular pathway out of numerous metabolic pathways necessary to support a patient with liver failure.

TABLE 1 provides a brief comparison of "first generation" BLSSs that are either in clinical evaluation or have shown sufficient evidence of safety and efficacy in preclinical large animal model evaluations that they are ready for Phase I safety evaluation in a clinical setting. These first generation systems[7–17] operate in a manner

**TABLE 1.** Comparison of bioartificial liver assist devices at clinical or preclinical stages of development

| Device: Features: | Demetriou *et al.*[7–10] | Gerlach *et al.*[11–13] | Kelly *et al.*[14,15] | Patzer *et al.* | Cerra *et al.*[16,17] |
|---|---|---|---|---|---|
| fluid: | plasma | blood | blood | blood | blood |
| hepatocytes: | primary porcine | primary porcine | human Hep2 cell line | primary porcine | primary porcine |
| amount: | 100–500 g | 100–500 g | 100–500 g | 100 g | 10–30 g |
| attachment: | beads | collagen matrix | | collagen matrix | collagen matrix |
| cartridge: | hollow fiber | tri-partite hollow fiber | hollow fiber | hollow fiber | hollow fiber |
| other: | charcoal filter | oxygenation in cartridge | ultrafiltration | blood oxygenator | cells in fiber lumen |
| | plasma oxygenator | nutrient supply to hepatocytes | | nutrient supply to hepatocytes | nutrient supply to hepatocytes |
| | cryopreserved hepatocytes | | | no net ultrafiltration | no net ultrafiltration |
| Advantages: | Phase I clinical trial success | Separate flows for oxygen | Human tissue | Simple design | Simple design |
| | Distribution system known | and hepatocyte nutrients | | | Simple scalability |

similar to hemodialysis. Patient blood is drawn from the body by veno-venous access, circulated to the BLSS, and returned to the body. The BLSS may have a plasma separator[7–10] in order to treat the plasma only. Perceived advantages of plasma separation are lessening of clotting potential in the BLSS hollow fiber cartridge and the ability to run plasma at high recycle rates, thus providing greater processing per unit volume of blood drawn. All systems provide oxygenation capacity for maintenance of hepatocyte viability, either indirectly through use of an oxygenator for blood or plasma prior to the bioreactor[7–10,14–17] or directly to the hollow fiber cartridge.[11–13]

The heart of each system is a hollow fiber cartridge housing an active liver cell culture on one side of the hollow fibers while plasma or whole blood flows on the other side. A patient's blood is protected from direct contact with the liver cells by the hollow fiber membrane. Some systems use a microporous membrane with about 200 nm pore size[7–10] that permits potential passage of immunological response mediators such as immunoglobulins. Other systems use membranes with a molecular weight passage cut-off of about 100 kD that permit passage of blood-borne toxins or albumin-bound toxins (~60 kD) and other metabolic moieties, but prohibit passage of large immune response modulators such as immunoglobulins.[31,32] Molecules pass across the membrane by diffusion where they can be taken up by the cells and detoxified or metabolized. Likewise, hepatocyte metabolic products can diffuse from the cell space, across the membrane, and return to the patient. Additional excretory function (biliary) is provided by flow or ultrafiltration on the cell side of the hollow fiber cartridge. Excreted hepatocyte waste products that are too large to cross the membrane, nominally 200 nm for microporous membranes and 100 kD for ultrafiltration membranes, or have insufficient time to diffuse across the membrane will convect out of the reactor with the cell side flow. The systems are distinguished from each other primarily by how hepatocytes are housed in the hollow fiber cartridge, source of hepatocytes, methods for supplying nutrients to the hepatocytes, and whether they use whole blood or plasma.

## EXPERIMENTAL

### *Novel BLSS Specifics*

FIGURE 1 is a schematic block-flow diagram of the Excorp Medical BLSS. Blood is drawn by veno-venous access from the patient and passed through a blood warmer and oxygenator prior to entering the bioreactor. Blood flow rates are 100 to 500 mL/min depending upon patient hemodynamic tolerance for the extracorporeal circuit. Provision is made for heparin administration when the patient's activated clotting time (ACT) falls below specified values. A pH probe prior to the bioreactor is used to monitor blood pH entering the bioreactor. The oxygenator gas flows, $N_2$, $O_2$, and $CO_2$, are maintained by mass flow controllers adjusted to sustain desired oxygen tensions and blood pH for blood entering the bioreactor. From the bioreactor, blood flows to a bubble trap to remove any entrapped gases prior to returning to the patient. The system is equipped with pressure sensors that monitor functions such as venous access pressure and differential pressures across the bioreactor. Alarms sound when pressures vary beyond specified setpoints.

The heart of the system is a hollow fiber cartridge containing greater than 70 g of primary porcine hepatocytes embedded in a collagen matrix. The hepatocytes are greater than 80% viable by trypan blue exclusion before mixing with 20% vol/wt Vitrogen 100 (3.1% collagen) and infusing into the bioreactor. The hollow fibers have a nominal molecular weight diffusion cutoff of 100 kD. Blood-borne toxins and metabolic precursors are free to diffuse across the membrane to the hepatocytes where they can be metabolized. Metabolic products and detoxified toxins are free to diffuse back across the membrane to the flowing blood.

Also in the circuit is a flowing nutrient stream that directly perfuses the hepatocytes, providing hepatocyte specific nutrients. The hepatocyte nutrient stream is metered into and out of the bioreactor (at about 0.25% of the blood flow rate) to maintain no net flow and, thus, prevent ultrafiltration or active delivery of cell side constituents to the patient's blood. The nutrient stream flow also provides a secondary mechanism for elimination of hepatocyte waste products that may be excreted by the cells and that are too large to cross the membrane back to the blood stream.

### *Canine D-Galactosamine Liver Failure Model*

The lethal canine D-galactosamine liver failure model is considered to be an appropriate large-scale animal model for preclinical evaluation of BLSSs.[22,17,23] The intervention protocols for the model, limited to supportive care consisting of electrolyte and glucose replacement and fluids management to maintain vascular pressures, are intended to highlight the safety and potential efficacy of a support device. The study protocol, reviewed and approved by the University of Pittsburgh Institutional Animal Care and Use Committee (IACUC), meets institutional and national standards for the humane care of research animals for minimization of pain and discomfort to the animals. The experiments were conducted in the Central Animal Facility of the University of Pittsburgh.

Fifteen purpose-bred male hounds, 1–3 years old, 25–30 kg, were administered a lethal dose, 1.5 g/kg, of D-gal. The animals were divided into three treatment groups: (1b) no BLSS treatment ($n = 6$); (2b) BLSS treatment starting at 24–26 h post D-gal ($n = 5$); and (2c) BLSS treatment starting at 16–18 h post D-gal ($n = 4$). While maintained under isoflurane anesthesia, canine supportive care was guided by electrolyte and invasive monitoring consisting of arterial pressure, central venous pressure, extradural intracranial pressure (ICP), pulmonary artery pressure, urinary catheter, and end-tidal $CO_2$. All animals were treated until death or death-equivalent, or euthanized at 60 hours. *Death equivalent* was defined as inability to sustain systolic blood pressure > 80 mmHg for 20 minutes despite maximal fluids and 20 μg/kg/min dopamine infusion. Comprehensive data collection included survival to voluntary termination, hemodynamic stability, cerebral perfusion pressure, ICP, cardiac output, time to anesthetic recovery, and laboratory parameters.

Assignment to groups was not random, but rather sequential. Group 1b animals generally preceded Group 2b animals, which preceded Group 2c animals. The decision to intervene at 16–18 hours post D-galactosamine with Group 2c was made after reviewing results of Group 2b animals in comparison with Group 1b. Another statistically confounding factor in the experimental design is that improvements in the hepatocyte isolation and bioreactor preparation procedures were made over time.

### *Porcine Hepatocyte Isolation*

Hepatocytes were isolated by a modified Seglen technique[24–27] under an IACUC-approved protocol. Briefly, 8–18 kg pigs were anesthetized with ketamine, 20 mg/kg im, and xylazine, 2 mg/kg im, induced with thiopental, 5 mg/kg iv, intubated and maintained under 1–1.5% isoflurane in oxygen. Working under sterile conditions, the abdomen was entered through a chevron incision, the infrahepatic inferior vena cava (IVC) isolated and encircled, and the suprahepatic IVC above the diaphragm isolated and encircled. The portal triad was dissected, ligating and dividing all structures except the hepatic artery and portal vein, which were isolated and looped. Sodium heparin (300 U/kg) was infused, followed by ligation of the infrahepatic IVC, cannulation of the portal vein, division of the hepatic artery, venting of the suprahepatic IVC, and removal of the liver from the pig. Several liters of a calcium chelating, balanced salt solution were perfused through the liver at a rate of about 100 mL/kg/min and discarded. Subsequently, a second, collagenase containing solution was recirculated through the liver until it was soft and well digested by palpitation and inspection. The pig was euthanized by KCl, 10 mL iv.

Immediately following digestion, the liver was quenched by submersion in cold Williams E wash media. Working under sterile conditions, the capsule was then ruptured and the hepatocytes gently raked from the liver tissue. The hepatocytes were filtered through a porcelain filter funnel to remove large tissue aggregates. The hepatocytes were then centrifuged at 50 g for three minutes followed by aspiration of the supernatant. The hepatocytes were washed by resuspension in cold Williams E me-

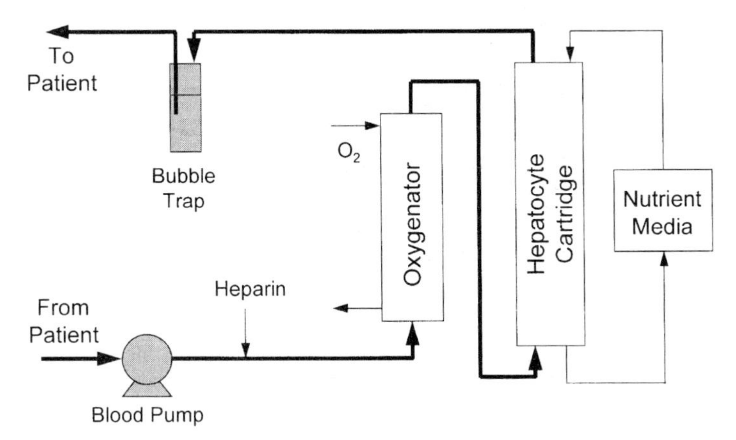


**FIGURE 1.** Block schematic diagram of the Excorp Medical bioartificial liver support system (BLSS).

dia, centrifugation, and aspiration of the supernatant until the supernatant appeared clear. The final hepatocyte pellet had a cell density greater than $10^7$ cells/mL. Hepatocyte viability by trypan blue exclusion was 70–85%.

### *Bioreactor Preparation*

The hepatocyte pellet was blended with 15–25% (vol/wt) collagen. At least 70 g of hepatocytes were infused into a hollow fiber cartridge containing cellulose acetate fibers with approximately 100 kD pore size cutoff. The bioreactor was then placed in an incubator in a flow system comparable to that of FIGURE 1 for 16 to 30 hours prior to use. Williams E media supplemented with insulin and glucagon[17] was used in the blood flow path during incubation. At time of use, the bioreactor was removed from the incubator and transported to the canine-care site under sterile conditions. The total time between disconnection from the incubator and reconnection into the BLSS system was typically less than 30 minutes.

## RESULTS

All of the animals in the study presented evidence of profoundly progressing liver failure at 12–24 hours as evidenced by blood pressure lability, elevated intracranial pressure (ICP), marked hepatocellular enzyme elevation (AST and ALT), rising blood ammonia levels, elevated prothrombin times (PT) and ACTs, and metabolic acidosis. Descriptions of the D-galactosamine canine liver failure model with respect to blood chemistries, hemodynamic stability, ICP, cerebral perfusion pressure (CPP), and survival are reported elsewhere.[22,23] TABLE 2 reports blood chemistry results for the experimental groups at 0, 24, and 48 hours post D-galactosamine as mean ± standard error of the mean (SE). Survival times are also included. Apart from thrombocytopenia and transient hypotension at the onset of BLSS treatment, the BLSS was well tolerated.

**TABLE 2.** Survival and blood chemistry results at 0, 24, and 48 h post D-galactosamine adminstration (mean ± SE)

| Parameter | Group 1b ($n$ = 6) | | | Group 2b ($n$ = 5) | | | Group 2c ($n$ = 4) | | |
|---|---|---|---|---|---|---|---|---|---|
| Treatment | No BLSS | | | BLSS @ 24–26 h | | | BLSS @ 16–18 h | | |
| Survival to 60 h, N | 0/6 (0%) | | | 2/5 (40%) | | | 2/4 (50%) | | |
| Survival time, h | 43.7 ± 4.6 | | | 53.2 ± 3.3 | | | 54.5 ± 4.3 | | |
| (time post D-gal:) | 0 h | 24 h | 48 h | 0 h | 24 h | 48 h | 0 hr | 24 h | 48 h |
| ICP, mmHg | [a]25 ± 6 | 31 ± 8 | 51 ± 16 | [a]29 ± 6 | 22 ± 4 | 29 ± 5 | [a]24 ± 1 | 30 ± 4 | 40 |
| CPP, mmHg | [a]82 ± 5 | 51 ±14 | 29 ± 9 | [a]95 ± 11 | 55 ± 8 | 43 ± 11 | [a]63 ± 5 | 47 ± 7 | 15 |
| ALT, µmol/L | 32 ± 2 | 1199 ± 460 | 9740 ± 2661 | 37 ± 3 | 1056 ± 33 | 10974 ± 3340 | 38 ± 4 | 266 ± 20†,‡ | 3837 ± 1829‡ |
| AST, µmol/L | 26 ± 3 | 1141 ± 388 | 5977 ± 1052 | 24 ± 1 | 693 ± 171 | 5778 ± 2249 | 30 ± 6 | 370 ± 86† | 2812 ± 1231 |
| $NH_3$, µmol/L | 19.8 ± 4.2 | 14.8 ± 2.9 | 85.3 ± 27.8 | 11.0 ± 1.8 | 11.0 ± 2.7 | 45.0 ± 7.5 | 10.0 ± 3.4 | 7.0 ± 1.4 | 37.0 ± 15.1 |
| Lactate, mmol/L | 2.80 ± 0.20 | 4.07 ± 0.79 | 4.63 ± 1.33 | 2.44 ± 4.58 | 4.58 ± 0.56 | 7.03 ± 0.67 | 2.60 ± 0.58 | 3.08 ± 0.70 | 3.87 ± 0.74** |
| PT, s | 8.7 ± 0.1 | 20.1 ± 3.0 | 46 ± 0 | 9.5 ± 0.4 | 19.1 ± 2.9 | 46 ± 0 | 8.4 ± 0.1 | 13.7 ± 0.1*,** | 46 ± 0 |
| Platelets, 1000/mL | 195 ± 43 | 121 ± 23 | 56 ± 6 | 167 ± 27 | 103 ± 13 | 13 ± 2* | 161 ± 19 | 89 ± 15 | 46 ± 6‡ |

[a]At 12 h post D-galactosamine. *$p < 0.05$ vs Group 1b; **$p < 0.05$ vs Group 2b; † < 0.10 vs Group1b; ‡ $p < 0.10$ vs Group 2b

Pairwise log rank survival analysis comparing BLSS treatment commencing at 24–26 hours post D-galactosamine with no treatment, Group 2b versus Group 1b, indicates treatment commencing at 24–26 hours marginally prolongs survival time ($p = 0.096$). Similar analysis for BLSS treatment commencing at 16–18 hours post D-galactosamine versus no treatment, Group 2c versus Group 1b, indicates an improving trend in survival ($p = 0.064$) with earlier BLSS intervention. Log rank survival comparison of the BLSS treatment groups, Group 2b with Group 2c, indicates no significant difference between the two groups ($p = 0.694$) with respect to survival. Since the two treatment groups are statistically equivalent with respect to survival, they can be combined to look at the overall effect of BLSS treatment versus no treatment on survival. Survival times for the combined active treatment groups are significantly prolonged versus no treatment ($p = 0.047$).

Kruskal-Wallis analysis of variance by ranks,[28] a nonparametric method to compare small sample sizes, was used to evaluate comparisons between the treatment groups at 0, 24, and 48 hours post D-galactosamine for ICP, CPP, ALT, AST, ammonia, lactate, PT, and platelet count. Statistical significance was defined as $p < 0.05$ and a strong trend was defined as $p < 0.10$. The two BLSS treatment groups, 2b and 2c, were compared against the untreated group, 1b, and against each other. The results are provided in TABLE 2.

Treatment starting at 24–26 hours post D-galactosamine, Group 2b, while providing a strong trend in survival time, appears to have had little effect in altering the course of progressing liver failure. Increasing blood chemistries generally associated with liver failure are only marginally lower for the Group 2b animals, the difference not rising to a strong trend. The only statistically significant difference between Groups 2b and 1b is found in the platelet levels at 48 hours: the Group 2b animals have significantly fewer platelets than Group 1b. This effect is attributed to extracorporeal blood circuits generally, which are known to deplete platelets upon start of perfusion, although the platelet fraction generally recovers within a couple of hours to preperfusion levels.

BLSS treatment starting at 16–18 hours post D-galactosamine administration, Group 2c, is more efficacious. Several of the rising blood chemistry values show strong trend or statistically significant reduction in comparison with the untreated cohort, Group 1b, and the cohort receiving BLSS treatment starting 24–26 hours post D-galactosamine administration, Group 2b. The general trend appears to be that, in addition to a strong trend in prolonging survival time, BLSS treatment commencing at 16–18 hours post D-galactosamine delays the onset of the progression of increasing blood chemistry values associated with liver failure.

The effect of BLSS treatment for the combined Groups 2b and 2c in comparison with the untreated Group 1b on ICP and CPP is shown in FIGURES 2 and 3, respectively, which plot the mean ICP or CPP values for each cohort. Rising and unstable ICP is an important clinical feature of fulminant hepatic failure that is also seen with the D-galactosamine canine liver failure model.[22,23] The mean ICP for the BLSS-treated canines is comparable to that of the untreated canines for the first 40 hours and is statistically indistinguishable by analysis of variance. After about 45 hours, the untreated mean ICP starts to rise in comparison with the BLSS-treated mean ICP. Too few animals remain alive at this juncture however to attribute any statistical significance to the difference.

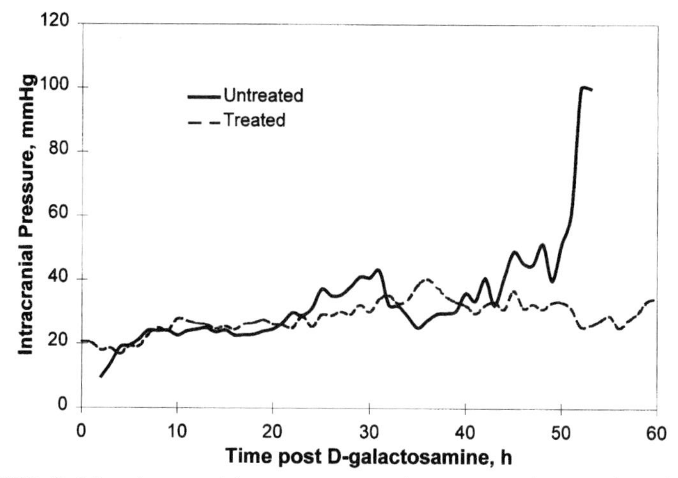


**FIGURE 2.** Mean intracranial pressure versus time post D-galactosamine administration for untreated and BLSS-treated dogs.

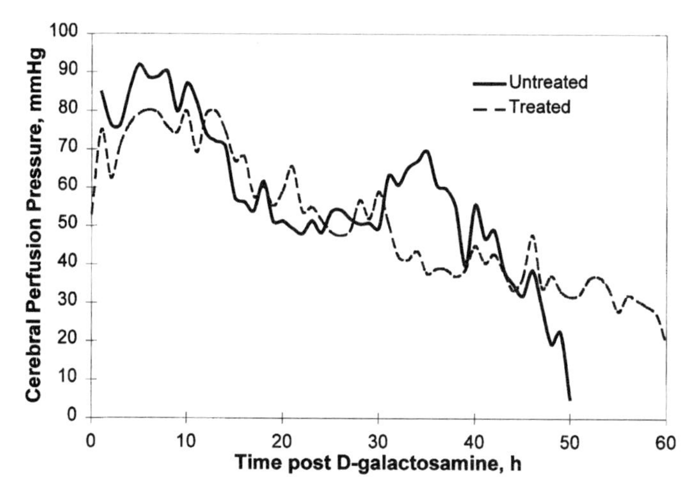


**FIGURE 3.** Mean cerebral perfusion pressure versus time post D-galactosamine administration for untreated and BLSS-treated dogs.

Clinically, CPP is a more crucial issue than ICP. Maintenance of adequate CPP in the face of rising ICP is necessary to prevent potential neurological damage. Inadequate maintenance of CPP is a feature of the D-galactosamine canine liver failure model.[23] As shown in FIGURE 3, the combined BLSS-treated cohort mean CPP trends with the untreated cohort until about 40–45 hours post D-galactosamine administration in a manner similar to the ICP trends. At about 45 hours, however, the mean CPP for the untreated cohort drops precipitously while that for the BLSS-treated cohort maintains its lesser, but steady, decline.

## DISCUSSION

Based upon the results of this study, the Excorp Medical BLSS appears safe in support of canines with D-galactosamine–induced liver failure (TABLE 2). Aside from some transient thrombocytopenia and transient hypotension at device initiation, the device was well tolerated by the animals. The cohort of animals receiving BLSS treatment had significantly longer survival times than those that did not receive treatment.

Qualitatively, the animals receiving BLSS treatment were deemed more stable by attending caregivers. The BLSS-treated animals required lesser amounts of potassium and calcium electrolyte replacement. They were also less likely to exhibit sudden changes in vascular tone that required quick fluid administration responses. The more stable hemodynamic response is reflected in the ICP and CPP data in FIGURES 2 and 3, respectively.

Time of intervention post D-galactosamine administration seems to be an important factor in treatment of D-galactosamine canine liver failure. Group 2c, which received BLSS treatment commencing 16–18 hours post D-galactosamine, had marginally longer survival times in comparison with the untreated cohort, Group 1b, than did Group 2b, which received BLSS treatment commencing 24–26 hours post D-galactosamine. Additionally, increasing blood-borne markers of progressing liver disease, such as ALT, AST, and ammonia occurred later in Group 2c than in Groups 1b and 2b. This observation may have important clinical implications for deciding when to intervene in the course of progressing liver failure with a BLSS-type treatment.

The Excorp Medical BLSS is one of a new generation of bioartificial liver assist devices that rely on viable, active liver cells in a biochemical tissue culture reactor to replace biochemical function for patients with acute liver failure. The liver is a complex organ that provides many functions and numerous metabolic pathways, many of which are poorly understood, in normal maintenance of life. Acute and progressing liver failure can involve alterations or failure in one or several of the liver functions and/or metabolic pathways, making therapies tailored to an individual function or metabolic pathway of limited value. Hence comes the interest in using viable liver cells to replace any or all functions and pathways that may be affected in the course of progressing liver failure.[29]

Numerous model compounds are available to evaluate generic (*in vitro*) BLSS metabolic activity, e.g., lidocaine, testosterone, 4-methylubelliferone, acetaminophen, cyclosporin, and other drugs can be used to evaluate the drug detoxification (P450) pathways of hepatocyte-based systems. Ammonia conversion to urea can be used to evaluate the urea cycle pathway both *in vitro* and *in vivo*. Protein synthesis can be evaluated by the appearance of albumin.

Many of these reaction systems have been studied intensively in batch tissue culture systems and are well understood.[33–36] However, the rates of reaction measured in such systems may be misleading because they are typically integral measurements rather than differential measurements.[30] Actual point reaction rates are likely to be much higher. BLSS systems, with flowing reactant streams, should be able to take advantage of the higher reaction rates with a concomitant reduction in the mass of liver cells required to perform a given level of metabolite conversion.

A confounding effect in the design of BLSS systems is that little is understood about the role of mass transfer. Metabolic species must diffuse a boundary layer in the flow stream, cross a membrane with poorly understood transmission characteristics, diffuse (or slowly convect) to a hepatocyte, be taken up by the hepatocyte for conversion, and then repeat the path back to the blood stream. Reactive conversion in the hepatocyte will most certainly depend upon other nutrient or cofactor availability, in particular, oxygen availability.

The current generation of BLSS devices had been developed heuristically based upon known analogies to other systems and with the belief that such systems will be able to provide the metabolic function required by patients with liver failure. The systems have been shown to provide levels of metabolic support to patients in clinical trials or animals in preclinical trials as has been shown by the results reported here. The next generation of BLSS devices, however, should be developed using formal reaction engineering principles that account for the roles of transport phenomena and reaction kinetics in the design of devices that provide maximum metabolic support with minimal hepatocyte requirements.

## SUMMARY

Overall, the authors found the Excorp Medical BLSS to be safe in the treatment of canines with D-galactosamine–induced liver failure. Treated animals tolerated the treatment well and have significantly prolonged survival times compared with untreated animals. Treatment with the device positively affects blood chemistry markers typically associated with progressive liver failure. The BLSS is ready for Phase I clinical safety evaluation in patients with acute and progressing liver failure.

## ACKNOWLEDGMENTS

Partial funding for this work was provided by Excorp Medical, Inc. Ladd Research Industries provided the Ladd-Steritek ICP monitor. Datex Medical Instruments provided the Datex-Engstrom Ultima Svi Gas Analyzer for respiration monitoring. Clinical Technology, Inc. provided the Hemochron Jr ACT analyzer. Additional experimental support from Joan Rosenberger, Frank McSteen, Jennifer Seng, Marek Rybek, Micheal Januszko, Julie Kovall, James Beall, and Jason Joy is appreciated.

## REFERENCES

1. AMERICAN LIVER FOUNDATION. 1997. http://gi.ucsf.edu/alf.
2. LUCEY, M.R., K.A. BROWN, G.T. EVERSON, J.J. FUNG, R. GISH, E.B. KEEFFE, N.M. KNETEMAN, J.R. LAKE, P. MARTIN, S.V. MCDIARMID, .J RAKELA, M.L. SHIFFMAN, S.K. SO & R.H. WIESNER. 1997. Minimal criteria for placement of adults on the liver transplant waiting list: a report of a national conference organized by the American

Society of Transplant Physicians and the American Association for the Study of Liver Diseases. Liver Transplant. Surg. **3:** 628–637.

3. United Network for Organ Sharing (UNOS) 1997 Annual Report. 1997. http://www.unos.org. See http://www.unos.org/Frame_default.asp?Category=Newsdata for current data on listed patients.
4. ASH, S.R., D.E. BLAKE, D.J. CARR & K.D. HARKER. 1998. Push-pull sorbent based pheresis for treatment of acute hepatic failure: the BioLogic-detoxifier/plasma filter system. ASAIO J. **44:** 129–139.
5. ASH, S.R., D.J. CARR, D.E. BLAKE, J.B. RAINIER, A.A. DEMETRIOU & J. ROZGA. 1993. Effect of sorbent-based dialytic therapy with the BioLogic-DT on an experimental model of hepatic failure. ASAIO J. **39:** M675–M680.
6. STANGE, J. & S. MITZNER. 1996. A carrier-mediated transport of toxins in a hybrid membrane. Safety barrier between a patients blood and a bioartificial liver. Int. J. Artif. Organs **19:** 677–691.
7. CHEN, S.C., C. MULLON, E. KAHAKU, F. WATANABE, W. HEWITT, S. EGUCHI, Y. MIDDLETON, N. ARKADOPOULOS, J. ROZGA, B. SOLOMON & A.A. DEMETRIOU. 1997. Treatment of severe liver failure with a bioartificial liver. Ann. N. Y. Acad. Sci. **831:** 350–360.
8. WATANABE, F.D., C.J. MULLON, W.R. HEWITT, N. ARKADOPOULOS, E. KAHAKU, S. EGUCHI, T. KHALILI, W. ARNAOUT, C.R. SHACKLETON, J. ROZGA, B. SOLOMON & A.A. DEMETRIOU. 1997. Clinical experience with a bioartificial liver in the treatment of severe liver failure. A phase I clinical trial. Ann. Surg. **225:** 484–491.
9. CHEN, S.C., W.R. HEWITT, F.D. WATANABE, S. EGUCHI, E. KAHAKU, T. MIDDLETON, J. ROZGA & A.A. DEMETRIOU. 1996. Clinical experience with a porcine hepatocyte-based liver support system. Int. J. Artif. Organs **19:** 664–669.
10. DEMETRIOU, A.A., F. WATANABE & J. ROZGA. 1995. Artificial hepatic support systems. Prog. Liver Dis. **13:** 331–348.
11. GERLACH, J.C. 1997. Long-term liver cell cultures in bioreactors and possible application for liver support. Cell Biol. Toxicol. **13:** 349–355.
12. BORNEMANN, R., M.D. SMITH & J.C. GERLACH. 1996. Consideration of potential immunological problems in the application of xenogenic hybrid liver support. Int. J. Arti. Organs **19:** 655–663.
13. GERLACH, J.C. 1996. Development of a hybrid liver support system: a review. Int. J. Artif. Organs **19:** 645–654.
14. ELLIS, A.J., R.D. HUGHES, J.A. WENDON, J. DUNNE, P.G. LANGLEY, J.H. KELLY, G.T. GISLASON, N.L. SUSSMAN & R. WILLIAMS. 1996. Pilot-controlled trial of the extracorporeal liver assist device in acute liver failure. Hepatology **24:** 1446–1451.
15. SUSSMAN, N.L., M.J. FINEGOLD, J.P. BARISH & J.H. KELLY. 1994. A case of syncytial giant-cell hepatitis treated with an extracorporeal liver assist device. Am. J. Gastroenterol. **89:** 1077–1082.
16. SIELAFF, T.D., S.L. NYBERG, M.D. ROLLINS, M.Y. HU, B. AMIOT, A. LEE, F.J. WU, W.S. HU & F.B. CERRA. 1997. Characterization of the three-compartment gel-entrapment porcine hepatocyte bioartificial liver. Cell Biol. Toxicol. **13:** 357–364.
17. SIELAFF, T.D., M.Y. HU, B. AMIOT, M.D. ROLLINS, S. RAO, B. MCGUIRE, J.R. BLOOMER, W.S. HU & F.B. CERRA. 1995. Gel-entrapment bioartificial liver therapy in galactosamine hepatitis. J. Surg. Res. **59:** 179–184
18. DIXIT,V. & G. GITNICK. 1996. Artificial liver support: state of the art. Scand. J. Gastroenterol. **220** (Suppl): 101–114.
19. DIXIT, V. 1994. Development of a bioartificial liver using isolated hepatocytes. Artif. Organs **18:** 371–384.
20. BHATIA, S.N., U.J. BALIS, M.L. YARMUSH & M. TONER. 1998. Microfabrication of hepatocyte/fibroblast co-cultures: role of homotypic cell interactions. Biotechnol. Prog. **14:** 378–387
21. BHATIA, S.N., M.L. YARMUSH & M. TONER. 1997. Controlling cell interactions by micropatterning in co-cultures: hepatocytes and 3T3 fibroblasts. J. Biomed. Mater. Res. **34:** 189–199.

22. SIELAFF, T.D., M.Y. HU, M.D. ROLLINS, J.R. BLOOMER, B. AMIOT, W-S. HU & F.B. CERRA. 1995. An anesthetized model of lethal canine galactosamine fulminant hepatic failure. Hepatology **21:** 796–804.
23. BLOCK, G.D., J.F. PATZER II, A. KHANNA, W.Y. YIN, E. MOLMENTI, D. GERBER, D.J. KRAMER, R.A. WAGNER, Y. CHEN, M.L. FULMER, B.P. AMIOT & G.M. MAZARIEGOS. 1998. Unpublished data.
24. SEGLEN, P.O. 1972. Preparation of rat liver cells. I. Effect of $Ca^{2+}$ on enzymatic dispersion of isolated, perfused liver. Exp. Cell Res. **74:** 450–454.
25. SEGLEN, P.O. 1973. Preparation of rat liver cells. II. Effects of ions and chelators on tissue dispersion. Exp. Cell Res. **76:** 25–30.
26. SEGLEN, P.O. 1973. Preparation of rat liver cells. 3. Enzymatic requirements for tissue dispersion. Exp. Cell Res. **82:** 391–398.
27. SEGLEN, P.O. 1976. Preparation of isolated rat liver cells. Methods Cell Biol. **13:** 29–83.
28. Statistica™ for Windows, 2nd edition. 1995. StatSoft, Inc. Tulsa, OK.
29. SUSSMAN, N.L. & J.H. KELLY. 1997. Extracorporeal liver support: cell-based therapy for the failing liver. Am. J. Kidney Dis. **30:** S66–S71.
30. CATAPANO, G. & L DE BARTOLO. 1996. Importance of the kinetic characterization of liver cell metabolic reactions to the design of hybrid liver support devices. Int. J. Artif. Organs **19:** 670–676.
31. NYBERG, S.L., J.L. PLATT, K. SHIRABE, W.D. PAYNE, W-S. HU & F.B. CERRA. 1992. Immunoprotection of xenocytes in a hollow-fiber bioartificial liver. ASAIO J. **38:** M463–M467.
32. NYBERG, S.L., R.A. SHATFORD, M.V. PESHWA, J.M. WHITE, F.B. CERRA, W-S. HU. 1993. Evaluation of a hepatocyte-entrapment hollow-fiber bioreactor: a potential bioartificial liver. Biotechnol. Bioeng. **41:** 194–203.
33. KEENAGHAN, J.B. & R.N. BOYES. 1972. The tissue distribution, metabolism and excretion of lidocaine in rats, guinea pigs, dogs and man. J. Pharmacol. Exp. Ther. **180:** 454–463 .
34. IMAOKA, S., K. ENOMOTO, Y. ODA, A. ASADA, M. FUJIMORI, T. SHIMADA, S. FUJITA, F.P. GUENGERICH & Y. FUNAE. Lidocaine metabolism by human cytochrome P-450s purified from hepatic microsomes: comparison of those with rat hepatic cytochrome P-450s. J. Pharmacol. Exp. Ther. **255:** 1385–1391.
35. TEPHLY, T., M. GREEN, J. PUIG & Y. IRSHAID. 1988. Endogenous substrates for UDP-glucuronosyltransferases. Xenobiotica **18:** 1201–1210.
36. HU, M.Y., M. CIPOLLE, T. SIELAFF, M.J. LOVDAHL, H.J. MANN, R.P. REMMEL & F.B. CERRA. 1995. Effects of hepatocyte growth factor on viability and biotransformation functions of hepatocytes in gel entrapped and monolayer culture. Crit. Care Med. **23:** 1237–1242.

# Three-dimensional *in Vitro* Cell Culture Leads to a Marked Upregulation of Cell Function in Human Hepatocyte Cell Lines—an Important Tool for the Development of a Bioartificial Liver Machine

CLARE SELDEN,[a] ALI SHARIAT, PASCHAL McCLOSKEY, TIM RYDER, EVE ROBERTS, AND HUMPHREY HODGSON

*The Liver Group, Gastroenterology Unit, Division of Medicine, Imperial College School of Medicine (Hammersmith Campus), W12 0NN, England, UK. and Division of Gastroenterology, Hospital for Sick Children, University of Toronto, Toronto, Canada*

**ABSTRACT: Upregulating hepatocyte function in proliferating human liver cell lines could provide cells for a bio-artificial liver. Ideally, a means of mimicking the biological extracellular matrix with a relatively inert, bio-compatible matrix is required. Alginate encapsulation of primary hepatocytes is biocompatible. This study aimed to characterize cells grown in a 3D configuration in alginate. A human-derived liver cell line encapsulated in 1% alginate was assessed for synthetic and detoxification functions. Secreted proteins measured (e.g., albumin, fibrinogen, α-1-antitrypsin etc.) were increased in alginate compared with monolayers. Cytochrome P450 1A1 activity increased three- to fourfold, whilst urea synthesis, undetectable in monolayer cultures, was synthesized by cells in alginate at levels approaching *in vivo* production. TEM revealed good ultrastructure reminiscent of normal hepatocytes. Alginate promotes 3D colonies of proliferating cells with upregulated liver functions. Rapid recovery of function of cryopreserved cells (< 18h) provides added advantages for this system to support the biological component of an artificial liver for patients with fulminant hepatic failure.**

## INTRODUCTION

Human hepatocytes grown in culture undergo rapid loss of differentiated function and do not readily proliferate making them unsuitable as a source of liver function in an artificial liver. Several hepatocyte derived cell lines of both normal and tumor origin do proliferate and retain a degree of differentiated function in culture, but at levels considerably lower than the liver *in vivo*. The ability to upregulate hepatocyte specific function in these cell lines could provide a source of liver cells for a bio-artificial liver. When cells are grown as monolayers on substrates providing extra-

[a]Corresponding author: The Liver Group, Gastroenterology Unit, Division of Medicine, Imperial College School of Medicine (Hammersmith campus), Hammersmith Hospital, Du Cane Road, London, W12 0NN, England, UK; +44-181-383-8066 (voice); +44-181-749-3436 (fax); c.selden@rpms.ac.uk (e-mail).

cellular matrix there is increased survival and improved function at the transcriptional level compared with monolayers on tissue culture plastic. For practical purposes a means of mimicking the biological extracellular matrix with a relatively inert but bio-compatible matrix is required. Alginate encapsulation of primary hepatocytes has been shown to be biocompatible and to support cell survival. This study has explored the hypothesis that allowing cells to grow in a three dimensional (3D) configuration in vitro would mimic the hepatocyte architecture *in vivo* and thereby lead to improved cell-cell contact, interaction and communication, resulting in improved levels of hepatocyte-specific function, e.g., secreted protein synthesis, cytochrome P450 function, and urea synthesis.

## METHODS

### *Cell Culture*

The human liver cell line HHY41 was derived as described previously.[1] This line has been in continuous monolayer culture for more than three years. Cells were cultured in fully supplemented modified MEM alpha with 10% fetal bovine serum (complete medium), in 5% $CO_2$ /95% air and 95% humidity, and passaged once a week using 0.25% trypsin in glucose-citrate-saline, pH 7.8 solution.

### *Cell Encapsulation*

Alginate encapsulated hepatocyte (0.5 million/ml) beads were prepared in 1% sodium alginate/culture medium by extrusion through a 23 gauge cannula with a concentric air flow (1200 ccs/min) at 1.5 ml/min into 0.102 M $CaCl_2$ in 0.15M NaCl, pH7.4. Beads were washed twice with culture medium prior to incubation at 37°C in a 5% $CO_2$/95% air humidified incubator. Spherical beads had an average 400 μm diameter. A typical experiment assessed 375 μl of beads in a volume of 5 ml supplemented culture medium; medium was changed every 48 h. Alginate was a medium viscosity High M grade isolated from *Macrocystis perifera*.

### *Release of Cell Spheroids from Alginate Beads*

Alginate beads were removed from culture medium rinsed in HBSS, and incubated in 4 mM EDTA, 0.15 M NaCl, pH 7.4 at 37°C, for 30 min. The cell spheroid suspension was disrupted by repeated passage through a 23 gauge hypodermic needle. The cell suspension was pelleted at full speed in a microfuge, washed with 0.15M NaCl, pH 7.4, and the pellet resuspended appropriately either for protein estimation or nuclei estimation.

### *Cell Quantitation*

The number of cells were estimated from the number of nuclei. Cell pellets were incubated in 1% crystal violet dissolved in 0.1M citric acid containing 0.2% Triton X-100, at 37°C for 1 hour with shaking prior to counting in a Modified Neubauer haemocytometer counting chamber (Philip Harris, London UK).

### *Synthetic Function*

*Secreted Protein*

Twenty-four hour conditioned medium from 6-well plates was collected for secreted-protein synthesis of 5 liver specific proteins, namely, albumin, α-1-antitrypsin, α-1-acid glycoprotein, fibrinogen, and prothrombin. Samples were frozen at –20°C until assay by the indirect sandwich ELISA technique using a primary capture antibody and a secondary detection antibody linked to horseradish peroxidase. Detection at 492 nm was made in the presence of $H_2O_2$ and 4 mg OPD/12 ml 0.1M citrate, pH 5.0. Quantitation was achieved by comparison with standard curves for each protein in culture medium performed on each ELISA plate, utilizing the "Biolise" software package (Labtech International, Uckfield, UK). Only values on the linear part of the standard curve were used. Albumin, fibrinogen, prothrombin, α-1-antitrypsin and α-1-acid glycoprotein were measured all using antibodies provided by Dako Ltd, High Wycombe UK. Lower detection limits of the ELISA assays were 25 ng/ml for all proteins except fibrinogen, which was 52.5 ng/ml. There was no cross-reactivity between any of the assays. Comparisons were made with 24 h conditioned medium from monolayer cultures.

*Cryopreservation*

Cell spheroids encapsulated within Alginate beads in freezing mix (10% DMSO, 90% FCS) were frozen in liquid nitrogen for 7 days. Beads were thawed by rapid addition of 5 ml of warm culture medium and incubation at 37°C for 30 minutes, followed by washing twice in fresh warm serum-free culture medium, prior to incubation in fully supplemented culture medium at 37°C in a humidified 5% $CO_2$/95% air incubator. Conditioned medium was collected after 6 h, 18 h, 24 h and 48 h for analysis of secreted protein by ELISA.

*Cytochrome P450*

The isozyme of the P450 family (1A1) was assessed utilizing the fluorescent products produced by addition of ethoxyresorufin (EROD) metabolized by the enzymes ethoxy- resorufin-O-dealkylase. Cells were exposed to the enzyme inducer, dibenzanthracene at 13 μm for 24 h in culture medium on days 7 and 17. Monolayer cultures of the same cells served as a control. EROD enzyme activity was determined as previously described by Donato *et al.*[2] on intact cultured cells in alginate beads in 6-well plates. Briefly the reaction was started by addition of 3 ml of serum-free (supplemented) medium containing 8 μM 7-ethoxyresorufin. After a 1 hour incubation at 37°C in a humidified incubator, a 375 μl aliquot of cell medium was withdrawn from each well and transferred to a 24-well plate. At this stage the beads were washed and the cells harvested for determination of total cellular protein. To allow hydrolysis of potential resorufin conjugates β-glucuronidase (75 Fishman units) and arylsulfatase (600 Roy units) dissolved in 125 μl of 0.1M sodium acetate buffer pH 4.5 were added to each well containing 375 μl of sample, and incubated in a shaking incubator at 37°C. After 2 h, 1 ml of ethanol was added to each well and plates were centrifuged at 3000 rpm for 10 minutes. Fluorescence of supernatants was measured using a Cytofluor 2350 (Millipore) with 530 nm excitation and 590 nm emission filters. A standard curve of resorufin was prepared in culture medium and was pro-

A

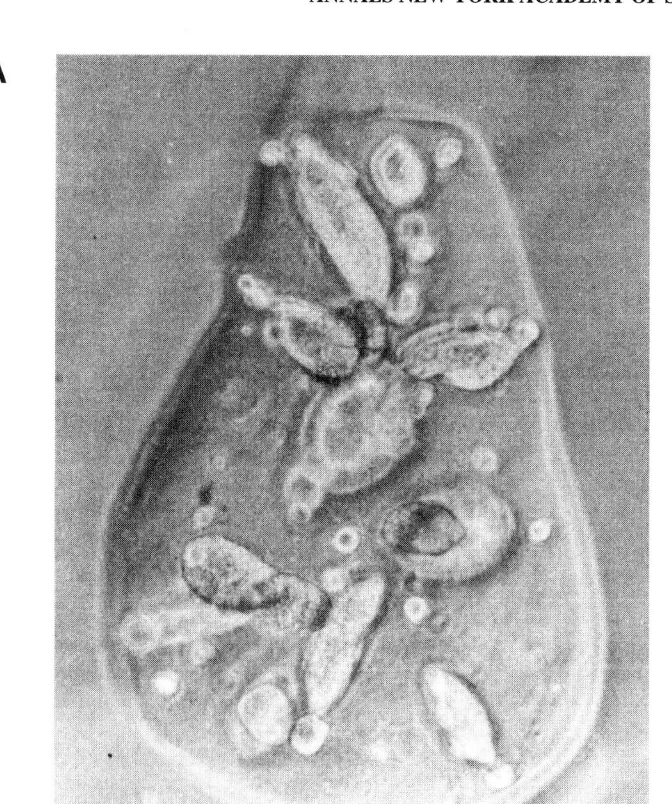

**FIGURE 1.** **(a)** Phase contrast observation of colonies of cells formed within alginate beads from a single cell suspension at day 0. Note the proliferating heads towards the periphery of the beads. **(b)** H&E staining of 3 μm sections of typical colony within alginate beads.

cessed as described for samples. Spheroids were released from alginate by the addition of 4 mM $Na_2EDTA$ in 0.1M NaCl at 37°C for 30 min. The cell pellet was dissolved in 0.3M NaOH. 1% SDS at 37°C for 1hour. Protein content was measured by a microplate Lowry assay, analyzed at 620 nm using BSA as a standard. Results were expressed as pmol/h/mg cell protein.

*Urea Synthesis*

Urea in 24 h conditioned medium was analyzed using a routine clinical assay based on urease reduction of urea to ammonia and subsequent reaction with 2-oxoglutarate to form glutamate and NAD.[3] Cells were released from the alginate beads as described above for estimation of nuclei number. Results were expressed as mmol urea/$10^6$ nuclei/day. To confirm specific urea synthesis the urea cycle substrate $^{14}C$-guanido arginine (5 μCi, NEC453, 51.5 mCi/mmol, Dupont NEN, Hounslow, UK) was added to 5 ml culture medium for 48 h prior to collection and separation on cel-

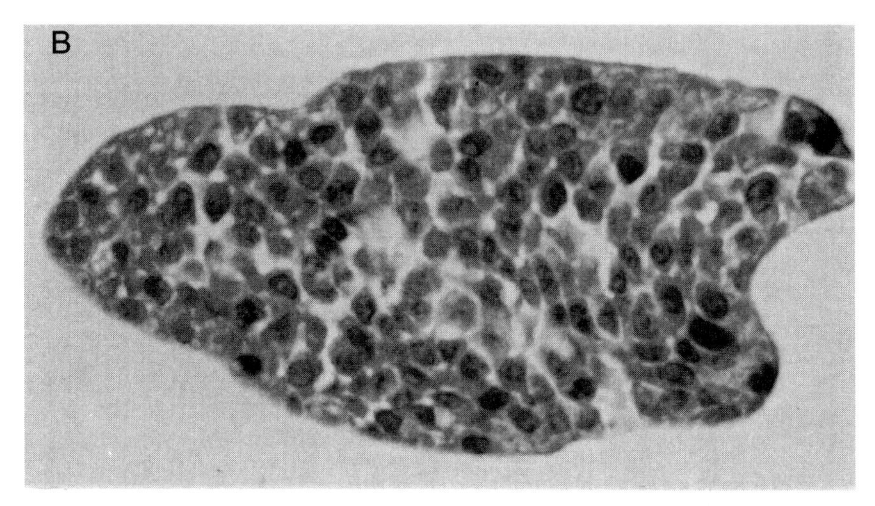


**FIGURE 1 (continued).**

lulose acetate TLC plates in the mobile phase butanol:acetone:glacial acetic acid: $H_2O$ (35:35:10:20). The flexible plates were cut into 3 mm strips and counted for radioactivity in a β scintillation counter $^{14}C$ arginine and $^{14}C$ urea were used as standards to identify rf values. A portion of the conditioned medium was treated with urease at 1000 units/ml in for 30 min at 37°C. The treated sample was also subjected to TLC to confirm specific urea production.

*Cell Appearance*

Alginate beads were observed by phase contrast microscopy during culture. For normal histology beads were set in 1% low gelling temperature agarose in 0.15 M NaCl, prior to fixation in 10% neutral buffered formalin. Paraffin sections (3 μm) were stained with hematoxylin and eosin. For transmission electron microscopy, beads were fixed in osmium tetroxide and glutaraldehyde.

## RESULTS

Cells in alginate proliferated from single cells entrapped within the beads to form colonies of several hundred cells; typically approximately 50–70% of the bead was filled with colonies, which had a proliferating leading edge towards the periphery of the bead within the alginate. The rate of proliferation was markedly reduced compared with the same cells on monolayers (alginate doubling time ~4 d, monolayer ~24 h). H&E staining of 3 μm sections demonstrated cohesive colonies with occasional mitoses and apoptotic cells (FIG.1, a and b).

Cell production of each of the secreted proteins measured was increased markedly in alginate compared with the same cells at the same cell density in monolayer. Five liver specific proteins exhibited marked increases as shown in FIGURE 2 (albumin, fibrinogen, prothrombin, α-1-antitrypsin, and α-1-acid glycoprotein).

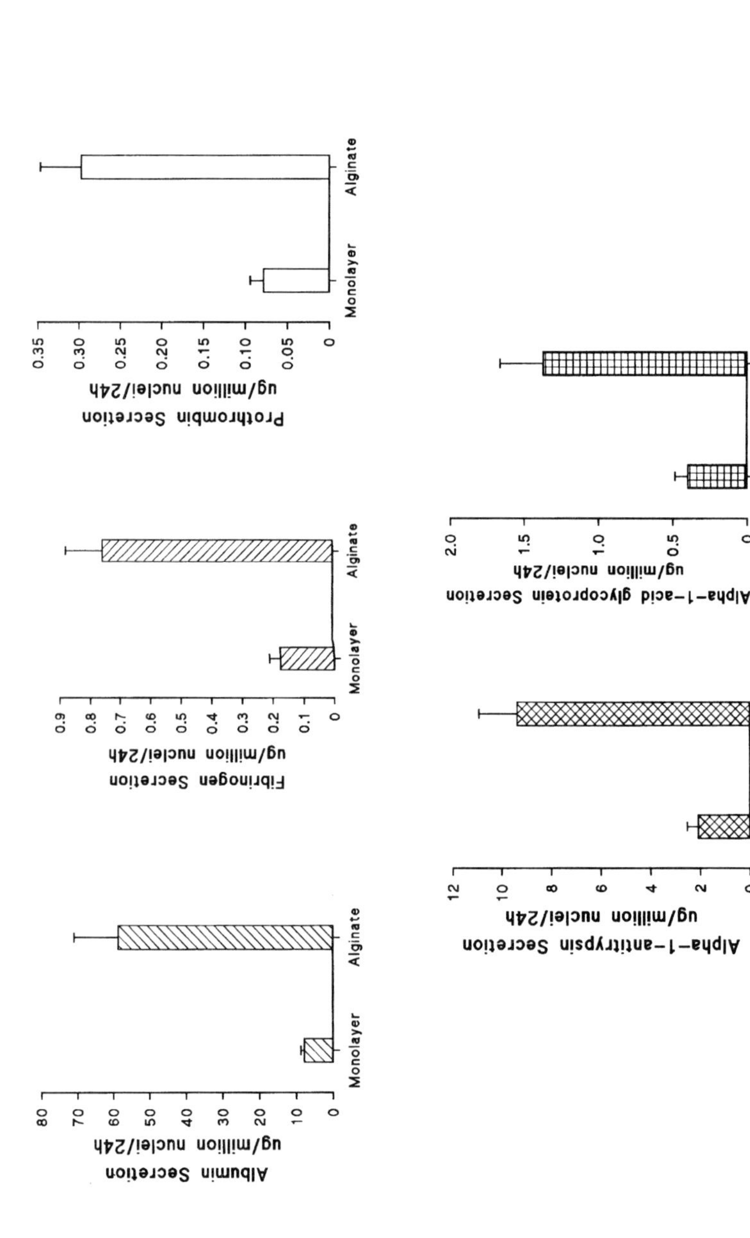


**FIGURE 2.** Comparison of secreted protein levels in alginate beads at 8 days, as compared with monolayer cultures at similar cell density. All five liver specific proteins measured, albumin, fibrinogen, prothrombin, α-1-antitrypsin, and α-1-acid glycoprotein, were increased markedly in alginate culture, to levels approaching those seen *in vivo*.

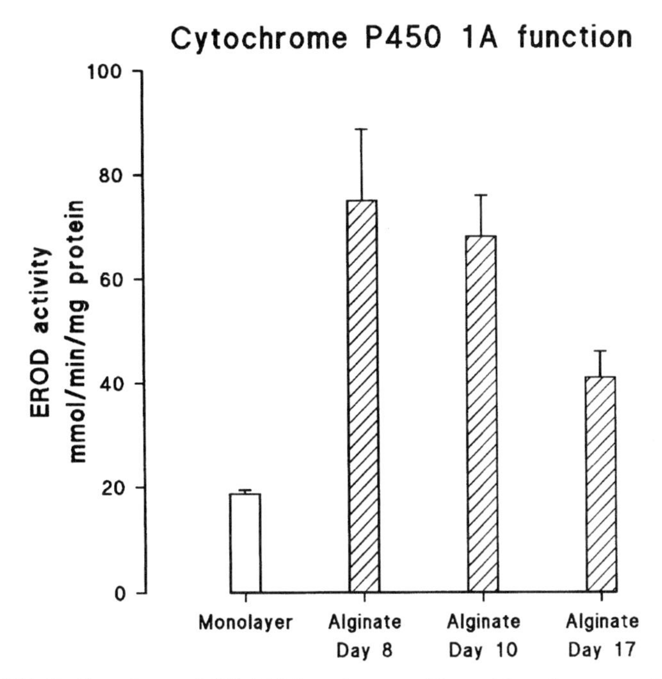


**FIGURE 3.** Cytochrome P450 1A1 function, as evidenced by ethoxyresorufun metabolism. Comparison was made between optimal monolayer cultures (*open bar*) and alginate encapsulated cell colonies at 8, 10, and 17 days (*hatched bars*).

A three- to fourfold increase in cytochrome P450 1A1 activity in alginate-entrapped cell colonies was observed compared with cells cultured as monolayers (FIG. 3). Peak levels in alginate were observed at 8 to 10 days; thereafter there was a decline in activity, however even at the later time point there was considerably more activity than in monolayer culture.

Urea synthesis was completely undetectable in monolayer cultures seeded at 0.5 $\times 10^6$/ml, was produced at very low levels (0.136 $\pm$ 0.08) in very high density monolayer (15 $\times 10^6$/ml—cells piled up), but was produced at 1.408 $\pm$ 0.22 mmol/l/$10^6$ nuclei/48 h, by colonies of cells in alginate. Conversion of $^{14}$C arginine into urea, as assessed by TLC chromatography confirmed there was arginase activity, an enzyme of the urea cycle pathway; destruction of the putative urea peak separated on TLC with urease confirmed the presence of urea (FIG. 4).

Low power views of TEM illustrated cohesive colonies with apparent secretion of extracellular matrix between individual cells (FIG. 5a). TEM at higher power revealed good ultrastructure reminiscent of normal human hepatocytes with abundant ER, golgi and mitochondria, with canaliculi and a remarkable network of microvilli; desmosomes and junctional complexes were prominent, illustrating that the cells were polarized within the colonies (FIG. 5, b, c , d).

Using the secreted protein $\alpha$-1-antitrypsin, as a representative measure of liver-specific function, activity after cryopreservation in liquid nitrogen could be recov-

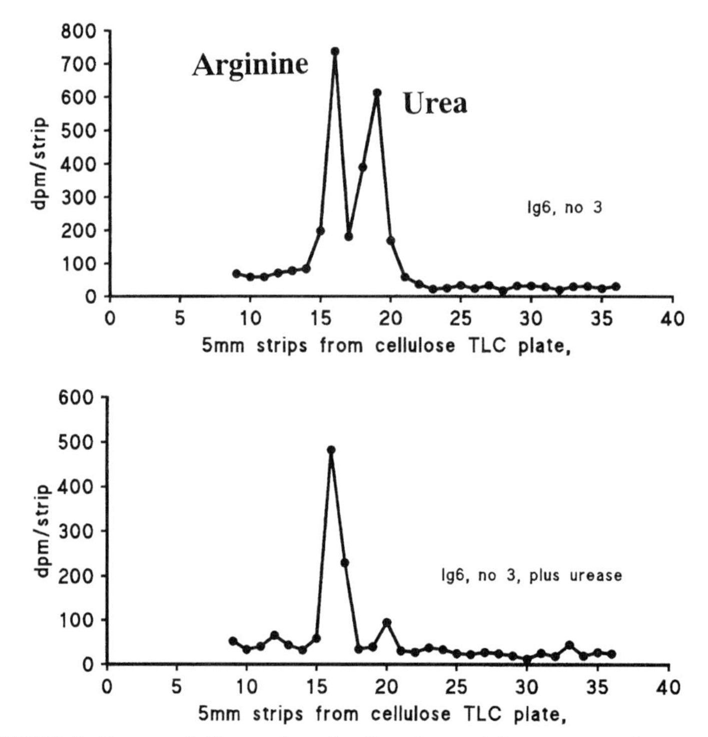


**FIGURE 4.** *Top panel*: Conversion of radioactive arginine to urea and separation by TLC; *bottom panel*: its specific destruction by urease confirmed the synthesis of urea.

ered within 18 hours. At 6 h post thawing, the cells secreted less protein per cell compared with pre-cryopreservation levels; however, at 18 and 24 h the per cell secretion had returned to pre-cryopreservation values. Indeed by 48 h, levels were almost double pre-cryopreservation values, indicating that some cells had started proliferating (FIG. 6).

## DISCUSSION

The data presented here illustrate the feasibility of upregulating in vitro function of proliferating cell lines derived from human liver, by forcing 3-dimensional colony growth. Unlike other reports of 3D colonies induced by collagen sandwich gels or thick EHS gels, both of which have an extracellular matrix component which is of itself capable of upregulating liver specific transcription,[4] the alginate system is relatively bio-inert. There are reports of a cellular immune response to alginate preparations used *in vivo*;[5] however, with the use of highly purified preparations of alginate[6] in an extracorporeal liver support device such an immune response is unlikely.

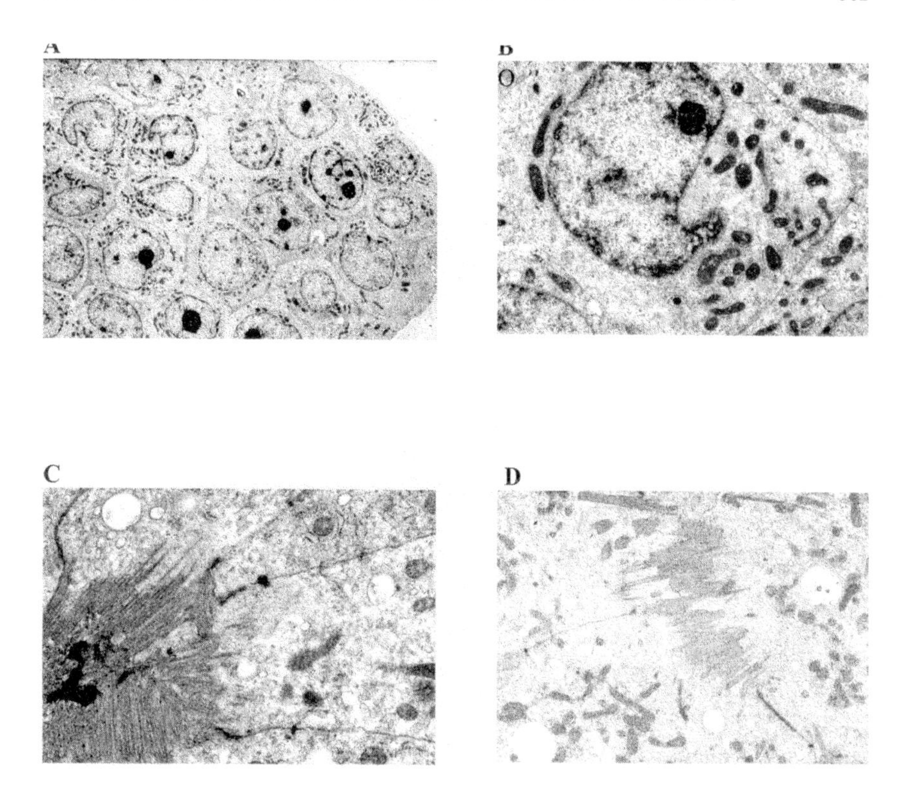

**FIGURE 5.** **(a)** low power TEM illustrates cohesive colonies of cells with an apparent extracellular matrix deposition between the cells; **(b, c, d)** high power TEM demonstrate hepatocyte-like cells containing nuclei with prominent nucleoli, a transcriptionally active cytoplasm with rough and smooth endoplasmic reticulin, mitochondria and Golgi apparatus. Note also the very prominent microvilli forming canaliculi and the desmosomes.

Transmission electron microscopy observations at both low and high power provide substantial evidence of a cellular communication system of desmosomes, tight junctions, junctional complexes, microvilli and canaliculi reminiscent of that seen *in vivo* but not observed in monolayer culture and only rarely in collagen gel sandwich or thick EHS culture. There could be two explanations for these findings. One possibility is that the restriction forcing the cells to grow three-dimensionally provided by geometric encapsulation, is sufficient of itself to upregulate transcription, as has recently been demonstrated in HELA cells when a mechanical force applied to the culture surface increased transcription via integrin receptor signaling.[7] A second is that the same restriction has allowed the deposition of secreted extracellular matrix to remain in close association with the cell colonies, and thereby to exert a bio-active response within the cells; it is well known that extracellular matrix components can upregulate cell function. To resolve this further we are currently measuring extracellular matrix components secreted into the alginate and surrounding medium; we are also making various preparations of alginate with higher and lower viscosities.

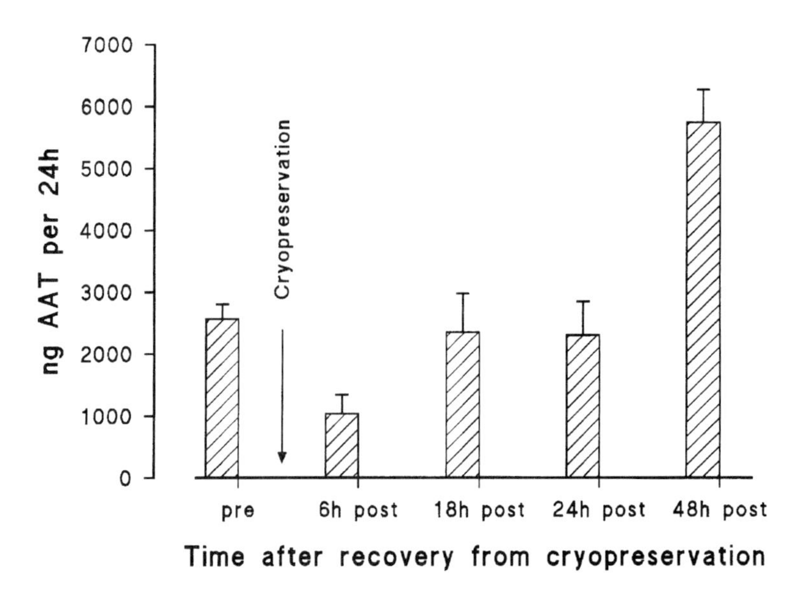


**FIGURE 6.** Recovery of α-1-antitrypsin activity after cryopreservation of alginate beads containing 3D colonies of cells. Note the 6 h time point which shows loss of function, which is restored by 18 and 24 h. The increased activity at 48 h suggests some cells within the beads are proliferating.

That urea synthesis was measurable in alginate culture but not in monolayer cultures at the same cell density was an interesting observation since it supports the notion that functions can indeed be induced and not simply upregulated by 3D growth. The radiotracer data can only be used to establish that at least one of the urea cycle enzymes, arginase, is active; unfortunately there is a lack of appropriate ammonium radioactive substrate for the earliest part of the urea cycle. Studies are underway, however, with radiolabeled ornithine, to test an earlier urea cycle enzyme, ornithine carbomoyl transferase. The clinical assay measures total urea whether it be from glutamine or detoxification of ammonia, hence the need for clarification of the usefulness of this urea production.

Protein secretion of a variety of liver specific proteins encompassing a range of liver function was improved by 3D culture. Albumin, a major carrier protein in the blood and involved in the maintenance of oncotic pressure, two proteins involved in the blood clotting, fibrinogen and prothrombin, and an antiprotease, α-1-antitrypsin, as well as an acute phase response protein, α-1-1acid glycoprotein, were all significantly upregulated by the 3D colonies resulting from alginate encapsulation. This global improvement is of importance, since it is unclear exactly what is missing or non-functional in patients with acute liver failure. In the absence of exact identification of what is absolutely required of an extracorporeal liver support system, one must strive to provide a full repertoire of liver function.

Recovery of cell function rapidly after cryopreservation is of utmost importance if such a system is to be useful in eventual clinical use. A patient with fulminant hepatic failure can be in grade 4 coma within 24–48 h of being admitted to hospital feeling unwell. Any cell support system needs to be readily available "off the shelf", to treat such patients. Similarly, the ability of these cells to continue proliferating in 3D culture is important for the provision of sufficient extracorporeal liver function to temporarily support a patient in liver failure. Data not shown here have indicated the survival of these colonies in human plasma, with continued function at similar levels to that demonstrated in supplemented cell culture medium.

In summary, the use of alginate to both support the growth of liver cells lines and to promote the formation of 3-dimensional colonies of cells leads to upregulation of liver specific function. In some cases, e.g., urea synthesis, it restores levels of function from undetectable levels in monolayer to values approaching *in vivo* production. The survival of cells in plasma and the rapid recovery of function of cells cryopreserved within alginate provides added advantages for using this system to support the biological component of extracorporeal liver support of patients with fulminant hepatic failure.

## REFERENCES

1. KONO, Y., S. YANG, M. LETARTE & E.A. ROBERTS. 1995. Establishment of a human cell line derived from primary culture in a collagen gel sandwich culture system. Exp. Cell. Res. **221**(2)**:** 478–485.
2. DONATO, M.T., M. JOSE GOMEZ-LECHON & J.V. CASTELL. 1993. A microassay for measuring Cytochrome P450IA1 and P450IIB1 activities in intact human and rat hepatocytes cultured on 96-well plates. Anal. Biochem. **213:** 29–33.
3. TALKE, H. & G.E. SCHUBERT. 1965. Enzymic determination of urea in blood serum, by the Warburg optical test. Klin. Wochshr. **43**(3)**:** 174–175.
4. BERTHIAUME, F., P.V. MOGHE, M. TONER & TH.L YARMUSH. 1996. Effect of extracellular matrix topology on cell structure, function, and physiological responsiveness: hepatocytes cultured in a sandwich configuration. FASEB J. **10**(13)**:** 1471–1484.
5. SOON-SHIONG, P., M. OTTERLIE, O. SMIDSROD, R. HEINTZ, R.P. LANZA & T. ESPEVIK. 1991. An immunologic basis for the fibrotic reaction to implanted microcapsules. Transplant. Proc. **23**(1)**:** 758–759.
6. KLOCK, G., A. PFEFFERMANN, C. RYSER, P. GROHN, B. KUTTLER, H.J. HAHN & U. ZIMMERMANN. 1997. Biocompatibility of mannuronic acid-rich alginates. Biomaterials **18**(10)**:** 707–713.
7. CHICUREL, M.E. 1998 Integrin binding and mechanical tension induce movement of mRNA and ribosomes to focal adhesions. Nature **392:** 730–733.

# Cultivation and Characterization of a New Immortalized Human Hepatocyte Cell Line, HepZ, for Use in an Artificial Liver Support System

A. WERNER,[a,d] S. DUVAR,[a] J. MÜTHING,[a] H. BÜNTEMEYER,[a] U. KAHMANN,[b] H. LÜNSDORF,[c] AND J. LEHMANN[a]

[a]*Institute of Cell Culture Technology, University of Bielefeld, D-33501 Bielefeld, Germany*

[b]*Institute of Botany, University of Bielefeld, Germany*

[c]*GBF, National Institute of Biotechnology Research, Department of Microbiology, Braunschweig, Germany*

**ABSTRACT: The new human hepatocyte cell line HepZ was investigated with regard to use it for a mass cell cultivation. The cells were originally derived from a human liver biopsy and immortalized through lipofectamine-mediated transfection of albumin-promotor–regulated antisense constructions against the negative controlling cell cycle proteins Rb and p53 (pAlb asRb, pAlb asp53). Furthermore, plasmids including genes coding for the cellular transcription factor E2F and D1 cyclin (pCMV E2F, pSV2neo D1) were cotransfected to overcome the G1-restriction point. Cell cultivation was performed in a 2-liter bioreactor with a working volume of 1 liter. With CultiSpher G microcarriers used in a concentration of 3 g/l a maximal density of 7.1 $\times$ $10^6$ cells/ml was achieved in a cultivation period of 20 days. The cells exhibited a maximal specific growth rate of 1.0 per day in the first 4 days. After 9 days of cultivation the stationary growth phase was reached with an average cell density of 5.5 $\times$ $10^6$ cells/ml. The viability status of the culture was determined indirectly by measuring of the lactate dehydrogenase activity (LDH) at 37°C. During the growth phase the activity rose slightly up to a value of 200 U/l. The cells were flat after first attachment on the gelatine microcarriers and spherical after growing into the three-dimensional inner matrix—both of which characteristics were verified by scanning electron microscopy (SEM) and transmission electron microscopy (TEM). The liver-specific cytochrome P450 activity was challenged with a pulse of 7 μg/ml lidocaine at a cell density of 4.5 $\times$ $10^6$ cells/ml. After an induction period of 3 days with 50 μg/ml of phenobarbital, 26 ng/ml MEGX were generated within one day compared to 5 ng/ml without induction. The new cell line HepZ has proven to retain liver-specific qualities and to be appropriate for mass cell cultivation for bioartificial devices.**

[d]Corresponding author: Institute of Cell Culture Technology, University of Bielefeld, POB 100131, D-33501 Bielefeld, Germany; ++49-521-106-6338 (voice); ++49-521-106-6023 (fax); awe@zellkult.techfak.uni-bielefeld.de (e-mail).

## INTRODUCTION

The current therapy to treat acute liver failure is immediate transplantation. Owing to a shortage of donor organs, 10 to 30% of the patients awaiting a liver die before one becomes available.[1] Nonbiological liver support trials such as hemodialysis, hemoperfusion and plasma exchange have failed to demonstrate any survival benefit.[2] A promising technique seems to be the application of an extracorporal liver support system, which could be used to bridge the time period until transplantation. This system should have the capability to detoxify the patients' blood plasma as well as to produce liver-specific proteins. Primary cells meet these requirements best, but unfortunately they divide poorly, whereas transformed cells such as hepatoma cell lines show a high proliferation rate but poor liver-specific performance. Cell-based devices containing primary pig cells,[3] rat cells,[4] and rabbit cells [5] were applied in several trials; however, primary cells lose most of their liver-specific biotransformation capability within the first week after isolation, thus immortalized cells may be a better solution. To ensure a mass cell production and to minimize immunological problems, non-tumorigenic, genetically stable human hepatocytes have to be propagated. These cells should steadily exhibit liver-specific performance and be able to provide a liver support device with the $2.5 \times 10^{10}$ to $5 \times 10^{10}$ cells needed for clinical application.

## EXPERIMENTAL

### *Cell Line*

The growth behavior and metabolic function of a new human hepatocyte cell line, HepZ, was investigated. The cell line was immortalized at the Max Delbrück Center for Molecular Medicine (Berlin)[6] through lipofectamine-mediated transfection of albumin-promotor-regulated antisense constructions against the negative controlling cell cycle proteins Rb and p53 (pAlb asRb, pAlb asp53). Furthermore, plasmids including E2F and D1 genes (pCMV E2F, pSV2neo D1) had been cotransfected to overexpress these positive cycle factors to overcome the G1-restriction point. The cells were used in their 40th passage for cell cultivation in the bioreactor.

### *Cell Cultivation*

The cells were cultivated in a 2-liter bioreactor (B. Braun Biotech International, Germany) filled with 1 liter of a 3 g/l glucose and 292 mg/l glutamine-supplemented 1:1 mixture of DMEM/F12 media containing 5% FCS. For cell attachment, macroporous CultiSpher G gelatine microcarriers (Percell, Sweden) were used in a concentration of 3 g/l. The medium was exchanged every day from day 7 after a sedimentation period of 5 min to let the microcarriers settle.

The dead cell concentration was measured indirectly by determination of the LDH activity with an Uvikon 933 photometer (Kontron, Germany) using a NADH-dependent assay. The supernatants were diluted 1:10 in 30 mM PBS and 10 mM pyruvate at pH 7.4. The samples were measured at a wavelength of 340 nm and a temperature of 37°C.

### *Cell Morphology*

Cell morphology was investigated with scanning electron microscopy (SEM) after fixation in glutaraldehyde at a concentration of 2.5% (v/v). Samples were examined with a digital scanning microscope DSM 982 Gemini (Zeiss, Germany). The inner cores of the microcarriers were investigated after cutting them into slices of 120 nm thickness. Ultrathin sections were examined with a CEM 902 transmission electron microscope (Zeiss, Germany).

### *Protein Secretion*

The protein secretion capability was investigated using fluorescence-labeled antibodies against human albumin. In addition, α2-macroglobulin was determined in a sandwich ELISA.

### *Cytochrome P450 Activity*

MEGX quantification was carried out by use of fluorescence polarization immunoassay (FPIA) using the TDx Fluorescence Polarisation Immunoassay System (Abbott, Germany).

### *Metabolism*

The amino acid metabolism profile was investigated with a HPLC system (Kontron, Germany).

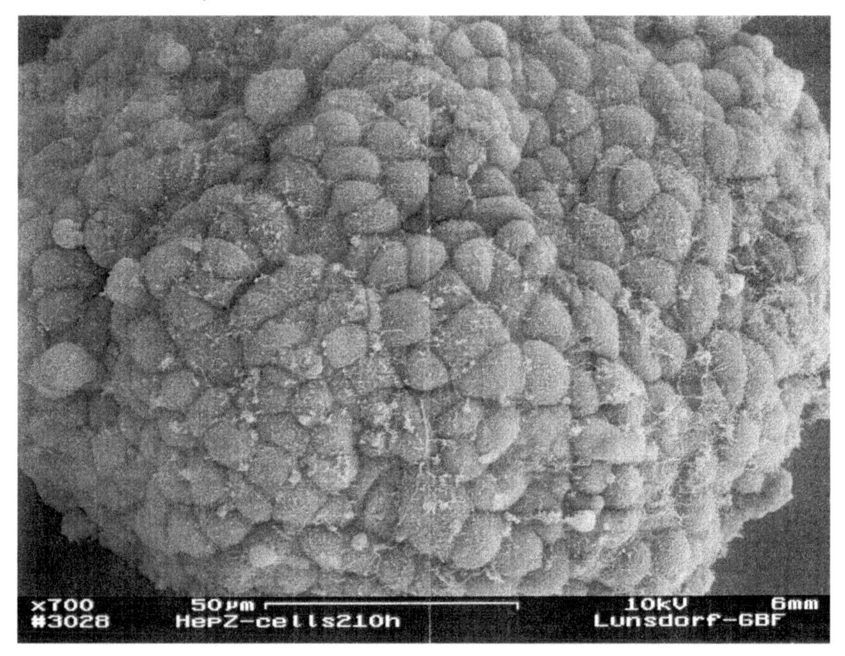


**FIGURE 1.** Confluent layer of HepZ cells on a CultiSpher G microcarrier after 210 h of cultivation.

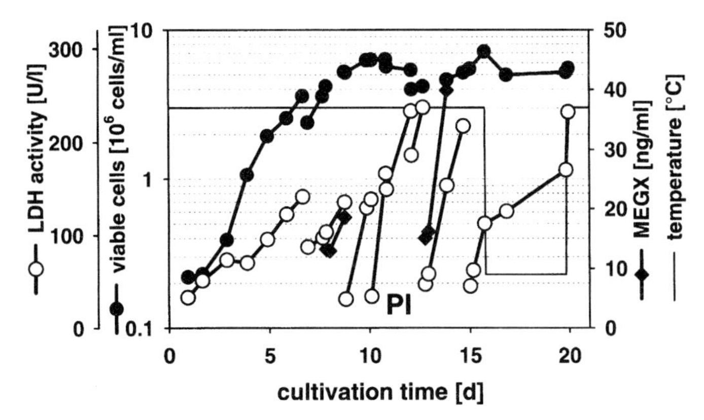


**FIGURE 2.** LDH (lactate dehydrogenase) activity, cell density, MEGX (monoethylglycinexylidide) kinetics, and temperature profile. LDH activity increased when cells reached confluency. Maximum cell concentration was $7.1 \times 10^6$ cells/ml. The cells survived a 4-day cooling period at 9°C. The cytochrome P450 system activity was tested with a 7 μg/ml pulse of lidocaine. The biotransformation to MEGX was found to be 5 times higher when preceded by 3-day induction with phenobarbital (PI).

## RESULTS AND DISCUSSION

Hepatocytes formed single round cells as well as spheroids of about 10 to 50 cells and flattened after attachment to the carriers (FIG. 1). At the end of cultivation, the macroporous carriers were completely filled with cells. Vesicle transport and lipid droplets were observed with transmission electron microscopy (TEM). Maximal cell concentration was determined to be $7.1 \times 10^6$ cells/ml using a bubble-free aeration in the bioreactor at a microcarrier concentration of 3 g/l in a repeated batch mode. The cells exhibited an average specific growth rate of 0.5 per day and a maximum of 1.0 per day in the first 4 days of cultivation. In the growth phase, the LDH activity rose slightly, but an increase was observed when the cells reached confluency.

The cells tested positive for secreting albumin and α2-macroglobulin. The cytochrome P450 system was induced with a 7 μg/ml pulse of lidocaine. Five ng/ml MEGX were generated in one day without phenobarbital induction compared to 26 ng/ml after a preceding 3-day induction period with 50 μg/ml of phenobarbital (FIG. 2).

## CONCLUSION

Within 9 days the cells grew to a cell mass of $5.5 \times 10^9$ in a 1-liter bioreactor. Therefore, a 10-liter bioreactor could provide the cell mass of $2.5 \times 10^{10}$ to $5 \times 10^{10}$ needed for one clinically usable bioartificial liver device.

## ACKNOWLEDGMENTS

We wish to thank Dr. Gerlach and his group for kind advice and support. This work was supported by a Max Buchner grant (MBFST 1847) and the University of Bielefeld.

## REFERENCES

1. KASAI, S.I., M. SAWA & M. MITO. 1994. Is the biological artificial liver clinically applicable? A historic review of biological artificial liver support systems. Artif. Organs **18:** 348–354.
2. YARMUSH, M.L., J.C.Y. DUNN & R.G. TOMPKINS. 1992. Assessment of artificial liver support technology. Cell Transplant. **1:** 323–341.
3. GERLACH, J., T. TROST, C.J. RYAN, M. MEIßLER, O. HOLE, C. MÜLLER & P. NEUHAUS. 1994. Hybrid liver support system in a short term application on hepatectomized pigs. Int. J. Artif. Org. **17:** 549–553.
4. NYBERG, S.L., R.A. SHATFORD, M.V. PESHWA, J.G. WHITE, F.B. CERRA & W.S. HU. 1993. Evaluation of a hepatocyte-entrapment hollow fiber bioreactor: a potential bio-artificial liver. Biotechnol. Bioeng. **41:** 194–203.
5. MATTHEW, H.W.T., S. BASU, W.D. PETERSON, S.O. SALLEY & M.D. KLEIN. 1993. Performance of plasma-perfused, microencapsulated hepatocytes: prospects for extracorporeal liver support. J. Ped. Surg. **28:** 1423–1428.
6. KIRILLOWA, I. 1996. Etablierung teilungsfähiger differenzierter Hepatozyten der Maus und des Menschen durch genetische Beeinflussung der Zellteilungsregulation. Ph.D. thesis, Humboldt University, Berlin, Germany.

# rhBMP-Collagen Sponges as Osteoinductive Devices: Effects of *in Vitro* Sponge Characteristics and Protein pI on *in Vivo* rhBMP Pharmacokinetics

H. ULUDAG,[a] W. FRIESS,[b] D. WILLIAMS, T. PORTER, G. TIMONY, D. D'AUGUSTA, C. BLAKE, R. PALMER, B. BIRON, AND J. WOZNEY

*Genetics Institute Inc., One Burtt Road, Andover, Massachusetts 01810, USA*

**ABSTRACT: Osteoinductive devices, comprised of biodegradable collagen scaffolds and recombinant human Bone Morphogenetic Proteins (rhBMPs), are being currently pursued for local bone induction. To better understand the biological performance of such devices, we have carried out a series of studies to investigate the effects of sponge properties and protein structural features on the pharmacokinetics of implanted rhBMPs. The results indicated little dependence of the rhBMP-2 pharmacokinetics on the *in vitro* determined sponge properties. The protein isoelectric point (pI), on the other hand, was found to significantly affect the initial implant retention of rhBMPs, but not the subsequent pharmacokinetics. A 100-fold difference in the implant-retained dose could be observed depending on the type of rhBMP implanted. We conclude that protein structural features are important variables controlling *in vivo* pharmacokinetics of rhBMPs, and possibly the osteoinductive potency of the devices.**

## INTRODUCTION

Osteoinductive proteins, members of Bone Morphogenetic Protein (BMP) family, are capable of forming *de novo* bone by acting on the osteoprogenitor cells and differentiating them into mature osteoblasts. The BMPs are being currently produced by recombinant means and they are pursued as a component of implantable devices for local bone regeneration.[1,2] Biomaterials are utilized in the osteoinductive devices for local delivery of the proteins. The devices are typically prepared in an operating room by soaking a BMP solution into a biomaterial scaffold and they are implanted in the wet state. The biomaterial provides a 3-dimensional scaffold for the mesenchymal cell invasion and retains the protein at the site of implantation. Recently, at Genetics Institute investigators have concentrated on the development of one of the BMPs, recombinant human Bone Morphogenetic Protein-2 (rhBMP-2), in combination with an absorbable collagen sponge (Helistat®/ACS).[3,4] The ACS is

[a]Corresponding author. Current address: Department of Biomedical Engineering, University of Alberta, Edmonton, Alberta T6G 2G3, Canada; 403-492-0988 (voice); 403-492-8259 (fax); hasan.uludag@ualberta.ca (e-mail).

[b]Current address: Department of Pharmaceutical Technology, University of Erlangen-Nurnberg, Cauerstrasse, 91058 Erlangen, Germany.

fabricated from a bovine tendon–derived collagen by processing it into a tissue-compatible macroporous sponge and is currently marketed as an implantable hemostatic agent. The interaction of rhBMP-2 with the ACS and rhBMP-2 retention within the implants (i.e., local rhBMP-2 concentration) were believed to contribute to the osteoinductive activity of a device. We have recently began to explore this critical issue in more detail[5] and preliminary results have indicated a positive correlation between the rhBMP retention and the osteoinductive activity; i.e., proteins with a higher implant-retention gave a more robust osteoinductive activity. This raises the important issue of exploring the factors affecting protein retention or local pharmacokinetics for better understanding the factors contributing to the osteoinductive activity. Such an understanding will facilitate the design of next-generation devices with improved potency.

In the first part of this study, the effects of collagen sponge properties on rhBMP-2 pharmacokinetics were investigated. The sponges were first characterized by using *in vitro* assays and then well-characterized sponges were used for implanting rhBMP-2. In the second part, the effects of protein structural features on protein pharmacokinetics were investigated by implanting different types of rhBMPs.

## MATERIALS AND METHODS

### *Proteins*

The rhBMPs used in this study were rhBMP-2, rhBMP-4, and rhBMP-6. The rhBMP-2 was obtained from both CHO and *E. coli* expression systems, whereas rhBMP-4 and rhBMP-6 were from CHO cells only. The proteins were initially formulated in different buffers and all were buffer exchanged into a glycine buffer (2.5% Glycine, 0.5% Sucrose, 5 mM Glutamic Acid, 5 mM NaCl, 0.01% Tween-80, pH = 4.5).

For some studies, succinylation and acetylation were used to substitute carboxyl and acetyl groups, respectively, on the amino groups of CHO-derived rhBMP-2. These modification reactions by acetic anhydride and succinic anhydride are well-established techniques in the field.[6,7] Briefly, rhBMP-2 was buffer exchanged into 50 mM $Na_2HPO_4$ (pH = 7.5) using microdialysis cassettes (PIERCE). Succinic anhydride and acetic anhydride were dissolved in anhydrous dimethylformamide (all reagents from SIGMA) at 0.5 M and added to 2 mg/mL of rhBMP-2 in phosphate buffer to give a final anhydride concentration of 10 mM. After a 30-minute incubation at room temperature, the reaction was stopped by dialysis against the glycine buffer. The modified proteins were not soluble in this buffer and, accordingly, the pH of the dialysis buffer was gradually increased using 1N NaOH. The succinylated rh-BMP-2 became soluble at pH of 7.5 and acetylated rhBMP-2 at pH 9.0, so that the final solution of these proteins was in glycine buffer at pH 7.5 and 9.0, respectively. Both acetylated and succinylated rhBMP-2 was purified by a chromatographic procedure (see below).

$^{125}$I-labeled rhBMPs were obtained by the Iodo-Gen method.[9] The microcentrifuge tubes were first coated with Iodo-Gen reagent according to manufacturer's instructions (PIERCE). 10 μg of protein (in glycine buffer) was then added to the tubes, followed by addition of 1 mCi carrier-free $^{125}$I (New England Nuclear). After a 25 minute incubation, the labeled protein was purified on a NAP-5 Column (Pharmacia) using the glycine buffer (pH = 4.5 for all proteins except for acetylated and succinylated rhBMP-2 for which the pHs were 7.5 and 9.0, respectively). Trichloroacetic acid (TCA) precipitation of the labeled protein routinely indicated a labeling efficiency of > 95%.

### *Protein Characterization*

(1) *Amino Acid (AA) Sequencing.* The N-terminus of the proteins were sequenced by gas phase Edman degradation using a HP G1005A Protein Sequencer. Only the terminal 15 AA residues were sequenced, the remaining residues being deduced from the cDNA sequence.
(2) *Isoelectric Focusing (IEF).* The polyacrylamide gels were employed for the protein isoelectric point (pI). The gel composition was: 14.4g urea, 12 mL water, 5 mL acrylamide/bis, 0.64 mL pH 5–7 ampholyte, 0.64 mL pH 6–8 ampholyte, 0.64 mL pH 8–10.5 ampholyte (ampholytes form Pharmacia), 30 μL TEMED and 100 μL ammonium persulfate. The gels were cast in between two glass plates immediately before use. The cathode and anode solutions were 50 mM NaOH and 25 mM phosphoric acid, respectively. The gels were typically pre-focused for 1 h at 600 V.h. Approximately 30–40 μg protein was loaded in each lane and the gels were run for 2 hours at 2800 V.h. The gels were then stained with 0.5% methylene blue and destained with 5.4% glacial acetic acid, 40.5% methanol and 10% isopropanol.
(3) *Reverse-Phase High Pressure Liquid Chromatography (RP-HPLC).* The RP-HPLC was used as the final purification step for buffer-exchanged proteins and for chemically modified rhBMP-2. Briefly, an aliquot of protein solution was injected onto a C-4 Vydec column (4 cm) connected to an HP-1090. The proteins were eluted with a linear gradient of 0.1% Trifluoracetic acid (A) and 90% acetonitrile (B) (0–100% B in 14 minutes). The area under elution curves were used to determine the concentration of the proteins for implantation (CHO rhBMP-2 served as the reference standard).

### *Collagen Sponges*

Helistat® sponges (Integra Life Sciences, Plainsboro, NJ) were used as the rhBMP-2 carrier. In the course of a typical sponge preparation, lyophilized collagen (bovine tendon–derived) sponges are first exposed to formaldehyde for crosslinking and then to ethylene oxide for sterilization. Succinylated sponges were prepared for some experiments by treating the sterilized sponges with 10 mM succinic anhydride,[7] removing the unreacted reagents by washing the sponges in excess water and lyophilizing the sponge. The sponges were characterized for:

(1) *Protein Incorporation* (%Inc). A 1.5 mg/mL rhBMP-2 solution was absorbed into a sponge strip and allowed to equilibrate for 30 min at 37°C. The sponge was then squeezed and the amount of rhBMP-2 in the

expressate was quantitated by the RP-HPLC method. The amount of rhBMP-2 retained was expressed as %Inc of the applied rhBMP-2. Sponges with > 90 %Inc (i.e., < 10% of added rhBMP-2 in the exudate) were designated as High %Inc sponges. Sponges with ~60 %Inc were designated as Low %Inc sponges;

(2) *Collagenase Sensitivity.* The collagenase sensitivity of the sponges was determined by incubating a 50 mm × 12.5 mm sponge strip with a collagenase solution (Type H, Sigma; 2 mg/mL in TES buffer) and determining the amount of soluble protein using PIERCE's BCA Assay. Sponges that were relatively resistant to collagenase degradation were designated as collagenase insensitive and sponges that were collagenase degradable were designated as collagenase sensitive;

(3) *Amino Groups.* The amount of free-$NH_2$ on sponges was determined by 2,4,6-trinitrobenzenesulfonic acid (TNBS).[10] Briefly, a sponge sample in 0.1 M borate buffer (pH = 9.3) was mixed with 0.1% w/v TNBS solution (Fluka) and incubated at 40°C for 2 hours. The reaction was stopped by adding 12N HCl and the absorbance was read at 346 nm.

### In Vivo *rhBMP-2 Pharmacokinetics*

The rat ectopic assay[11] was used as the *in vivo* implantation model. The housing and the care of the animals were in accordance with the institutional guidelines. For implant preparation, 200 μL rhBMP solution was added onto 14 × 14 mm sponges (thickness: 3.5 mm) and allowed to soak for 30 minutes. The wet sponges were implanted subcutaneously at central thorax in Long-Evans rats (2 implants/rat) though a small incision (~5 cm). The protein solutions contained a trace amount of $^{125}$I-rhBMP (typically hot:cold = 1:1000). At the indicated times, 2 rats were sacrificed, the implants retrieved and the implant associated radioactivity was determined. The explants were routinely homogenized in 4 M guanidine by a high-speed blender and the homogenate was precipitated by 10% cold TCA solution (to ensure the protein-bound nature of the radioactivity).

The pharmacokinetics of the proteins was analyzed by WinNonLin software (Scientific Consultants Inc., Apex, NC) non-compartmentally and compartmentally using a bi-exponential model. A difference greater than ±20% between two parameters was considered significant.[12] The pharmacokinetics parameters computed were: Area Under Curve (AUC), Area-Under-Moment-Curve (AUMC), Mean Residence Time (MRT = AUMC/AUC) and bi-exponential half-lives ($t_{1/2}$).

## RESULTS

### *Sponge Properties and Pharmacokinetics*

*In vitro* assays indicated some variability in the sponge characteristics investigated. The results for two sponge Lots are shown in FIGURE 1. The sponges were susceptible to collagenase to a variable degree, some sponges being degraded rapidly (within 5 h; Absorbance > 0.5), whereas others did not degrade at all. The protein

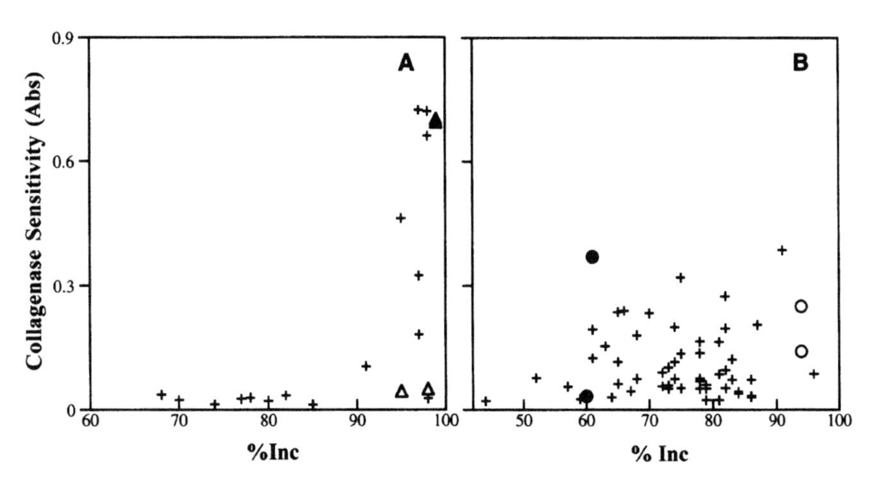


**FIGURE 1.** Collagenase sensitivity and %Inc for two sponge lots (shown separately in **A** and **B**). The larger symbols represent sponges used for the pharmacokinetics studies.

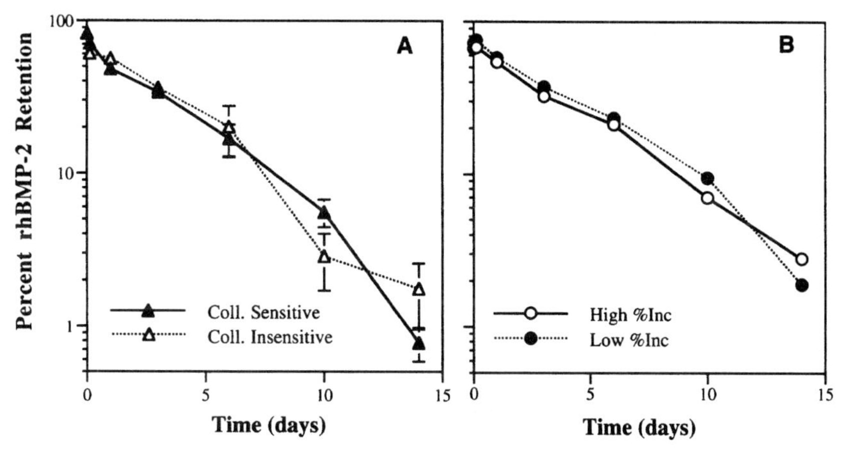


**FIGURE 2.** Pharmacokinetics of rhBMP-2 implanted with different sponge types. (**A**) Collagenase sensitive vs. collagenase insensitive sponges. (**B**) Low %Inc vs. high %Inc. sponges. The rhBMP-2 concentration was 0.4 mg/mL and 1.5 mg/mL in **A** and **B**, respectively.

incorporation (%Inc) was also variable among the sponges, ranging from 45 to 99%. The variability in collagenase sensitivity in %Inc was present within the individual Lots of ACS. A correlation between the collagenase susceptibility and the %Inc was not immediately apparent.

We compared the pharmacokinetics of rhBMP-2 implanted with (i) collagenase sensitive vs. insensitive (total vs. no degradation in 24 h) sponges, and (ii) Low vs. High %Inc (60% vs. 90%) sponges. FIGURE 1 shows the individuals sponges used in these studies. The explants were homogenized and TCA precipitated to ensure

**TABLE 1.** Summary of pharmacokinetic analysis for collagenase sensitivity and %Inc Groups[a]

| Group | Partial AUC (%total AUC) | MRT | Bi-Exponential Model | $t_{1/2}$ |
|---|---|---|---|---|
| Coll. Sensitive | 265.6 (99%) | 3.48 days | $30.7e^{-84.4t} + 69.3e^{-0.254t}$ | 0.01 & 2.73 days |
| Coll. Insensitive | 277.6 (98%) | 3.36 days | $34.5e^{-70.4t} + 65.6e^{-0.212t}$ | 0.01 & 4.09 days |
| Low %Inc | 294.8 (96%) | 3.89 days | $32.2e^{-1112t} + 67.8e^{-0.220t}$ | <0.01 & 3.16 days |
| High %Inc | 329.8 (98%) | 3.92 days | $26.2e^{-1024t} + 68.7e^{-0.213t}$ | <0.01 & 3.26 days |

[a]Data from Figure 2.

that the recovered radioactivity was protein-bound. Decalcification of explants before homogenization (by incubating them in 2–3M formic acid) did not release a significant amount of radioactivity. The counts retained in the decalcified matrix were > 95% precipitated with TCA after homogenization (not shown), indicating the protein-bound nature of the recovered counts. No difference in the time course of rhBMP-2 retention between the collagenase sensitive and insensitive sponges was noted (FIG. 2A, TABLE 1). A small difference appeared to develop between Days 10 and 14 (given by a higher $t_{1/2}$ in TABLE 1); however, a subsequent study, in which the rhBMP-2 pharmacokinetics was determined between Day 6 and Day 22,

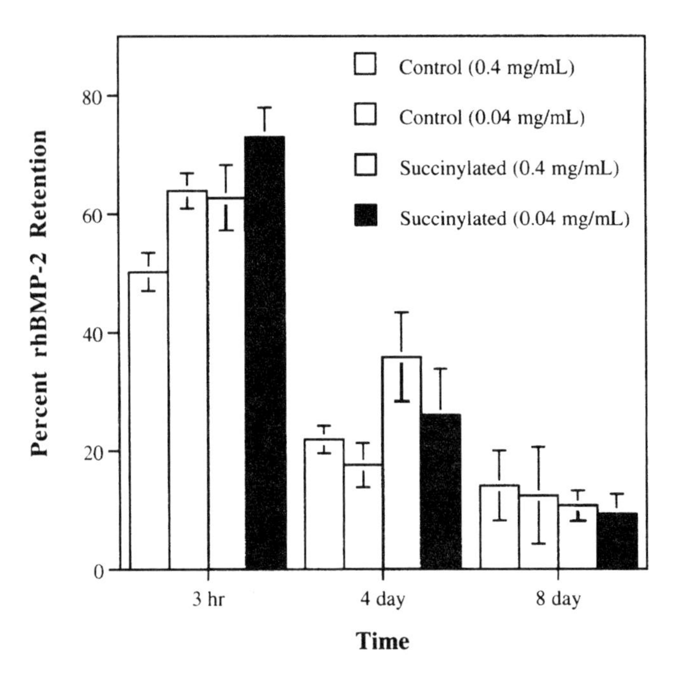


**FIGURE 3.** Pharmacokinetics of rhBMP-2 implanted with control and succinylated sponges. The rhBMP-2 concentration was either 0.4 mg/mL or 0.04 mg/mL.

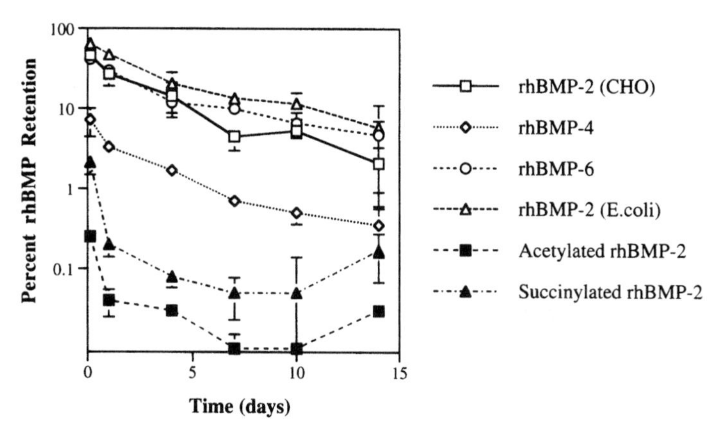


**FIGURE 4.** Pharmacokinetics of different rhBMPs implanted with ACS. The protein concentration was 0.05 mg/mL for all implants.

did not indicate such a difference between the two sponge types (not shown). The results from the Low %Inc and High %Inc sponges indicated no significant difference between the two sponge types as well (FIG. 2B, TABLE 1).

As an additional sponge type, succinylated sponges were prepared. Our preliminary experiments indicated that formaldehyde/ethylene oxide treatment did not consume all of the free -$NH_2$ groups. Successful succinylation was confirmed by a ~50% reduction in free -$NH_2$ groups of the sponges. *In vivo* rhBMP-2 pharmacokinetics was determined at a protein concentration of 0.4 mg/mL and 0.04 mg/mL (FIG. 3). A small difference in the rhBMP-2 retention was present at the first time point (3 h); however, the long-term rhBMP-2 retention was not affected by the sponge succinylation at either of the doses tested.

### *Protein Properties and Pharmacokinetics*

The IEF of the proteins indicated a pI of 9.0 for CHO rhBMP-2 and rhBMP-6, ~8.5 for *E. coli* rhBMP-2 and 5.0–7.0 for rhBMP-4. There were 5 distinct bands in rhBMP-4 sample but N-terminal sequencing indicated only two species (differing in only one AA). N-neuraminidase digested rhBMP-4 gave only a single band on IEF, suggesting that sialic acid residues might be present on the protein. The pI of acetylated and succinylated rhBMP-2 was ~3.5 and there was only a single band on the IEF gel for these proteins, indicating a relatively uniform rhBMP-2 modification. The pharmacokinetics of different rhBMPs is shown in FIGURE 4. The differences among the proteins were evident in the first hours of implantation. The proteins with higher pIs (rhBMP-2 and rhBMP-6) were retained the most, whereas the proteins with lower pI (acetylated/succinylated rhBMP-2) were retained the least. Based on the pAUC, the total dose retained at the implant site ranged a 100-fold (2.0 to 256.0 arbitrary units) and it correlated with the initial protein retention. The rate of rhBMP-2 loss (given by the slope in FIG. 4) for CHO and *E. coli*–derived protein was similar.

## DISCUSSION

The purpose of this study was to investigate the factors contributing to the local pharmacokinetics of an implanted rhBMP. A relatively simple and robust animal model, namely the rat ectopic assay, was used to study the pharmacokinetics of the implanted proteins. Irrespective of the rhBMP and the biomaterial implanted, the protein loss from the carriers was in two phases: an initial phase of rapid protein loss within hours of implantation, followed by a secondary, more gradual phase of protein loss.

### In Vitro *Sponge Properties and rhBMP-2 Pharmacokinetics*

The sponges were characterized *in vitro* for their collagenase sensitivity and %Inc. The *in vitro* results indicated some degree of heterogeneity in the physicochemical characteristics of collagen sponges in an individual Helistat® lot. The collagenase assay measures the ability of a collagenase enzyme to degrade the sponges. The initial (i.e., 0–3 h) and the subsequent (> 3 h) rhBMP-2 loss *in vivo* was not affected by the collagenase sensitivity. We expected the collagenase sensitivity to be an indicative of *in vivo* implant degradation rate, however the wet weight data on the explants (not shown), which is used as quantitative measure of implant size, did not indicate a difference between the collagenase sensitive and insensitive sponges. This is consistent with a similar rate of rhBMP-2 loss for the two types of sponges. It is possible that *in vitro* degradation by yet to be determined enzyme might be a better indicator for *in vivo* sponge degradation.

The %Inc is believed to reflect the amount of rhBMP-2 retained within a sponge, a higher %Inc indicating a higher retention of rhBMP-2 in a sponge. A higher retention is presumably due to a higher rhBMP-2 binding to the collagen or a higher physical entrapment of rhBMP-2 within the sponge. Surprisingly, rhBMP-2 loss kinetics did not correlate with the *in vitro* determined %Inc. Lower rhBMP-2 recovery was expected for sponges with lower %Inc, yet initial retention data did not support this. The implanted sponges were probably not exposed to as excessive mechanical forces as the *in vitro* squeezing test for %Inc; hence, the relatively gentler *in vivo* conditions might not have allowed the differences in rhBMP-2 incorporation to be manifested. The long-term (i.e., between 3 hours and 14 days) rhBMP-2 loss was not affected by the %Inc. It is possible that the factors contributing to *in vivo* rhBMP-2 retention in a sponge are different than the factors contributing to rhBMP-2 retention in the *in vitro* %Inc assay (e.g., other proteins in the interstitial fluid). Alternatively, the microenvironment in the sponges (e.g., ionic strength, pH etc.) *in vivo* is expected to be different from the conditions in the %Inc assay (likely initially, most definitely after longer time periods).

In an attempt to increase rhBMP-2 retention, we prepared succinylated sponges. The rhBMP-2 has a net positive charge (especially at the N-terminus[13,14] at physiological pH). The interaction of the such residues with a negatively charged surface (such as carboxyl residues from succinylation) was expected to give a better rhBMP-2 retention; however, the modified sponges gave the same retention profile as the unmodified sponges. This indicates either (i) an inadequate degree of modification, (ii) a mechanism of rhBMP-2 release independent of sponge-rhBMP-2 interactions, or (ii) a weak affinity of introduced carboxyl groups towards rhBMP-2. Further experiments will be needed to clarify this point.

### *Protein Characteristics and rhBMP Pharmacokinetics*

The rhBMPs comprise a family of proteins of similar AA sequence and with a characteristic 7-cystine motif[1,15] and presumably a 3-D structure. The rhBMP-2 (both CHO and *E. coli*) and rhBMP-6 was retained the most within the implants, followed by rhBMP-4. The acetylated and succinylated rhBMP-2 was retained the least. The descending order of retention among the proteins (rhBMP-2 ~ rhBMP-6 > rhBMP-4 > acetylated/succinylated rhBMP-2) was the same as the protein pI order, suggesting a correlation between the protein pI and the initial recovery. Among the likely reasons for the pI effect are differential adsorption to biomaterials, solubility profile in biological milieu or interaction with other biomolecules at the implant site. Our experimental system does not allow us to distinguish among these possibilities.

Two rhBMP-2 preparations in this study were derived from *E. coli* and CHO cells, the former giving an unglycosylated protein whereas the latter giving a glycosylated protein (at Asp-338: an average of 9 mannose residues per rhBMP-2[10]). Since the pharmacokinetics of both proteins were similar, the mannose residues on the CHO protein did not seem to affect the overall protein retention. On the other hand, sialic acid residues on rhBMP-4 might have been the reason for faster clearance of this protein from the implant site. The evidence for this stems from the fact that (i) the experimental rhBMP-4 pI was lower than its expected value based on the protein's on AA sequence,[9] (ii) there were at least 5 distinct rhBMP-4 bands on the IEF gel but N-terminal sequencing did not indicate such variations, and (iii) neuraminidase treatment reduced the protein bands on IEF into a single band. The sialic acid residues may affect the clearance of proteins in systemic circulation,[16] but no information has been published to-date on the effect of sialic acids residues on pharmacokinetics of implanted proteins. It will be interesting to find out if our observation on sialic acid of BMPs holds for other types of proteins as well.

The concentration of CHO rhBMP-2 in this part of the study (0.05 mg/mL) was lower than the concentration used in the collagenase sensitivity and %Inc experiments (0.4 and 1.5 mg/mL, respectively). Despite a slightly lower initial recovery at the lower dose (43%), the subsequent pharmacokinetics was not dependent on the protein concentration. This was also observed with the experiments with the succinylated sponges. This lack of concentration effect again argues against the physical adsorption of rhBMP to carrier surfaces as the primary mechanism controlling the protein pharmacokinetics.

### *Relationship between rhBMP Pharmacokinetics and Osteoinduction*

An important issue for the design of osteinductive devices is the relationship between the local rhBMP-2 retention and the final osteoinductive activity. Our recent observations have shown a positive correlation between the two parameters (i.e., higher the retention higher the osteoinductive activity) in the rat ectopic model. This result suggests that the osteopotency of bone-regeneration devices can be improved by using engineered BMPs with superior implant-retention. This is a viable alternative to using BMP heterodimers (e.g., BMP-2/-4 and BMP-4/-7) for improving device potency.[17,18] A critical issue is the applicability of the results obtained from the ectopic system to clinically relevant sites. The ectopic site may be an appropriate model for clinical sites where the osteoinductive devices will be implanted intramuscularly (e.g., in spinal fusion). The validity of the ectopic site as a model for intraosseously implanted devices (e.g., in fracture healing) remains to be seen. In the latter site, additional factors might contribute to rhBMP-2 loss from an implant (e.g., interaction with proteins in a hematoma). More studies will be needed to establish the relationship between the rhBMP pharmacokinetics and the osteoinductive activity at osseous sites.

## REFERENCES

1. WOZNEY, J.M. *et al.* 1988. Novel regulators of bone formation: molecular clones and activities. Science **242:** 1528–1534.
2. WINN, S. *et al.* 1998. Sustained release emphasizing recombinant human Bone Morphogenetic Protein-2. Adv. Drug Del. Rev. **31:** 303–318.
3. Boyne, P.J. *et al.* 1997. A feasibility study evaluation rhBMP-2/absorbable collagen sponge for maxillary sinus augmentation. Int. J. Periodont. Restor. Dent. **17:** 125–2139.
4. HOWELL, T.H. *et al.* 1997. A feasibility study evaluating rhBMP-2/absorbable collagen sponge device for local alveolar ridge preservation or augmentation. Int. J. Periodont. Restor. Dent. **17:** 11–25.
5. ULUDAG, H. *et al.* (abstract). 1998. A correlation between osteoinductive activity and local retention of recombinant human bone morphogenetic proteins. Transactions of the Society for Biomaterials Meeting (San Diego, CA), p. 140.
6. KLOTZ, I.M. 1967. Succinylation. Methods in Enzymology **11:** 576.
7. HERMANSON, G.T. 1996. Bioconjugate Techniques. Academic Press. San Diego, CA, pp.93–94, p128.
8. KINLEY, R.A. *et al.* 1993. Biotechnology and bone graft substitutes. Pharm. Res. **10:** 1393–1401.
9. FRAKER, P.J. & J.C. SPECK. 1978. Protein and cell membrane iodinations with a sparingly soluble chloroamide, 1,3,4,6-tetrachloro-3a,6a-diphenylglycoluril. Biochem. Biophys. Res. Commun. **80:** 847-857.
10. FRIESS, W. & G. LEE. 1996. Basic thermoanalytical studies of insoluble collagen matrices. Biomaterials **17:** 2289–2294.
11. SAMPETH, T.K. & A.H. REDDI. 1983. Homology of bone inductive proteins from human, monkey, bovine and rat extracellular matrix. Proc. Natl. Acad. Sci. USA **80:** 6591–6595.
12. STEINIJANS, V.W. & D. HAUSCHKE. 1993. International harmonization of regulatory bioequivalence requirements. Clin. Res. Reg. Aff. **10:** 203-220.
13. RATHORE, S. *et al.* (abstract) 1995. N-terminal isoforms of recombinant human Bone Morphogenetic Protein-2 (rhBMP-2) are active in vitro and in vivo. Prot. Sci. **4:** p140.
14. RUPPERT, R. *et al.* 1996 Human bone morphogenetic protein 2 contains a heparin-binding site which modifies its biological activity. Eur. J. Biochem. **237:** 295–302.
15. CELESTE *et al.* 1990. Identification of transforming growth factor beta family members present in bone inductive protein purified from bovine bone. Proc. Natl. Acad. Sci. USA **87:** 9843–9847.
16. WIDNESS, J.A. *et al.* 1996. In vivo $^{125}$I-erythropoietin pharmacokinetics are unchanged after anesthesia, nephrectomy and hepatectomy in sheep. J. Pharmacol. Exp. Therap. **279:** 1205–1210 (and references therein).
17. ISRAEL, D.I. *et al.* 1996. Heterodimeric bone morphogenetic proteins show enhanced activity in vitro and in vivo. Grow. Fac. **13:** 291–300.
18. AONO, A. *et al.* 1995. Potent ectopic bone inducing activity of bone morphogenetic protein 4/7 heterodimer. Biochem. Biophys. Res. Commun. **210:** 670–677.

# Tissue Engineering of Bone in the Craniofacial Complex

JEFFREY O. HOLLINGER[a] AND SHELLEY R. WINN

*Division of Plastic and Reconstructive Surgery, Oregon Health Sciences University, Portland, Oregon 97201-3098, USA*

**ABSTRACT: Tissue engineered therapies to regenerate bone in the craniofacial complex will probably include combinations of BMP-like molecules, a BMP-responsive set of cells (both endogenous and exogenous), and packaging in a surgically convenient format. In this report we have described our work with OPCs, BMP, and polymer: components suitable for tissue engineering.**

## CRANIOFACIAL BONE DEFICIENCIES: TRADITIONAL TREATMENTS

Craniofacial deficiencies caused by oncologic resection and trauma most frequently are restored with autografts.[1–3] In a series of 80 patients with gunshot wounds of the face, 89% required autografts.[2] Manson *et al.* reported that of 314 patients with midface fractures incurred from trauma, 34% needed autografts[4] and in a retrospective study, Manson and colleagues determined that of 4,468 trauma patients, 25% involved the craniofacial complex.[5] There is an unacceptably high failure rate for autografts (13–30%),[6] and an even greater level of failure for allogeneic preparations (20–35%).[7] Unacceptable clinical outcomes, as well as issues of pathogenic transmissions and immune responses (from allografts),[8–10] warrant developing and fielding safe, rational, and efficient alternatives offering predictable outcomes.

## A TISSUE ENGINEERED ALTERNATIVE: COMPONENTS

### *Bone Morphogenetic Proteins*

Bone morphogenetic proteins (BMPs) 2–15[11–16] are categorized within the transforming growth factor β superfamily[17–19] and direct the progression of cells and their organizational format to tissues and organs in the embryo;[20–23] influence body patterning, limb development, size and number of bones;[24–28] and modulate post-fetal chondro-osteogenetic maintenance.[18,29] Meriting consideration in bone engineering therapies, is the ability of BMPs, such as BMP-2, to promote undifferentiated mesenchymal cells into osteoblasts,[30–32] thus leading to bone formation. This property has been exploited in preclinical studies with recombinant human (rh) BMP-2 to regenerate calvaria[33–35] and long bone[36,37] in the rat, rabbit

[a]Author for correspondence: Division of Plastic and Reconstructive Surgery, Oregon Health Sciences University, 3181 SW Sam Jackson Park Rd., L352A, Portland, OR 97201-3098; 503-494-8426 (voice); 503-494-8378 (fax); hollinge@ohsu.edu (e-mail).

ulna[38] and radius,[39,40] sheep long bone,[41] the mandible[42] and premaxilla[43] of the dog, and the ulna of the African green monkey.[44] Furthermore, rhBMP has been applied for spine fusions in dogs[45] and rhesus nonhuman primates.[46,47] In these studies, the rhBMP prompted regeneration of critical-sized defects that ordinarily would not have healed by new bone formation.[48] To date, there have been two clinical studies with rhBMP-2: maxillary sinus floor augmentation[49] and alveolar ridge preservation.[50] In the first report, the authors concluded rhBMP-2 plus absorbable collagen sponge may be an acceptable alternative to traditional treatments. The second report focused on feasibility and safety, noting rhBMP-2 and an absorbable collagen sponge were convenient and safe. However, in both studies, massive doses of rhBMP-2 were needed for effect, and only the highest dose range of 1.7–3.4 mg suggested efficacy.

### *Osteoblast Precursor Cells*

BMP-mediated strategies to regenerate bone depend on responsive osteoblast precursor cells (OPCs)[51,52] and there must be a sufficient quantity of these cells whose response(s) will produce the desired outcome: restoring form and function to bone. We have developed an OPC cell line that responds favorably to BMP and therefore, can be exploited in craniofacial bone engineering.[53] Consistent with this strategy, was a study where rhBMP and a nonspecific phenotype population of marrow cells promoted a superior bone regenerative response in segmental defects in rats than rhBMP alone.[54] A similar mixture of marrow cells and a ceramic material were combined (without BMP) to treat segmental defects in rats and dogs, and the authors reported a regeneration of bone.[55,56] Polymers and transformed cell lines have been explored by others.[57–59]

We hypothesize that a characterized population of OPCs would minimize the therapeutic dose of rhBMP (currently, milligram quantities are required for effect) and augment a locally responsive cell stock that would differentiate into osteoblasts. This notion is especially valuable for the geriatric patient plagued with a limited number of functionally challenged precursor cells.[60–64] Furthermore, we hypothesize local BMP can be supplemented by genetically bolstering the capacity of OPCs to express this molecule. This novel approach to local BMP regulation by OPCs could be accomplished with a plasmid expression vector containing the rhBMP-2 gene, a genetic engineering procedure we have accomplished with human CNTF.

### *Development of the OPC Cell Line*

A conditionally immortalized OPC cell line was derived from human fetal bone tissue. The primary cultures were transfected with a plasmid in which the MX-1 promoter drives the SV40 large T antigen (when activated by A/D interferon).[53] We derived several clones based on phenotypic characterization and expression of osteoblast markers (e.g., alkaline phosphatase, mRNA for osteocalcin, osteonectin, parathyroid hormone receptor, and procollagen type I). We selected the OPC clone 1 as a consequence of its superior osteoblast-like characteristics. TABLE 1 lists the osteoblast markers that were measured. A striking characteristic for one of the clones was the capacity to promote *in vitro* mineralization.

**TABLE 1. Osteoblast markers**

| OPC clone | Doubling times (days) | APase (control) | APase (50 ng/ml BMP-2) | Mineralize |
|---|---|---|---|---|
| 1 | 1.8 | 15.9 ± 1.9 | 218.7 ± 17.7 | +++ |
| 2 | 1.9 | 13.6 ± 2.3 | 65.6 ± 6.8 | ++ |
| 3 | 1.6 | 14.5 ± 2.1 | 83.3 ± 9.5 | ++ |
| 6 | 2.2 | 14.4 ± 2.4 | 96.2 ± 10.3 | ++ |
| 7 | 2.9 | ND[a] | ND[a] | – |
| Nontransformed cells | 2.4 | 12.8 ± 1.8 | 36.5 ± 5.6 | + |

[a]ND = not determined.

### *The Polymer Delivery System*

Bone regeneration with a tissue engineered therapy should be formulated to permit surgical convenience, as well as localization of the cells and BMP at the surgical site. Consequently, the notion that a delivery system merely is a transit vehicle must be dispelled. It is correct the delivery system must fulfill a pivotal role as a "delivery system";[65] however, the "system" also must fulfill stringent macrophysiological requirements consistent with bone regeneration.[66,67] Therefore, we have engineered a unique polymer delivery system for the craniofacial complex.

The options for the design could include various poly(α-hydroxy acids), such as poly(lactide-co-glycolide) (PLG) and poly(lactide) (PL), as well as hydrogel scaffolds to support and promote the dynamics of the bone healing cascade.

PLG has enjoyed a 30-year history of clinical safety and FDA approval, thereby encouraging relatively rapid clinical approval for the polymer system (reviewed in ref. 68). Moreover, PLG can be engineered by post-synthesis technologies to encourage cell attachment and combined with BMP and OPCs, it can support and promote the bone healing cascade, thus offering advantages over the ceramic-based materials.

PLG and PL have delivered rhBMP-2 to restore long bone and skull defects in rats,[34–36] long bone in sheep[41,69] and rabbits,[40] and alveolar cleft defects in dogs.[43] However, in these studies and others with rhBMP-7, superphysiological doses of rhBMP were necessary in dogs,[70] sheep,[41,69] and rhesus.[44] Massive doses were needed in two clinical studies.[49,50] The superphysiological dosing issue raises clinical concerns. What are the systemic risks from superphysiologic doses of rhBMP? Rational engineering of a unique polymer delivery system will position OPCs and rhBMP[65] at desired surgical sites, thus selectively localizing these agents and decrease dosing requirements.

A design feature of the system is its property as a *substratum*. This feature is significant since it is highly unlikely either OPCs or rhBMP-2 or a combination of the two will be effective without the polymer substratum.[67] The impact of an extracellular matrix-substratum (or *scaffold*) in tissue wound repair has been emphasized repeatedly.[64,65,67,71] As a substratum, the system should provide a haven for attachment of host pluripotential cells and support their conversion to osteoblasts, as well as shuttle the cargo of rhBMP and OPCs to the bone defect. This functional con-

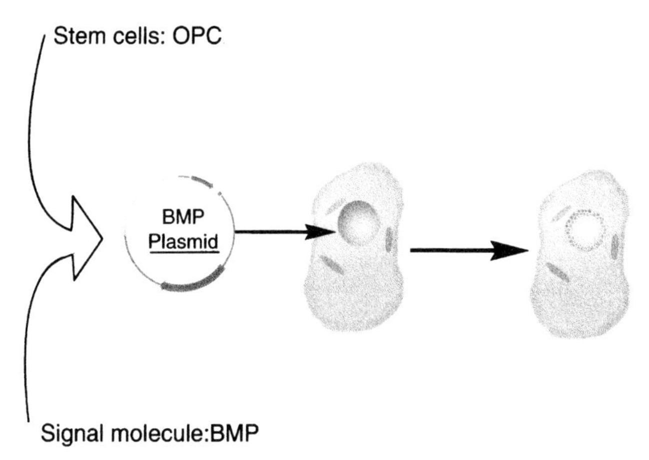


FIGURE 1a.

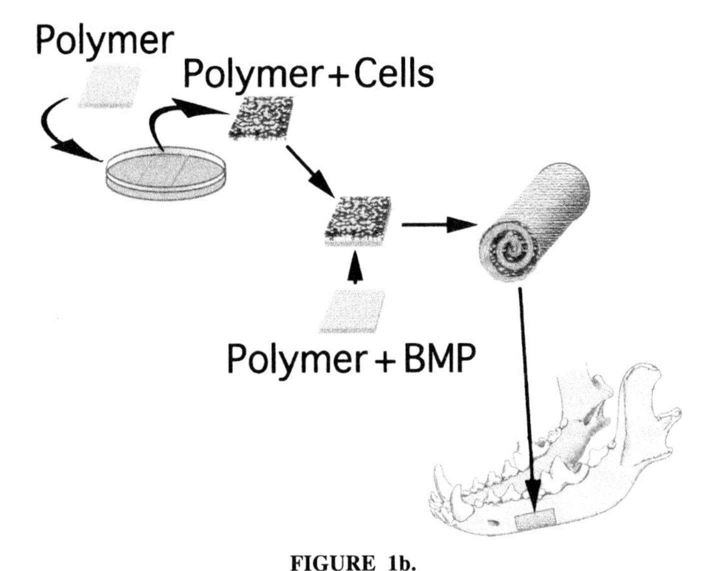


FIGURE 1b.

cept is consistent with an extracellular matrix-substratum,[71,72] the regulatory role of BMP,[12] and clinical demands.[67]

## ASSEMBLY OF THE TISSUE ENGINEERED BONE COMPONENTS

Porous polymer as a "cortex" and "sheet" formats (FIG. 1, a and b) can be fabricated by a multiple solvent/thermodynamic procedure involving dissolution of the poly(α-hydroxy acid) (e.g., PLG) into methylene chloride/cyclohexane or dioxane/water mixed solvents, freezing the solutions at 0 to –4°C, and sublimating under vacuum. The post-synthesis engineering procedure with two miscible solvents enforces control of the polymer solution thermodynamics, chain extension and aggregation, and predictably yields a solid-state post-synthesis product with a pore volume ≥ 90% and a size optimized for osteoconduction (≥ 350 μm).[73] Moreover, preliminary results have validated polymer products with predictable crystalline and amorphous fractions, capacity to delivery OPCs, rhBMP-2,and biocompatibility and degradation characteristics consistent with tissue engineered devices for bone regeneration.[65,74]

## REFERENCES


1. KELLY, J.K. 1973. J. Oral Surg. **31:** 438–445.
2. GRUSS, J., O. ANTONYSHYN & J. PHILLIPS. 1991. Plastic Reconstr. Surg. **87:** 436–450.
3. MANSON, P. 1994. Facial bone healing and bone grafts. A review of clinical physiology *In* Bone Repair and Regeneration. A.E. Seyfer & J.O. Hollinger, Eds. : 331–348. W.B. Saunders. Philadelphia.
4. MANSON, P., W. CRAWLEY, M. YAREMCHUK, G. ROCHMAN, J. HOOPES & J. FRENCH. 1985. Plastic Reconstr. Surg. **76:** 1–10.
5. MANSON, P., B. MARKOWITZ, S. MIRVIS, M. DUNHAM & M. YAREMCHUK. 1990. Plastic Reconstr. Surg. **85**: 202–212.
6. GREGORY, C.F. 1972. Clin. Orthop. Rel. Res. **87:** 156–166.
7. ENNEKING, W.F. & E.R. MINDELL. 1991. J. Bone Joint Surg. **73-A:** 1123–1142.
8. BUCK, B.E., L. RESNICK & S.M. SHAH. 1990. Clin. Orthop. Rel. Res. **251:** 249–252.
9. DELUSTRO, F., J. DASCH, J. KEEFE & L. ELLINGSWORTH. 1990. Clin. Orthop. **260:** 263–279.
10. HOROWITZ, M.C. & G.E. FRIEDLAENDER. 1991. J. Bone Joint Surg. **73-A:** 1157–1168.
11. CELESTE, A.J., R. TAYLOR, N. YAMAJI, E. WANG, J. ROSS & J. WOZNEY. Keystone Symposium, 1992.
12. WOZNEY, J.M. 1992. Molecular Reproduct. Develop. **32:** 160–167.
13. CELESTE, A.J., J.J. SONG, K. COX, V. ROSEN & J.M. WOZNEY. 1994. J. Bone Miner. Res. **9:** S137.
14. CELESTE, A.J., A.J. ROSS, N. YAMAJI & J.M. WOZNEY. 1995. J. Bone Miner. Res. **10:** 334.
15. DUBE, J.L. & A.J. CELESTE. 1995. J. Bone Miner. Res. **10** (Suppl.)**:** 333.
16. INADA, M., T. KATAGIRIR, S. AKIYAMA, M. NAMIKI, M. KOMAKI, A. YAMAGUCHI, K. KAMOI & T. SUDA. 1996. Biochem. Biophys. Res. Commun. **222:** 317–322.
17. WOZNEY, J. 1993. Cellular and Molecular Biology of Bone. : 131–165.
18. KINGSLEY, D.M. 1994. Genes Develop. **8:** 133–146.
19. YAMAGUCHI, A. 1995. Cell Biol. **6:** 165–173.
20. TOMIZAWA, K., H. MATSUI, E. KONDO, K. MIYAMOTO, M. TOKUDA, T. ITANO, S. NAGAHATA, T. AKAGI & O. HATASE. 1995. Molec. Brain Res. **28:** 122–128.
21. IWASAKI, S., A. HATTORI, M. SATO, M. TSUJIMOTO & M. KOHNO. 1996. J. Biol. Chem. **271:** 17360–17365.
22. REISSMANN, E., U. ERNSBERGER, P.H. FRANCIS-WEST, D. RUEGER, P.M. BRICKELL & H. ROHRER. 1996. Development **122:** 2079–2088.
23. ZHAO, G.Q., K. DENG, P.A. LABOSKY, L. LIAW & B.L. HOGAN. 1996. Genes Develop. **10:** 1657–1669.
24. DUBOULE, D. 1992. Bioessays **14:** 375–384.
25. DUBOULE, D. 1994. Science **266:** 575–576.
26. LAUFER, E., C.E. NELSON, R.L. JOHNSON, B.A. MORGAN & C. TABIN. 1994. Cell **79:** 993–1003.
27. TICKLE, C. 1994. Nature **368:** 587–588.

28. WINNIER, G., M. BLESSING, P. LABOSKY & B.L.M. HOGAN. 1995. Genes Develop. **9:** 2105–2116.
29. KINGSLEY, D. 1994. Trends in Genetics **10:** 16–21.
30. THIES, R.S., M. BAUDUY, B.A. ASHTON, L. KURTZBERG, J.M. WOZNEY & V. ROSEN. 1992. Endocrinology **130:** 1318–1324.
31. BODEN, S.D., K. MCCUAIG, G. HAIR, M. RACINE, L. TITUS, J.M. WOZNEY & M.S. NANES. 1996. Endocrinology **137:** 3401–3407.
32. YAMAGUCHI, A., T. ISHIZUYA, N. KINTOU, Y. WADA, T. KATAGIRI, J.M. WOZNEY, V. ROSEN & S. YOSHIKI. 1996. Biochem. Biophys. Res. Commun. **220:** 366–371.
33. KENLEY, R., L. MARDEN, T. TUREK, L. JIN, E. RON & J. HOLLINGER. 1994. J. Biomed. Mater. Res. **28:** 1139–1147.
34. MARDEN, L.J., J.O. HOLLINGER, A. CHAUDHARI, T. TUREK, R. SCHAUB & E. RON. 1994. J. Biomed. Mater. Res. **28:** 1127–1138.
35. SMITH, J., T. TUREK, J.O. HOLLINGER, L. MARDEN, J. WOZNEY & R. KENLEY. 1995. J. Controlled Rel. **36:** 183–195.
36. YASKO, A.W., J.M. LANE, E.J. FELLINGER, V. ROSEN, J.M. WOZNEY & E.A. WANG. 1992. J. Bone Joint. Surg. **74-A:** 659–671.
37. STEVENSON, S., N. CUNNINGHAM, J. TOTH, D. DAVY & A.H. REDDI. 1994. J. Bone Joint Surg. **76-A:** 1676–1687.
38. COOK, S.D., G.C. BAFFES, M.W. WOLFE, K. SAMPATH, D.C. RUEGER & T.S. WHITE-CLOUD. 1994. J. Bone Joint Surg. **76A:** 827–838.
39. HOLLINGER, J.O., M. MAYER, D. BUCK, H.D. ZEGZULA, E. RON, J. SMITH, L. LIN & J. WOZNEY. 1996. J. Controlled Rel. **39:** 287–304.
40. ZEGZULA, H.D., D. BUCK, J. BREKKE, J. WOZNEY, & J.O. HOLLINGER. 1997. J. Bone Joint Surg. **79-A:** 1778–1790.
41. GERHART, T.N., C.A. KIRKER-HEAD, M.J. KRIZ, M.E. HOLTROP, G.E. HENNIG & E.A. WANG. 1993. Clin. Orthop. Rel. Res. **293:** 317–326.
42. TORIUMI, D.M., H.S. KOTLER, D.P. LUXUNBERG, M.E. HOLTROP & E.A. WANG. 1991. Arch. Otolaryngol. Head and Neck Surg. **117:** 1101–1112.
43. MAYER, M.H., J.O. HOLLINGER, E. RON & J. WOZNEY. 1996. Plastic Reconstr. Surg. **98:** 247–259.
44. COOK, S.D., M.W. WOLFE, S.L. SALKELD & D.C. RUEGER. 1995. J. Bone Joint Surg. **77-A:** 734–750.
45. MUSCHLER, G.F., A. HYODO, T. MANNING, H. KAMBIC & K. EASLEY. 1994. Clin. Orthop. Rel. Res. **308:** 229–240.
46. BODEN, S.D., J.H. SCHIMANDLE & W.C. HUTTON. 1995. J. Bone Joint Surg. **77-A:** 1404–1417.
47. SCHIMANDLE, J.H., S.D. BODEN & W.C. HUTTON. 1995. Spine **20:** 1326–1337.
48. SCHMITZ, J.P. & J.O. HOLLINGER. 1986. Clin. Orthop. Rel. Res. **205:** 299–308.
49. BOYNE, P.J., R.E. MARX, M. NEVINS, G. TRIPLETT, E. LAZARO, L.C. LILLY, M. ALDER & P. NUMMIKOSKI. 1997. Int. J. Periodontal Restor. Dent. **17:** 11–25.
50. HOWELL, T.H., J. FIORELLINI, A. JONES, M. ALDER, P. NUMMIKOSKI, M. LAZARO, L. LILLY & D. COCHRAN. 1997. Int. J. Periodontal Restor. Dent. **17:** 125–139.
51. ROSEN, V. & S. THIES. 1992. Trends in Genetics **8:** 97–102.
52. SAMPATH, T.K. & D.C. RUEGER. 1994. Complications Orthopaed. **Winter:** 101.
53. WINN, S.R., G. RANDOLPH, H. ULUDAG, S. WONG, Z. HU & J.O. HOLLINGER. J. Bone Mineral Res. In press.
54. LANE, J.M., A. TOMIN, M. BOSTROM, V. ROSEN & V. WOZNEY. First International Conference on Bone Morphogenetic Proteins, 1993. Baltimore, MD.
55. BRUDER, S.P., N. JAISWAL & S.E. HAYNESWORTH. 1997. J. Cell. Biochem. **64:** 278–294.
56. KADIYALA, S., R.G. YOUNG, M.A. THIEDE & S.P. BRUDER. Cell Transplant. **6:** In press.
57. VACANTI, J.P., J.C. STEIN, J.C. GILBERT, C.A. VACANTI, D.E. INGBER & R. LANGER. 1991. Polymer Preprints **32:** 227.
58. VACANTI, C.A., R. LANGER, B. SCHLOO & J.P. VACANTI. 1991. Polymer Preprints **32:** 228–229.

59. VACANTI, C.A., W. KIM, J. UPTON, B. SCHLOO & J.P. VACANTI. 38th Annual Meeting, Orthopedic Research Society, 1993. San Francisco.
60. SHIROTA, T., K. OHNO, K. SUZUKI & K. MICHI. 1993. J. Oral Maxillofac. Surg. **51:** 51–56.
61. CAPLAN, A.I. 1994. Clin. Plastic Surg. **21:** 429–435.
62. QUARTO, R., D. THOMAS & T. LIANG. 1995. Calcif. Tissue Int. **56:** 123–129.
63. FLEET, J.C., K. CASHMAN, K. COX & V. ROSEN. 1996. Endocrinology **137:** 4605–4610.
64. CAPLAN, A.I. & S.P. BRUDER. 1997. *In* Principles of Tissue Engineering. R. Lanza, R. Langer & W. Chick, Eds. : 603–618. Academic Press, Inc. San Diego, CA.
65. WINN, S.R., H. ULUDAG & J.O. HOLLINGER. 1998. Advanced Drug Deliv. Rev. **31:** 303–318.
66. HOLLINGER, J.O. & J.P. SCHMITZ. 1997. Ann. N.Y. Acad. Sci. **831:** 427–437.
67. BURGESS, E.A. & J.O. HOLLINGER. *In* Frontiers in Tissue Engineering. A.G.M., C.W. Patrick & L.V. McIntire, Eds. Elsevier.
68. HOLLINGER, J. 1995. Biomedical Applications of Synthetic Biodegradable Polymers. CRC Press, Inc. Boca Raton, FL, pp. 1–257.
69. KIRKER-HEAD, C.A., T.N. GERHART, S.H. SCHELLING, G.E. HENNING, E.A. WANG & M.E. HOLTROP. 1995. Clin. Orthop. **318:** 222–230.
70. COOK, S.D., G.C. BAFFES, M.W. WOLFE, T.K. SAMPATH & D.C. RUEGER. 1994. Clin. Orthop. **301:** 302–312.
71. REDDI, A. 1984. Extracellular matrix and development. *In* Extracellular Matrix Biochemistry. K.A. Piez & A.H. Reddi, Eds.: 375–412. Elsevier. New York.
72. RAGHOW, R. 1994. FASEB J. **8:** 823–831.
73. ROBINSON, B., J.O. HOLLINGER, E. SZACHOWICZ & J. BREKKE. 1995. Arch. Otolaryngol. Head and Neck Surg. **112:** 707–713.
74. WINN, S.R., J.M. SCHMITT, D. BUCK, Y. HU, D. GRAINGER & J.O. HOLLINGER. J. Biomed. Mater. Res. In press.

# Computer Controlled Bioreactor for Large-scale Production of Cultured Skin Grafts

J.E. PRENOSIL[a,c] AND M. KINO-OKA[b]

[a]*Department of Chemical Engineering, ETH-Zurich, CH-8092 Zurich, Switzerland*
[b]*Department of Chemical Science and Engineering, Osaka University, Toyonaka, Osaka 560, Japan*

**ABSTRACT: KERATOR—an automated membrane bioreactor—was developed to produce Autologous Wound Dressing (AWD) at significantly reduced cost and time of transplantation down to two weeks time. At the same time, the risk of human error is largely eliminated. The computer-controlled reactor is modular, allowing the production of up to 0.5 m$^2$ AWD at one time. A special feature of the reactor is a hydrophilic polymeric support membrane on which the human keratinocytes attach and proliferate. Recently developed serum-free medium is used to culture keratinocytes as a monolayer without a feeder layer of murine fibroblasts. The use of composite skin grafts consisting of a subconfluent keratinocyte layer on a polymeric support film is a very promising method for skin transplantation owing to the high activity of non-differentiated keratinocyte cells and reduction of the time needed to prepare the skin grafts. A microscopic video system with image analysis was developed for on-line monitoring of the cell growth and morphology in the KERATOR. The computer uses the obtained information to control medium change and to predict the end of cultivation.**

## INTRODUCTION

Looking at the field of biotechnology, currently in a state of rapid flux, you will find one exception: the prices of biotechnological products remain high. This fact is, at least in part, responsible for the sluggish growth of the biotechnology market.

Several problems, listed in FIGURE 1, contribute to this predicament. Obviously, the R & D costs attached to almost every new product are enormous. The raw materials are usually rare or expensive, and the final product is usually produced only in small quantities. This leads to the false idea that a laboratory procedure can be used for commercial production with only small modifications. The production processes become too complicated or labor intensive, and the applied unit operations are either inefficient or inadequate.

Examining individual costs, it becomes clear that the process and unit operation problems can and must be addressed by chemical and biochemical engineers together with the equipment manufacturers. To do that, several requirements may be identified (FIG. 2). New equipment should be developed only after a careful scrutiny of the existing equipment to determine whether it can be adapted for a new process,

[c]Author for correspondence: Swiss Federal Institute of Technology, ETH-TCL, Chemical Engineering Department, CH-8092 Zurich, Switzerland; 41-1-632-3080 (voice); 41-1-632-1082 (fax); prenosil@tech.chem.ethz.ch (e-mail).

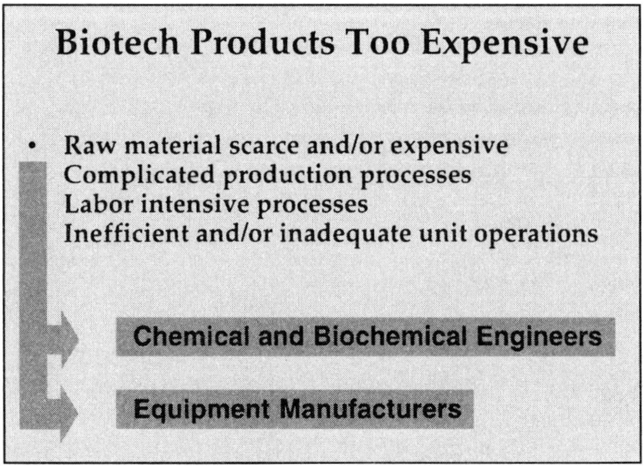

Biotech Products Too Expensive

- Raw material scarce and/or expensive
- Complicated production processes
- Labor intensive processes
- Inefficient and/or inadequate unit operations

Chemical and Biochemical Engineers

Equipment Manufacturers

**FIGURE 1.** Biotechnology products are too expensive.

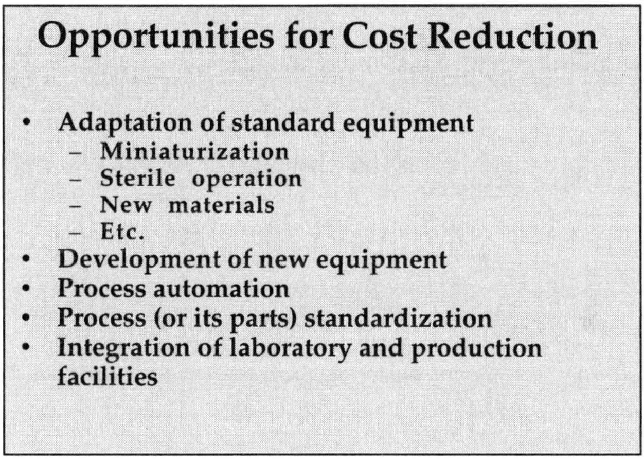

Opportunities for Cost Reduction

- Adaptation of standard equipment
  - Miniaturization
  - Sterile operation
  - New materials
  - Etc.
- Development of new equipment
- Process automation
- Process (or its parts) standardization
- Integration of laboratory and production facilities

**FIGURE 2.** Possibilities for cost reduction.

e.g., scale down, sterility features, new construction materials, etc. A new process should be highly automated, and high priority should be given to its standardization. Responsibility for use of standard elements lies largely with equipment manufacturers. Owing to similar production scale and other factors, the laboratory and production environments must be integrated. Ideally, they should be located very near or together and have personnel with both research, and production skills. Production of skin grafts by human cell culture is an example of such a process and a description of the procedure is given here.

Cultivation of human keratinocytes is one of the most important tissue culture operations used not only in the basic investigations in toxicology, pathology and im-

**TABLE 1.** Cost of burn wound therapy using autografts[a]

| | Cultured autografts | Split-skin autografts |
|---|---|---|
| Average total cost of hospitalization [$] | 318,874 | 107,235 |
| Average daily cost of hospitalization [$] | 4,454 | 3,311 |
| Average cost of cultured skin/patient [$] | 20,280 | |

[a]Adapted from: A.M. Munster.[5]

munology, but mainly in the clinical application of the skin transplantation, which is the most advanced and widely used human organ transplantation so far.[1] Cultured keratinocytes are used as multilayer skin grafts (cultured epithelial autografts or allogeneic skin grafts), including layers of basal keratinocytes for proliferation and differentiated keratinocytes for structure integrity. Laboratory production of skin grafts was developed soon after a breakthrough in the multilayer keratinocyte culture using serum-containing medium and murine fibroblast cells (3T3) as a feeder layer.[2] This technique was commercialized, leading to clinical availability of skin grafts for burn wounds and chronic leg ulcers.[3,4] This traditional method using serum and 3T3 cells has been successful; however, it is complicated and has a number of problems, both biological and clinical.

Production of multilayer skin grafts requires a period of 3–4 weeks, and is extremely costly (TABLE 1[5]). In addition, the wounds covered with the skin grafts often show blisters due to serum antigen in the cells and immunogenic rejection after transplantation.[6,7]

Boyce and Ham[8] developed a serum-free medium in which keratinocytes can grow without serum and a feeder layer of murine fibroblasts, resulting from the addition of growth factors and hormones. Growth of keratinocytes can be further improved by coating the bottom surface in the culture vessel with attachment and matrix factors such as collagen and fibronectin.[9]

On the basis of these developments, a promising protocol for novel skin grafts for skin transplantation emerged. The skin grafts consist of subconfluent proliferative keratinocytes attached to a support film. The main advantages are the high activity of non-differentiated subconfluent keratinocytes and the shorter preparation time of such skin grafts, only 2 weeks, resulting in reduction of production costs.[10,11] A support film on which keratinocytes can grow is needed to provide the necessary mechanical strength for handling and transplantation. The foil must fulfill a number of requirements, summarized in TABLE 2.

The Teflon® membrane FEP hydrophilic film (Type C-20, DuPont Co.) was found to fulfill such requirements. Insufficient pliability was offset by using the film only 12 μm thick. Its non-toxicity was demonstrated by Bonnekoh *et al.*[12]

In the present study, the culture of keratinocytes on the FEP support film in a serum-free medium, and large-scale production of skin grafts in a modular bioreactor are described.

**TABLE 2.** Support film requirements

| Biological properties | Physical-mechanical properties |
|---|---|
| Non-toxic, inert | Transparency |
| Good affinity for fast cell attachment | Gas and/or liquid permeability |
| Cell growth rate same as on tissue culture plastic | Sterilizability:<br>Thermal and/or radiation stability<br>Mechanical strength<br>Flexibility and pliability |

## MATERIALS AND METHODS

### *Isolation of Keratinocytes and Primary Culture*

Keratinocytes were isolated by enzyme digestion from the skin biopsies taken from a patient and treated with 0.2% trypsin 1:250 (Sigma) for 13 h at 4°C.[1] As a primary culture, keratinocytes were incubated in a T-flask (Nunclon Delta Flask, Nunc Co.) in the modified DMEM medium with 10% fetal calf serum described by Rheinwald and Green.[2] The cultures were maintained without a feeder layer at 37°C in an atmosphere of 5% $CO_2$ in air using a $CO_2$ incubator. The initial concentration of cells was approximately $10^5$ cells/cm$^2$ and the medium was kept at a depth of 4 mm in the culture vessel. After 72 h the medium was changed to the serum-free medium for keratinocytes (Keratinocyte-SFM, Life Technology Co.). After that, the medium was changed every 72 h until reaching confluence, which was found to be optimal for the medium change.[13]

### *Culture in T-Flask and Petriperm*

The keratinocytes were subcultivated further in 170 cm$^2$ T-flasks (Nunclon Delta Flask, Nunc Co.) with the serum-free medium. During a series of subcultures lasting 2 months, neither a decline in the cell growth rate nor a change in cell morphology was observed.

For the culture experiments, 25 cm$^2$ T-flasks (Nunclon Delta Flask, Nunc Co.) or 20 cm$^2$ Petri dishes with polymeric films of hydrophilic polyfluoroethylene (Petriperm, Heraues Co.) were used. The culture conditions were set as follows: medium depth = 4 mm (serum-free medium for keratinocytes, Life Technology Co.), temperature = 37°C, initial cell concentration = ca. $1.0 \times 10^4$ cells/cm$^2$, medium change = 72 h, $CO_2$ concentration in atmosphere = 5%.

### *Bioreactor System*

FIGURE 3 shows a schematic drawing of the bioreactor system, named KERATOR. The KERATOR is a further development of a computer-controlled bioreactor described eaerlier.[14] The culture module consists of special growth chambers stacked together. Each chamber contains a polymeric support film (Teflon® FEP Fluorocarbon Film Type C-20, DuPont Co.) of 660 cm$^2$ in size, on which the keratinocytes attach and proliferate. The bottom of the Petriperm culture dish is made of the same material. The culture module can be mounted on the mounting stage using

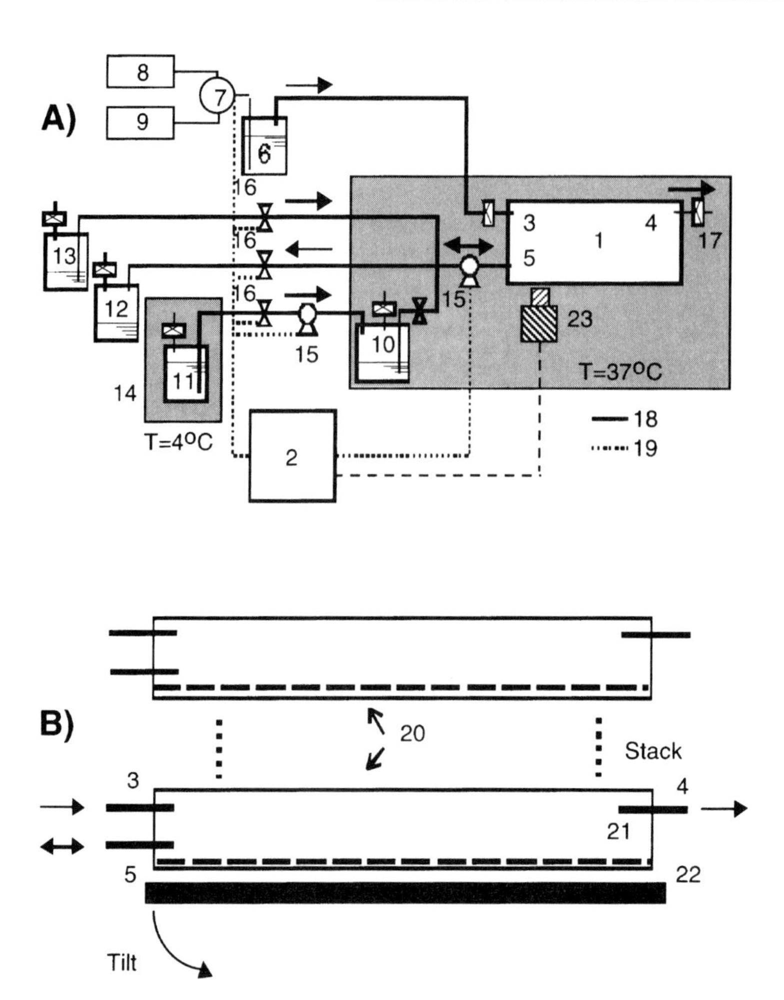


**FIGURE 3.** Schematic drawings of (**A**) bioreactor system, KERATOR and (**B**) culture module: 1, Culture module; 2, Personal computer with data acquisition system; 3, Gas inlet; 4, Gas outlet; 5, Medium port; 6, Humidifier; 7, Mass flow controller; 8, $CO_2$ cylinder; 9, Air cylinder; 10, Temperature equilibration of fresh medium; 11, Fresh medium reservoir; 12, Waste medium reservoir; 13, Seeding bottle; 14, Refrigerator; 15, Multichannel peristaltic pump; 16, Computer automated pinch valve; 17, Filter; 18, Medium and gas lines; 19, Control line; 20, Growth chamber; 21, Hydrophilic film; 22, Module stage; and 23, CCD camera system.

as many growth chambers as needed. In this way, up to 5280 $cm^2$ of skin grafts can be produced in one batch. The $CO_2$ concentration in the gas phase of the growth chamber was maintained at 5% $CO_2$ by a mass flow controller (Type 5850S, Brooks Instrument).

The CCD camera (GP-US502E, Matsushita Electronic Industrial Co.) with a specially developed optical system was attached to the mounting stage for monitoring the culture growth in the KERATOR. With the current optics, the total observation area is 2.1 $mm^2$ of the culture surface. Using a remote control unit, the CCD camera can be moved horizontally to choose various observation positions and vertically to adjust the image focus. Two observation positions can be pre-selected using electric microswitches.

For inoculation, the cell suspension was prepared manually in a laminar flow hood, and from there it was pumped into each growth chamber using a multichannel peristaltic pump. The medium was changed every 72 hours. For this purpose, a given amount of fresh medium was warmed up to 37°C from the stock medium, which was preserved at 4°C. In the meantime, the module stage was tilted and the old medium was sucked out from the growth chambers by the pump into the waste medium reservoir. To fill up the chambers with fresh medium again, the direction of fluid flow was switched with the pinch valves and by changing the pump direction. All culture operations, including inoculation and medium change, were performed automatically and controlled by the computer (Macintosh Quadra 840AV, Apple Computer, Inc.) with a data acquisition board (NB-MIO-16, National Instruments Corp.). LabVIEW (National Instruments Corp.) was used as the operation software.

### *Image Analysis Procedure*

For image analysis in the T-flask or Petriperm, a phase contrast microscope (TMS-F, Nikon Corp.) with CCD camera (ICD-44AC, Ikegami Tsushinki Co.) was used. The original image was captured with a video digitizer card (Image Grabber 24, Neotech Ltd.) in the computer (Macintosh Quadra 840AV, Apple Computer, Inc.). The captured area of an original image was 0.83 $mm^2$. The values of confluence at several positions in T-flask and Petriperm were determined by using the LabVIEW software (National Instruments Corp.) with the add-on image processing software IMAQ Vision (Graftek SA.) as follows.

To evaluate the confluence degree, the original image was converted into the binary image (gray level of projected area being 1 and gray level of non-projected area 0) through the processes of the cell edge detection by the non-linear high pass filter and the intensity thresholding. To remove noise from this binary image, the primary morphological transformation was processed by combination of erosion and dilation, and particles were removed by area thresholding (object area < 2.2 $\mu m^2$). The confluence degree [–] in the processed image was obtained after that by filling the holes inside the cells:

$$\text{Confluence degree} = \frac{\text{Number of pixels with their level being 1}}{\text{Total number of pixels in the image}} \quad \textbf{(1)}$$

Owing to the small area of the original image (< 1 $mm^2$), the average confluence degree in each T-flask was determined as the arithmetic mean of the calculated confluence degrees of images taken from 9 positions. In the case of Petriperm, three images were taken from "center," "middle," and "out" positions and the average confluence degree [–] was determined.

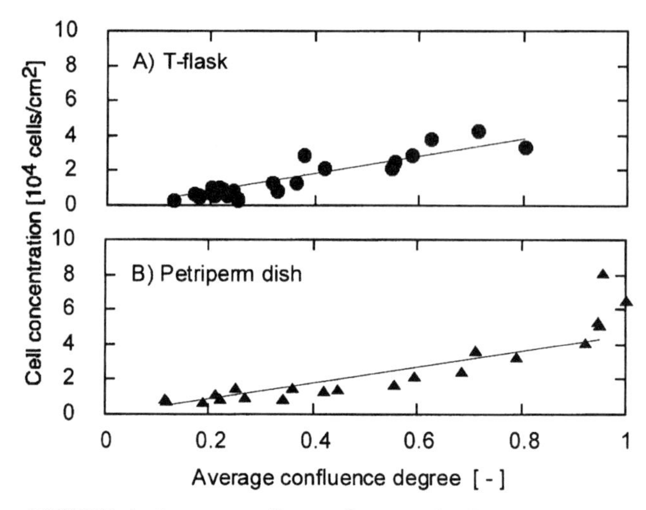


**FIGURE 4.** Average confluence degree and cell concentration.

### *Cell Concentration by Cell Counting*

The cell concentration in the T-flask or Petriperm was determined by direct cell counting using a hemocytometer after harvesting cells from the bottom of the culture vessel by enzymatic digestion using a solution of 0.1% trypsin 1:250 (Sigma) and 0.02% EDTA solution.[1] In the bioreactor, the cell concentration at a given culture time was obtained using the average cell counting value of three pieces (3 cm × 3 cm) cut from the film in one growth chamber.

## RESULTS AND DISCUSSION

### *Confluence Degree and Cell Concentration*

A linear relationship between average confluence degree and cell concentration in T-flask or Petriperm was found experimentally (FIG. 4). It can be expressed by the following equation holding within broad limits (TABLE 3):

$$\text{(Cell concentration)} = \alpha \text{ (Average confluence degree)} \qquad \textbf{(2)}$$

**TABLE 3.** Values of constant $\alpha$ and range of confluence degree in Equation **(2)**

| | T-flask | Petriperm |
|---|---|---|
| $\alpha$ [cells/cm$^2$] | $4.87 \times 10^4$ | $4.61 \times 10^4$ |
| Available range of average confluence degree [–] | 0.13 < value < 0.80 | 0.12 < value < 0.95 |
| Correlation factor [–] | 0.90 | 0.93 |

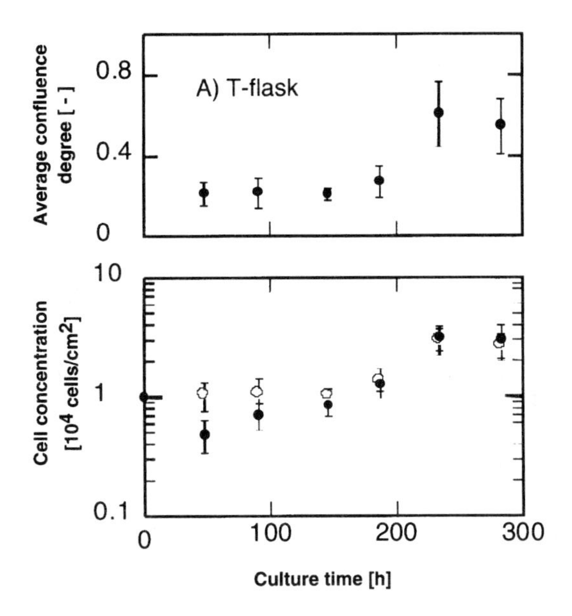


**FIGURE 5.** Calculated and experimental cell concentrations in T-flask and in Petriperm cultures: (**A**) T-flask; (**B**) Petriperm.

The values of the slope α [cells/cm$^2$] and correlation coefficients in T-flask and Petriperm were determined by fitting the experimental data (FIG. 4) by linear regression (TABLE 3).The equation was valid for the average confluence degree ranging from 0.13 to 0.8 in the T-flask and 0.12 to 0.95 in the Petriperm, respectively.

To check validity of the on-line monitoring of growth by image analysis, the cell concentration values calculated by the image analysis method were compared with the values obtained experimentally by direct cell counting. FIGURE 5 shows a very good agreement between the calculated and experimental cell concentrations in T-flask as well as in Petriperm cultures.

### *Keratinocyte Culture on Hydrophilic Film*

The time profiles of cell adhesion in the T-flask and Petriperm were compared using the cell adhesion ratio defined by

$$\frac{\text{Number of adhesion cells}}{(\text{Number of adhesion cells}) + (\text{Number of floating cells})}$$

As shown in FIGURE 6, with increasing culture time, the adhesion cell ratio in the T-flask increased sharply to 0.63 at 4 h of culture time. After that, the adhesion cell ratio slowly approached its asymptotic value. In the Petriperm, the rate of adhesion was higher than in the T-flask, and within 6 h the adhesion cell ratio number was 0.84.

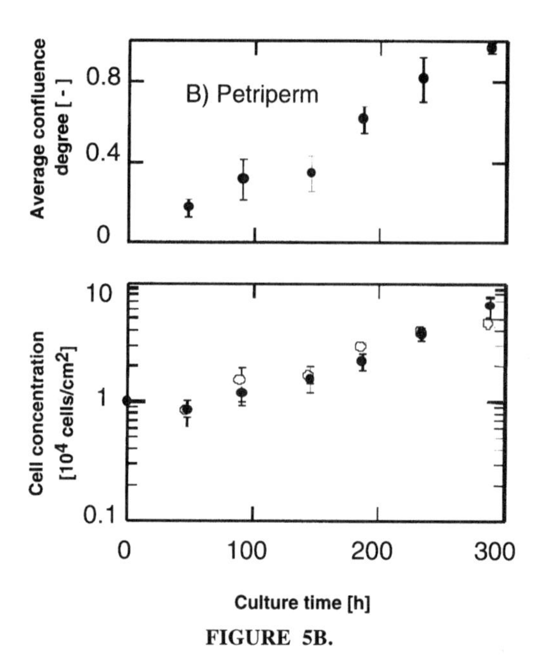


FIGURE 5B.

The cell growth cycle consists of cell adhesion, spreading, and mitosis. High cell-adhesion affinity leads to the enhancement of growth rate caused by an increase in adhesion and spreading rates[9] and the hydrophilic surface was considered to improve adhesion of the keratinocytes without coating, e.g., by collagen or fibronectin.[15,16] In general, the hydrophilicity of the surface increases with the decrease in contact angle of water on the surface. In the present work, the contact angles of water on the bottom surfaces in the T-flask and the Petriperm were measured as 50.4° and 45.6°, respectively, under conditions of temperature = 25°C and relative humidity = 60%.

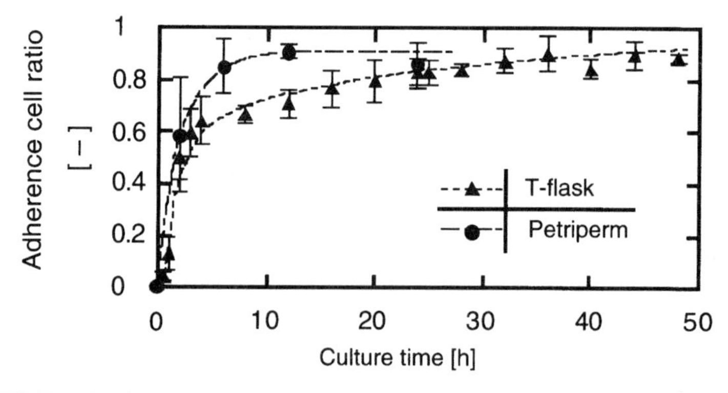


**FIGURE 6.** Time profiles of cell adhesion on bottoms of T-flask and Petriperm.

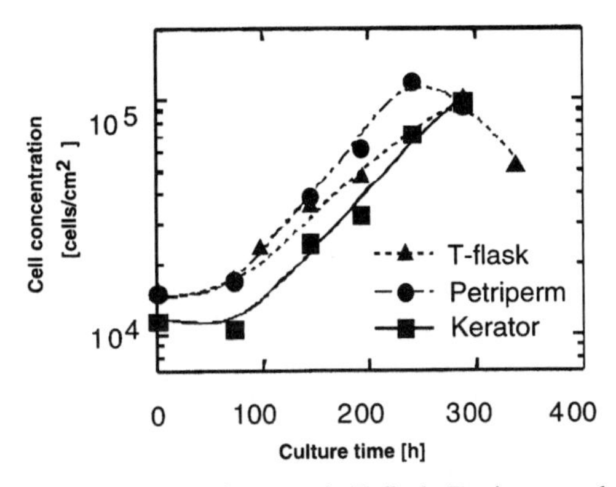


**FIGURE 7.** Keratinocyte growth curves in T-flask, Petriperm and the bioreactor.

The hydrophilicity of the bottom surface in the Petriperm was higher than that in the T-flask; consequently, the growth rate in the Petriperm was found to be higher.

From the clinical point of view, a subconfluent monolayer of keratinocytes is useful for skin transplantation because of good cell proliferation and low or negligible differentiation. However, the keratinocyte monolayer is not strong enough to be harvested, let alone to prepare skin grafts like conventional culture epithelial autografts, which have adequate mechanical strength due to the differentiated multilayer.[10]

In our procedure, the polymeric film on which the cells grow provides the necessary mechanical strength. The support film becomes an integral part of the skin graft, and for clinical applications the skin graft is turned upside down with the keratinocyte layer facing the wound.

The advantages of this strategy are shortening of the total culture time to 2 weeks and high activity of undifferentiated cells in the subconfluent culture. In our study, the skin grafts consisting of a subconfluent monolayer of keratinocytes on the FEP hydrophilic film were used for the skin transplantation. Several patients with burn wounds or chronic leg ulcers were treated with such autologous skin grafts.[11,17] Generally, the wounds responded well and started to form a new epithelium; however, more clinical evidence is needed to ultimately demonstrate the utility of such skin grafts.[11]

### *Culture in Bioreactor*

FIGURE 7 shows the growth profiles in a 25 $cm^2$ T-flask, in a 20 $cm^2$ Petriperm with hydrophilic film bottom, and in the bioreactor. In all three cultures, cell concentration started to increase exponentially after 72 h of culture time, and the average specific growth rates in the range of culture time from 72 h to 240 h were $7.2 \times 10^{-3}$ $h^{-1}$ for T-flask, $9.0 \times 10^{-3}$ $h^{-1}$ for Petriperm, and $8.8 \times 10^{-3}$ $h^{-1}$ for the Kerator. The maximum cell concentration in the Petriperm culture was $1.2 \times 10^5$ cells/$cm^2$ at 240 h, which was 1.7 times higher than in the T-flask at the same time. Therefore, growth in the Petriperm was superior to that in T-flask. For the culture of other cell lines, the Petriperm was reported to also be a suitable culture vessel owing to incorporation of the hydrophilic film.[18]

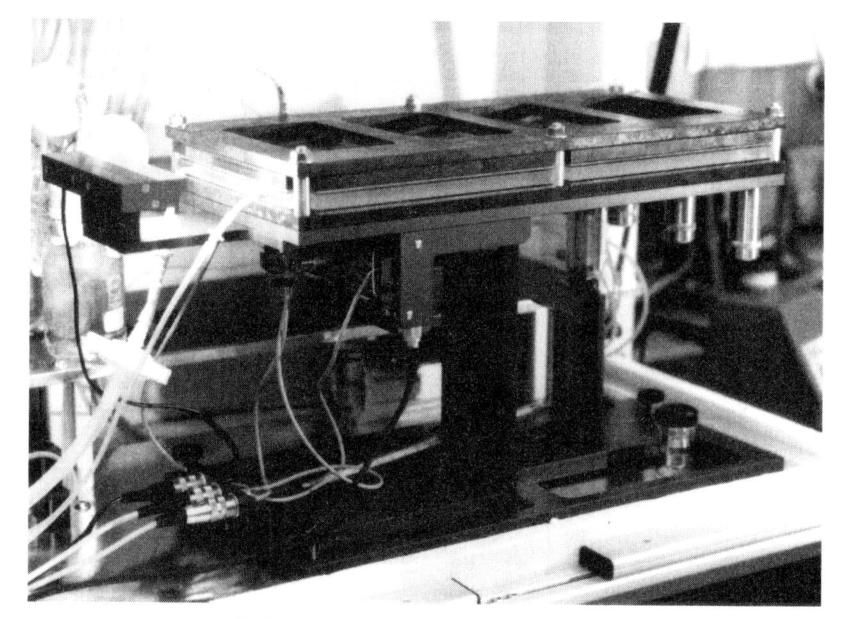

**FIGURE 8.** Photograph of the Kerator.

For large-scale production of skin grafts, a culture of keratinocytes on the hydrophilic film was conducted in a bioreactor with up to five growth chambers. As shown in FIGURE 7, the average specific growth rate was similar to that in the Petriperm. This showed the automated culture operations of cell seeding and medium change had no adverse effects on cell viability in the bioreactor.

Several designs of culture vessels for the culture of keratinocytes have been presented in the past.[19] However, they were designed only with respect to their form and not as an integral system including control and all the operation steps of the culture. Moreover, the size of these culture vessels was too small to prepare the skin grafts for large burn wounds. This was critical in assessing the ultimate usefulness of a bioreactor for production of skin grafts. The presented bioreactor represents a significant step toward complete automation of the production of skin grafts with greatly reduced costs and labor and a lower risk of human error. Its application can be easily extended to cultivation of other types of anchorage-dependent cells. A photograph of the Kerator with one growth chamber mounted, is shown in FIGURE 8.

## ACKNOWLEDGMENTS

The work presented here was supported by the Swiss National Foundation (No.5002-37967). The authors wish to thank Miss Sabina Mazza for her careful experimental work. The authors also thank Dr. Meyer, Dr. Burg, and their staff in the sections of surgery and dermatology of University Hospital Zurich for the supply of skin material.

## REFERENCES

1. FRESHNEY, R.I. 1997. Culture of Animal Cells, 3rd edit. 1997. Wiley-Liss, Inc. New York.
2. RHEINWALD, J.G. & H. GREEN. 1975. Serial cultivation of strains of human epidermal keratinocytes: the formation of keratinizing colonies from single cells. Cell **6:** 331–343.
3. O'CONNOR, N.E., J.B. MULLIKEN, S. BANKS-SCHLEGEL, O. KEHINDE & H. GREEN. 1981. Grafting of burns with cultured epithelium prepared from autologous epidermal cells. Lancet **1:** 75–78.
4. HEFTON, J.M., D. CALDWELL & D.G. BIOZES. 1986. Grafting of skin ulcers with cultured autologous epidermal cells. J. Am. Acad. Dermatol. **14:** 399–405.
5. MUNSTER, A.M. 1996. Cultured skin for massive burns—a prospective, controlled trial. Annals Surg. **224:** 372–377.
6. WOODLEY, D.T., H.D. PETERSON, S.R. HERZOG, G.P. STRICKLIN, R.E. BURGESON, R.A. BRIGGAMAN, D.J. CRONCE & E.J. O'KEEFE. 1988. Burn wounds resurfaced by cultured epidermal autografts show abnormal reconstruction of anchoring fibrils. J. Am. Med. Assoc. **259:** 2566–2571.
7. SHERIDAN, R. L. & R. G. TOMPKINS. 1995. Cultured autologous epithelium in patients with burns of ninety percent or more of the body surface. J. Trauma **38:** 48–50.
8. BOYCE, S. T. & R. G. HAM. 1985. Cultivation, frozen storage, and clonal growth of normal human epidermal keratinocytes in serum-free media. J. Tissue Cult. Methods **9:** 83–93.
9. DANIELS, J. T., J. N. KEARNEY & E. INGHAM. 1997. An Investigation into the potential of extracellular matrix factors for attachment and proliferation of human keratinocytes on skin substitutes. Burns **23:** 26–31.
10. BARLOW, Y.M., A.M. BURT, J.A. CLARKE, D.A. MCGROUTHER & S.M. LANG. 1992. The Use of a polymeric film for the culture and transfer of sub-confluent autologous keratinocytes to patients. J. Tissue Viability **2:** 33–36.
11. HAFNER, J, M. KINO-OKA, P.E. VILLENEUVE, J.E. PRENOSIL, G. SENTI & G. BURG. 1997. Autologous pancellular skin culture (pasc) in the treatment of leg ulcers: preliminary report. Dermatology **195:** 199.
12. BONNEKOH, B., R.P. MULLER, G. MAHRLE & G.K. STEIGLEDER. 1988. Wound treatment with autologous epidermal cell expansion culture. Dtsch. Med. Wschr. **113:** 1748–1752.
13. KINO-OKA, M. & J.E. PRENOSIL. 1998. On-line monitoring of human keratinocyte growth by image analysis and its application to bioreactor culture. Biotechnol. Bioeng. In press.
14. PRENOSIL, J.E. & P. VILLENEUVE. 1998. Automated production of cultured epidermal autografts and sub-confluent epidermal autografts in a computer controlled bioreactor. Biotechnol. Bioeng. **59:** 680–683.
15. KOTTKE-MARCHANT, K., A.A. VEENSTRA & R.E. MARCHANT. 1996. Human endothelial cell growth and coagulant function varies with respect to interfacial properties of polymeric substrate. J. Biomed. Mater. Res. **30:** 209–220.
16. DEWEZ, J.-L., Y.-J. SCHNEIDER & P. G. ROUXHET. 1996. Coupled influence of substratum hydrophilicity and surfactant on epithelial cell adhesion. J. Biomed. Mater. Res. **30:** 373–383.
17. VILLENEUVE, P., J. HAFNER, J.E. PRENOSIL, P. ELSNER & G. BURG. 1998. A novel culturing and grafting system for the treatment of leg ulcer. Br. J. Dermatol. **138:** 849–851.
18. PAUWELS, P.J., J. ABARCA & A.C. TROUET. 1983. Cultivation of rat cerebellar cells under conditions of optimal oxygen supply. Neurosci. Lett. **43:** 309–314.
19. LYMAN, G., G. MATHUS & D. ROOT. 1995. U.S. Patent No. 5466602.

# A Method for Tissue Engineering of Cartilage by Cell Seeding on Bioresorbable Scaffolds

RONDA E. SCHREIBER,[a] NOUSHIN S. DUNKELMAN, GAIL NAUGHTON, AND ANTHONY RATCLIFFE

*Advanced Tissue Sciences, Inc., 10933 North Torrey Pines Road, La Jolla, California 92037-1005*

**ABSTRACT: This chapter describes a method for the *in vitro* generation of a 3-dimensional cartilage matrix from articular chondrocytes seeded onto a bioresorbable polymeric scaffold. This particular growth system was chosen for the subject of this chapter owing to the relative simplicity of the methods required and the ease with which the necessary materials can be obtained. The tissue produced using this protocol is a cellular, metabolically active hyaline-like matrix, containing the major cartilage constituents: sulfated proteoglycan, collagen type II, and water. It serves as a useful *in vitro* tool for studying the influence of various mechanical and chemical factors on cartilage metabolism, as well as providing an implantable material for *in vivo* cartilage repair studies.**

## INTRODUCTION

Damaged articular cartilage has a limited capacity to repair. The degeneration of this tissue in diarthroidal joints contributes largely to the pathology of osteoarthritis and related diseases. Because the available treatments result in limited pain relief and/or tissue function, many patients must suffer pain and joint dysfunction until the joint has deteriorated to the point of necessitating replacement. Tissue-engineered cartilage implants hold promise for supporting biologically functional cartilage repair of focal defects.

This chapter describes a simple method for cartilage tissue engineering by *in vitro* culture of chondrocytes seeded onto bioresorbable scaffolds. After seeding, there is a period of cell proliferation, followed by matrix deposition. This growth phase can occur *in vivo*, after implantation of the seeded scaffold subcutaneously in nude mice,[1] or *in vitro*, either under static or dynamic growth conditions.[2–6] Several biodegradable scaffolds have been used, including poly (glycolic acid) and poly (L-lactic acid) polymers fabricated as non-woven, fiber networks (felt). Pluripotential bone marrow-derived cells, an alternative cell type and tissue source to that of fully differentiated chondrocytes, have recently been shown to synthesize and deposit a hyaline-like cartilage *in vitro.*[7] The macroarchitecture as well as the molecular components of a scaffold can influence the synthesis and deposition of tissue within the construct.[8,9] In addition, the amount and rate of tissue that is formed is dependent on the culture time and method, as well as the quality and quantity of cells applied

[a]Author to whom correspondence should be addressed: 619-713-7878 (voice); 619-713-7970 (fax); ronda.schreiber@advancedtissue.com (e-mail).

to the scaffold. The methods described here will result in the formation of a uniformly distributed tissue containing proteoglycan, collagen, and water comprising up to 2%, 0.9%, and 90%, respectively, of the total cartilage construct weight. These levels approach the lower levels of the corresponding matrix components of normal articular cartilage. The constructs grown in this manner consist of a smooth, hyaline-like cartilage containing uniformly distributed cells that are contained within lacunae. Cartilage constructs made from rabbit chondrocytes have been successful in repairing osteochondral defects *in vivo.*[10,11] In addition to its use in *in vivo* cartilage transplantation studies, tissue-engineered cartilage is a useful tool for conducting *in vitro* experimental studies of cartilage metabolism.

## MATERIALS AND METHODS

### *Tissue Harvest and Chondrocyte Isolation*

#### *Tissue Isolation*

The potential for chondrocytes to synthesize and secrete cartilage matrix *in vitro* is largely dependent on the quality of the tissue source. Chondrocytes isolated from the articular cartilage of the distal femoral joints of very juvenile, skeletally immature donors are optimal for growing a hyaline-like cartilage. Rabbits (≤ 1 year), sheep (≤ 3 weeks), cows (≤ 3 weeks), and foals (≤ 1 month) have been used to generate such tissue. Between 5–8 × $10^7$ cells per gram of tissue are typically obtained from this tissue.

To isolate chondrocytes, place the skinned femur(s), along with the equipment and reagents listed below, into a sterile tissue culture hood. Make a medial parapatellar incision in the distal femur to expose the articular surface of the condyle and patellar groove. Dissect the tissue within the patellar groove, patella, and condylar surfaces using scalpel blades (sizes 10, 15, and 20) and place in culture dishes (10 cm diameter). Collect chips about 1 cm in length and 2–4 mm in depth (depending upon the donor species and age), being careful to collect only the articular cartilage. Avoid collecting any tissue within 1 mm of or into the subchondral bone or any fibrous tissue (which has a distinct texture and is usually more yellow in color than that of the smooth, white, opaque cartilage). Place the tissue chips in 50 ml plastic tubes containing gentamycin (25 µg/ml phosphate-buffered saline).

#### *Tissue Digestion*

After the tissue dissection is complete, rinse tissue chips once with fresh gentamycin solution, then transfer the tissue into culture tube(s) containing freshly prepared digestion solution [bacterial collagenase Type II dissolved to a final concentration of 506.0 units/ml of culture medium: to Dulbecco's Modified Eagle's Medium (DMEM), add fetal bovine serum; FBS (10%), L-glutamine (2 mM), nonessential amino acids (0.1 mM), L-proline (50 µg/ml), sodium pyruvate (1 mM), and gentamicin (25 µg/ml)]. Close the tubes, secure tops with parafilm, place tubes on their sides on an orbital shaker set at 200–300 rpm and incubate overnight at 37°C, 5% $CO_2$.

After the tissue digestion is complete, filter the cells through a cell filter (70 μm), discard the trapped cells, and save the cell filtrate. Centrifuge the cell filtrate at 200–300 × g for 10 minutes between 4°–15°C (4°C is preferred). Discard the supernatant. Re-suspend the pellet in culture medium to obtain a single cell suspension of an estimated $5 \times 10^6$ cells per ml. Remove an aliquot of the final cell suspension and suspend in trypan blue (1:1 dilution). Dispense this into a hemacytometer and count the cells. These should be approximately 90–95% viable. Centrifuge the cell suspension as above, discard the supernatant, and re-suspend cell pellet in culture medium to obtain a single cell suspension of $2.5–9.5 \times 10^7$ cells/ml, depending on the desired cell seeding density of the scaffold (see below). Place the remaining cell suspension on ice or at 4°C until scaffold seeding is to occur.

## *Cartilage Construct Growth*

### *Scaffold Characteristics*

A commercially available entangled, non-heat plated, porous (97%) polyglycolic acid (PGA) mesh composed of fibers 14 μm in diameter is a rapidly degrading scaffold on which chondrocytes can synthesize and deposit cartilage matrix.[12] This mesh is available from Albany International Research Company (Mansfield, MA, USA) in the form of 20 × 30 cm sheets. Scaffold discs ranging from 2–3 mm in thickness and 8–10 mm in diameter have been used routinely to generate hyaline-like cartilage constructs.[12,13] Place the mesh (sheets or discs obtained with a mechanical punch) in foil pouches (Georgia Packaging, Inc., Columbus, GA) and vacuum seal or sparge the pouches with dry nitrogen and seal. Store the sealed pouches at room temperature for short-term storage (8 weeks or less), or in a non-thaw cycling freezer at –20°C to –70°C for longer term storage.

### *Seeding and Culture of Cartilage Constructs*

Pre-wet the scaffold discs by submerging them in 100% ethanol for 15 minutes at room temperature. Rinse the scaffolds 3 times with large volumes of PBS to remove residual ethanol, then submerge them in culture wells containing approximately 5 mls of culture medium per scaffold (10 mm × 2 mm) and incubate at 37°C and 5% $CO_2$ for 5–16 hours. To hasten wetting, draw culture medium bidirectionally through the scaffold several times with a 1 or 5 ml pipette.

Prior to scaffold seeding, withdraw excess medium from scaffolds with a pipette and transfer each scaffold disc into an individual well of a 24 well dish. Suspend the chondrocytes in culture at $4–15 \times 10^6$ cells/ml of culture medium and dispense $2.5–9.4 \times 10^7$ cells/ml scaffold. Pipette the cell suspension slowly onto scaffold, using a 1000 μl pipetter with a pipette tip to draw the suspension bidirectionally several times through the scaffold. Place the scaffolds in dishes on an orbital or vibrational shaker set at 300 rpm, and incubate overnight at 37°C and 5% $CO_2$. The efficiency of cell seeding is between 80–90%.

Chondrocyte-seeded scaffold constructs can be cultured statically, by culturing constructs in petri dishes, or dynamically, in a recirculating bioreactor system through which culture medium is perfused by a peristaltic pump.[12,13] Both methods result in substantial levels of hyaline-like matrix. For ease of use, only the static method is described in this paper. To culture the seeded constructs, transfer them to

6 well dishes to which 10 ml of culture medium containing freshly added insulin (50 µg/ml) and ascorbate (50 µg/ml) have been added. Incubate statically at 37°C and 5% $CO_2$. Culture the cartilage constructs for 2 weeks or more, changing culture medium every 3–4 days (with freshly added insulin and ascorbate), and culture plates once a week to prevent an overgrowth of chondrocytes in monolayer.

The described methods will routinely result in a homogeneous tissue containing up to 2% S-GAG, 0.9% total collagen, and 90% water of the total construct weight, when constructs are cultured between 4 and 6 weeks. These are levels that approach the lower levels of normal articular cartilage.

### *Cartilage Construct Analyses*

To evaluate the composition of cartilage constructs, routine histologic, biochemical, and molecular analyses are performed. Since these conventional techniques are well described elsewhere, this section includes general methods and references only.

#### *Histological Analyses*

*Tissue Fixation and Embedding.* Immerse the tissue-engineered constructs in 10% buffered formalin, incubate at room temperature for 24 hours, and dehydrate through graded concentrations of ethanol (0%, 70%, 90%, 100%). Embed the fixed, dehydrated tissue in paraffin. Cut sections with a rotary microtome to 4 or 5 µm and place onto microscope slides. Deparaffinize the sections with xylene, then rehydrate by 5 minute sequential incubations in 100%, 90%, and 70% ethanol. Incubate sections in water for 5 minutes. (If preservation of newly seeded cartilage constructs with negligible levels of extracellular matrix is desired, embed tissue in methacrylate).

*Histochemical Staining for Extracellular Matrix Components.* To examine cell and tissue morphology, total collagen, and sulfated-glycosaminoglycan (S-GAG), stain with Hematoxylin and Eosin, Trichrome,[14] and Safranin-O,[15] respectively, as described.

To detect collagen type I and II, obtain antibodies specific for either collagen type I or II and appropriate enzyme-conjugated secondary antibodies and substrate. If no signal is detected, enzymatically pretreat the sections with chondroitinase A,B,C,[16] with or without subsequent treatment with pepsin, trypsin, or a combination of these enzymes, as recommended by a histochemical vendor.

To detect chondroitin-4-sulfate and chondroitin-6-sulfate, use monoclonal antibodies 2B6 and 3B3, respectively, as described.[16,17]

#### *Biochemical Analyses*

*Construct Sample Preparation.* Record the total construct weight (wet weight), as well as the dry weight of the constructs after drying with a SpeedVac (Savant Instruments, Holbrook, NY) or by lyophilization. Enzymatic digestion of dried cartilage constructs with papain is recommended, since it renders the samples amenable to the evaluations described below. Follow the procedure described by Kim *et al.*[18]

*Cell Number.* The total cell number in cartilage constructs can be calculated after performing a DNA dye binding assay on papain digested cartilage constructs.[18]

*Total Collagen.* The total collagen in cartilage constructs can be calculated after determination of the hydroxyproline content from acid-hydrolyzed, papain-digested cartilage constructs.[19]

*Total S-GAG.* The total S-GAG content in cartilage constructs can be determined after performing a dye-binding assay on papain-digested constructs.[20]

## RESULTS AND DISCUSSION

This section describes the characteristics of ovine tissue-engineered cartilage, synthesized in our laboratory using the culture method described above. Cartilage constructs were generated by culturing freshly isolated primary ovine articular chondrocytes at a sub-scaffold saturating density ($2.5 \times 10^7$ cells/cc scaffold) on PGA scaffolds in culture wells, statically, for 4 weeks.

Safranin-O–stained histological sections of constructs cultured for 4 weeks demonstrated a smooth matrix rich in S-GAG, similar to that of native articular cartilage from 2-to 3-week-old sheep (FIG. 1).

Quantitation of the major constituents of the tissue-engineered cartilage cultured statically for 4 weeks was determined by the assays referred to in the MATERIALS AND METHODS section of this chapter. The water content of these constructs was slightly higher than that measured in native juvenile ovine articular cartilage; 89.8% and 76.6%, respectively. The S-GAG content of the cartilage constructs, 21.6% of its dry weight and 2.2% of the total tissue weight, was similar to that of native ovine articular cartilage, which was 21.8% of its dry weight and 5.0% of the total tissue weight (FIG. 2). The collagen content in the tissue-engineered cartilage was 8.2% of its dry weight and 0.8% of the total construct weight, as compared to that of the native tissue, which was 31.8% of its dry weight and 8.5% of the total tissue weight. Although these cartilage constructs contained less collagen than that observed in native ovine articular cartilage from young sheep, this is unlikely to impede the ability of the tissue-engineered cartilage to support the repair of cartilage defects, since we

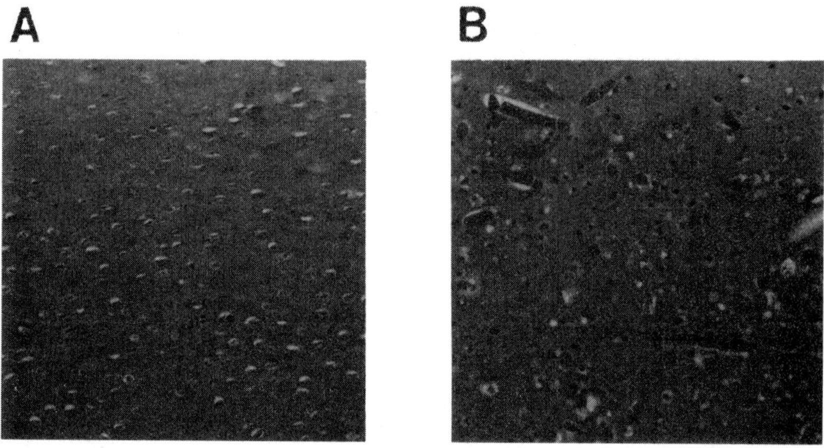


**FIGURE 1.** Photomicrographs showing S-GAG distribution in histological sections of native ovine articular cartilage from 3-week-old sheep (**A**) and ovine cartilage constructs cultured statically for 4 weeks (**B**). Residual PGA fibers in the cartilage construct are visible.

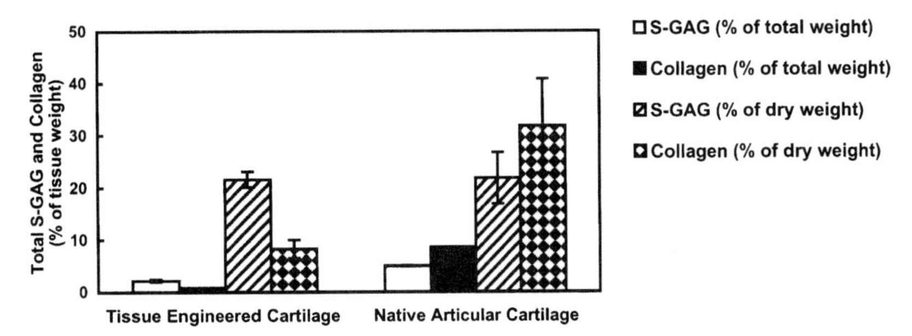


**FIGURE 2.** Biochemical composition of tissue-engineered ovine cartilage and native articular cartilage from 3-week-old sheep. Total collagen and S-GAG of papain-digested cartilage constructs or juvenile ovine articular cartilage were determined as described in MATERIALS AND METHODS and expressed as a percentage of the total tissue weight or the dry weight of the tissue. Replicate samples of the cartilage constructs and articular cartilage were measured; $n = 4$ and 14, respectively.

have shown that tissue-engineered rabbit cartilage constructs containing even lower collagen levels supports successful tissue repair when implanted into rabbit osteochondral defects.[11] Furthermore, we routinely grow tissue-engineered ovine constructs with collagen levels within the range measured in the native tissue, 18.0% of the construct's dry weight and 2.0% of the total construct weight, when cultured dynamically for 8 weeks.

In summary, ovine tissue-engineered cartilage cultured statically in tissue culture wells for 1 month is composed of a hyaline-like cartilage qualitatively similar to that of articular cartilage from juvenile sheep. The ease with which functional tissue-engineered cartilage can be made from chondrocytes of a variety of species using the static culture technique enables researchers to use tissue-engineered cartilage as an *in vitro* tool to investigate both normal and pathological cartilage metabolism.

## REFERENCES

1. CIMA, L.G., J.P. VACANTI, C. VACANTI, D. INGBER, D. MOONEY & R. LANGER. 1991. Tissue engineering by cell transplantation using degradable polymer substrates. J. Biomech. Eng. **113:** 143.
2. FREED, L.E. & G. VUNJAK-NOVAKOVIC. 1995. Tissue engineering of cartilage. *In* Biomedical Engineering Handbook. J.D. Bronzino, Ed.: 1788. CRC Press. Boca Raton, FL.
3. PUELACHER, W.C., J.P. VACANTI, N.F. FERRARO, B. SCHLOO & C.A. VACANTI. 1996. Femoral shaft reconstruction using tissue-engineered growth of bone. J. Oral Maxillofac. Surg. **3:** 223.
4. FREED, L.E. & G. VUNJAK-NOVAKOVIC. 1997. Microgravity tissue engineering. In Vitro Cell Dev. Biol. Anim. **33:** 381.
5. FREED, L.E., H.A.P., I. MARTIN, J.R. BARRY, R. LANGER & G. VUNJAK-NOVAKOVIC. 1998. Chondrogenesis in a cell-polymer-bioreactor system. Exp. Cell Res. **240:** 58.
6. VUNJAK-NOVAKOVIC, G., B. OBRADOVIC, I. MARTIN, P.M. BURSAC, R. LANGER & L.E. FREED. 1998. Dynamic cell seeding of polymer scaffolds for cartilage tissue engineering. Biotechnol. Prog. **14:** 193.

7. MARTIN, I., P.R.F., G. VUNJAK-NOVAKOVIC & L.E. FREED. 1998. In vitro differentiation of chick embryo bone marrow stromal cells into cartilaginous and bone-like tissues. J. Orthop. Res. **16:** 181.
8. GRANDE, D.A., C. HALBERSTADT, G. NAUGHTON, R. SCHWARTZ & R. MANJI. 1997. Evaluation of matrix scaffolds for tissue engineering of articular cartilage grafts. J. Biomed. Mater. Res. **34:** 211.
9. SITTINGER, M., D. REITZEL, M. DAUNER, H. HIERLEMANN, C. HAMMER, E. KASTENBAUER, H. PLANCK, G.R. BURMESTER & J. BUJIA. 1996. Resorbable polyesters in cartilage engineering: affinity and biocompatibility of polymer fiber structures to chondrocytes. J. Biomed. Mater. Res. **33:** 57.
10. FREED, L.E., J.C. MARQUIS, A. NOHRIA, A. EMMANUAL, A.G. MIKOS & R. LANGER. 1993. Neocartilage formation in vitro and in vivo using cells cultured on synthetic biodegradable scaffolds, J. Biomed. Mat. Res. **27:** 11.
11. SCHREIBER, R.E., B.M. ILTEN-KIRBY, N.S. DUNKELMAN, K.T. SYMONS, L.M. REKETTYE, J. WILLOUGHBY & A. RATCLIFFE. 1999. Repair of osteochondral defects with allogeneic tissue-engineered cartilage implants, Clin. Orthop. & Related Res. Accepted for publication.
12. FREED, L.E., G. VUNJAK-NOVOKOVIC, R.J. BIRON, D.B. EGLES, D.C. LESNOY, S.K. BARLOW & R. LANGER. 1994. Biodegradable polymer scaffolds for tissue engineering., Biotechnology **12:** 689.
13. DUNKELMAN, N.S., M.P. ZIMBER, R.G. LEBARON, R. PAVELEC, M. KWAN & A.F. PURCHIO. 1995. Cartilage production by rabbit articular chondrocytes on polyglycolic acid scaffolds in a closed bioreactor system. Biotechnol. Bioeng. **46:** 299.
14. SHEEHAN, D. & B. HRAPCHAK. 1980. Theory and Practice of Histotechnology. Batelle Press. Columbus, OH.
15. ROSENBURG, L.C. 1971. J. Bone Joint Surg. **53:** 69.
16. COUCHMAN, J.R., B. CATERSON, J.E. CHRISTNER & J.R. BAKER. 1984. Mapping by monoclonal antibody detection of glycosaminoglycans in connective tissues. Nature **307:** 650.
17. SORRELL, J.M., *et al.* 1988. J. Immunol. **140:** 4263.
18. KIM, Y.-H., R.LY. SAH, J.Y. DOONG & A.J. GRODZINSKY. 1988. Fluorometric assay of DNA in cartilage explants using Hoescht 33258. Anal. Biochem. **174:** 168.
19. WOESSNER, J.F. 1961. The determination of hydroxyproline in tissue and protein samples containing small proportions of this amino acid. Arch. Biochem. Biophys. **93:** 440.
20. FARNDALE, R.W., D.J. BUTTLE & A.J. BARRETT. 1986. Improved quantitation and discrimination of sulphated glycosaminoglycans by use of dimethylmethylene blue. Biochem. Biophys. Acta **883:** 173.

# Bioreactor Development for Tissue-Engineered Cartilage

FLORENCE WU,[a] NOUSHIN DUNKELMAN, AL PETERSON, TWANA DAVISSON, REBECCA DE LA TORRE, AND DEEPAK JAIN

*Advanced Tissue Sciences, Inc., 10933 N. Torrey Pines Road, La Jolla, California 92037-1005, USA*

**ABSTRACT: The development of tissue engineered cartilage is emerging as a potential treatment for the repair of cartilage defects. By seeding chondrocytes onto poly-glycolic acid (PGA) biodegradable scaffolds within a convective-flow bioreactor, the synthesis of tissue-engineered articular cartilage has been recently demonstrated. The ability to cultivate and manipulate this cell-polymer construct to possess specific dimensions, as well as biochemical and biomechanical properties is critical for potential application as an *in vivo* therapy of damaged articular surfaces. Bioreactor design requirements for stages from research to development to commercialization are discussed. Advantages and limitations to various bioreactor designs are critiqued. These studies illustrate the ability to synthesize tissue-engineered cartilage under convective-flow conditions for potential human tissue repair.**

## INTRODUCTION

In the United States alone, over 250,000 knee arthroscopies were performed in 1997 on patients suffering from joint pain and loss of mobility due to articular cartilage defects.[1] This loss of function is often the result of idiopathic or primary osteoarthritis, as well as from trauma and sports injuries which destroy the articular cartilage surface. It has been widely accepted that adult articular cartilage has a limited capacity to heal. Once damaged, either by disease or by injury, articular surfaces of joints will often progressively degenerate and can lead to the need for a total joint replacement. Joint prostheses provide a satisfactory treatment for extensive joint diseases in individuals over 60 years of age. However, there is presently no suitable treatment modality for younger, active individuals. This patient population is often consigned to tolerating progression in disease, with decreased function, until joint replacement is appropriate.

In the last thirty years, there have been many attempts to develop clinically useful cartilage repair procedures, as reviewed recently.[2] Despite recent technological advances, the degree of success to date of a purely cell- or biological-based approach has been modest. Consequently, prosthetic joint replacement remains the standard clinical approach for treatment to restore pain-free mobility. However, significant short-term and long-term problems still persist. Hence, the opportunity exists to develop a hybrid strategy, whereby living cells are combined with an artificial support

[a]Corresponding author: 619-713-7929 (voice); 619-713-7400 (fax); flo.wu@advancedtissue.com (e-mail).

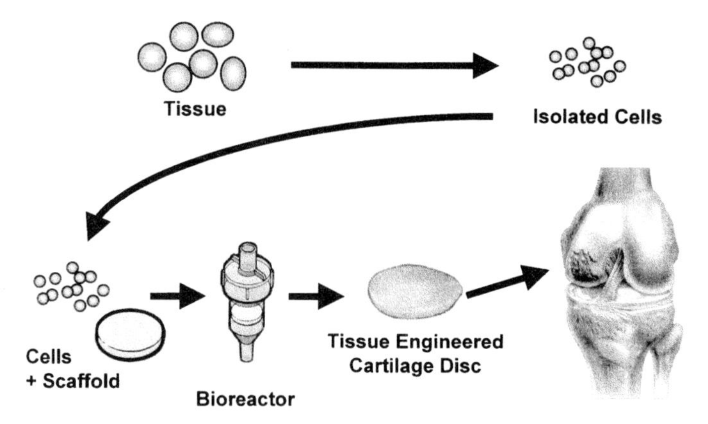


**FIGURE 1.** Process for cultivation of tissue engineered cartilage. Cartilage tissue is aseptically harvested and chondrocytes isolated by enzymatic digestion. Cells are then seeded onto polymer scaffolds and cultured within a bioreactor system. During cultivation, cells proliferate and deposit matrix, resulting in a construct that can be implanted to treat articular surface defects.

to provide a tissue-engineered approach for successful repair or replacement of articular cartilage defects.

### *Tissue Engineering of Cartilage*

The development of tissue engineered cartilage is emerging as a potential treatment for the repair of cartilage defects. Isolated chondrocytes are seeded onto three-dimensional, bioresorbable, porous scaffolds,[3,4] and cultured *in vitro* within a recirculating bioreactor.[5,6] A schematic of the process is shown in FIGURE 1. By using this approach, allogeneic rabbit cartilage constructs have been recently cultured and a preclinical study conducted.[7] Allografts were implanted into the medial patellar grooves of rabbits for healing of osteochondral defects. Results at 9 months post-surgery have shown that defect sites treated with cartilage implants contained significantly greater amounts of hyaline-like cartilage with high levels of proteoglycan, compared to untreated defects.[7] For large animal and clinical studies, a scale-up in size and quantity of constructs is necessary. Reaching this goal depends upon attaining a better understanding of the design and operating parameters that affect construct growth.

To gain a better understanding of the parameters that affect construct growth, a characterization of the kinetics of ovine chondrocyte proliferation and matrix deposition was performed for constructs cultured in the recirculating bioreactor. As described previously, cartilage from the patellar groove of young Rambouillet sheep was aseptically excised, and chondrocytes were isolated by digestion in collagenase (Worthington, Freehold, NJ).[7] Biodegradable poly-glycolic acid (PGA) scaffolds were cut into 2 mm thick × 10 mm diameter discs and placed within recirculating flow bioreactor systems. Each system consisted of five manifolded bioreactors connected to a medium reservoir, as was described previously.[5]

**TABLE 1.** Comparison of biochemical composition of tissue engineered ovine articular cartilage and native ovine articular cartilage tissue, after 1 week and 4 weeks of culture. Percentages are based on wet weight

| | | Tissue Engineered Ovine Cartilage | |
|---|---|---|---|
| Parameter | Native Ovine Cartilage | 4 days | 4 weeks |
| % water | 70–85% | 80–90% | 80–90% |
| Cellularity | 80–160 × $10^6$ cells/g | 10–50 × $10^6$ cells/g | 50–100 × $10^6$ cells/gm |
| % GAG | 6–9% | 0–2% | 2–5% |
| % Collagen | 7–15% | 0–1% | 1–3% |

## RESULTS

At the beginning of cultivation, cells attached to the fibers of the PGA scaffold and proliferated into a three-dimensional construct. Analysis of DNA content[8] within constructs over culture time indicated that chondrocyte cell number increased approximately threefold during a 4-week culture period, as summarized in TABLE 1. Safranin-O staining of histological sections showed that sulfated-proteoglycans were deposited uniformly throughout the thickness of the construct. Biochemical analysis of deposited matrix showed modest deposition of glycosaminoglycans and total collagens[9,10] throughout culture, with levels approaching those in native tissue.[7,11] Analysis of results shows that synthesis follows classical growth and product formation kinetics, allowing prediction of cell and matrix content as a function of culture time.[11] Results comparing the biochemical composition of native ovine tissue with tissue engineered constructs at early and late culture times are summarized in TABLE 1. These findings support the development of tissue engineered cartilage for tissue repair applications.

## DISCUSSION

### *Bioreactor Design Requirements*

For large animal and clinical studies, a scale-up in both size and quantity of constructs is needed. In addition, reproducible production of constructs with uniform physical shape and dimensions, as well as with *in vivo*–like biochemical and biomechanical properties, will likely be required. In anticipation for developing a bioreactor system to provide tissue engineered cartilage for large animal and clinical production, defining the system requirements is essential. Listed in TABLE 2 are several general requirements for successful bioreactor design and how each requirement potentially relates to the production of tissue-engineered cartilage. Many of the parameters are inter-related and ideally should be investigated collectively. Advantages and limitations of specific proposed designs are discussed.

### *Modes of Operation*

Selecting the mode of operation of the bioreactor system will depend highly upon the product dimensions needed for clinical application. Based on the general physi-

**TABLE 2.** Summary of bioreactor design requirements for tissue engineered cartilage

| General Bioreactor Design Requirements | Potential Bioreactor Design and Operating Parameters for Tissue Engineered Cartilage |
|---|---|
| Capability to produce product of clinically relevant size and shape | Evaluation of modes of operation, e.g.:<br>• Static system<br>• Dynamic system<br>• Combination system |
| Capability to produce product with clinically relevant structural and functional properties | Identification, characterization and control of key chemical and physical factors, e.g.:<br>• Oxygen, nutrients, growth factors, cytokines<br>• Fluid shear, mechanical loading, hydrostatic pressure |
| Marketable | Specification of requirements for end-user satisfaction, e.g.<br>• Storage and preservation<br>• Shipping and packaging<br>• Preparation and handling |
| Manufacturable | Evaluation of scalability and robustness, e.g.<br>• Quantity<br>• Quality |

ology of human articular cartilage, a final product with uniform and substantial dimensions (>2 mm thickness) is likely required. The simplest bioreactor design is a static system. Though a static culturing system may have the advantage of simplicity in design and operation, one limitation is that it may not provide a sufficiently homogenous culture environment to produce a construct of uniform composition. Depending upon the relative rates of chondrocyte metabolism and transport of key nutrients, diffusion barriers may prove this system inadequate. To overcome this, a dynamic system may offer solutions. A dynamically stirred system rather than a static culture system has been shown to increase significantly construct dimensions as well as matrix accumulation of proteoglycans and collagens when primary bovine articular chondrocytes were cultured on PGA scaffolds.[12,13]

A system that combines different modes of operation within one unit may also be advantageous if different phases of the culture period have different requirements. For example, a convective-flow system may prove optimal for achieving uniform and efficient cell seeding of porous materials,[14,15] after which a shear flow system may be preferential during the culture phase to promote matrix synthesis.[16]

### *Product Structure and Function*

Chondrocytes have been demonstrated to respond to both soluble mediators such as cytokines and growth factors, as well as to physical modulators of chondrocyte activity, like mechanical loading, fluid shear, and hydrostatic pressure, as previously reviewed.[17] Capitalizing on these signals for tissue formation will greatly impact the defining of requirements for bioreactor design and development. Volume, concentration and frequency of introduction of key chemical components during culture will determine whether systems should operate under traditional modes like batch, fed-batch, recirculating or perfusion modes, or whether a novel design will be better suited. Dynamic compression of cartilage has been shown to stimulate chondrocyte synthetic activities.[18–20] Incorporating such modulators will likely require novel designs. However, the contribution of this and other physical parameters on stimulating cartilage synthesis *in vitro* will need to be balanced by the added complexity in design and operation of the bioreactor system. Ability to monitor and control these chemical and physical modulators of cartilage synthesis will allow characterization and optimization of the process to yield a reproducible product.

Selecting the appropriate scaffold or support may also play a critical role. The scaffold ideally should be structured to withstand deformation due to hydrodynamic forces within the bioreactor system. Depending upon culturing conditions, chondrocytes cultured on bioresorbable scaffolds can be stimulated to deposit matrix, thereby providing the biochemical and biomechanical properties required at time of implantation. Alternatively, depending upon the rate of degradation and other intrinsic material properties, the scaffold itself can be chosen to supplement the structural and functional properties of the construct.

### *Marketability*

Incorporated within the bioreactor design for construct growth may be the requirement to also satisfy storage, shipping, packaging and end-user handling. This integrated packaging design will reduce operator handling and risk of contamination, but also may complicate the design of the bioreactor system itself. Opting for aseptic re-packaging after construct growth may allow greater flexibility and scalability during the growth, storage and shipping phases. However, the risk of compromising sterility is also increased.

### *Manufacturability*

Ultimately, for commercialization, the product must be manufacturable. The bioreactor system and the production process must pass quality system regulations, and do so reproducibly and in large quantities. In progressing down the pipeline from research towards commercialization, the bioreactor system will need to adapt to changing applications and requirements.

At the research and preclinical stages, the bioreactor is generally inexpensive to fabricate, and the assembly is predominantly manual. Designs are relatively unrefined, but easily modified to accommodate testing of alternate designs. The bioreactor system is also generally highly monitored for analysis of key design and operating parameters. In the stages of development and pilot clinical trials, a moderate (i.e., typically 10-fold) scale-up in quantity is conducted. A more refined design and some permanent tooling for fabrication of parts are often implemented. Failure rates are lower, and quality control is more prominent. For pivotal clinical trials, pre-production bioreactors are designed to test reproducibility and robustness of product and process, while also increasing volume. A high level of quality control is in place, and failure rates should be low. High expenses are expected for fabrication using permanent tooling and automation. Few modifications can be made at this stage. In the commercial stage, there is large-scale market volume production. Fabrication and assembly of production units are predominantly automated. Designs are very refined, and aesthetic and ergonomic features are incorporated. Full quality control specifications are in place, and a history of low failure rates has been demonstrated.

For tissue-engineered cartilage, most bioreactor systems are currently in the research and pre-clinical stages. The microgravity bioreactor has been utilized predominantly to understand the effects of dynamic mixing and nutrient utilization on construct growth.[21] Besides providing preclinical material as described earlier, the recirculating system has been utilized for investigating the role of perfusion on cell proliferation and matrix synthesis and accumulation during construct growth.[22] This system has also been designed to consider scale up in quantity, as it can be manifolded to allow parallel and simultaneous operation of several bioreactor systems.

## SUMMARY

Once damaged, either by disease or injury, articular surface joints have only a limited capacity for repair. By developing a hybrid strategy whereby chondrocytes, the cells of cartilage, are combined with a biocompatible scaffold as a support, tissue engineering of cartilage *in vitro* followed by transplantation into articular cartilage defects may provide a successful long-term treatment modality. A first generation recirculating bioreactor has been recently developed for the synthesis of tissue engineered cartilage. During cultivation cells deposit modest amounts of matrix, with levels approaching that of native tissue. This bioreactor has thus far been successful in allowing characterization of the synthesis process and for providing implant material for preclinical studies. In anticipation of large animal and clinical trials, the product and process specifications will need to be further evaluated and defined. To accommodate these requirements, a re-evaluation of the bioreactor design is recommended such that design requirements are addressed and well-integrated into an effective system for tissue engineering.

## ACKNOWLEDGMENTS

This work was funded by an Advanced Tissue Sciences–Smith & Nephew joint venture.

## REFERENCES

1. Medical Data International.
2. BUCKWALTER, J. & H. MANKIN. 1997. Articular cartilage Part II: degeneration and osteoarthrosis, repair, regeneration, and transplantation. J. Bone Joint Surg. **79-A:** 612–632.
3. VACANTI, C.A. & J.P. VACANTI. 1994. Bone and cartilage reconstruction with tissue engineering approaches. Otolaryngol. Clin. North Am. **27:** 263–276.
4. FREED, L., D. GRANDE, L.A., J. EMMANUAL, J. MARQUIS & R. LANGER. 1994. Composition of cell-polymer cartilage implants. Biotechnol. Bioeng. **43:** 605–614.
5. DUNKELMAN, N.S., M.P. ZIMBER, R.G. LEBARON, R. PAVELEC, M. KWAN & A.F. PURCHIO. 1995. Cartilage production by rabbit articular chondrocytes on polyglycolic acid scaffolds in a closed bioreactor system. Biotech. Bioeng. **46:** 299–305.

6. SCHREIBER, R.E., N.S. DUNKELMAN, G. NAUGHTON & A. RATCLIFFE. A method for tissue engineering of cartilage by cell seeding on bioresorbable scaffolds. Ann. N.Y. Acad. Sci. **875:** 398–404. This volume.
7. SCHREIBER, R. & A. RATCLIFFE. 1998. Tissue engineering of cartilage. *In* Methods in Molecular Biology. C. Streuli & M. Grant, Eds. Humana Press. In press.
8. KIM, Y-H., R.L.Y. SAH, J.Y. DOONG & A.J. GRODZINSKY. 1988. Fluorometric assay of DNA in cartilage explants using Hoescht 33258. Anal. Biochem. **174:** 168–176.
9. FARNDALE, R., C. SAYERS & A. BARRETT. 1982. A direct spectrophotometric microassay for sulfated glycosaminoglycans in cartilage constructs. Connective Tiss. Res. **9:** 247–248.
10. WOESSNER, J.F. 1961. The determination of hydroxyproline in tissue and protein samples containing small proportions of this amino acid. Arch. Biochem. Biophys. **93:** 440–447.
11. WU, F., T. DAVISSON, N. DUNKELMAN, A. PETERSON, R. DE LA TORRE, M. APPLEGATE, R. SCHREIBER & D. APPLEGATE. 1997. Kinetics of cell proliferation and matrix deposition of tissue engineered cartilage on biodegradable polymer scaffolds. *In* Proceedings of the Topical Conference on Biomaterials, Carriers for Drug Delivery, and Scaffolds for Tissue Engineering. American Institute of Chemical Engineers, Los Angeles, CA.
12. FREED, L. & G. VUNJAK-NOVAKOVIC. 1995. Cultivation of cell-polymer tissue constructs in simulated microgravity. Biotechnol. Bioeng. **46:** 306–313.
13. VUNJAK-NOVAKOVIC, G., L.E. FREED, R.J. BIRON & R. LANGER. 1996. Effects of mixing on the composition and morphology of tissue-engineered cartilage. Bioengineering, Food, and Natural Products **42:** 850–860.
14. RAMIREZ, O. & R. MUTHARASAN. 1989. Physical immobilization characteristics of a hybridoma in a glass bed packed bed reactor. Biotechnol. Bioeng. **33:** 1072–1076.
15. VUNJAK-NOVAKOVIC, G., B. OBRADOVIC, I. MARTIN, P. BURSAC, R. LANGER & L. FREED. 1998. Dynamic cell seeding of polymer scaffolds for cartilage tissue engineering. Biotechnol. Prog. **14:** 193–202.
16. LANE SMITH, R., B. DONLON, M. GUPTA, M. MOHTAI, P. DAS, D. CARTER, J. COOKE, G. GIBBONS, N. HUTCHINSON & D. SCHURMAN. 1996. Effects of flow-induced shear on articular chondrocyte morphology and metabolism in vitro. J. Orthopedic Res. **13:** 824–831.
17. MANKIN, H.J., V.C. MOW, J.A. BUCKWALTER, J. IANNOTTI & A. RATCLIFFE. 1994. Form and function of articular cartilage. *In* Orthopaedic Basic Science. S.R. Simon, Ed.: 1–44. Rosemont IL. American Academy of Orthopaedic Surgeons.
18. SAH, R.L., Y. KIM, J. DOONG, A. GRODZINSKY, A. PLAAS & J. SANDY. 1989. Biosynthetic response of cartilage explants to dynamic compression. J. Orthop. Res. **7:** 619–636.
19. BACHRACH, N.M., V.B. VAHLMU, E. STAZZONE, A. RATCLIFFE, W.M. LAI & V.C. MOW. 1995. Changes in proteoglycan synthesis of chondrocytes in articular cartilage are associated with the time dependent changes in their mechanical environment. J. Biomech. **28**: 1561–1569.
20. BURTON-WURSTER, N., M. VERNIER-SINGER, T. FARQUAR & G. LUST. 1993. Effect of compressive loading and unloading on the synthesis of total protein proteoglycan, and fibronectin by canine cartilage explants. J. Orthop. Res. **11:** 717–729.
21. OBRADOVIC, B., L. FREED, R. LANGER & G. VUNJAK-NOVAKOVIC. 1997. Bioreactor studies of natural and engineered cartilage metabolism. *In* Proceedings of the Topical Conference on Biomaterials, Carriers for Drug Delivery, and Scaffolds for Tissue Engineering. American Institute of Chemical Engineers, Los Angeles, CA.
22. DAVISSON, T., F. WU, D. JAIN, R. SAH & A. RATCLIFFE. 1999. Effect of perfusion on the growth of tissue engineered cartilage. *In* Transactions of the Orthopaedic Research Society, Orthopedic Research Society, Anaheim, CA.

# Index of Contributors